Classics in Psychiatry

TEXTBOOK
OF PSYCHIATRY

BY

EUGEN BLEULER

ARNO PRESS

A New York Times Company

New York • 1976

Editorial Supervision: EVE NELSON

———◆———

Reprint Edition 1976 by Arno Press Inc.

Reprinted from a copy in
  The University of Virginia Library

CLASSICS IN PSYCHIATRY
ISBN for complete set: 0-405-07410-7
See last pages of this volume for titles.

Manufactured in the United States of America

———◆———

Library of Congress Cataloging in Publication Data

Bleuler, Eugen, 1857-1939.
  Textbook of psychiatry.

  (Classics in psychiatry)
  Translation of Lehrbuch der Psychiatrie.
  Reprint of the ed. published by Macmillan, New
York.
  1. Psychiatry. I. Title. II. Series.
[DNLM: WM100 B647L 1924a]
RC454.B5713 ~~1975~~ 1976 616.8'9   75-16685
ISBN 0-405-07417-4 1976

TEXT-BOOK OF PSYCHIATRY

TEXTBOOK
OF PSYCHIATRY

BY

Prof. Dr. EUGEN BLEULER
DIRECTOR OF THE PSYCHIATRIC CLINIC, ZÜRICH

AUTHORIZED ENGLISH EDITION
BY

A. A. BRILL, Ph.B., M.D.
FORMER ASSISTANT PHYSICIAN OF THE CENTRAL ISLIP STATE HOSPITAL AND ASSISTENZ-
ARZT OF THE CLINIC OF PSYCHIATRY, ZÜRICH. LECTURER ON PSYCHOANALYSIS
AND ABNORMAL PSYCHOLOGY, NEW YORK UNIVERSITY

New York
THE MACMILLAN COMPANY
1924

Press of
J. J. Little & Ives Company
New York, U. S. A.

TRANSLATOR'S PREFACE

WHEN after about five years in the New York State Hospital I entered Burghölzli, the clinic of psychiatry at Zürich, I found a new spirit in psychiatry there. Having been accustomed to look at patients through the eyes of the German psychiatry, as notably represented by Kraepelin, Professor Bleuler's ways impressed me not only as more interesting but also as more instructive and farther reaching in scope and result. Professor Bleuler was the first noted psychiatrist who recognized the great value of Professor Freud's discoveries and impressed his feelings on his co-workers.[1] In Burghölzli the psychoanalytic methods were applied to all accessible patients, and the Freudian mechanisms were investigated even in the organic psychoses. This resulted in many works of great importance which have exerted much influence on psychiatry and psychopathology in general.[2]

It was while I was Professor Bleuler's assistant, in 1907, that he spoke to me about writing a textbook on psychiatry, and I volunteered to put it into English. Since then I have translated a number of Professor Freud's works and became closely identified with the psychoanalytic movement, but my interest in psychiatry, through which I first became acquainted with psychoanalysis, has remained just as deep. It is therefore with a strong feeling of satisfaction that I present this work to English readers.

This translation was made of the author's fourth German edition, and as far as was possible the German text was strictly followed. The only part omitted was the addendum dealing with forensic psychiatry. The author's ideas are based on the Swiss, German, and Austrian laws which are quite different from ours, and as ours are so numerous, so indefinite and so contradictory it was thought best to omit this subject for the present.

This book was primarily written to furnish the student and the general practitioner with a general knowledge of psychiatry. The author endeavors to present clear concepts, and whenever that is not

[1] The works of the Zürich school are too well known to be mentioned here.
[2] For a complete bibliography of Bleuler's works the reader is referred to Hans W. Maier's paper on Eugen Bleuler, Zeitschr. f. d. gesammte Neurologie und Psychiatrie, LXXXII.

v

possible he lucidly exposes the existing gaps. He lays stress on the understanding of psychology, because, to put it in his own words, "psychiatry without psychology is like pathology without physiology, and also because a good physician can be only he who understands the whole human being."

Dr. George H. Kirby, Director of the N. Y. Psychiatric Institute, and Professor of Psychiatry at the Cornell University Medical College, who is most qualified to judge the development of psychiatric instruction in the United States, has rendered a great service by writing the introduction. I am further indebted to him for many helpful suggestions in the work of translation.

I owe gratitude also to Dr. M. S. Gregory, Director of the Psychopathic Pavillions of Bellevue Hospital and Professor of Psychiatry at N. Y. University Bellevue Medical College, and Dr. M. B. Heyman, the Superintendent of the Manhattan State Hospital, New York City, the former for his encouragement and valuable suggestions, and the latter for a number of handwriting specimens of patients in his hospital.

A. A. BRILL.

November, 1923.

INTRODUCTION

THE appearance of a translation of Professor Bleuler's textbook will supply a need long felt by psychiatrists in English-speaking countries. During his twenty-five years' service as a teacher at the University of Zürich and Director of the Cantonial Hospital at Burghölzli Bleuler has been a most indefatigable worker and painstaking investigator in the field of psychopathology and his numerous scientific contributions and original observations have brought him international recognition as an outstanding leader in the progress of modern psychiatry.

At least two of Bleuler's monographic studies have already been translated into English. His description and illuminating analysis of negativistic phenomena was translated by Doctor William A. White in 1912 under the title of "The Theory of Schizophrenic Negativism." In the same year another of his important studies, entitled "Affectivity, Suggestibility, Paranoia," was translated by Doctor Ricksher. American psychiatrists also have had an opportunity to become acquainted with another of Bleuler's important contributions, a summary of which he gave in an address on "Autistic Thinking" delivered at the opening exercises of the Phipps Psychiatric Clinic, Johns Hopkins Hospital, in 1913. Those who had the pleasure of hearing and meeting Professor Bleuler on that occasion were immediately charmed by his pleasing personality and scholarly attainments, as well as impressed by his ability to present a complex subject in clear and simple language and to show by a penetrating analysis of symptoms how the ordinarily incomprehensible or illogical ideas and bizarre reactions of dementia præcox had very plainly their counterparts in normal day-dreaming and in childhood phantasy and play.

Of Bleuler's special studies, that on dementia præcox is generally conceded to be the most important. This monographic work of over 400 pages was published in 1911 as one of the volumes of Aschaffenburg's Handbook under the title of "Dementia Præcox oder Gruppe der Schizophrenien." Unfortunately this work has not been translated although the textbook which now becomes available in English contains a comprehensive chapter on Schizophrenia (dementia præcox) with an admirable symptom-analysis, and psychological interpretation of the development and course of the disorder.

The first edition of the textbook which appeared in 1916 was a crystallization of Bleuler's long experience as a teacher and investigator and contained a systematic presentation of his important psychopathological formulations and their application in clinical analysis. The warm reception accorded the book is attested by the fact that four editions have already appeared.

The book marks a notable advance in psychiatry in that it emphasizes sharply the contrast between the older descriptive psychiatry of Kraepelin and the newer interpretative psychiatry of the present time which utilizes the psychoanalytical principles and general biological viewpoints developed by Freud and his pupils in Europe and by Meyer, Hoch, White and others in this country. Bleuler was apparently one of the first psychiatrists to grasp the great importance of a psychodynamic viewpoint in the study of mental disorders and as early as 1906 he published a paper on Freudian mechanisms in the symptomatology of the psychoses. Although he became convinced of the value and importance for psychiatry of many of Freud's formulations, he has always preserved a well balanced and distinctly independent attitude toward psychoanalytic theories and in the course of his work he has not hesitated to criticize certain aspects of the Freudian psychology.

As an introduction to the study of clinical psychiatry the physician and the student will find the chapters dealing with the principles of psychology and psychopathology particularly helpful and stimulating. While Bleuler adheres to Kraepelin's general scheme of classification of clinical types, it will be found that unlike Kraepelin he does not stop with the mere enumeration of symptoms but seeks through the application of psychological principles to give an interpretation and explanation for the particular reaction type under consideration. This applies not only to the so-called functional mental disorders and psychopathic states but he also discusses most interestingly the psychology and affective reactions of the toxic and organic syndromes.

Bleuler's book will be of interest and help to all those who wish to advance beyond the formal descriptive psychiatry of a period now rapidly drawing to a close. Teachers, practicing neuropsychiatrists and state hospital physicians will find the book to be of great value and assistance in their clinical work, as it will furnish them a comprehensive presentation of the principles of modern psychiatry and their practical application in a form not hitherto available in a psychiatric textbook. It is a work which, as already intimated, marks a distinct advance beyond the boundaries of the Kraepelinian psychiatry. To Doctor Brill, a former pupil of Bleuler's, the profession is indebted for the successful completion of the difficult task involved in the translation.

GEORGE H. KIRBY.

Psychiatric Institute,
Sept. 1, 1923.

CONTENTS

ILLUSTRATIONS

TEXTBOOK OF PSYCHIATRY

TEXTBOOK OF PSYCHIATRY

CHAPTER I

PSYCHOLOGICAL INTRODUCTION

THE PSYCHOLOGICAL PRINCIPLES [1]

THE PSYCHE

The human psyche is so largely dependent in all its functions on the cerebral cortex and on this alone that it is said to be located there.[2] But not all functions of the cerebral cortex belong to the complex which we ordinarily call psychic.[3] Thus what has been called psychic fluctuations of the vascular tone or of the secretions are cortically directed functions, which though depending on the psyche in some manner are not psychic.

Like the reflex mechanism, the purpose of the psyche is to receive external stimuli and to react to them in a manner beneficial to the individual or the genus. There are, however, great differences between the two modes of reaction. The influence exerted upon a reflex through a stimulus other than the one initiating it (or the initiating and directing group of stimuli), is so limited qualitatively and quantitatively, that we ordinarily take no account of it. On the other hand, in the psyche this influence is qualitatively and quantitatively almost unlimited. It is particularly noteworthy that not only actual stimuli play an essential part in determining the reactions, but also former stimuli, especially "experiences" and "memories"; on the other hand, such memory effects play a very slight part in the reflexes. In other words, the reflex always reacts in the same manner to the same stimulus, while the psyche has infinite possibilities of reaction, which are highly complex and plastic, that is, they differ with the same stimulus according

---

[1] Comp. Bleuler Naturgeschichte der Seele, Springer, Berlin, 1921.

[2] In many vertebrates evidently not all psychic functions have gone into the cerebral cortex; that is particularly true of the lower ones. Even in man there is still some connection between basal ganglia and affectivity.

[3] Contrary to general assumptions, the line of demarcation between psychic and non-psychic cortical functions is quite indefinite. It is certain that only small parts of the cortical functions are conscious. (Cf. Section on "Unconscious.")

1

to the particular circumstances, while those of the reflexes are simple and very stable. Thus as far as objective conditions are concerned the difference between reflex and psychic reaction is enormous in degree, but none in principle. An absolute difference is ordinarily assumed on the subjective side, whether correctly or incorrectly no one can tell (Pflueger's spinal cord soul!) The assumption is that only psychic functions can become conscious but not reflexes.

CONSCIOUSNESS

Some authors consider consciousness as the very essential quality of psychic processes. It is an indefinable something, a *quality* of the same, in fact that quality which most clearly differentiates us from an automaton. We can imagine a machine which will perform complicated reactions but we will never ascribe consciousness to an apparatus constructed by us, that is, we cannot assume that it "knows" what it is doing, that it "feels" the influences of its environment, that it knows the "motives" of the reaction. The same idea is expressed by the word "conscious," when we inquire whether someone has consciously or unconsciously arranged his hair.

To compare consciousness with a form which has for its content conscious processes is misleading. Nor can one do anything in psychopathology with such a definition as "the sum of all real or simultaneously present ideas" (Herbart), which is about what one would call the actual psyche. We cannot get along, however, without differentiating between conscious and unconscious psychic processes on the one hand, and between psychic and physical on the other.[4]

Wundt defines consciousness as the "association of the psychic structures." This definition is also used elsewhere in the concepts referring to the "disturbances of consciousness," where it is merely a question of a disturbance in the association of the psychisms. *Consciousness in our sense cannot very well be disturbed; it is either present or absent.* On the other hand, *extent* and *clearness* of consciousness are relative terms. The extent of consciousness corresponds to the number of the (actually or possibly) simultaneously existing conscious ideas, and clearness of consciousness depends on the completeness of one conscious concept or on one idea of a partially forming concept, as well as on the degree of exclusion of irrelevant ideas.

The psychism itself and not a mere quality or form of it is involved in expressions like "consciousness of time and place" for which we had better substitute "orientation as to time and place."

4 See pp. 7-8.

The expression "dual consciousness" for "dual personality" is just as inappropriate.[5]

Furthermore, one is inclined to assume consciousness in our sense, when one observes purposive actions. This is not correct, for even reflexes may be purposive; even an automaton may react differently to different situations, as in the case of automatic scales in the mint. The *ability to remember* a certain experience has often been considered as a sign that consciousness had been present, and it has also been said that an action performed in a twilight state has been "without consciousness." This is also wrong.

Likewise one should not identify "conscious" and "voluntary." The act of dressing oneself is usually voluntary, but not conscious, whereas compulsive actions are conscious, but not voluntary, that is, they are contrary to our will. And neither of these holds good in automatic actions like scratching oneself, mimicking motions, etc.; and in pathological automatisms.[6]

Concerning the Theory of Cognition [7]

Consciousness is said to differentiate psychic from physical occurrences. Two fundamentally different series of experiences have been assumed, those that refer to the "inner life," to that which "takes place merely in time," the conscious or the psychic, and those experiences which refer to the outer world or to that which has extent, namely, the physical.

The relationship between these two forms of experiences is differently conceived. Most suitable for the naïve mind is the conception of *Dualism*, which assumes a carrier of consciousness independent of the body. One sees the body remaining after death, while all psychic manifestations disappear with the cessation of life. The "soul," used here according to the earlier views, representing not only the psychic, but a fusion with the term life, has separated itself from the body. That it has not simply been resolved into nothingness is shown by its reappearance in dreams, in waking hallucinations, and in the illusions of those who survived. And that the observer's own soul can free itself from his body is shown by his dream experiences, during which, regardless of time and space, he perceives things which are far removed from his motionless body.

[5] Disturbances of Personality, p. 137.
[6] The subject of "self-consciousness" will be discussed at the end of the chapter on personality, p. 50.
[7] Ziehen, Zum gegenwärtigen Stand der Erkenntnistheorie Wiesbaden, Bergmann, 1914.

Dualism is an essential constituent of religions; it has been attacked for thousands of years and is at present still rejected by most scientists. Its most important fundamental elements, the dream experiences, and the apparitions of spirits, have proven illusory, and what is more, it has been shown that the psychic functions of man are in all respects dependent upon the brain. On the other hand, it is self-evident, even if one does not always bear it in mind, that in reality the physical world cannot at all be as we perceive and imagine it, and finally, every certain proof is lacking that it even exists.

Thus *monistic* views have been formed regarding the relationship of the two series. They can be divided approximately into three categories:

The first of these categories, of which *Spinoza* is the foremost representative, assumes a "substance," whose two attributes are extension (physical series) and thought (psychic series). However, from the viewpoint of the cognitive theory, it is faulty. Substance, physical and psychic attributes (in modern terms matter, force and consciousness) cannot be placed side by side in this manner. For direct perception is possible only in regard to conscious (psychic) processes. From a part of these we form conclusions (with some probability) concerning external influences, which we call forces. From the grouping of forces we *construct* the idea of matter, which needs not necessarily have a corresponding reality. But there is still another difficulty in this theory: It has to conceive everything as conscious whereas we observe consciousness only in beings similar to us and cannot conceive of an elementary consciousness without content, which is really connected with a nervous center. To be sure, nowhere in evolution do we see a point where consciousness may be said to have appeared in man? in the amoeba? or in the atom?[8] And the ubiquity of consciousness is so readily accepted just because one cannot conceive of something principally new suddenly appearing in evolution. There is really no basis whatsoever for the assumption that the psychic and the physical are so very different. We neither know what the psychic nor what the physical processes are, and consequently nothing about their relationship or difference. *To be sure, for the being endowed with feeling, consciousness is something very special and the only thing of importance.* It is a matter of entire indifference to us whether the world exists, the only thing of importance being whether that which is conscious, our ego, is happy or unhappy.

The second form of monism starts from the idea that all proofs for the existence of an external world are false conclusions, and

[8] Cf. also Loeb's tropisms.

that consequently the physical world exists only in our ideas (Idealism)
or, in so far as we conceive it ("esse = percipi"). Even if this view
could be carried through with logical consistency, it would not be
able to acquire a more general acceptance. For in the first place,
it is incorrect to deny the outer world simply because it is impossible to prove its existence. Anyhow one is always forced to act
as if it exists. The philosopher who claims to believe in the existence only of ideas would have no reason for disseminating his
views if his pupils were only creations of his own imagination. No
matter how certain it were that a rock in the road had existence
only in my imagination, I would still have to go out of its way if
I wished to avoid something unpleasant. If I wish to get rid of
the feeling of hunger, there is nothing for me to do except to eat,
whether food has reality or not. Practically therefore, idealism
will lead to an impossibility. Theoretically, however, it leads to
a conclusion which no one likes to accept, to *Solipsism*. For our fellow
beings are part only of the outer world, and if the outer world
exists only in my ideas, then there are no other beings beside myself.
I am not only the whole world but also the only human being. This
conclusion is unavoidable. The attempt to escape solipsism through
the assumption of an absolute ego is a sophism. Even if an absolute ego were to imagine the world, it would not be *my* world, the
world which *I* imagine, not to mention the fact that such an absolute
ego cannot be imagined and that the whole assumption is entirely
without foundation.

Much more common than the idealistic monism is the materialistic
monism, the materialistic theory of cognition. It starts from the
fact that we always see psychic functions bound to matter, in particular to nervous centres, that they change with this matter, and
that the laws of the central nervous processes, so far as they come
into consideration, are also the psychic laws. From this it concludes that the psyche is a function of the brain. At present this
is the only view which can be carried out theoretically and practically without contradictions, in the form of the so-called *hypothesis
of identity*, which assumes that central nervous functions are "seen
from within" and become "conscious" if they occur in definite relationships. This view is almost the only one which modern science,
and in particular psychiatry, takes into consideration, in fact it is
even accepted by those who theoretically advance another view. Of
course, this theory, too, is impossible to prove, but the hypothesis that
the psychic functions are brain functions has a better foundation
than most assumptions which are accepted as self-evident in the sci-

ences. *But it is by no means necessary as a basis for any mental science, including psychiatry,* in so far as we are not concerned with studying the psychic functions in connection with the brain. This theory, too, is being zealously attacked, primarily on religious grounds. Perhaps with the exception of its earlier periods Christian thought has been altogether dualistic. But the essential content of the Christian doctrine could be just as easily reconciled with materialism as with dualism; as a matter of fact the more favored idealism would encounter more difficulties. Our confession of faith contains the doctrine of the resurrection of the body. If the theory of materialism is correct, then with the resurrection of the body the soul must also *eo ipso* be resurrected at the final judgment. Difficulties arise only in connection with secondary doctrines like those of purgatory, the existence of bodiless souls, etc. Moreover, partly as a result of unclear thinking and partly from rancor, the materialism of the cognitive theory is usually identified with ethical materialism, which, regardless of morality and consideration for other people, egoistically strives merely for "material" goods, by which is meant money, position, good food, drink, and women. But the materialism of the cognitive theory has nothing in common with such ideas except its name. One may accept any view of the cognitive theory and still be either good or bad. But on the basis of the materialistic view, one can deduct a utilitarian ethics by strict logical reasoning, which is superior to all other, which professes to have originated from revelation or the categorical imperative, or from other incomprehensible eternal laws, and which at the same time can be fashioned by every one according to his own desire.

Many modern scientists hold to the theory of *psycho-physical parallelism.* This theory starts from the idea that both series are so heterogeneous in principle that one cannot act upon the other. To explain this relationship nevertheless, Ceulincex assumed that if the psyche wished to perform a physical movement, it was accomplished in each case by an interposition of divine power, and that every time a stimulus strikes the sensory organs the corresponding sensation is produced in the psyche (*Occasionalism*). Leibniz, as is well known, held the view that these two series (which were complicated by his theory of monads) were so arranged by preestablished harmony, since the beginning of creation, that they run an entirely uniform course like two ideal watches, so that every act of the will has a corresponding equivalent movement, and every stimulus on the senses a corresponding equivalent sensation. But this theory of psycho-physical parallelism contains one great error: For if the physical series cannot react upon the psychic then it can reveal neither its existence nor its nature to our psyche. It is then quite useless to assume that the outer world exists, at any rate it surely does not exist as we think we perceive it, and then there is no perception, but only hallucination.

The concept of parallelism could still have some meaning within monistic conceptions (*Spinoza*) inasmuch as the conscious side of the substance has knowledge of the physical part which is really substantially identical with it.

Many view psycho-physical parallelism simply as a confirmation of our ignorance regarding the relationship which undeniably exists between the psychic and physical; sometimes,—and this is particularly true of experimental psychology,—with the secondary thought that we must examine what processes correspond to each other in the two series. This view is also possible, but the name, which is otherwise used quite differently, easily leads to confusion. Some clinicians, without realizing it, get still further away from the original idea, when, for instance, they consider hysteria as a disturbance of the psycho-physical parallelism, because the psychic reaction to the experiences becomes too strong or too weak. Here, of course, the physical "parallel processes" in the brain certainly correspond to the psychic phenomena. In this case therefore the expression is highly misleading.

Wundt has assumed a peculiar view concerning the psycho-physical parallellism. Like many others, he does not only limit the psychic series to the brain functions, but also makes the psychic go beyond the physical, by assuming that certain synthetic functions of our mind take place in the brain without parallel processes. This is an inconsistency which is not only impossible to prove, but which, among other things, is opposed by the fact that we have an analogous synthesis in the physical sphere. Many reflex processes are the result of a whole group of stimuli, which act only as a unit. Likewise the performance of a complicated machine is not equal to the simple sum of the effect of the individual constituents, at least if sum and constituents have the same meaning as in *Wundt's* synthesis.

In the dispute between idealism and materialism one senses an uncertainty regarding the *value of reality* of these two series. But if one only follows up the thought, this question can be very easily settled. Only its own psychic processes have absolute reality for every psyche (it is not in their "contents," i.e. we *perceive* the light or the rose, but not the light, the rose). If I feel a pain, I feel the pain. This is so certain that it can only be expressed tautologically. Since there are also hallucinated pains, this pain need not necessarily have a corresponding process in the aching part of the body. But if a skeptic does not wish to believe that I feel pain, it will be impossible for me to prove it. *The psychic series therefore has absolute, or better, indisputable reality, but only for the psyche in question. This reality is therefore subjective.* But for the existence of the external world there are no proofs. That the table which we see has existence is only an assumption, even if of practical necessity. But if I once take for granted the existence of the table, and that of other people, and the external world, then this table can be shown to these other people. Like myself they can perceive it with their senses. *The reality of the physical world is therefore uncertain and relative, that is, it is not possible to prove it, but on the other hand, it is objectively demonstrable.*[9]

THE UNCONSCIOUS

We perform many trivial actions, such as stroking our hair, undoing a button, shaking off an insect, without knowing it. To a large extent these are neither reflexes, nor subcortical actions, but actions which are performed by the cerebral cortex and are really analogous to conscious functions. Such acts also presuppose memories. "Automatic" actions in hypnotic experiments and in pathological states can be just as complex in thought and motility as any conscious act. The hand may write and the mouth speak without the person having the slightest feeling that these actions originate from his own psyche. In association experiments the train of thought often goes by way of ideas which are not conscious. The answer to "black" may be "star" without there being any conscious thought of "night" which forms the connecting link. As a matter of fact, the constellations which direct our thought are only conscious to a small degree, as a more detailed analysis shows; we often make slips in speaking which are based on unconscious thoughts accompanying it. Only a small part of what our senses perceive comes into consciousness, but the rest surely is not lost to our psyche. Thus, in walking we constantly guide ourselves by perceptions which do not become conscious. Many perceptions come into consciousness only later on. Thus, when one is very busy, he may not hear the striking of a clock, but when the attention is relaxed it is so well

[9] Psychoanalysts also differentiate a "psychic reality." This term is misleading, for they refer to ideas which are created by inner needs and are accepted and used as if they corresponded to what we call reality (the dead child continues to live, the fire of love really burns, or the mediæval personal God).

remembered that one can still count the strokes to about five. Other things become conscious in dreams and in the hypnotic state. Unconsciously a number of complex conclusions are drawn; the so-called intuition is partly based upon this. We may meet a person and feel certain that he is an 'acquaintance, but we are surprised that we do not evince the same feelings that we ordinarily have for him, only to ascertain shortly afterwards that it is not at all the expected person. Here, besides the conscious mistaken identification, there was also present an unconscious correct one. The physician automatically puts the correct key into the many different locks of his hospital; but as soon as he wishes to do it consciously there are difficulties. Signs of an affect are frequently seen in normal persons, and daily in pathological conditions, of which the person affected has no knowledge. And if we carefully observe ourselves and our fellowmen, we will frequently find that just in important decisions the decisive elements are unconscious. By post hypnotic suggestions we can also experimentally provoke actions, the motives of which remain hidden from the person performing them. Hysterical patients may respond to perceptions of which they do not become conscious.

Everything that occurs in our consciousness can therefore also take place unconsciously. In this sense there are unconscious psychic processes. They have absolutely the same value as the conscious psychisms, as links in the causal chain of our thought and action. It is therefore necessary to include them among psychic processes, not only because they have the same value as conscious ones, lacking only conscious quality, but principally, because psychology, and particularly psychopathology, can only be an explanatory science if such important causes of the phenomena are also taken into consideration.

The unconscious functions are best designated as *"the unconscious."* But in the above described psychisms this does not imply a definitely limited class of functions; the real facts, however, are that potentially any function whatsoever can manifest itself consciously as well as unconsciously. Neither are there special laws for unconscious thinking; there are merely relative differences in the frequency of the different forms of association.

To be sure one may place into a special unconscious the mainsprings of our strivings and actions which are also hidden from our introspection. This includes not only the congenital impulses but also the unconsciously acquired paths of the strivings.[10]

Such impulses are particularly striking when they are contrary

[10] Comp. The Collective Unconscious, p. 43.

to the conscious strivings through which they attain the same pathogenic meaning as the repressed tendencies.

The unconscious also contains the paths upon which the psyche
influences our secretions, the cardiac vasomotor and other activities,
even if exceptionally they sometimes become conscious and are accessible to the will in the same sense as we move our limbs consciously
and unconsciously.

Many authors, notably *Freud, Morton Prince* and others, include
among the unconscious functions also the "latent memory pictures"
("Engrams").[11] But these are principally altogether different from
what we have here described. Latent memory pictures, in so far as
we are concerned here, are dispositions without actual functions, but
our unconscious psychisms are actual functions just as valid as
those that are conscious. We can include among the psychic only
those functions which are conscious, or may become conscious under
different circumstances. It is for this reason also that we do not
designate the action of a machine as unconscious, although it has no
consciousness.

To understand the relationship between conscious and unconscious it is best to assume that a function becomes conscious only
when it is in direct associative connection with the ego complex; if
this is not the case, then it follows an unconscious course. This assumption fits in well with all observations; nor does it run counter
to the fact that there are all the transitions from consciousness to
semiconsciousness and to the unconscious. The greater the number
of associative connections at a given moment between the ego and
the psychism (idea, thought, action) the more conscious and at the
same time the clearer is the latter.

What we call "unconscious" is designated by some as "subcon-
scious." Philosophers define the term unconscious quite differently;
it also varies in meaning in different authors.

THE INDIVIDUAL PSYCHIC FUNCTIONS

While taking a walk I stop and take a rest. Then I see a well
and I go over and drink some water. What has taken place in
my psyche?

The light rays which strike my retina cause sensations, that is,
I see certain colors and lights in definite spatial arrangement. Some
of these groups I have already seen before in a corresponding combination. As related units of a higher order they acquire a certain

[11] See chapter on Memory.

independence and are rendered prominent as objects (trees, houses, wells), and from former experiences I know that there is something in the well which I call water which can quench my thirst. That is, the *"concept"* of the well with all its essential elements has been awakened in me, while the momentary experience has only given me a number of color spots. This awakening of former similar sensory complexes by the new sensation is a *perception*. *I have a sensation* of certain light arrangements but I *perceive* certain objects, I have a sensation of sounds but I *perceive* a speech or the bubbling of the spring, I have a *sensation* of an odor, but I *perceive* the scent of violets.

As I am thirsty, I have an *"impulse"* to drink from the well. The thirst and the impulse to drink are evidently also responsible for the fact that the well was rendered more prominent than the numerous other objects striking the eye. But I have not only the impulse to drink, but I would also like to rest a little longer. It also occurs to me that the water might be infected, that I will get a better drink in the next inn, etc. Opposed to this is the thought that I don't know how long I will have to walk until I get there. The source region of the well does not look suspicious; the impulse to quench my thirst therefore becomes the stronger of the two. I decide to take a drink here, but to do it only after I have rested a little longer and am ready to continue my walk. The different impulses with the ideas accompanying them have provoked a play of thought, a *reflection*, which finally had as its resultant the decision which at the proper time led to action.

We have here as in other nervous functions a centripetal [12] reception of stimuli or of material, which we divide into sensations and perceptions, and then an elaboration and a partial transformation of the material into centrifugal functions (decision, actions). It is perhaps only to a very slight degree, if at all, that there is an elaboration sufficient to lead the incoming psychokym [13] by preformed mechanisms into centrifugal paths, a process surely not quite correctly assumed in the reflexes. Here the elaboration occurs in such

[12] I do not speak of "psychopetal" functions, because although there is a given "direction" yet both incoming and outgoing functions, as far as psychology is concerned, take place within the psyche. It is well, however, to understand by "center" and "direction" only symbols and as little as possible real space. On the other hand, the paths between sense organ and brain, and between brain and muscle, of course, must be understood in spatial sense.

[13] "Psychokym" is used to designate psychic processes conceived physiologically, namely, that which is conceived analogous to a form of energy, that something which flows through the central nervous system and which is at the basis of psychic processes. "Neurokym" is used to designate the nervous processes in general.

a way that even new processes are created. The perceptions arouse ideas which combine with the other according to definite norms (Thinking) and only the resultant of these processes as a whole determines the centrifugal action.

Besides these intellectual processes, we have also observed the effects of two other functions, which as qualities are peculiar to all psychic functions, or according to other views always accompany them, namely, *memory* and *affectivity*. In the process of perception we noticed residua of former experiences which somehow reproduce the latter in content and in association. And as a matter of fact, everything psychic leaves behind permanent traces ("Engrams") which later manifest themselves in the form of memories, routine actions and the like, by being revived ("ekphorized") again, and either reproduce the same experience, such as practiced movements or hallucinations, or represent it merely in a similar manner in the form of an image after perception.

The sight of the well aroused pleasant feelings, likewise the quenching of the thirst; the idea of the possibility of infection aroused unpleasant ones. Thus every psychic act is "accompanied by a feeling tone (affectivity), which is at the same time the decisive element in decisions.

We have also seen that any psychic process arouses memory images of former experiences, that through simultaneous occurrence, these are combined in such a manner that they again are ekphorized together and as a whole, or as a unit, that different ideas, feelings and strivings, influence, inhibit, or enhance each other, and finally are combined into one resultant. These different kinds of combination among individual psychisms we call *association*.

a)   The Centripetal Functions

Sensations. The sensations are the most elementary psychic process which we can observe, nevertheless they are already quite complicated. Every sensation of light possesses quality in two directions. There is the quality contrasted with sensations of other senses (light, not sound), and quality within the same sensory region (color). It further includes quantity, as the intensity of the light, the saturation (mixture of the color with white), and the local mark of direction, as well as size and shape.

Perceptions. Perceptions arise from the fact that sensations, or groups of sensations, ekphorize memory pictures of former groups of sensations within us. This produces in us a complex of memories of sensations, the elements of which, by virtue of their simultaneous occurrence in former experiences, have a particularly fine coherence and are differentiated from other groups of sensations.[14] In perception therefore we have three processes: sensation, memory, and association. The latter should be taken in the sense that the sensation, as of certain color spots, or the bubbling noise, has ekphorized a concept, like in the case of the well, and in the sense, that the individual sensory engrams, contained in the concept of the well, have been combined with each other before and now appear simultaneously as a unit.

The act of perception is not sharply defined. A statue may be perceived merely as a statue, or as a Statue of Shakespeare, or as a certain statue of Shakespeare. A word may be perceived as a word, or as an English word, and finally as a word with its meaning and all its relations to a definite situation. This identification of a homogeneous group of sensations with previously acquired analogous complexes, together with all their connections, we designate as *"apperception."* It also embraces the narrower term of perception.

b) CONCEPTS AND IDEAS

Concepts. Let us suppose that we see ripe strawberries for the first time, either a number of them at the same time, or several at different times. With our sight we have sensations of certain shades of color, certain shapes and certain proportions of size. Touch and kinæsthetic senses give us sensations of roughness, hardness, and weight, while the senses of taste and smell give us the taste and odor of the fruit. Among the berries there are similarities and differences. The dissimilar sensations occur only in seeing one or a few berries, while those that are similar appear again and again. These are combined in the psyche into a firm complex, so that more or less vivid memory pictures of the whole concept appear whenever a few sensations somewhat characteristic of the strawberry are experienced. This whole structure of memories of constantly repeated sensations produced in us by the strawberries is the *concept of the strawberry,* or the "strawberry" as a genus. This can now be supplemented by further experiences, for instance, by seeing that the strawberry grows on a plant, that it is a fruit, that it has certain botanical relationships. The process of concept formation is therefore similar to that of type photography.

We also speak of the "concept" of an individual thing or person, an individual strawberry, an individual person seen at different

[14] See below "Concepts."

times, at different distances and perspectives, and from different sides. The residua of the repeated sensations become elaborated into a unified picture containing only that which is common to all, and this forms the concept of this certain thing, this certain person.

On the other hand, the concept formation can also become complex, if more and more individual experiences participate in it. Besides the strawberry we see many other things which grow on plants and are capable, with suitable treatment, to produce new plants. Everything that these things have in common again forms a somewhat firmer engram structure, that of the concept "fruit."

Concepts of activity or quality are, of course, formed in the same manner. "To go" is composed of similarities in observing many processes together; "blue" emphazises a certain form of visual sensations which are frequently repeated. The highest abstract concepts are also formed in this manner without anything new in principle being added. One person rescues his enemy, another becomes a martyr for a good cause, and a third does not steal in spite of great temptation. All these occurrences have something in common which lies in our feeling tone, as well as in the significance that these acts or omissions have for the community. What they have in common, if rendered prominent, gives us the concept of "virtue." In ourselves and in the external world we observe that certain events always follow upon certain others. What is common to them we call "cause" and "effect" or in connection with the other relations of the things and events among themselves, "causal relationship."

A very important task which must partly precede and partly accompany concept formation is the *selection of the material*. We do not form a picture of a tree with the different perspectives of its location and the other simultaneous experiences which were present when we saw it, nor do we see it with all its different fronts, but only the tree in particular in an aspect which is especially suitable to our view. Everything else that was part of the experience in forming the concept tree is eliminated in the concept-formation. The particular associations which were necessarily formed by the coincidence of the experience, and the existence of which can be shown by occasional tests, are *inhibited*. This is only a slight indication of the enormous work our psyche must perform in putting together and separating the individual engrams, even in the simplest functions. As a rule, only the positive process, the putting together, is noticed. The inhibition, or the elimination, is underestimated or even entirely ignored.[15]

[15] See Oligophrenia.

Simultaneously with the perception of a thing or a process we very frequently also hear the word which designates the thing. This, then, must also be combined with the concept in a manner similar to its individual components, though the association is distinctly not as close. In every person who knows the fruit, the word "strawberry" also evokes the concept of the strawberry. Language, however, is of still greater importance for concept formation, inasmuch as with the help of the word it transmits to others the definitions of concepts once formed. The individual may easily come to form the concept "tree," but without the cooperation of former generations it would be somewhat more difficult to form that of "plant." The different language groups therefore have different concepts. The French *"manger"* embraces the German *"essen"* and *"fressen."* The English "fish" is a much wider concept than the German *"Fisch."* The German *"Brunnen"* resolves itself in French into *"fontaine"* and then *"puits."* However, the importance of language for concept formation has also been overestimated. The child was thought to be unable to differentiate men from each other as long as it called each one "papa," but it can be easily shown that this is usually wrong. Likewise, the extent of a person's vocabulary was thought to indicate the number of his concepts and consequently the concepts of an English laborer of the lowest grade were supposed to number only a few hundred. But any idiot, if he is only able to express concepts, and any dog have many more than that. Untrained deaf mutes form not only many concrete but also abstract concepts. There are also people who are as rich in words as poor in concepts (higher forms of dementia), or poor in words and rich in concepts. It was also asserted that one can only think in words. The actual facts are that in ordinary thought one uses abbreviated symbols instead of concepts. Words are frequently used as such symbols, but there are also very different kinds of symbols. Different individuals prefer different ones. Thus for numbers some use the word, others the figure, still others conceive them in form of a colored spot or in regard to their mere position in a numerically schematized scale, etc.

Concepts are not fixed; they are easily supplemented or transformed by new experiences. The concept "God" is not only different in the savage and the civilized person, but also in the child and the adult, the educated and the uneducated. The concept of electricity is changed when one begins to study it through higher mathematics, etc.

In every concept formation, even the simplest, we see the activity of the process of *abstraction,* that is, certain classes of sensations and memory pictures are pushed aside, and others are rendered prominent.

Abstraction does not represent a special or even "higher" faculty, but it is inherent in the nature of the nervous centre and hence belongs to psychic activity. For in both of these activities there are no identical experiences, but only similar ones. One must, therefore, not take too literally the statement in physiology that the same reactions follow the "same" stimuli. In reality, the nervous centres respond to *similar* processes in the same manner; unessential differences do not noticeably influence the reaction, that is, the centre or the reaction makes use of the process of abstraction. If memory images with associatively connected processes, such as thoughts or actions, take the place of preformed or reflex mechanisms, then the abstraction from these differences becomes more diversified but not different in principle. This is already the case in perception. The infant sees its mother at different distances, in different projections and different clothes, and yet recognizes her as the same being, by abstracting from these differences. It is also the same kind of abstraction as in concept formation, when in his general perception the child raises its mother from the environment. Although the infant never sees the mother alone, he always observes her together with the room, yet he is able to abstract and emphasize the mother concept. That this is an important function can be seen in those cases where it fails. Children frequently behave very differently toward the same persons in a different environment. In the case of cats, one regularly observes that they act as strangers outside of the house to persons of their home.

That the abstraction does not merely take away from a number of engram groups some components and combines the rest into one sum but forms thereby a *new psychic structure* is self evident and is in no way peculiar to the psyche. Thus a clock work is as little the mere sum of its little wheels as a human being is the sum of his cells and molecules ("mere sum" is precisely an abstraction, which exists as little in reality as the "sum" two).

Ideas. Everything that has been perceived by the senses, such as qualities, things and processes, is imagined as an ekphorized memory picture. In addition, the ideas contain also psychic structures which have never been perceived by the senses. Among these we have all possible combinations of sensory images, phantasies, wishes and possibilities, as well as the abstractions and their combinations with ideas; indeed, it comprises everything *in so far as it can become actual in time by ekphorization and not by sense perception.*[16]

c)   THE ASSOCIATIONS.   THOUGHT.

Combinations of Psychisms We Call Associations.

We see them in different forms; they may also combine with each other and cannot really be sharply separated from one another.

(1) Two synchronous functions may modify, enhance or inhibit each other. The perception of the road as well as the obstacles direct our steps. A moral reflection inhibits a reproachable act. Two motives acting in the same direction promote the reaction. Physical functions such as reflexes may be influenced in all three directions by accidental secondary stimuli.

(2) Simultaneous or successive experiences are connected with each other, in so far as they have a tendency to appear together in memory, or in so far as the revival of one of these experiences recalls the others. We may add to this the fact that our ideas and concepts, with many or all of their components, simultaneously appear in memory or thought, or follow in immediate succession. If we hear the word rose or think of a rose, we also have a more or less clear idea of the individual psychisms red, beautiful, fragrant, all of which form the general concept of flower.

(3) One idea generates another. We think of roses, and this in turn suggests a verse we learned about tulips and carnations. We set out to write our name, whereupon follow the different movements in the accustomed and successive order. This also explains why a certain action is performed after a given signal. In the psychological selection experiment we perform the required reactions, thus to the bell signal we react with the right hand, to the optic signal with the left. This function already resembles much the reflex process which is also no simple transition of the sensory stimuli to the motor apparatus, but a setting in motion, or generating the function of a performed mechanism.

(4) The forms mentioned may occur in any combination. In the sense of the progressive association (Form 3), the perception of an apple generates in the child the impulse to eat it, but also the memory picture of the thrashing formerly provoked by stealing it, and these later inhibit the acquisition impulse as a simultaneous function (Form 1).

Ordinarily, however, we do not think of all these forms but only of the following phenomena:

[16] For the differences between ideas and perceptions, see p. 66.

(1) Through temporal connections in experience, associations are created in the corresponding engrams (associations are formed). (2) These connections remain in existence with the engrams of the experiences (engrams are associated). (3) A new event may ekphorize the engrams of memory images which (a) have somehow become connected at its origin or which (b) refer to the same experiences, or which (c) refer to similar experiences. In the same manner a whole idea is likewise associated to a former one. In the same manner as in simple concepts whole ideas form associations among one another.

Association is a *state* so far as engrams are connected with one another. But it is also a *process*, through the connection of simultaneous experiences, through the generation of one idea by another, as in thought, and above all through the influence of one psychism upon another.

Associations in the sense of permanent connections originate when several psychisms take place simultaneously or in immediate succession, as can be seen in the act of perceiving the association of lightning and thunder. We must assume that everything simultaneous and successive is connected in the psyche, not only because such functions very frequently influence each other, but because they appear connected in memory, as shown by every'day experiments. If something has eluded us, we can frequently recall it, by going to the place where the thought or experience took place, indeed, even if there is no logical connection between the place and the forgotten content of the ideas. And yet the associations accessible to us evince a certain selection. Primarily we recall only experiences which in themselves or through their connections have a certain importance for us. In reference to the capacity to ekphorize there are thus important differences in the associations, and perhaps also in the elaboration of memory images. Unfortunately we cannot enter here into the investigation of these differences; at any rate affective mechanisms cooperate in them.

Moreover, as seen in every other function, there is also something negative in the formation of associations. If we have once been accustomed to write a letter of the alphabet in a certain manner, there will be a tendency always to write it the same way, even if we did not write for a long time. But if we have later acquired a different form of writing, then there is difficulty in reproducing the earlier ones, even if we think of it in due time. The present medical training does not make psychological thinking difficult because it ignores it, but mainly because it forms associations in other directions and thereby virtually inhibits psychological thinking.

If we consider the associations as a process of memory, we see that what has been experienced simultaneously or in immediate succession is ekphorized with relative frequency. Furthermore, for evident reasons, this is also true of similar and analogous experiences.[17] The child having burned itself by a candle, is afraid of all fires.

Most associations, particularly those obtained by simultaneousness, may take either the course a—b or b—a. In related individual experiences, as in the details of a lawsuit, direction plays no part whatever, as a single component associates the main concept, which connects them all and from it other details can result in any series of succession.

But under certain conditions direction is not a matter of indifference. This is particularly true of associations which are important only as they follow each other. No matter how fluently we can recite the alphabet or a verse, to say it in reverse order can at first be done only with difficulty. Many associations of motion we can never reverse. For even if we are able to draw a letter, by starting from the front or back, we have two different motions in which the muscles do not simply contract in reverse order. But even associations formed by simultaneousness may obtain a one sided direction through practice. Most people who can read the printed Gothic letters have not necessarily the capacity to form an image of them by hearing them. For reasons easily understood, the direction from the special to the general has a relative preference over, and against the reverse. A name very easily arouses the idea of the person designated by it, while it frequently happens that the idea does not call forth the name. The latter element is of importance in pathological disturbances of memory.

Logical thinking is at first a repetition, an ekphoria of associative connections, that were once experienced, or of similar or analogous connections.

Every time we dig around a tree we see the roots. An association is therefore formed between the idea of the tree and the root. If we see a tree and the concept root comes into consideration, it is associated with the tree, and what is more, it has an added feeling of belonging together. In the subsequent abstracted laws of

---

[17] Similar or analogous experiences have in common partial psychisms. Furthermore, the sensibility of the psyche and possibly of the central nervous system for differences is limited. Whatever has differences below a certain limit appears and acts as being identical.

logic we express it as follows: Every tree has roots; this is a tree, therefore it has roots. But we only think in this way in exceptional circumstances, when the correctness of the inference is questioned, as in "proving" something. The millions of inferences, which are daily made in thought and action, are accomplished in a much simpler way. If one wishes to percuss a person's heart, one does not say: Every man's heart is on the left side; this is a man, therefore his heart is on the left side, but one simply associates the customary place with the idea, to percuss the patient's heart.

Conclusions, therefore, like thought in general, are repetitions of identical or analogous associations as we see them in life.

One can prove the Pythagorean proposition through four experiences which every person has gone through; from two special experiences (hypothetical lines drawn for this purpose) and from nine analogous associations, wherein, however, generally existing concepts such as triangle, right angle, parallels, and multiplication are assumed, and hence not enumerated.

Causal thinking is only an analogy of the regular sequence of two ordinary events, or of the general sequence of two unusual events. When it gets warm, the snow melts. An otherwise incurable disease is cured as a result of a new remedy.[18] Of course, the terms "regular sequence" and "unusual event" are very indefinite. Thus, for the savage, many things are *propter hoc* which for us are only *post hoc.* Moreover, it must be determined through further experience, whether one event depends directly upon the other, or whether both can be traced back to the same cause. The rotation of the earth is the common cause of both day and night, although for children and in myths, day arises from the night. A falling barometer and rain have a common cause. Nevertheless we frequently see a desire to smash the falling barometer in order to force good weather. But causal concepts contain also inner experiences. We ourselves are very often a link in the causal chain. Through our own actions we can set up causes and therefore effects. We even permit our actions to be influenced by these considerations. We see *causes* outside of us and *motives* within us. But these two relationships can only be differentiated by the viewpoint from which they are seen, and possibly through the greater complication of the apparent motives as compared with the apparent causes.

---

[18] As a matter of fact no occurrence has only *one* cause. The main difficulty in causal investigation lies precisely in the manifold preconceptions connected with every single occurrence. However, in psychological reflection it is not necessary to solve the causal concept in the sum of conditions, as useful as it would be in medicine to apply it with greater clearness than is usually the case.

Many persons have recently attached great importance to the differentiation between "causal" and "final" thinking. There is no difference as regards logical forms. In final thinking determinants referring to the future are taken into consideration, as in the case of calculating in advance an eclipse of the sun. But there is a certain difference in the goal of thinking; the final operation determines our action, while in causal thinking the explanation obtained satisfies our need. To be sure, the final function is the original and usual one. The causal function acquires greater importance only in the civilized person, who satisfies his growing need for theoretical explanation and who, at the same time, has learned to value the great advantage offered him by a causal understanding of the associations of future achievements.

Judgment consists in a repetition of associations acquired through experience. "Snow is white," "Kant was a great man," are expressions of direct and indirect experiences. *But it is important to note that the word "judgment" signifies two things.* In logic, judgment is "the form in which cognitions are thought and expressed." But if we speak in psychiatry and jurisprudence of the capacity to judge, we mean the ability to *form* judgments, that is, the capacity to draw correct conclusions from the material acquired by experience.

In tracing back the individual thought processes to external associations we have, of course, not completely explained "thought." When the concept "tree" is awakened in us, we do not always associate its roots with it. We only do this when this direction is determined by a certain *constellation*, as in observing that the wind may uproot the tree, or by the trend of thought, as when we think about the nutrition of the tree. For every single idea has countless others which are associatively connected with it. Which of these paths is followed in a concrete case depends upon broader determinants, among which the trend of thought and the constellation are most important.

The **aim of thought** is not something simple but a whole hierarchy of a trend of ideas systematically arranged. If I wish to write now about associations, I must constantly have this aim before me more or less consciously, but besides this I must also view the plan as a whole, as far as I have worked it out, the basic thought of a chapter and of a sentence, what I have said before, etc.

Even in such mental trends which are seemingly very much connected, the momentary and general **constellation** plays a noticeable part. It was momentary constellation which suggested to me the **example** just used in illustration. The course of ideas is not only determined by immediate, but also by former experiences. The con-

stellation also becomes an essential factor in loose or aimless thinking. A person who is hungry, or vice versa one whose stomach is
overfilled, starting from any idea at all, is much more likely to hit
upon an association or an idea concerning food (dream!). A person
who is just coming from a lecture on chemistry and hears of "water"
will not easily think of water in connection with scenery or with
commercial uses.

*Besides the positive effect, mental trends and constellations have
also a pronounced negative effect.* Every psychic process like every
other central nervous process, not only promotes the minor selection
of like-minded functions, but it also inhibits the infinite number of
other psychisms. The development of thinking is therefore also
in this 'respect entirely parallel to that of motility, which must not
only learn to contract the necessary muscles in proper sequence,
but must also learn *not* to put tension in all the others.

If we free the associations as far as possible from ideas of a
special trend by instructing a test person to repeat as quickly as
possible the first word flashing through his mind when a word is called
out to him, we then find that the simple associations of experience
and constellation come to the surface very clearly. We thus find
associations of spatial and temporal contiguity, of similarity and contrast, of coordination and subordination, and of conceptual and sound
similarities. Some pretend to see in the grouping of these different
kinds of associations the "laws of association." But from what has
been said above, it is self-evident that they are only a fractional
part of the determinants of our natural thinking.

The principal trend of thought is determined by the impulses and
the affects. We wish to reach a definite aim. But even in the individual elements of thought we can see the influence of affective
needs. It accounts for daily disturbances and even direct falsifications of logic, which manifest themselves to a slight degree in normal
persons and to a much greater extent in the insane.[19]

The material taken up forms new combinations in **phantasy**,
whereby different degrees of detachment from experience become
possible. The *inventor* has set for himself new aims which he endeavors to attain by analogy to the familiar. The poet assumes
greater freedom of movement, and in fairy tales and in mythology he
is thus able to put himself in an attitude contradictory to reality,
to be sure, in a senseful manner.[20]

The associations are not peculiar to the psyche alone, but they

[19] See affectivity; delusions.
[20] Cf. Dereistic thinking, p. 45.

can be experimentally demonstrated in the other central nervous processes, in all their qualities except the quality of consciousness. It is true that *Pawlow's* "association reflexes" (conditioned reflexes) go via the cerebral cortex, which alone is capable of such plastic functions to a high degree, but this does not mean that they must go via the psyche, and particularly beyond the conscious psyche.

The mechanism of association, the possibility that parallel psychisms may or may not influence each other, and that of the infinite number of possible paths a particular one is taken by choice, can best be understood by comparing it with the switches in an electrical plant. These switches may connect different machines with one another or let them run independently of each other; they can switch them on or off. The constellation determined in our example by the lecture on chemistry decreases something, which in the electrical plant would correspond to the resistance in the direction of "chemistry," and it increases the resistance in other paths. That is the reason why the idea "water" evokes associations of chemical ideas of this concept rather than others. The comparison with electrical switches also makes it possible for us to understand a number of other phenomena, such as flight of ideas, schizophrenic disturbance of association, hypnotic phenomena, the existence of different personalities in the same psyche either simultaneously or side by side, the phenomena of the unconscious, and a number of pathological symptoms which are either denied or reluctantly admitted. One must be careful, however, not to connect the concept of association and switching with any idea of cerebral localization. According to our present day knowledge it is quite possible that the individual concepts are partially (or wholly) "localized" in the same anatomical structure.

d)   THE INTELLIGENCE

The foundations of **intelligence** lie in the process of association. It is a complex of many functions which can be differently developed in every individual. There is no uniform intelligence. It would be a praiseworthy task to elucidate once for all the whole concept of intelligence. Besides the faculty of intelligence, it would be important to abstract correctly the following points: (1) the capacity to understand what is perceived or explained by others, (2) the capacity to be able to act in such a manner as to achieve what one is striving for, and (3) the capacity to make correct combinations of new material (logical power and phantasy).

All these achievements are primarily dependent upon the *number of possible associations.* The greater the number of stones at our disposal, the greater the number of ideas and the finer the shades that we can express in the mosaic of our thinking. In the animal series, or from the idiot to the genius, the scale of intelligence depends principally upon an increase in the possibilities of association. Of secondary importance we consider the *speed* and *ease* in the flow of associations. For the scholar in his study it may not be very important how much time he takes for his reflections. But a person in active life must be able to survey a situation rapidly and to draw the conclusions necessary for action. Intelligent achievement also includes the *proper selection* of the material to be associated. I only enumerate this in the third place because this function is comparatively satisfactory to the average person. It is relatively rare to find many irrelevant associations; one observes this mostly in oligophrenics lacking mental clearness whom we shall discuss later. To select the appropriate material it is necessary to differentiate between the important and the unimportant. This is a complicated function and depends on the survey of the whole subject and therefore, in the final analysis, again on the number of associations. In order to make new combinations and not merely to follow in the old grooves, there must be a certain capacity to split up the associations into their components,[21] but one also needs a special activity of the will and thought in the direction of controlling the circumstances.

The greater the intelligence, the more use is made of elaborated thought material. The intelligent person makes far less use of concepts which are still closely related to perceptions than of inferences drawn from them, and often enough he is altogether unable to reproduce the original experiences. He follows his judgment of a person without thinking how he came to this judgment. He also thinks his concepts with their relationships. On the other hand, he also resorts to short cuts; this is partly accomplished through the arrangement of details into a uniform main concept which is already a short cut, and partly by changing complex ideas into symbols, which are not only used in intercourse with others but also in thinking (e.g. mathematical signs like π, sin, etc.).

A schoolgirl asks her mother for some money for a poor friend, so that the latter may join in a school picnic. The mother refuses, since she has no money herself. The girl observes that her playmate frequently earns a few nickels for running errands. She now conveys to her the idea that all she has to do, in order to get enough money for the picnic, is to save this money instead of spending it, and for

[21] Cf. Concept formation, p. 14, and the oligophrenias.

this purpose she gives her a small, improvised, savings bank. Besides she keeps on inquiring how much money the child has earned and what she has done with it. This proved to be quite successful.

Here we deal, in the first place, with a characterological function on which all that follows is dependent. The girl was not satisfied with her mother's answer and tried to find another solution. But pure intelligence also had a share in this first step. The girl had to recognize the possibility of providing help, before she found the solution, while a feeble-minded person would have faced an impossibility from the very beginning. The next step was seemingly very simple, but only seemingly, for often enough it fails in reality, in spite of the fact that it is so frequently drilled in; we refer to the application of the thought that twenty nickels make a dollar, that is, that one has to save only twenty nickels in order to have a dollar. To seek a way out of a difficulty, in spite of the fact that the nearest solution is impossible and the application of this mathematical principle is what differentiates civilized people from those that remain primitive. After giving the advice to save, many a sage would have considered the matter settled. But here we have besides, the important idea of the small savings bank. This required the "feeling" which many moralists lack, and which is of course, a purely intellectual process, that mere advice was not sufficient, that is, it requires a complex of associations regarding the fickleness of her friend and the desire to make it harmless. For this purpose a means was invented, with the help of imagination, to interest the spendthrift in another direction. That this solution was sought and found, of course again presupposes the possession of a great number of ideas regarding the psychology of her friend, and, in the long run, of people in general. Furthermore, there was the capacity to utilize all these ideas at the proper moment, and at the same time to sift the experiences into what is important and what is unimportant for this particular case. This latter selection requires among other things the constant presence of the psychological ideas about the motives of action, for it is with the guidance of these ideas that the sifting must be done. Intellectual as well as characterological functions are involved in the subsequent supervision of saving and in the *detachment from the usual associations*. The latter is particularly important when it is not merely a question of understanding, but of acting, or finding new solutions. The usual thing is the idea of obtaining money from parents; if this is impossible thousands of young girls will resign themselves to what is apparently unavoidable. Our heroine detached the thought of procuring money from the idea of the usual source and sought a different one. The classical witticism of the egg of Columbus is a very striking example for the significance of this detachment. Columbus could count on the fact that his narrow-minded rivals would not be able to detach themselves from the stereotyped ideas of the undamaged egg. If it were not for the strong resistance of ordinary minds against the unaccustomed, as represented by the broken end, the solution would instinctively have had to force itself upon them. One need merely call to mind an egg of wax.

A fundamentally different grading of intelligence is that according to *clearness* of ideas. This does not depend on the number of possible associations; on the contrary, in those who lack clearness one often gets the impression that there are too many associations, or that not enough are inhibited. On the other hand, there is not much that is unclear in those concepts which are formed by the ordinary oligophrenics themselves. Idiots do not go very far beyond the material existence in forming concepts and that alone relatively protects them against a want of clearness. Lack of clearness will appear at most if concepts are forced upon them from the outside, for the understanding of which they are too feeble. On the other hand, there are intelligent and even highly gifted people who utilize many confused concepts. Under some circumstances this may have a certain advantage for discoverers: they can deduce a hypothetical concept from any experience without great difficulty and if it does not properly conform to subsequent experiences, they can without noticeable effort, or even without knowing it, transform it in accordance with the new conditions, that is, they can use it in a somewhat different sense. It is self-evident that this quality is very dangerous and can only be rendered harmless by very great intelligence. What we mean here by confused concepts can be best explained by using the illustration of the constellations. The astronomer knows every star belonging to Orion; to him that is a very sharply defined concept. The layman, however, knows only a few stars of it or only the celestial region where it is located. But he is conscious of his weakness. He has an incomplete but not a confused concept of it. Conscious of his ignorance he will not make the mistake of suddenly taking an entirely different group of stars for Orion and will not say that a comet has just entered Orion, when in reality it does not touch Orion at all or is just leaving it. But the unclear person may express himself in this manner, because there are no definite and constant limits to his concepts; he speaks of Orion when it is simply a question of that legend; at times he will add to it stars which at another time he does not include; what the unclear person lacks particularly is the conscious and vivid distinction of related concepts. He who calls all psycho-motor difficulties inhibitions may have a clear concept of them, even if it is unsuitable for our diagnosis. But a person who speaks of inhibition and blocking and does not see the difference between these two terms, that are now current in psychiatry, has an unclear conception of them.

There are people whose more complex concepts are all unclear in this manner. Many conceal this defect by a clever way of expression, but in life they fail like all the other feeble-minded.

Intelligence in any sense whatsoever is never a unit. There is no one who is eminent in all psychic fields, while most idiots naturally fail in all directions. Practical intelligence does not necessarily imply theoretical intelligence and vice versa. The great difference between school intelligence and worldly intelligence depends only partly on the fact that pedagogues with their one-sided standards are deceiving themselves regarding the abilities of their pupils.[22] A number of highly gifted people were poor in school. Alexander von Humboldt, for instance, "was unfit for study" according to the judgment of his teachers. And even after the school period "worldly wisdom" is something quite different from intelligence in general. The particular gifts for mathematics, languages, engineering, psychology, philosophical thinking, etc., are well known. This specialization may go to very great lengths. Indeed there are people with one-sided genius for figuring out on what day of the week a certain date will come, or for playing chess, etc.

Even in such cases we do not merely deal with abstract intelligence. The good mathematician not only has the ability to think mathematically but also the *impulse* to occupy himself with it. But the intellectual effects depend also in other ways on their interplay with other functions, principally the *affects*. We have seen in the case of the schoolgirl how the impulse to think and act cooperated in controlling the circumstances. A people without a thirst for knowledge, like most of the Orientals, even though it had the greatest intelligence and perhaps a vivid phantasy, would nevertheless be unable to accomplish anything in the sense of our occidental technique. The abulic schizophrenic and the over-labile organic dement both appear demented as a result of their affective disturbances.

[22] Unfortunately one still observes quite frequently that the result of education and school training, the mere acquisition by memory of the subject matter of education, is mistaken for intellectual accomplishments.

Mere clearness of thinking, likewise, is considerably improved if one has the patience and the impulse to think a matter through. Logic falsified by affects is constantly seen in the insane. A failure of the intellectual functions may be due to a disturbance of the equilibrium between reflective power and affectivity (apathy on the one hand, and proportionate dementia on the other). Important above all, is the influence of the feelings relating to the ego which only too readily cause an entirely different standard to be applied to one's own interests than to other things. Furthermore, a large part of worldly prudence is due to perseverance. The ability to concentrate the attention in understanding and elaborating things may have an important influence upon intelligence. The ability to find new material is favored by a certain degree of phantasy or is perhaps identical with it, if by "new" we do not merely mean the correct "new" material. That a good *memory* considerably aids intelligence, that it may even replace intelligence and conceal the weakness of it, is self-evident. For, the more intelligent a person is, the less need he has for primary memory, which reproduces experiences exactly as they have been experienced. For the intelligent person uses deduced concepts; a "fish" does not call to his mind a collection of all the fishes he has ever seen, but he has for it a very abbreviated formula which is of a zoological-scientific content.

e) MEMORY

Everything that has been psychically experienced leaves behind a lasting trace, or *engram*. We recognize this by the facts, that the more often a process has been repeated (practice) the easier it runs off, that past experiences act in a modifying way on some actual processes, that repeated experiences are recognized as repetitions, and above all that one *remembers* psychic processes. What modification the engram represents we do not know. In remembering something there must be a recurrence of a function resembling a previous experience, like an idea of something perceived, or of a function almost like it, like the repetition of a practiced motion. We designate this as an *ekphoria* of the engrams. That every experience, including unconscious ones, really leaves behind engrams, cannot be directly demonstrated, but it seems very probable from off hand tests, furnished us by chance memories. In dreams, hypnosis, and in diseases, and sometimes also in the normal states, experiences are recalled which would otherwise be considered as impossible of recollection.

A young woman who could neither read nor write reproduced in a feverish state Latin, Greek and Hebrew verses, of which she knew nothing in her normal state. During her childhood she lived with a clergyman, who was in the habit of reciting such sayings.[23] A person hypnotized in a drug store may, under certain conditions, reproduce a great many of the inscriptions on the glass jars, even if he understands nothing about them.

Although every experience leaves an engram, those memories which we usually utilize are really products of very complicated elaborations. We do not form an image of a momentary vision of a certain region by confining it within the limits of the field of vision at that particular time, but we image a tree, a meadow, a meadow with trees, mountains, etc. In short, in the available engrams, the experiences are analyzed and synthesized according to the rules of concept formation.

The ability to form engrams, the engraphia, was designated by *Wernicke* as "impressibility" (*Merkfähigkeit*)—and this has been hazily contrasted with "memory." Memory in this connection no longer means the whole memory, a designation for which is clumsily lacking, but the retention of the ability to ekphorize the engrams. It is still unknown in what respect the latter may be regarded as a special quality. The only thing definite is that under certain conditions many engrams cannot be ekphorized, and that, if a cause for it is found at all, it has so far always been in something entirely different from the nature of the engrams; it was mostly in affective obstacles. So far then the mere inability to remember has thus far not shown us why the engrams are lost. A more detailed discussion will be given in the chapter on pathology of memory.

The engrams seem to *last* as long as the brain is not very extensively and markedly injured. It is not very rare that apparently long lost memories from childhood reappear in old age with great vividness. All things being equal, the older an engram the greater is its resistive capacity to ekphorization. *Forgetting* therefore is not as a rule due to a disappearance of the engrams, but to an inability to revive them as memories or to ekphorize them by association.

The apparent paling of those pictures of perception which are tangibly vivid is really only a substitution of the same by elaborations which are more suitable for the idea and hence more capable of recollection. Another way of weakening by age the capacity to recall an engram was shown by Ranschburg.[24] Material learned by heart consisting of similar components is more difficult to reproduce

---

[23] Carpenter, Mental Physiology, p. 437, Trubner, 1896, London.
[24] Ranschburg, Ueber Wechselbeziehungen gleichzeitiger Reize usw. Zeitschrift für Psychologie 67, 1913.

than that which is altogether dissimilar. In self-observation we find that to a large extent memories disappear in a manner that one is at first uncertain which of several similar memory pictures is the correct one, and that gradually so many possibilities offer themselves that one is no longer able to choose, or that one is altogether unable to grasp the correct engram out of the great number of others. Other disturbances and falsifications of memory are determined by the affect.

There are facts, however, which could, in the first place, be explained by a change in the engrams. Thus, rooms which we saw in childhood often seem much smaller in later life than we had expected. We have enlarged the image with the growth of the size of our body. Whoever studies the testimony of witnesses in court proceedings will be surprised how, even in very simple matters, people will make the most contradictory statements in good faith; this naturally occurs most frequently in the case of precipitated or excited events. But even without any particular reason the errors are often very great. The experiments regarding the giving of evidence, particularly those made by *Stern's* school,[25] have furnished us much unexpected information concerning this. Every one who observes himself, even if only a little, is familiar with the daily irregular falsifications which reproduce a memory not only incompletely but change it also in other ways. Thus the memory image of a somewhat unfamiliar person, garden, or of an event is frequently quite different from the reality of it, and in time also loses regularly in correctness and in clearness.

In all such cases, however, the original correct engram continues to exist together with the modified one. For the error is often subsequently corrected, either through reflection or through the fact that the correct memory involuntarily appears on some occasion. In pathological conditions we can frequently demonstrate that the correct and the falsified idea exist at the same time.

Such occurrences prove that in falsifications of memory we do not deal with alternations of the engrams, but with a complex process which is analogous to the creation of new ideas. How much of this has taken place in the unconscious during the apparent latency of the engrams and how much during the act of recalling is unknown.

Even in a sober-minded normal person the falsifications which correspond to an affect, namely, to the wishes of the individual, are very marked. It is very instructive to reread one's diary after the lapse of a number of years. One finds a great deal which he no longer

[25] *Stern,* Beiträge zur Psychologie der Aussage. Barth. Leipzig, 1903.

believes even though it is written in his own handwriting. But on closer examination one finds that the version of the diary fits least the person concerned.

Ekphorization of engrams can be either conscious or unconscious. Unconscious memories of ideas can only be demonstrated in a round-about way, but well-grounded capacities, particularly of the motor type, very easily take place unconsciously. If we were once able to swim, we make the correct swimming motions as soon as we get into deep water.

The ekphorias that are most frequently spoken of are the conscious memories. Without exception they are probably generated by way of associations. The laws of memory are therefore the laws of association. The better drilled an association, the more associative paths lead to an engram, the easier it is to remember. It is therefore relatively easy to remember what has been brought into many relationships, or what has been understood. An unintelligible chaos, as for instance a story heard in a foreign language, cannot be reproduced. Likewise it is just as impossible, in the ordinary conscious course of thought, to revive all those innumerable engrams which we take up unconsciously as all the faces of the unfamiliar people we meet on a walk.

The faculty of memory is very easily disturbed through such a constellation as recalling something otherwise familiar in a new relationship; we are often unable to do so. The affects, however, as we shall see, are particularly important as factors inhibiting and facilitating memory. Pleasurable experiences are particularly easy to remember. In unpleasant experiences there is a struggle between two antagonistic tendencies; on the one side we have the one belonging to the affect in general, which makes the memories more vivid, and on the other side there is the tendency which strives to shut out everything unpleasant, hence also a disagreeable memory. Unpleasant events are frequently crowded out of memory, especially if they somehow depreciate the personality. Thus the lapse of many decades creates the idea of "the good old times." Most important of all, however, are the actual affects, which cause only those memories to come to the surface which are suitable for them.

Recognition is a special form of memory. If we hear or see something for the second or third time we regularly recognize it as a former experience. One speaks of a "quality of familiarity" in the repeated sensation, but one is unable to describe it. It is more important to know that recognition is easier than spontaneous recollection. Thus, even if one is absolutely unable to remember the oriental name of Alexander, one will easily recognize it, if among other names Iskander is mentioned. Not every one is able to form a clear image of a person, but is able to recognize him as soon as he sees him.

f) ORIENTATION

Present and former perceptions combine into *orientation as to time and place,* so that one always thinks more or less conspicuously of being at a certain place and at a certain period of time, and connects his memories with these dates. It is self-evident that orientation depends on memory (for it is impossible when memory is lacking), on perceptions (for hallucinations can produce an entirely different place), and on attention (for if we are absorbed in thought or in conversation while walking or riding in a vehicle, we may suddenly find ourselves at a different place than we had expected). But as pathology shows, there is besides this also an independent function of orientation, the disturbances of which are not necessarily proportional to the disturbances of other functions.[26] Nevertheless we find no anomalies of orientation without a disturbance of other functions.

Orientation as to space, which is constantly controlled by the eyes, is of course much surer than orientation as to time, which requires an uninterrupted memory record and has only a linear dimension.

Something entirely different is the *orientation as to situation,* which tells us why we are at a certain place, what relationship we have to the other people, etc. This is of course a function of reflection, as far as it depends on the understanding of complex conditions.[27]

g) AFFECTIVITY

Every psychism can be divided into two sides, an intellectual and an affective. The latter often remains unnoticed, but is never altogether lacking, as can be demonstrated through comparisons. For instance, most people can immediately answer the question whether they like better a trapezoid or a square. It can be concluded that the mere sight of such simple figures is associated with a feeling of pleasure or displeasure.

Under the term affectivity we comprise the affects, the emotions, and the feelings of pleasure and displeasure. The expression "feel-

[26] E.g., following an alcoholic delirium, orientation as to time and place sometimes remains disturbed a few days longer, while the other functions appear quite normal.

[27] Regarding Wernicke's classification of orientation into autopsychic somatopsychic and allopsychic, see the disturbances of orientation, p. 110.

ing," which is frequently used for this whole group of phenomena, is misleading. For it is also used to designate sensations in the lower sensory qualities, such as feelings of warmth, somatic feelings, and Munk's sphere of feeling, as well as indefinite perceptions such as the feeling of someone approaching. It is furthermore used to designate the result of inferences originating in the unconscious, such as reaching a diagnosis by a "diagnostic feeling," and finally it is used to designate complex processes of cognition, the elements of which are not clear to us, such as the feeling of familiarity. The terms "affects" and "emotions" are too limited in their application, and they really do not embrace the simple feelings of pleasure and displeasure.

Affectivity includes somatic as well as psychic manifestations, which are sometimes conceived as symptoms and sometimes as effects of the same.

It influences gestures in the broadest sense; this includes the emphasis in speech, the attitude of the body and muscular tone; it also influences the vascular system, as in blushing, turning pale, and in palpitation of the heart; and it also affects all secretions, such as tears, saliva, urine and faeces; finally it influences also the whole trophic system of the body.

On the other hand, affectivity is markedly dependent on physical influences. We note this in anxiety of endocarditis, in depressive irritability of dyspeptics, in the euphoria of tubercular patients or alcoholics, and in the affective manifestations of inner secretions.

In the *psychic field* we must first mention the undescribable subjective sensations of pleasure, displeasure, joy, sadness, anger, and similar feelings.

Affectivity also determines our actions. We strive to procure and retain pleasure, that is, pleasurably accentuated experiences, and we keep away from displeasure. If we take upon ourselves displeasure, it is only to avert a still greater one or in order to obtain some pleasure which we value higher than the assumed displeasure.

Affectivity has a determining effect upon action also by way of *thought* which is more influenced by it than is ordinarily imagined. In regard to its content this is shown in two ways:

(1) The path is cleared for associations corresponding to an actual affect, i.e. these associations are favored, while all the others, particularly those incompatible with the affect, are hindered (the dominating force of the affects). From this one may conclude: (a) There is a compulsion to occupy oneself with the emotionally accentuated subject. (Actual emotionally accentuated experiences can only be ignored in exceptional cases, and under certain conditions they absolutely prevent

any thought in other directions.)   (b) Logic becomes falsified.   (In a state of euphoria, a person is unable to take into account all the poor chances; they do not even "occur to him," or they are deliberately disregarded in the logical operation.   One ignores his own faults.)

(2) The valuation, or the logical weight of the ideas which are in accord with an affect, become enhanced, whereas the value of irrelevant and especially of opposing ideas is depreciated.   From this again one may infer on the one hand, that there is a tendency to occupy oneself with those ideas which seem important, and on the other hand, that there is a broader alteration in the logical operations.   A timid person puts too high a value on the dangers involved and too low a value on the good chances, if he considers them at all.   An investigator whose ambition depends on one of his formulated theories will continually find corroborations for it, and he is unable to give full weight to the arguments against it.

The effects of an affect manifest themselves differently and have a different significance, particularly in psychopathology, depending on whether they are caused by a general mood, such as euphoria, sadness, anxiety, etc., or whether they only emanate from a single affective idea. On the whole, one can be in a different mood and yet have a complex of ideas, which, whether it is conscious or unconscious at the moment, is endowed with anxiety or joy or chagrin.   In the latter case not all associations are influenced in the sense of this affect, which controls the idea, but only those which in any way touch the "complexes." [28] Our thinking may be quite correct in all other respects, but it is very one-sided in regard to some one who has angered us, or some one with whom we are in love. As a rule, all complexes have a tendency to establish a relationship between themselves and the other experiences (The onanist imagines that every one is looking at him because of his vice), and thus lead to the formation of false self references in both normal and pathological people.   If the thought is difficult to bear, the whole complex can more or less be split off from consciousness and merge into the unconscious but it does not always lose its influence upon the psyche as a result.   The effects of an affectively accentuated complex are designated as *katathymic* by *Hans. W. Maier.*

The influence of affectivity upon thought and action becomes re-enforced by its *tendency to spread*. In point of time the affects quite generally outlast the intellectual process at their basis, and what is more, they frequently continue for a long time.   Besides, they easily "irradiate" to other psychic experiences which are associated in some way with the idea having an affective tone.   Thus we love the place

[28] See the following page.

where we have experienced something beautiful and we hate the innocent bearer of bad news. Love often is "transferred" from the originally beloved person to another who bears some analogy to the former
or it may be transferred to an object, such as a letter, etc. Even in
normal conditions it may happen that the transferred affect detaches
itself from the original idea, so that the latter seems indifferent, while
the secondary idea carries the affect which does not properly belong
to it (*Displacement* of the affect).

If a definite affect persists and dominates for some time the whole
personality with all its experiences, we speak of a *mood*. The tendency
of an affect, which has once appeared, to continue and to become transferred to other experiences, as well as its influence upon thought, facilitate the occurrence of permanent moods. But the latter may also be
the result of physical causes, based on constitutionally determined
moods or as partial symptoms of temperaments, alcoholic euphoria,
mania, melancholia and similar states.

Positive or pleasurably accentuated affects accelerate the train of
thought, while negative ones retard it. As a result of acceleration,
thought sometimes becomes changed even in content, it becomes more
superficial; in a high degree of retardation it never reaches its object.

The affects possess great *associative power*. An unpleasant affect
has a tendency to ekphorize former affects of a similar nature. Thus
an event, not very important in itself, may produce a great effect by
reviving affects from former situations of similar quality of much
greater emotional tone. It is remarkable that the former events often
remain unconscious in this process. In other cases the very experiences
are recalled to memory in the first place, and then reenforce and modify
secondarily the original affect. These peculiarities are of great significance in the pathology of the neuroses.

By inhibiting the ideas which do not belong to them the affects
also exert a limiting influence upon the complexes of ideas accentuated
by them. In some connections such complexes form a whole category
and between them and the other psyche there exists not only an *association readiness* for ideas that can be utilized compatibly, but there is
also a certain *association-hostility* to anything not belonging to them.
They are therefore only slightly influenced by new experiences and are
not easily accessible to criticism. If the affective tone is unpleasant,
they are even readily repressed into the unconscious.

If such bundles of ideas, which are held together by an affect, exert
a permanent influence upon the psyche, we call them briefly "complexes."

A complex may thus be formed in regard to a person who has disappointed us, so that everything connected with him is not only burdened with the unpleasant feelings, but it also participates in the association readiness or in the repression which adheres to the idea of this person. The memory of the place where he lives produces an irritable mood and reaction; distant ideas which would ordinarily never be associated with the person call him to mind, or, the opposite occurs, the whole complex is forgotten, repressed, so that we find it difficult to recall even the names of his friends. The complexes are mostly either vividly conscious, or later repressed and unconscious. In both cases they influence our thinking, striving and mimicry. The most common complexes are connected with the instincts and many are recognized in the attitude and in the whole behavior of the individual. Feelings of inferiority in any sphere (insufficiency complex) which contribute to the formation of many neuroses are very important and especially those with an ambivalent feeling tone.[29] Such complexes may even acquire a kind of independence as far as certain voices may represent a "greatness" that the patient would like to attain and others may personify a weakness, which hinders him in the success of his plans.[30]

An intellectual process, a perception, an action in response to a stimulus, and a thought, are all in a certain respect partial functions. We could imagine that only a part of the psychic organism participates in these processes. In contradistinction to this, the affective processes signify an *assumed attitude of the whole person.* They participate in the affective changes of all psychic activity, in the creation of uniform striving for an aim on the part of all associations, in a general facilitation or restraint of the psychic processes, in the changing of the blood supply in the brain, and in similar mechanisms. Intellectual and affective processes are related parallel manifestations; they represent the local and the general side of the same psychism. Nevertheless, they can subsequently separate so that each process may proceed independently or become associated with other processes of the other series. As a result of irradiation an affect may become connected with ideas to which it was not originally related, and still remain in contact with the original idea, but it may also be completely separated from it. Under certain conditions we may form a distinct image of the death of a beloved person, either while the event actually takes place or later from memory, without experiencing with it the corresponding affect. On the other hand, the idea of mourning may be attached to a secondary

[29] See p. 125.
[30] Cf. The classical self-portrayal of *Staudenmaier,* Die Magie als experimentelle Naturwissenschaft, Leipzig, Akademische Verlagsgesellschaft, m. b. H. 1912.

idea indifferent in itself, as to the perception of the place where we last saw the deceased or to a song. In such a case we are frequently unable to understand the significance of the affect (displacement). Or the affect may become detached from the idea it belongs to without associating itself with any other idea. There is, for example, *"a freely floating anxiety"* which originally belonged to a fearful idea and was repressed into the unconscious; one feels anxiety but does not know why. There is, however, an anxiety which cannot be differentiated from this one, which may be of physical origin, as in circulatory disturbances or in melancholia. In both cases it may attach itself under certain conditions to some secondary idea, which in itself need not at all be endowed with anxiety.

The affects show more clearly than anything else how the psyche as a whole is always the decisive factor, and how the individual ideas, concepts, and affects which we emphasize are only artificial classifications. The taste of a certain food may be very pleasant to one hungry and very unpleasant to one who has over-eaten. Music, which in itself would be considered pleasant, may be very disagreeable if it is not in harmony with the mood of the listener, or if he is disturbed by it, or if he happens to have very sensitive nerves, or if he is in a state of melancholy. If a lunatic gives us a box on the ear it produces no affect in us, but under different circumstances it may fill us with the greatest anger or despair. *Careful observation impels us to make the general statement, that in reality we never react to a single experience or idea with a definite affect, but that the affect is always merely a part of the whole complex of functions which forms the actual psyche.*

In human beings endowed with memory who do not merely live for the moment, but form ideas from the past and have ambitions for the future, the tendency to manifest themselves on the part of the ideas and strivings, carrying a negative affect, conflicts with the opposite tendency to keep away from the unpleasant. Thus if one has a feeling of revenge or sexual love for one's mother, which is intolerable to a moral person, he usually solves this conflict by shutting the idea out of consciousness in *statu nascendi*. Notwithstanding this, the idea continues to exist and may influence his actions in a roundabout way, or it may provoke symptoms. The idea has simply been repressed into the unconscious. Repression naturally plays a great part in psychopathology.

Every affect has a tendency to act in a definite direction. Because some one has insulted me an apparatus (chance apparatus) results in my psyche which seeks to avenge me, just as the accommodation in the psychological experiment creates a kind of transient reflex apparatus, which, without any further exertion on the part of my will, responds to the appearance of a red light with a pressure of the right forefinger on the button, or like any resolution when formed incites one to put it into execution. The apparatus is shut off, e.g., through the fact that it has accomplished its purpose. I have revenged myself, or the experiment is finished, or it stops because it has lost its purpose, as when I become reconciled with the person who offended me. According to the strength of the affect it has a motive power which can be compared with physical tension of energy. If the motive power is too weak, or if the function of the apparatus is restrained by external circumstances of inner opposing forces, then the apparatus with its *"tension,"* remains inactive. But if new impulses are added to the same or even to a similar action, the "tension of the apparatus then becomes reenforced, so that, under certain conditions, it finally overcomes all obstacles in an explosive manner and like an inhibited reflex it may even shoot extensively and intensively beyond the aim. One then conceives the impression of an *"accumulation of affects."* Qualitative departure from the original purpose, in the form of simple mimetic expressions, such as exultation, screaming, or smashing of an innocent object, may also occur and they suffice to put the apparatus out of action. One then speaks of a discharge or *abreaction* of the affective tension, while the real process consists in the dismantling of the apparatus in question.

For, if the apparatus is not actually put out of function, it remains throughout life and may cause in normal people some sort of an incomprehensible readiness to react explosively to certain experiences; in sick people it may provoke a variety of symptoms without losing any energy thereby. This is particularly true if the affective complex has been repressed. In that case it cannot be shut off by the conscious personality and may continue unrestricted in the same condition; indeed, through similar new experiences the complex may even acquire more and more tension. Exaggerated sensitiveness to fear in an adult may thus be traced back to a repressed terrifying experience of childhood which has been furnished with tension from all similar later experiences, without any knowledge of it on the part of the patient. Indeed, such an occurrence may produce the tendency to experience similar things over and over again.

Chance apparatus occur also without any special affects, wherever there is an intention to do something, even if it is simply a question of finishing some thought. Secondary experiences and thoughts of the previous day to which one often pays no attention and which appear in dreams also belong here. *Habit* too creates chance mechanism which are particularly difficult to abolish, because they are not set for a definite aim happening but once and the attainment of which automatically stops the machine.

Affectivity varies greatly in different individuals and frequently even in the same person at different ages. While every normal person must call a cat a cat and observe the general rules of logic in order to get along with his fellow-men and the external world in general, he may love the cat or consider it a monstrous animal. The individual's mode of reaction, which primarily expresses itself in affectivity, is not tied to such narrow standards as logic. It is for this reason that one may argue, for example, whether or not the isolated absence of feeling tone in moral concepts is to be looked upon as pathological.

The *character* of a person is almost exclusively determined by affectivity: Animated and easily changeable feelings constitute the sanguine temperament, while persistent and profound feelings the phlegmatic character; a person who does not accentuate the concepts of good and evil with pleasure or displeasure, or who puts a weaker accent on them than on egotistical ideas "has a bad character." Next to the quality of reactions we must also consider the rapidity and force of the affects and hence of the impulses. Jealousy, envy, vanity are characteristics as well as affects. Affectivity is also responsible for laziness, energy, steadiness, diligence and carelessness.

From what has been said above, the function of affectivity in our psyche is evident. It determines the direction and force of action, and through its endurance and irradiation, as well as through its influence upon the logical functions, it provides uniformity and emphasis for this action. It especially regulates social intercourse with our fellowmen. Here it is important to note that we constantly apprehend and respond instinctively to the most delicate fluctuations of affects in our fellow-men.

We strive for the pleasurable, which on the whole consists of what is useful to the individual or the genus. The reverse is true of the displeasurable. Exceptions to this are concerned with experiences which are quite rare and therefore do not endanger the existence of the genus, or with occurrences to which the race has not yet adapted itself because of lack of time. Thus we find the taste of the beneficial cod liver oil disagreeable, but that of harmful alcohol pleasant.

That *excessive* affects may be harmful (paralyzed with fear, blind rage) is quite obvious. Compared with the daily and hourly occurrences in which, for example, a very slight anger or slight fear is a help in overcoming an obstacle, they are rare exceptions which cannot threaten the existence of the genus.

Physical *pain* assumes a special position. It accompanies destructive processes in the body and is localized like a physical sensation. At the same time it is also a feeling or an affect and has the same significance. It forces us to direct our attention to injuries of the body and to ward them off energetically. There are also other "primitive feelings" (*v. Monakow*), which cannot be clearly separated from our conception, as for instance hunger.

h) ATTENTION

Attention is a manifestation of affectivity. It consists in the fact that certain sensory perceptions and ideas which have aroused our interest are facilitated and all others inhibited. If we are performing an important experiment, we only observe what is relevant to it; everything else is entirely lost to our senses.

If we wish to concentrate on a certain theme we call to our assistance all appropriate associations and exclude the others. The greater "clearness" of observation and thoughts to which we direct attention is merely the expression of the fact that everything relevant is observed and considered while the irrelevant is eliminated. Hence in attention the "interest" inhibits and facilitates the associations in the same way as is ordinarily done by the affects. The more successfully this is done, the greater is the intensity or the *concentration,* and the greater the number of useful associations put in operation, the greater the *extent* of attention.

A distinction is also made between *tenacity* and *vigility* of attention which are usually, but not always antagonistic to each other. Tenacity is the ability to keep one's attention fixed on a certain subject continuously, and vigility the capacity to direct one's attention to a new object, particularly to an external stimulus.

We must also differentiate between *maximum* and *habitual* attention. Many patients habitually observe very little, they do not orientate themselves when they go to an unfamiliar place, etc. But if they are induced to exert their maximum of attention, they can do this without any difficulties and sometimes particularly well.

If attention is directed by the will, we designate it as *active:* if by external occurrences, we call it *passive.* Maximum attention will always be active while habitual attention may be either active or passive. The latter plays a special part in recording the daily happenings of one's environment.

The success of attention is, of course, not merely dependent on the affect, but also on the *general disposition of the psyche.* Some people are not capable of great concentration although they seem to possess a sufficiently strong and stable affect. Exhaustion, alcoholic effects, and many pathological states hinder concentration and tenacity. The extent of attention is, of course, also dependent on the general capacity to form associations, and it is therefore not as great in people of lesser intelligence.

The opposite of attention is *distraction*, which shows two contrasting forms. On the one hand, if a pupil shows a lack of tenacity in hypervigility he may be designated as distracted if he is disturbed by every noise, whereas hypertenacity and hypovigility are characteristics of the absent-minded scholar. A third form, which is pathological in its more pronounced manifestations, is due to an insufficient capacity to concentrate. The latter may have an affective basis, as in the case of neurasthenia, or it may be due to disturbances in association, as in schizophrenia and certain deliria, or it may depend on more complicated conditions, such as exhaustion.

Temporary distraction usually originates in a definite situation. It is self-evident that an affect will hinder the attention from being focused on something of quite a different nature, as in the case of a schoolboy who is about to make a trip and has to do his lessons. But an affect of fear may just as easily transcend beyond the mark and interfere with even an adequate reflection. In a critical situation attention often fails us, the ability to concentrate is usually entirely lacking and frequently also the tenacity, one continually wanders away from the individual idea, or, like the pupil who is anxiously trying to complete his lesson, one is distracted by every fly. Frequently, however, tenacity becomes too great, and the individual is dominated by one single idea.

A process quite analogous to attention, which is a sort of unconscious and permanent situation of the latter, is the *association readiness*. If something occupies us affectively, then the most various experiences will remind us of it. All kinds of ideas will find associative connection with this idea, even if it has not become actual in thought. A person who is afraid of being arrested will easily be frightened by any one who might in some way remind him of a detective. The association readiness, like attention, can also be intentionally fixed on certain things. Thus I may be searching for something in a book, but I am also interested in many other things in the book and therefore read at random, but as soon as I strike the passage upon which I have fixed, or even something that is only similar, I associate it with the desired subject.

Mere habit may also produce a sort of association readiness, even if in a somewhat different sense. Thus a person who is occupied with much proof reading will easily notice typographical errors in other reading.

Even in normal persons the association readiness often produces deceptions which are very much like delusions, thus a person with a bad conscience thinks that he is everywhere the subject of observation.

There is also a negative fixation of attention which plays an important rôle in pathology. Here one does not wish—usually unconsciously—to consider certain things, or one refuses to take them into consideration in reflections. The *association hostility* makes itself felt in attention.

i) SUGGESTION [31]

Uniformity of action is not only necessary for the individual with his various strivings, but even more for a community of individuals. Animals, even those living in herds, are apparently unable to communicate to one another ideas of a predominantly intellectual content. Most of their communications are about the approach of prey or of danger and, as observation shows, this is done mainly through affective display, which evokes the same affects in the other members of the herd. It is only through the movement of flight or attack of the animal first seized with the affect that the others learn the direction of the prey or danger. This is entirely sufficient for most cases.

This affective suggestibility is still fully present also in man, in spite of his language which has been more and more developed for intellectual needs. Even the infant reacts appropriately to affective manifestations, and the adult cannot remain cheerful when he is among sad people, not because of the ideas at the basis of the sadness, but because of the affective display which he perceives. Because of the close connection between the affect and the ideas to which it belongs and because of the influence of the affect upon logic, it is self-evident that the ideas are very easily suggested along with the affect, quite apart from the fact that the object of this arrangement is surely also to transmit the ideas. Ideas without an accompanying affect do not act suggestively. "The greater the emotional value of an idea, the more contagious it is." [32] In conscious suggestion, to be sure, we usually deal with a "pair" of affects instead of a uniform affect; in the sug-

[31] Forel, Der Hypnotismus, 6th Ed., Stuttgart, Enke, 1911. Moll, Der Hypnotismus, 4th Ed., Berlin, Fischer, 1907.

[32] The affect, however, may be present merely in the person subject to suggestion as when a remark, indifferent in itself, touches an affectively toned complex. A person with an incurable disease hears about a miraculous cure spoken of in an indifferent or even disparaging tone, and is immediately enthused to try it himself.

gestor there is the affect of domination, while in the person subject to suggestion the affect of being dominated or of submissive. Moreover, in natural suggestions, and even in animals there are also identical as well as similar reciprocal relationships of affects. Among enemies the fear of the one increases the courage of the other and vice versa.

Not only thoughts are accessible to suggestion but also perceptions, such as suggested hallucinations, and all functions controlled by the brain, i.e. by the affects, such as the "involuntary muscles," the heart, the glands, etc. *The influence of suggestion is therefore much greater than that of the conscious will,* but it corresponds with that of the affects.

However, the individual suggestion is not of great importance in the ordinary life of man. Infinitely more important is the suggestion of the mass, which even the most intelligent person cannot escape. The swaying of the masses in political and religious movements is principally done by suggestion, and not by logical persuasion; frequently it is even quite contrary to logic. A whole nation is quite incapable of viewing critically, or resisting suggestions which deal with the instincts and impulses of preservation, greatness, power, and position.

The psychology of the masses has laws which are quite different from those of individual psychology. A feeling of community is set in motion only by impulses possessed by most individuals. The finer feelings which are developed individually only, cannot come to expression; thus the masses possess another more primitive morality in the good as well as in the bad sense. Whereas the feelings become enhanced through agreement, the individual's logic not only remains without any unified connection of the mass, but it is hindered by it; at most the mass permits it only a subservient part. Reflection, reasoning, and the creation of great intellectual and spiritual values of the mass or of a people originate more from dereistic thinking. Due to elementary suggestibility the "leader" in the crowd attains great power in the discovery and accomplishment of ideas. But sometimes he is only the one who most definitely, most consciously, or most forcibly perceives the chaotic ideas created by the people, he is merely the focus of the mass psyche. The more the community increases in numbers, the more and more does the guiding force become impelled by obscure instincts, which are not clear to any individual and of which the majority never becomes conscious. They are likewise difficult to grasp objectively and resemble much more the evolutionary tendencies of the vegetative or animal organism, or sudden migrations of animal species, than actions with a conscious aim. Each individual of a certain race or period possesses the same tendencies, which burst forth with irresistible power and stubborn persistency from the *"collective uncon- scious,"* of which the generally known *"spirit of the age"* is a partial manifestation. In chronological succession crowd psychology expresses itself in *traditions,* legends, and similar mechanisms; only what is common to the various generations is selected and retained.

Suggestion has the same significance for a community as the affect for the individual. It makes for a uniform striving and provides it with power and endurance.

Simple *habits,* as well as examples, can exert very much the same influence as actual suggestion. One does what one is accustomed to do without any other reason; one likes to do as other people do without much thought or feeling in the matter. In the latter case, to be sure, suggestion, particularly mass suggestion, may easily be a contributing factor. Viewed from another angle, habit also appears in the form of *Pawlow's* association of reflexes (conditioned reflexes), in which, for instance, secretion of saliva is associated with the sounding of a certain tone, by letting this note sound a few times at the time of nourishment. These mechanisms must theoretically be clearly differentiated from suggestion, although in reality they are frequently mixed.

We also speak of *autosuggestion,* but this is merely a name for the effects of affectivity upon one's own logic and bodily function. It is of greater importance in pathology.

Suggestibility is artificially increased in states of hypnosis which are themselves produced by suggestion. In hypnosis the associations are so limited that one only perceives and thinks what the suggestor wishes, that is, as far as the test person is able to understand his wishes. On the other hand, the psyche has far more power over the voluntary associations than ordinarily. The hypnotized person will guess what is expected of him far better than the normal person. He can utilize sensory impressions which would be too weak for him in the ordinary state. He can imagine things so vividly that he hallucinates them, but on the other hand, he is able to shut off completely from his psyche actual sensory impressions ("negative hallucinations"). He has memories at his disposal of which he ordinarily does not know anything. He frequently also controls in a striking manner the vegetative functions, such as heart action, the vasomotors, the intestinal movement. All these processes may also be continued beyond the time of hypnosis, if desired (posthypnotic effects).

Negative suggestibility is the counterpart of the positive. Just as we have an impulse to follow the suggestion of others, we have as primary an impulse not to follow or to do the opposite. Children at a certain age often manifest this negative suggestibility in pure form.

In general, we see it very distinctly in people who have a strong positive suggestibility, one reason perhaps being that both kinds of suggestibility are two sides of the same characteristic, but also because one is in greater need of protection through the negative suggestibility, the greater the danger of becoming a prey to the positive. The appearance of negative impulses beside the positive is of the greatest importance. It prevents us from too easily beccming the sport of suggestions, it protects the child in particular against an excess of influences, it forces the adult to reflect, and it makes self-assertion possible at every stage of life.

k) DEREISTIC [33] THINKING

Whenever we playfully give free reign to our phantasy, as happens in mythology, in dreams or in some pathological states, our thoughts are either unwilling or unable to take cognizance of reality and follow paths laid out for them by instincts and affects. It is characteristic of this "dereistic thinking," "the logic of feeling" (Stransky), that it totally ignores any contradictions with reality. Thus the child and sometimes the adult fancy themselves in their day dreams as heroes or inventors or something else great; in one's night dreams one can realize the most impossible wishes in the most adventurous manner; and in his hallucinatory state the schizophrenic day laborer marries a princess. Mythology finds it quite natural to allow the Easter rabbit to lay eggs simply because it happens that rabbits and eggs have one thing in common, namely, they are both sacred to the goddess Ostara as symbols of fruitfulness. The paranoid finds a piece of thread in his soup which proves his relationship to Miss Threadway. Reality which does not fit in with such modes of thinking is frequently not only ignored, but actively split off, so that, in these connections at least, it is no longer possible to think in terms of reality. Thus the day laborer as the fiancé of the princess, is no longer a day laborer, but the Lord of Creation or some other great personage.

In the sober-minded forms of dereistic thinking, particularly in day dreams, there is very little disregard or transformation of actual situations, and only few absurd associative connections formed. On the other hand, dreams, schizophrenia, and to some extent mythology, exercise far greater freedom in dealing with the thought material, where, for example, a God may give birth to himself. In these forms dereism goes so far as to destroy the most common concepts: Diana of Ephesus is not Diana of Athens, Apollo is split into several personalities, now he blesses and now he kills, he is a fructifier and he is an artist; indeed,

[33] Derived from *de* and *reor* (away from reality, unrealistic).

he may even be a woman although he is ordinarily a man. The interned schizophrenic demands damages in a sum of gold which would exceed the mass of our entire solar system a trillion times. A female paranoid calls herself free Switzerland, because she should be free. Similarly in other cases, symbols are treated like realities, and different concepts are condensed into one. Persons appearing in dreams of normal people usually have features of several acquaintances; a normal woman without being aware of it speaks of the "hind-legs" of her small child, which was due to the fact that she had fused it with a frog.

Dereistic thinking realizes our wishes, but also our fears. It makes the playing boy a general, and the girl with her doll a happy mother. In religion it satisfies our longing for eternal life, for justice and joy without sorrow. In the fairy tale and in poetry it gives expression to all our complexes. In dreams it serves to represent the person's most secret wishes and fears. For the abnormal person it creates a reality which is far more real to him than what we call reality. It makes him happy in his delusion of greatness, and absolves him from blame if he fails in his aspirations, by attributing the cause to persecutions from without, rather than to his own short-comings.

If the results of dereistic thinking seem to be sheer nonsense when measured by realistic logic, still, as an expression or fulfilment of wishes, as a provider of consolation, and as symbols for other things, they possess a kind of realistic value, a "psychic reality" in the above defined sense.[34]

Besides the affective needs, the intellectual ones may also be satisfied in dereistic thinking; but as yet we know very little about them. Thus in mythology, the sun which travels across the sky has feet or rides in a carriage. In a certain sense, however, all "needs" are affective. At any rate, affectivity plays an important rôle in dereistic thinking when it attempts to give us information regarding the origin of the world and the structure of the universe.

In its full development dereistic thinking seems to be different in principle from empirical thinking. But in reality one finds all the transitions, from the slight deviation from acquired associations as is necessary in every conclusion drawn by analogy, to the wildest phantasy.

For, within certain limits, independence of habitual trends of thought is a preliminary condition of intelligence, which strives to find new paths. And the effort to fancy oneself into new situations, day dreams and similar occupations are indispensable exercises of the intelligence.

[34] Cf. p. 7.

*To be sure, the contents and aims of such unbridled mental ac-
tivities always represent strivings which most deeply touch our inner-
most nature. It is therefore quite obvious that dereistic aims are valued
much higher than real advantages, which can be replaced.*[35] This not
only explains the peculiar barbarities of religious wars, but we can also
understand why primitives are fettered with taboo rules, and similar
superstitions, and why they exert the most painstaking efforts not to
leave a particle of their food which could give an enemy the chance
to practice harmful magic on them. We can also see why we find it
difficult to understand how the savage is willing to bear such burdensome regulations, even if we compare them with Chinese or European
rules of etiquette.

It will be interesting to trace the circumstances which determine
so marked a deviation of thinking from reality:

1. We think dereistically wherever our knowledge of reality is insufficient for practical needs or our impulse for knowledge urges us to
keep on thinking; this happens in problems referring to the origin and
purpose of the world and of mankind, in problems dealing with God,
the origin of diseases, or evil in general, and how it can be avoided. The
greater our knowledge of the actual relationships, the less room there
remains for such forms of thinking. Questions, such as how winter
and summer come about, how the sun traverses the sky, how the
lightning is flashed, and a thousand other things, which were formerly
left to mythology, are now answered through realistic thinking. 2.
Wherever reality seems unbearable it is frequently eliminated from
our thinking. Delusions, dreamlike wish fulfilments in twilight states,
and neurotic symptoms, which represent a wish fulfilment in symbolic
form, originate in this way. 3. If the different co-existing ideas do not
converge in the one point of the ego to form a logical operation, the
greatest contradiction can exist side by side, there is no question of
any critique. Such conditions are present in unconscious thinking and
perhaps also in some delirious states. 4. In the forms of associations
prevailing in dreams and in schizophrenia the affinities of empirical
thinking are weakened. Any other associations directed by more accidental connections, such as symbols, sounds, etc., obtain the upper
hand, but this is especially true of those guided by affects and all kinds
of strivings.

1) Belief, Mythology, Poetry, Philosophy

Belief is closely related both to suggestion and to dereistic thinking.
The word "to believe" has two meanings: "To accept something as true

[35] Cf. the next chapter on "Belief."

without logical proof," and "to consider something as probable." We'
confine ourselves here to the former concept.

The greatest creeds in religion, politics, theories of social position,
esthetics, etc., are maintained almost entirely through suggestion. Suggestion is above all responsible for the uniformity in forms and details,
and to some extent also for the motive power of belief. The origin of
belief always proceeds in accordance with the laws of the affective
mental stream in dereistic thinking. The several great creeds serve
as a definite gratification of general affective needs, and for this
reason they are so easily suggestible and possess such great power
that in most cases one assumes these ideas without any logical
realitic value. We wish to know that something happens after death;
we wish to feel that we can influence fate. The *beatus possidens*
who, in the face of misery, wishes to establish his position on moral
grounds, acts in the same way; and the sick person who wishes
to become well and therefore believes in the quack follows the same
mechanism.

We also differentiate between belief and superstition; the latter
contains a great deal of magic which operates with unknown forces,
while belief has to do more with religion which deals with our relations
to a higher being. But viewed psychologically, there is principally no
difference between them; the main difference lies in the valuation which
is measured by different standards. Belief becomes pathological only
when it dominates the psyche far too much and when it glaringly conflicts with the logical faculties and eventually also with the views of
the individual. But from this alone, and without other supporting
points I should not like to make a diagnosis. The name of *prejudice* is
applied to false belief or to superstition, when it does not refer contently
to matters of religion, or to one's relationship to fate. This varies from
the prejudices of the people in the recent war to the prejudice of one
individual for another. Prejudice may at first actually be based on a
mere hasty judgment; but it can only derive its power from affective
sources by way of dereism or suggestion.

Poetry and *mythology* satisfy the same need as belief, with the
difference that the former lays no more claim to direct realistic value
than the day dreams of normal people. *Philosophy* differs very little
from it, in so far as it actually is pure philosophy. (For there are some
real sciences classified under this name, such as the deduction of logical
and esthetic laws, the theory of cognition, etc.) The current explanations of the optimistic and pessimistic theories as a characteristic expression of the philosophers originating them, perhaps most clearly
demonstrate the subjectivity of philosophy.

m) THE PERSONALITY, THE EGO

Most of our psychic functions have a continuity, in so far as the experiences become connected with one another through memory, and in so far as they unite with a very firm and constantly present complex of memory pictures and ideas, namely, the ego, or the personality. To be exact, the ego consists of the engrams of all our experiences plus the actual psychism. By this, of course, we must not merely understand passive experiences, but also all our former and present volitions and strivings; the ego thus really comprises our entire past in a very abbreviated form. Still, not all of these constituents have the same value. At a given moment most of them recede until they lose all effectiveness, that is, they are not ekphorized; others are usually, or always present. The composition of the ego of individual memory images, may be compared to the "public" in a certain restaurant; individual frequenters may come and go, some are constant visitors, others come frequently, and still others have visited the place only a few times. It is true that I have learned to extract square roots but in my present activity this knowledge is almost altogether latent. Certain ideas, however, such as who we are, what we have been, and what we are now, what we strive for in life, must be constantly more or less clearly present. They are part of the directive power of our daily actions. The fact that a student goes to the class at the right time is not merely determined by the idea of the hour and his schedule, but among other things also by that of wishing to study, and by the point at which he has arrived in his study.

Thus personality is not something changeable. The component parts of its ideas change constantly in accordance with momentary aims, but also in accordance with experiences. There is still a greater distinction between the *strivings* of the man and those of the child; and the destinies of life such as depression determined by inner causes and even toxic influences (alcohol) may, within a very short time completely transform the affective part of the personality, which in some respects is the more important. In a similar manner as in severe psychoses, the personality may go to pieces in the dream. Some parts of it fall away and are replaced by others that are quite foreign to it. Thus a dreamer who in ordinary life is unassuming may feel himself as being King David, a gentle person may commit a murder, and a hard-hearted man may wallow in benevolence.

We also often attribute to the person a special *personal consciousness* or a *"self-consciousness."* [36] These two expressions contain two

[36] In popular psychology the expression "self-consciousness" has a different but important meaning, namely, estimation of oneself.

sets of ideas, the former represents the continuity of the person,—the ego of a normal person has the feeling of being the same through life— the latter deals with the fact of rendering the person prominent and distinguishing him from the environment, and particularly from other people. It was assumed that the child had no self-consciousness, and to prove this it was argued that the child does not correctly distinguish its own person, in so far as it speaks of itself in the third person. This is wrong. In principle the child differentiates itself from everything else and also from other people just like the adult. That it speaks of itself in the third person has its obvious reasons which may be sought in the manner of teaching language to the child.

n) THE CENTRIFUGAL FUNCTIONS

To assert oneself or the genus in accordance with the *aim* of the psychic apparatus, to make use of the environment or to defend one-self against it, is expressed in every psychism in a tendency to react, or in a striving. In a more complicated being this finds expression in the form of affectivity. If we perceive something beautiful, we would like to enjoy it, and if it is unpleasant we would like to ward it off. Besides this we have a number of strivings which become effective even without any external cause. Among these we may mention the impulse to live, the activity impulse, the self-assertion impulse, the impulse for knowledge, hunger, and the sex impulse. The activities in the sense of these strivings are also connected with pleasure. The instincts of animals evidently represent the same thing. Principally there is really no line of demarkation between these two kinds of strivings.

In the countless strivings and exciting experiences many conflicts and inhibition must frequently arise. One would like to rest and at the same time drink some water which must be brought from the well; one would like to be virtuous and at the same time get rid of his sexual tension. Even for physical reasons one cannot do many things at the same time. The inhibiting effect exerted by contrary impulses upon one another represents only another special case of the general law, namely, that central functions not having a similar aim inhibit each other. But if the force of one impulse is not very much stronger than that of the other, there results a competition, whereby in the "reflection" or in the "choice between good and evil" each impulse attracts associatively the material resembling it, intellectually and affectively. And under certain conditions it may also attract that which is contrary to it, in the sense of negative suggestion. Thus arise different functional complexes which act as a whole, and of which one finally asserts itself and dominates in such a manner that the other is "suppressed." We designate this as the *decision* or the *act of volition.*

In a serious struggle of impulses, as for instance in a decision between good and evil, the material brought into play includes our virtues and vices, our entire ethical training, former decisions to be good or to disregard moral standards, as well as our experiences in former violations of ethics; in brief, it involves *the whole personality;* "the decision belongs to it."

Thus we see that the *"will"* is entirely dependent on the affects, and not merely as regards its direction, but also quantitatively. He has a strong will, who possesses energetic feelings which are not swayed by every new impetus. By a *weak will* we understand quite different dispositions: (1) it may represent a weak affectivity without motive power (Abulia),[37] (2) it may evince an affectivity that is lively but too labile, too easily changeable, one who follows the crowd and paves the road to hell with good intentions, or (3) for various reasons one is unable to form any decisions.

The much mooted question whether there is a *"free will"* in the sense that a decision can be reached without any reason, does not exist in natural science. We see that the actions of living beings are determined by the inner organization and the external influences reacting upon them in exactly the same manner as any other happening. There is no decision which does not have a complete causal basis in motives and strivings. But motives and strivings are either a complex of nervous functions, which is subject to the ordinary psychic laws of cause and effect, or something analogous to these nervous processes, which depend on physical as well as psychic causes. "Motives" are causes even though they are complicated. Science is therefore *deterministic* even in those cases where it is not fully admitted. To be sure, we assumed that one acts badly "because he is a bad fellow," but we also know that he himself has not selected his own organization but that he has inherited it when he came into the world, or that it has been changed by some influences or other exerted on the brain.

Nevertheless, the subjective feeling of being free in one's decisions is not an illusion in the real sense. Our actions are the outcome of our own strivings, but as some of these contradict each other, the reaction follows exactly our feelings in the direction of our strongest impulse. The act of volition is therefore in harmony with the momentary aims of the psyche as a whole, that is, with the personality, with the complex, which comprises all strivings and in which the latter can form a resultant. *We do what we wish because we wish what we do,* or to

[37] Abulia as a consequence of inability to reach decisions, see p. 143.

express it objectively: Volition and action is one process, the two sides of which are individually rendered prominent. This has an analogy in the physical sphere, namely, when all the conditions of a process or a state are present, then the result or the state is also present. It is a mistake to think that one could wish, that is, act, something else. However, one can covet only something else. We make this mistake wherever we form an insufficient estimate of the causes, even in the physical realms; the concept of *accident* is based on this. If a brick falls from the roof and strikes the ground near a person, he says, "I could have been struck by it."

The dispute concerning the conception of the will is a striking example of the power of emotions. Scientifically viewed, determinism is the only possible conception. And yet many people cling to indeterminism although they cannot even follow the thought to any clear conclusion, the moralist, because he has falsely based his ethics thereon, the theologian because in spite of the contradiction with God's omnipotence he needs it for his actual ideas, the jurist because he thinks that otherwise his laws, particularly the penal code, will be shaken. As a matter of fact it makes no difference in practice which point of view one holds. The penal code, for instance, would not have to change a single one of its provisions, but only a few expressions, if it accepted the theory of determinism.

Among the various impulses of man the *nutritive impulse,* which is a part of the self-preservation impulse, is greatly denatured in our present condition and therefore difficult to study. But the *sexual impulse* is still clear to us. It shows us how tendencies of pleasure and displeasure impel us to actions whose natural aim (in this case the preservation of the species) may be unwelcome to us, or not become conscious at all. This is the case, for instance, in the choice of clothing and most of the other preparatory actions in the approach of the sexes. It also teaches us to understand the *instincts,* which are defined as a capacity to act in such a manner that certain aims will be fulfilled without becoming known or without being considered, and without the necessity of any particular training, acquisition, and practice.

The *ethical impulses* are of particular importance for every being living in society. They preserve the community, and hence they often conflict with the interests of the individuals; they also have a great many points of contact with sexuality. But it is just as wrong to create the impression that ethics deals with sex only, as it is incorrect to follow an ethics of "to sow one's wild oats" and to ignore altogether the sexual restraints which are originally determined by nature. Nevertheless it is certain that the existing sexual ethics is not adapted to the demands of modern civilization. Indeed, our form of society on the one hand and the sexual impulse on the other often conflict in such a way that even a theoretical solution seems impossible. *As a result conflicts are created which not only are of great importance socially, but also medically.*

Other definitions of the word "impulse" will be discussed at the end of the section on Psychopathology.

An effect similar to that of the congenital impulses is exerted by *chance apparatus* and *habits.*[38]

The other centrifugal functions, such as "psychomotility" and "motility" we shall pass over as being self-evident.

[38] See p. 50.

CHAPTER II

GENERAL PSYCHOPATHOLOGY

The symptoms of psychic diseases show such an infinite variety of manifestations that one is forced to put them into a certain scheme and to select what is most important in them. For it must be borne in mind that although superficially two phenomena may look alike, they may nevertheless have entirely different meanings, depending on their psychic environments and on their genesis. Moreover, and this is even more true here than in physical pathology, every symptom is really only a special part of a general process. What we, for example, described in the spheres of association, is not simply a disease of the associations, but a general psychic disturbance, from which we pick out one part, namely, that which concerns the associations.

For a scientific study of the psychoses it is necessary to distinguish between *primary* and *secondary* symptoms. Thus a paralysis of the abducens nerve is a primary symptom, whereas the subsequent contracture of the internal rectus and the diplopia are secondary symptoms. A certain disturbance of mental function in dementia praecox is a primary symptom while the resulting twilight state following it under the influence of an unpleasant experience is a secondary symptom. If a paronoic conceives an indifferent experience in the sense of a delusion of reference, it is in a certain relation a primary symptom, but the reaction following it, in the form of an insult which is normal in itself, is a secondary symptom. The last example also shows that these concepts are only relative, inasmuch as a fundamental disturbance often produces a whole casual chain; for the delusion of reference is already a derivative symptom, in the particular case.

In some diseases it is of value to differentiate between *principal* and *accessory symptoms*. The former appear in every one of these cases as soon as the disease reaches a certain height. One must therefore assume that *in nuce* they are also present even where we do not yet see them, that because of insufficient intensity they have not yet crossed the diagnostic threshold. Among these we have the organic symptom-complexes, in organic diseases, the association and affective disturbances in schizophrenics, and the manic and melancholic states in manic depressive psychoses. The accessory symptoms, like hallucinations and delusions, may be absent in these diseases, or they may appear and disappear at any time and in any combinations.

1. DISTURBANCES OF THE CENTRIPETAL FUNCTIONS

The centripetal functions may be disturbed through disease of the peripheral conducting or the central receptive organs. Under the latter one includes the central sensory fields as well as the whole cortex as the carrier of the psyche. The disturbances in the conducting organs can naturally only be disturbances of sensation, while those of the cortex (respectively the psyche) are almost only disturbances of perception and the first elaboration connected with it, namely, apperception.

DISTURBANCES OF THE SENSORY ORGANS

Disturbances of the sensory organs appear in part as accidental complications and in part as symptoms of individual psychoses, like paresis. On the whole they are of no importance in psychopathology, still, peripheral irritations may occasionally become important by producing hallucinations through as yet unfamiliar paths. The patient is often unable to recognize the origin of his paresthesias, and thinks that noises in his ear are bells, or what is most common, the false sensations are interpreted in the sense of illusions. Thus buzzing in the ears is conceived as rushing water or as words, shadows and light on the retina as visions of animals, and nervous pains as physical injuries.

Weakness of the sensory organs influences the psyche during its development and also later. Marked short-sightedness may lead to a deficiency of perspective or to a lack of consideration of a definite kind. Thus the miniature paintings of the poetess Annette von Drosta are supposed to be due to her myopia. *Absolute blindness*, naturally, exerts a very marked influence on the subjective view of the world, which in the normal person is in the first place optic; it does not, however, change the psyche in its relations to people.

It is quite different in the case of *deafness* or *disturbances of hearing*. With the exception of the modern way of teaching the deaf and dumb, we perceive the whole cultural achievement of older generations directly or indirectly through hearing and all our relations to human environment are regulated through language. (Writing presupposes language.) Hence the deaf person, without special instruction, remains a psychic cripple in the most important relations, even if he is intelligent; and as he is unable to put the correct value on the behavior of his environment, he becomes irritable, hot-tempered, and suspicious.

Even acquired difficulties of hearing change the psyche in both of these directions, wherein suspicion is most prominent and may even rise to the degree of delusions.

Central Disturbances of the Sensations and Perceptions. *Sensations* are seldom disturbed through psychotic processes. In melancholic and neurotic states we often encounter a more or less general *hyperesthesia*. The patients not only suffer much from the usual sensory stimuli, but they also falsely interpret the stimuli. Thus a dim light may seem glaring, knocking on the door may be conceived as shooting, and the sound of a fountain may be taken as the hissing of the escaping steam from a locomotive. Hysterical and hypnotized persons may, under certain conditions, react to the slightest sensory impressions in a manner unperceived by normals.

Hyperalgesia too, is present in the same conditions and also as a result of organic processes in the nervous system.

Hypalgesia and *Analgesia* are quite common; they are centrally determined and present a great many different types.

1. In coma of epilepsy and other diseases, it is assumed that there is an absence of consciousness and hence pain can be as little perceived as anything else. In *soporose* and *torpid* states the threshold of feeling is generally raised and the perceived stimulus, too, is of lesser value than in normal states.

2. In *strong* affects attention may be so one-sided that one may not feel even the most severe pain; thus the officer may first become cognizant of his shattered arm when he attempts to brandish his sword. Maniacal patients often injure themselves when in an excited state without noticing it; but when their attention is directed to the pain as in a minor operation, they evince great suffering. The complete analgesia which one often observes in alcoholic deliria, perhaps also belongs here.

3. *Hysterical mechanisms* can shut off altogether the feeling of pain or confine it to a circumscribed part of the body.[1] But in contradistinction to those evincing organic analgesia the hysterical patients do not injure themselves, for the feelings are only shut off from the conscious ego but continued to function in the unconscious orientation.

4. Peculiar is the analgesia in some *catatonic patients* which extends over the whole body and can be so absolute, that intentionally or accidentally, the patient may sustain the most severe injuries. It may come and go very rapidly and is thereby independent of conscious at-

---

[1] This is not to be confused with the *pleasure* in ɣαιɴ ɪn some hysterics and masochists.

tention. But even here, one perhaps deals with a blocking of feeling, of psychogenetic nature.

5. Hypalgesias and analgesias in *general paresis* are mostly confined to the skin, while the deeper structures remain sensitive. A paretic can bite out pieces of skin from his hand in order to tease the attendant, but he is extremely sensitive when an effort is made to move his ankylosed joint. The diminution or absence of sensations are to some extent mostly dependent (but not principally so) on attention. We have no comprehension for this form of analgesia.

Other *hypesthesias* and *anesthesias* are not common in the psychoses. Hysterical blindness, deafness, and similar afflictions are based on (auto-) suggestion. Depressed patients sometimes complain that their food has no taste, that it feels like chewing straw or paper, that all colors look equally grey as if covered with ashes, but when one examines their sensations they are found to be normal. The same phenomena may be produced in normal persons through a strong depressive affect.[2]

We omit here the aphasic and agnostic disturbances because they surely belong to the pathology of the cerebral cortex and not to the symptomatology of the psychoses, even if they sometimes accompany an organic mental disease.

Perception and **comprehension** show the following disturbances in *idiots*. Idiots cannot comprehend anything complicated. They see the elements of an object but not the whole thing. Or they recognize pictures with difficulty or not at all, while they can readily identify the same things in nature; they often lack the understanding for perspective imagery.

Perception may be *imperfect*. In a clouded state, catatonics and especially alcoholics, may perceive a green head of cabbage as a rose, a cucumber as a sausage, and an ear of corn as a fir-cone. All this is due to the fact that they do not comprehend the color or the size in the whole picture-complex. On the surface these disturbances resemble illusions, but they differ from them through the fact that the alteration of the picture has no meaning to the patient and is the same as falsification produced by carelessness. The mistake that brings about the illusions has a definite aim.

When apperception in the optical field is made difficult by exposing pictures for a very short time, the following will be noted: In *organic psychoses* the perception needs more time and even then the patient

---

[2] Cf. *Goethe* (Kanonenfieber bei Valmy): "The eyes lose nothing in force and clearness; but nevertheless it is as if the world assumed a distinct brown-reddish tone."

often makes mistakes.—In *epilepsy* the behavior is the same. There seems to be some difference but it cannot be definitely fixed. At all events the symptoms correspond with the general retardation of the psychic processes in the patient. *In both groups* the tendency to perseveration expresses itself in the fact, that a later image is mistaken for one seen before (paraphasic disturbances should here be excluded).—In *alcoholics* the answers mostly follow quickly and with subjective sureness; nevertheless mistakes are frequently made and sometimes they show that the real picture somehow reached the psyche. Thus mistaken objects are named which, although they show no optic similarity to the picture exposed, they nevertheless are in some way related to it. For example, the picture of an axe brings the answer shovel, or the image of a number may evoke an entirely different number. In all these diseases the results may be improved through exertion of attention, so that one is often inclined to ascribe such mistakes to inattention which would be incorrect.—In profound *melancholic states* the apperception must be given more time if one wishes to avoid an abnormal number of mistakes.—*Manic states* show nothing characteristic in the habitual perception of their environment, and in tests conducted without accurate measurements. In laboratory experimentation the patients perceive things incorrectly and make more mistakes than normal people: this probably does not depend on perception but on the flightiness of attention and similar factors. Nor are we aware of any real apperceptive disturbances in *schizophrenia;* the mistakes which occur here so often can be regularly explained by the state of complicated functions of attention, affects, and thinking.

Analogous disturbances, though not so easy to demonstrate, are also found in the *acoustic field.* In organic patients particularly, one is often struck by the fact, that questions must be often repeated before they are correctly grasped; this is especially true when one changes to another theme.

The most important psychopathic manifestations in the centripetal fields are the *sensory deceptions.* (Phantasms.) They are divided into **Illusions and Hallucinations.**

Illusions are real perceptions pathologically changed. The striking of the clock becomes an insulting remark or is conceived as a promise; the grasped hand is hurled back because it feels like a dead hand; people are seen walking on their heads; instead of the white color of the face, it looks black, and instead of the nurse one sees a waitress. *The real mistaking of personality* where some one of the environment is looked upon as a relative or acquaintance of the patient, or as the president, is rarely a pure illusion; often it is a delusion, as in schizophrenia, and occasionally it is a semi- or total conscious playfulness as in mania. Most frequently it is a process belonging to confabulations, as in organic psychosis.

The illusion is a caricaturing of a normal process. In ordinary perception it is only exceptional that we perceive all the qualities of a thing in question; the missing parts we unconsciously supplement and those that are falsely perceived are corrected in the sense of the whole thing. Thus even the normal perception is a sort of illusion. It is very difficult not to overlook a printer's errors, and the telephone certainly does not give us all the consonants with the required clearness; we supplement them without being aware of it. It is only a difference in quality, when during a markedly affective situation a tree stump is taken for a highway man, or a fog for an apparition of an angel, and yet the last examples can no longer be differentiated from the illusions of insane patients.

Hallucinations are perceptions without corresponding stimuli from without. Everything perceived can also be hallucinated, and indeed, this may be achieved in a manner, that the elements form free combinations; thus a lion may have wings, and a figure may be composed of attributes from different persons. Besides, morbid functions apparently produce inner feelings, which never occur in any other way.

The theoretical distinction between hallucinations and illusions is not always self-evident. No sense organ is ever quite without a stimulus ("Light, dust" of the dark fields; entotic noises, etc.), so that one can almost always speak of a false interpretation of a sensory impression. As a matter of fact, the so-called visual hallucinations of alcoholic deliria are illusions based on irritations of the sensory apparatus. But as the stimulus does not come from without it is counted among the hallucinations. In hallucinations of smell and taste one can hardly ever exclude sensations of smell and taste; the skin is constantly touched by the clothes, currents of air, as well as similar stimuli.

One cannot decide whether one deals with hallucinations or illusions in the case of voices coming "from" the whistling of the wind or the rattle of the wagon, which are perceived simultaneously with the noises causing them.

In most cases the differentiation is simple. Visions which are not connected with definite objects are undoubtedly hallucinations, the same is true of words which are heard as coming from the wall, and this is especially confirmed in both cases when the optic and acoustic nerves furnish beside a great many other stimuli.

Hallucinations may be graded according to three directions: the clearness of the projection to the outer world, the clearness of the perception, and the intensity. These qualities are independent of one another.

The projection to the outer world is usually perfect. What the patients see and hear they accept as impugnable reality, and when hallucination and reality contradict each other they mostly conceive what is real to us, as unreal and falsified. It is of no avail to try to convince the patient by his own observation, that there is no one in the next room talking to him; his ready reply is that the talkers just went out or that they are in the walls or that they speak through invisible apparatus.

However, hallucinations evince all gradations. There are hallucinations which are recognized as hallucinations but are none the less perceived with perceptible distinctness (Kandinsky's Pseudo-hallucinations); others concerning which the patient cannot say whether they are visions or vivid imaginations, whether they are voices or "inspired" thoughts ("psychic hallucinations"), and so they gradually shade off until they reach the usual thoughts and ideas.

The patients often localize in the body the voices, and sometimes also the visions (mostly in the chest, sometimes in the head, and occasionally even in any other part of the body).

Projection is facilitated through a high perfection of the image. Still hallucinations often show the vagueness of ordinary ideas; although the patient often sees, definitely, a "dog," he is nevertheless unable to tell anything about the breed, color, size and the position of the dog. While the patient himself is never conscious of this deficiency, it may furnish the physician important suggestions that we deal here with an illusion. One cannot, however, reason the other way, for there are also hallucinations endowed with the perfection of an actual perception.

Remarkable are the "extracampine" hallucinations which are localized outside of the sensory field in question. In the nature of the thing one deals mostly with visions, the patient sees with perfect sensory distinctness the devil behind his head, but it may also concern the sense of touch; thus the patient feels how streams of water come out from a definite point of his hand. Whether voices which seem to come from thousands of miles should be designated as extracampine or not, is arbitrary.

Sometimes, and this is most frequent in alcoholic deliria, the distinctness of the projection fluctuates with the intensity of the disease, instead of real things, the convalescent alcoholics see in the hallucinations only "images" which are shammed for their benefit; other patients maintain that the voices are only produced to deceive them or they are "dreams." Still such indistinct projections are also present at the height of the disease.

Intensity fluctuates from the loudest reports of a cannon to the hardly audible whispering, from the most glowing light to the dimmest shadow. During actual attacks, especially in schizophrenia, the intensity may rise and fall with the intensity of the attack.

The *distinctness* is sometimes extremely obtrusive; it may, however, sink to dissipating cloudlike figures, to confused voices and indistinct whispering, for the understanding of which the patient is forced to exert all his attention. At all events the patients seldom conceive the indistinctness, for they understand what the hallucination tells them.

Of other qualities of sensory deceptions the following may be mentioned: the visual hallucinations of alcoholic deliria which show a tendency to be moving, multiform, small, and without color; the visual hallucinations of touch, in cocaine insanity are often microscopically small. Visions showing a tendency to become greater and greater and which at the same time in most cases seem to come nearer and nearer are usually connected with anxiety.

Hallucinations may be changeable or stable. The voices are often abrupt and fragmentary. Auditory hallucinations put together in a dramatic fashion point to alcoholism, particularly alcoholic insanity. Connected hallucinations which fit together, accompanied primarily by visual illusions are found in hysterical twilight states, and also in other cases. Occasionally one finds one-sided hallucinations, particularly in one-sided lesions of the sensory organs or of the sensory fields and tracks in the brain.

The relation to the real perception varies. Voices can naturally be localized anywhere, in the next room, in the walls and in open spaces. Visions come in conflict with reality. Thus, behind the hallucinated man one cannot see anything of reality, or he appears transparent (ghosts). A hallucinated person can be placed in the midst of reality. Thus a skull may be seen over the shoulder of a neighbor, etc. In most cases, however, the manifestations are independent of reality. The whole environment may be changed hallucinatorily. Thus a patient imagines himself in heaven instead of the observation ward.

The patients are often cognizant of the hallucinations, not exactly that they are false sensations, but they feel that there is something strange about them. Thus they know them through their different content, they state that they have feelings that they have never experienced before, for the expression of which they have to coin new words.　They feel that they see remarkable images and scenes, abnormal localizations, voices in the walls or in their own arms, a light in their own body or in the uterus of a passing woman.　They also recognize the strangeness through indefinite projection to the outer world.　The patient believes that he hears through his leg and not in his ears; he does not know whether he touches an animal or sees it.

The relation of the hallucinations to the other mental content is remarkable.　At the height of the disease the hallucinations in most cases have not only the reality value which is unimpugnable to the patient but they also have contently a compulsive power.　Thus if a healthy person would hear a command ("Kill your child"), it would never occur to him to follow it, but the patient obeys it with or without resistance.　That has nothing to do with the form of the command, with the clouding of consciousness, or with the dementia, for the last named conditions are often absent, but it is due to the fact that the hallucinations originate from the strivings belonging to the personality of the patient.　It is for that reason that the patients find it so difficult to ignore their hallucinations.　Thus a paranoid patient suffering from pneumonia does not bother about the inflammation of the lungs, but occupies herself with the hallucinated prolapse of the rectum; a real misfortune is barely noticed while the hallucinated one lays claim to the whole personality.　On the other hand, patients in an alcoholic delirium often view their conditions like an audience in the theatre, and demented schizophrenics may even constantly hallucinate and apparently pay no attention to it.

Because the hallucinations really only express the thoughts of the patient, be they conscious or not, it is quite comprehensible how definite explanations are readily given to apparently incomprehensible hallucinations.　Thus a patient hallucinates the word "clean,"—nothing else, and becomes very excited over it because one means to tell her by this word that she has soiled the bed.　A great many definitely recognize poisons in hallucinated odors and tastes, the real odor of which they do not at all know.

This also shows the possibility of *teleologic hallucinations* which give the patient good advice or warn or prevent him from doing something which would harm him.　Thus the dead mother holds him back at the last moment from committing suicide, an hallucinated physical resistance prevents him from throwing himself out of the window.　The Maid of Orleans is told by the Holy Virgin what to do in order to conquer, but this only took place as long as the war situation was so simple that the girl's reason could grasp it.

A similar situation prevails when the so-called "voice of conscience" criticizes the actions and thoughts of the patient, be they just or evil. Sometimes warning and enticing, friendly and hostile voices, become separated into two persons which are endeavoring to persuade the patient.

Whereas in one case the hallucinations appear quite strange to the conscious personality of the patient,—a circumstance which he uses as a proof for the exogenous origin of the voices, "Such thing I really have never thought of,"—in another case they are intimately connected with the patient's thoughts. The latter case is most pronounced in the so-called *"thought-hearing"* (wrongly called "double thinking"), whereby the patient's own thoughts seem to be uttered by others. This occurs frequently during reading. It is remarkable that the voices can also utter what is contained in one or many lines perceived by the eye at the time.

Some patients are filled with their hallucinations and can talk of nothing else, while others either will not or cannot give any information about them. This is particularly true of schizophrenia where the hallucinations or the memories of them are easily blocked from the other content of consciousness.

Many patients assume as facts even the most nonsensical hallucinations. Others seek to explain them by machines, or by distant physical effects of all sorts. Nowadays one seldom hears of demoniacal influences. Some patients, who feel that their thoughts are read by others imagine themselves to be transparent. Still others believe that hearing voices signifies the attainment of a special faculty.

Causation of hallucinations. Hallucinations accompany many mental diseases, toxemias, marked exhaustions, and normal sleep. In the psychoses their appearance is facilitated by an absence of sensory stimuli, thus the darkness of the night favors visions, and the quietude of the prison auditory hallucinations. On the other hand, real stimuli sometimes act as exciting causes, thus auditory hallucinations may appear even during a noise. Many patients close their ears in order to hear the voices well, and others in order to rid themselves of them. Occupation (distraction of attention) sometimes hinders them and more seldom promotes them.

Exogenous experiences as well as thoughts may give rise to hallucinations and determine their content when it is more a question of heightening of the momentary disposition. Thus the patient seeing dishwater carried past him, hallucinates the insulting remark "food-spoiler," or seeing the grass cut, he feels himself cut with every stroke of the scythe. Other patients feel themselves "spooned in," if some one eats near them, or hearing a key turned in the lock they feel it painfully in their hearts. As a perception in one sensory field produces hallucinations in another field, one speaks in such cases of *Reflex hallucinations.* This is certainly an incorrect conception of the mechanism.

Visual hallucinations (visions) usually come in conflict with the surroundings and may also be corrected through other senses (touch, resistance). They are therefore rare during the day and in clear patients, but they easily dominate delirious and twilight states. At times they lack the third dimension, and more than any other hallucinations they show an indifferent content. Thus the patient imagines that he witnesses a theatrical performance which has nothing to do with him.

It is quite different with *auditory hallucinations.* In language they express as voices all things that move man: The patient is abused, insulted, threatened, and hears the wailing of maltreated relatives; on the other hand, he also receives joyous promises, orders, and other messages. He can enter into conversation with the voices, but in most cases he need not talk loudly to them, they answer even to his thoughts. The voices communicate with the patient from any distance, and through all possible hindrances by means of the most secret paths and through apparatus, especially invented for this purpose. "The voices" not only talk but electrify him, poison him, and make thoughts for him; they become embodied in the persons who have any dealings with him.

Auditory hallucinations without words are not so prominent. In ecstasies, fever deliria and especially in delirium tremens, one often hears music and singing but otherwise one rarely encounters this type of hallucination.

Hallucinations of smell and taste rarely appear alone. In ecstasies and occasionally in the later stages of manic paresis, they enhance the great pleasure; in schizophrenic delusions of persecution they reveal some disgusting and some poisonous substances, including also pitch and sulphur. Other tastes and smells are only very rarely hallucinated.

Cutaneous sense. The sense of touch (*"Haptic Sensory deceptions"*) hallucinates vividly only in delirium tremens, where small animals, bugs, tight bands, and mucous threads are felt. They are also found in connection with bodily hallucinations, inasmuch as snakes which crawl to the genitals, blows, stabs, and similar hallucinations are also felt by the sense of touch. The other qualities of the cutaneous hallucinations are still more difficult to differentiate from the following:

Hallucinations of *general sensations* of the bodily organs are wont to appear in great numbers in schizophrenia. The patients feel, how their liver was turned, the lung sucked dry, the intestines torn out, the brain sawn apart, and the joints stiffened, or how they are beaten, burned,[3] and electrocuted ("physical delusions of persecution").• Here belong also the very common sexual hallucinations, which seldom cause pure pleasure, but mostly great pain. The patient feels that his "nature" is drawn from him, his genitals are squeezed, and his semen is driven inside of him. Women feel themselves violated in the worst way.

The physical hallucinations can be differentiated from paresthesias mostly through the fact that the patients feel the former as "done" from without.

Some authors associate the physical hallucinations with the self-preservation impulse, with the affectivity; they are supposed to be in most intimate relation to the ego. There may be some truth in this, but what, is difficult to say.

Hallucinations of kinesthetic sensations are most frequently seen in delirium tremens, where the patients imagine that they are at work while they lie in bed. It also happens, that they suddenly feel their seat swinging under them, or see objects moving. Schizophrenics may have the feeling that one of their joints is moved. Instead of expressing themselves in voices, the thoughts sometimes manifest themselves in kinesthetic hallucinations of the speech organs,' so that the patients imagine that they say something while in reality their speech apparatus remains quiet. "Vestibular" hallucinations produce the feeling of floating and falling.

Also *pains* can be hallucinated, but it is not always easy to differentiate them from other functional pains.

The hallucinations of the various senses frequently *combine* with one another; thus one sees and hears a man and feels his influence, or one sees and touches objects.

As *elementary hallucinations* in the optic field we designate such unformed visions as lightning, sparks, and cloudlike partial darkening of the visual field, and in the acoustic field, the simple noises such as murmurs, knocks, and shooting.

Negative hallucinations, or not to perceive an object which is accessible to our senses, are rare occurrences in pathology but they can easily be produced in a state of hypnosis through suggestion.

"Retroactive hallucinations" is another name for hallucinations of memory.

Many authors include under the hallucinatory disturbances also the

[3] Continuous uncontrollable burning in the form of paresthesia is mostly a symptom of a brain lesion.

secondary sensations or *synaesthesias*. The peculiarity of the latter lies in the fact that sensations of one organ are accompanied by sensations of another sensory field. The most common form is "color hearing," that is, a feeling of color on hearing of sounds or the vowels ("photism"). However, the secondary sensations have nothing to do with hallucinations and in any case they have as yet no meaning in pathology.

The *theory of hallucinations* is very instructive. There are still psychiatrists who cannot think of an hallucination,—that is, a projection of ideas with perceptible distinctness into space,—without the cooperation of the peripheral sense organs. For they maintain that under normal conditions only those processes can be projected to the outer world which are accompanied by the corresponding sensory stimuli. But since, as far as we know, we only perceive processes in the cortex, directly "through consciousness," this conclusion is not binding, and, aside from other reasons, is false, because one can also hallucinate when the peripheral sensory organs are destroyed.

It is then assumed that there are perception cells or perception centres in the cortex; and that when they are normally put into "strong" activity by the periphery they produce sensations and perceptions in the organ of thought (the whole cerebral cortex), and when put into "weak" activity they give rise to ideas. If we could speak at all about the "strength" of such processes we would say that it has nothing to do with the difference between perception and ideas. And principally it has just as little to do with localizations. Even the simplest psychic element, as, for example, the sensory sensation of blue, is a far reaching psychic *elaboration* of the mere incoming stimulus; just let us imagine the process of singling out the individual color feeling from the chaos of all synchronous sensations and psychic processes in general. The pure sensory element of perception, as the most vivid idea or hallucination, must perforce be something just, or nearly, as diffuse as the "idea." Nor is the most essential part in the "projection to the outer world," in the "reality judgment," which lies in perception, or in the substantiality of the latter. In the case of artists or in pseudo-hallucinations, "ideas" may be so clear, so sharp, so detailed and vivid in color, tone, and in all other sensory qualities that in this regard they differ in no way from perceptions, but they, nevertheless, lack the reality character of hallucinations or perceptions. Conversely, the accuracy and substantiality of the psychic structure may be absent in sensory perceptions (in fogs, dawn, etc.), and hallucinations may show so much resemblance to the most flighty ideas, that the patient could not say definitely in what words a hallucinated thought was heard,—

and nevertheless it máy have such an unshakeable reality judgment, as if I saw my own hand in front of me in broad daylight. *The reality judgment, the substantiality of a true or hallucinated perception, depends almost altogether on the psychic environment.* The difference between perceived and imagined space is an invention of speculative psychology. If I looked at the table and then turned my back on it, it still exists for me in the same true reality, and in the same place as at the moment before, when I looked at it. The same holds true when I look at a coin on the table and then cover it.

At all events, the ideas represent reality to the naïve consciousness just like the perceptions, although one soon learns to make a certain distinction between them. One also reacts to them as to perceptions—they have the meaning of timely prolonged perceptions. If I run away from a persecutor, I need not see him or hear him every moment. Thus we understand the continuous scale from the most abstract idea to the one with sensory distinctness of the pseudo-hallucination. The more one abstracts from the sensory components and from the details of a physical idea, the lighter is the "sensory distinctness." The latter does not, however, altogether determine the reality judgment and the substantiality, although it naturally may contribute to the conclusion that a manifestation is "real." Besides this there is another scale, which can more or less definitely furnish substantiality to an idea regardless of whether the latter has sensory vividness or not. However, the distinction is less delicate here, in most cases one is simply confronted with the absolute question, "real or not?" The appearance of a saint is conceived by the normal minded modern person as a vision (= pseudo-hallucination), whereas the devout may consider it as a real manifestation of the saint.

We must distinguish two types of hallucinations. The first represents ideas projected to the outer world; this is the hysterical type. The second type represents illusionally misinterpreted paresthesias. Thus the irritations of the optic organs in delirium tremens produce visions of animals while those of the cutaneous nerves, perceptions of threads or needles; in schizophrenia the processes of the brain lead at first to paresthesias and hypochondriacal sensations, and then change to physical hallucinations as the disease progresses. It is noteworthy that the relations of the hallucinations to the ego are very close in schizophrenia and in dreams and very weak in alcoholic insanity and even in some organic diseases. Delirious patients often regard their hallucinations as a moving-picture show. Another remarkable thing is the fact that the manifestations in alcoholic deliria are mostly colorless, while similar appearances in paresis and other organic insanities more frequently show color; the patients speak of variegated butterflies, red powder spread all over, and blue threads. Hence the second type belongs to hallucinations only insofar as its basic sensory stimulus originates in the body itself, whereas if conceived in the pure psychic sense one deals with simple illusions.

Most of the *elementary hallucinations* are likewise misinterpretations of irritating states of the sensory apparatus, nevertheless it is naturally also possible that the hallucination of shooting, of running water, or lightning could sometimes also result from an idea.

2. DISTURBANCES OF CONCEPTS AND IDEAS

Persons who are congenitally blind or deaf mute naturally lack the respective sensory components in their concepts. Even shortsighted people must perforce perceive many things somewhat differently from those who have full vision. Some assume that one cannot remember odors and tastes, still in many persons such memory pictures form a part of the concepts of foods, flowers, and similar articles smelt and tasted. Whether this or that sense predominates, undoubtedly depends largely on individual idiosyncrasy. In some it is the optic memory pictures which constitute the most important components of their concepts and hence of their thinking, in others it is the acoustic, and in still others it is the motor memory pictures. These differences are of importance in the pathology of cerebral localization, for a person belonging to the extreme "visual" type having a lesion in the occipital lobe is deprived of the most important components of his concepts and hence sustains a greater loss in his psychic functions than one of the extreme "auditif" type.

Due to a poverty of associations congenital defectives cannot make full use of their experiences in the formation of concepts, and consequently are less able to connect and combine the individual memory pictures. What is even of much more importance is the fact that they do not sufficiently comprehend the concepts which others convey to them through speech. In this respect deaf persons are worse off, even if they are endowed with good intelligence. Both classes therefore form less concepts than normal people, and they are very apt to put an incorrect limitation on them. They act like little children who may put into the same concepts, let us say, the duck and the hornet because both fly, and regard the caterpillar and butterfly as different animal species. They also form *insufficient, unclear,* and *inaccurate limitations;* they cannot, for instance, distinguish between "state" and "country," or even between "sparrow" and "finch." These wrong and insufficient differentiations are, of course, much more common and more profound in idiots than in deaf people, for the former do not note small differences and are unable to discriminate between essentials and unessentials. Nevertheless most concepts formed by idiots are not at all unclear; this is not only due to the fact that they form only simple concepts, but chiefly because they do not go far from things tangible, and form few abstract thoughts.

However, there are types of congenital defectives, in whom the most essential deficiency is a lack of clearness in concept formation, but they have not as yet been sufficiently studied. Thus an erethic imbecile defines the concept "valuable" as: "When you knock it higher (raise the cost), it will cost even more." [4]

The more complicated a concept and the more remote its components are, the less possible is it for an imbecile to form or to grasp the same; he might in some case understand the idea of "family" but not that of "state." *However, it would be incorrect to state that idiots and imbeciles form no abstract concepts, but it may be said that they do not form complicated abstract ideas, and that frequently their abstract concepts are falsely construed.* Those of a lower order may grasp the concept of "father" and "mother," but no longer the concept of "parents"; they can thoughtfully state: "John hit me and I hit John," but they are unable to comprise this reciprocal activity under the term "each other" or "one another."

Here, however, the difficulties of language must be distinguished from those of concepts. This is not always easy, even in normal people. The differences of personal disposition, of education and especially those of race are very great. The disposition and education of the French is such, that a schoolboy there may talk very nicely about things, of which he has at most a very meagre understanding. In the German part of Switzerland with its clumsy expression, the intelligence of foreigners is at first frequently overestimated; in our Swiss clinic Germans, who are more fluent in speech, are not unfrequently diagnosed as manic cases, and real manic patients often seem much richer in concepts than they are.

A good fluent speech, congenital or acquired, often disguises real deep defects of intelligence, be it in society, in school, or even in the highest examinations, which only goes to show how imperfect these organizations are. In such cases one speaks of higher dementia,[5] and persons so afflicted sometimes play a great part in life. Thus a famous "Nature Healer" belonging to this category, reduced everything to the

[4] Cf. Also below the "Nature Healer" with his "Principle of Contrasts."
[5] Cf. below Oligophrenia.

"Principle of Contrasts," but he could not distinguish between "contrast" and "difference," between "power" and "stimulus," between "health" and "feeling of health." In more difficult matters such confusions of ideas may be encountered even in the most intelligent class; the frequent confusions in the deductive sciences are mostly due to the fact that two somewhat differing concepts are connected by a common designation and are then interchanged.

Thus one may admit, that behind the properties of the psyche, there must be a carrier of the properties, a "being." But if one then deducts from the concept of the "being," that the psyche is punctiform, lacking space and time, one finds suddenly that instead of the above concept of the "being" or the carrier of the observed psychic properties, another concept has been substituted, the origin of which one does not know and concerning which it must be proven that it is applicable to the relationships of the psyche. Another excellent false deduction can also be seen in the following reflection: Cancer may be caused by a cold; for all physiological reactions, hence also those leading to cancer are conditioned by an "irritant," and cold is surely an "irritant."

Symbols or concepts having one or many common components, are also used by normal people, but more so by patients. This gives rise to many coarse errors of thought, for instead of conceiving something as a mere figure, it frequently takes the place of the original concept, thus the fire of love is seen as red-hot, or the patient actually feels it burning him.

In psychoses, concepts may be profoundly distorted. "Right" to a litigious paranoiac is usually what suits him, and "justice" becomes hypertrophied in the epileptic patient who feels justified in almost killing another patient, because the other brushed against the attending physician in passing. A conglomerate of concepts, as well as markedly distorted concepts are found only in schizophrenia and in states of clouded consciousness. Nevertheless one observes nothing here that cannot occasionally be found everywhere to a lesser extent.

Many patients experience things which are unknown to normal persons, for which the patient must create new concepts. Thus a paranoid praecox said that the "Double polytechnic" is her highest intelligence and accomplishment which she claimed as her due reward, or another patient speaks of the "Dossierpath," meaning the path of the hallucinatory influences. New concepts are sometimes created through the process of "condensation" in so far as attributes of many persons are fused in one.

The mental elaboration of concepts is frequently imperfect, especially in dementia praecox, which causes temporary mistakes, thus barrel and hoop, or even father and mother, may be identified with one another. The boy who played sexually with the patient in her childhood, her lover, her seducer, two physicians in the asylum to whom she transferred her love,—all these are thought of by the patient as one person. In most of these cases we do not deal with a permanent injury. That an advanced paretic can no longer think of a complicated concept like "logarithm" or even "state," in its totality, is naturally the result of a disturbance in his associations. *Nevertheless, an actual destruction of the concept has not yet been demonstrated in the psychoses.* If a patient looks upon the attendant as his sister, it is not the result of a disturbance of a concept, but it is due to an illusion or delusion.

At all events, the anomalies in the formation, retention, and in the transformation of concepts have not yet been sufficiently studied.

Disturbances of ideas naturally exist insofar as the psychic processes in general are disturbed. Disturbances of perceptions, of memory pictures, and of the mental stream, must secondarily lead to disturbances of ideas. Moreover, it actually happens that the specific quality of ideas becomes blurred by the fact that the ideas become transformed into hallucinations, or they are mistaken for earlier experiences.

3. DISTURBANCES OF ASSOCIATIONS AND OF THOUGHT

GENERAL FACILITATION OF THE PSYCHIC PROCESSES. FLIGHT OF IDEAS.

Even normal persons who are "in good humor," or "stimulated" sometimes give the subjective and objective impression as if their thinking process ran with particular ease. Such people have more to say, and sometimes utter thoughts which are not habitual to them, especially jokes, even quite daring ones. To be sure, such performances cannot always stand the test of criticism. In pathological states, mostly in connection with euphoria and exalted self-reliance, we often find a morbid exaggeration of the afore-mentioned state, which is designated as *flight of ideas*. Here the most striking phenomenon is the exaggerated *distractability*, which at first comes from within but later also from without. The patients change their objective idea with abnormal frequency, and in the most serious cases it follows every thought uttered or indicated. Thus a patient wishes to tell about a trip to the Righi Mountains and he suddenly thinks of the donkeys which were used there before the construction of the railroad, then of salami sausage supposed to be made of donkey meat and then of Italy where these sausages come from. In less severe cases the patient is able to revert to the original theme, or he merges into a thousand and one things, being unable to bring a single thought to completion. But, except in the most difficult cases where the patient's thoughts can no longer be followed, or where the intermediate connecting thoughts are not uttered, one can understand how thought is distracted. The secondary associations which also appear in normal persons but which they suppress, absorb the patient to the same extent as the principal theme.

The reenforced *distractability* from without may be lacking, but in most cases it is very noticeable, in so far as every sensory impression which impedes the flight of ideas is immediately elaborated into the patient's garrulous talk. Thus seeing the doctor's watch chain he speaks about it, or hearing the jingling of coins he immediately talks of dollars. This enhanced distractability may also be described as a disturbance of attention in the form of hypotenacity with hypervigility.

Both subjectively and objectively one gains the impression that the flighty patients think more rapidly. However, the correctness of this cannot be demonstrated experimentally. There is no doubt that the patient spends much less than the normal time on the individual ideas, which also accounts for the fact that they are insufficiently elaborated.

Thus flighty thinking is not aimless in content, although its aim is forever changing. It shows a preponderance of external and word associations at the expense of inner associations, which connect the ideas according to logical sequence following the actual mental trend in the form of associations of super-order, sub-order, or causality.[6] In place of inner associations there may be accidental connections, as Salami, Italy, instead of the journey to the Righi, which do not even emanate from the sense of the word but from its sound, as seen in association types of rhyme and word completions. Thus to the word "bird" a manic patient answered: "Birds of a feather, flock together."

The following example taken from the production of a patient showing flight of ideas will serve as an illustration: Question, "Who is the president of the U.S.?" "I am the president, I am the ex-president of the United States, I have been a recent president. Just at present I was present, president of many towns in China, Japan and Europe and Pennsylvania. When you are president you are the head of all, you are the head of every one of those, you have a big head, you are the smartest man in the world. I do testory and all scientist of the whole

----

[6] One of the main headings in the classification of associations is "Coordination" which includes associations of co-order, super-order, sub-order, or contrast. Examples of super-order are "fly," "insect"—"water," "ocean." Examples of sub-order are "forest," "trees"—"animals," primates," etc. (*Editor.*)

world. The highest court of doctoring, of practicing, I am a titled lady by birth of royal blood of rose blood (pointing to another patient), he has black blood, yellow blood, he is no man, a woman, a woe-man, etc." [7]

The stimulus word "key" elicited the following: "Oh you can have all the keys you want, they broke into the store and found peas, what's the use of keys, policeman, watchman, dogs, dog shows, the spaniel was the best dog this year, he is Spanish you know, Morro Castle what a big key they have (refers to a visit in Cuba) Sampson, Schley, he drowned them all in the bay, gay, New York bay, Broadway, the White Way, etc." [8]

One can always note a weakness in the patient's reflection and judgment. Even if they bring to the surface some ingenious thought and are able to utter truths which would not occur to normal persons or which they would suppress, such productions are in most cases extremely superficial in judgment, they are one sided and hasty, and are deficient in some of the necessary factors. Wherever the choice of impressions and ideas are inadequate there is also a lack in orderly arrangement. Whenever one gets the impression that the patient's achievements are above the average it is usually due to *cessation of inhibition* and not to an acceleration of his mental facilities. The average person cannot say some things, he cannot even think of them, because of consideration for others or himself or because an inner critique keeps him back, the flighty patient, however, ignores such reflections or they never occur to him, he knows no embarrassment.

Sometimes, especially before merging into a depression or into a manic depressive mixed state, the patients firmly adhere to an apparent aim but leave out all logical connections. Such persons limit their productions to a series of names of persons, places, offices, etc., some individual parts of which besides being linked through the general superordination of the ideas, are also associated through sound similarities.

Flight of ideas is an essential component of the *manic* symptom-complex. Similar mental disturbances also occur in *exhaustion* and perhaps also in *toxemias*. In all probabilities there are distinctions between the individual forms, but we do not know them as yet.

Flight of ideas does not represent a simple acceleration of associations. Liepmann endeavored to explain it on the basis of a disturbance of attention, but one gains nothing by it as one can just as lief reason the other way and explain disturbances of attention through flight of

[7] Given by editor.
[8] Given by editor.

ideas. We might venture the following conception: Regulated thinking is conditioned by the fact that the hierarchy of the leading thoughts inhibit all ideas not belonging to the theme. As we must also assume in other cases, the inhibiting resistance obtruding itself is relative in its action. As intrapsychic functions are only too easily stimulated in manic patients—the patients feel a bubbling over of thoughts—the stimulus threshold seems smaller and the relation between inhibition and function is disarranged. In view of all that, the resistance exerted by the leading thought no longer suffices to inhibit associations which are unrelated to it.

Melancholic Retardation of Associations (Inhibition)

A retardation of the train of thought, already noticeable in sad normal persons, is present in cases of morbid depressions; the entire process of thought proceeds slowly and in a laboriously subjective manner. It is difficult, and often impossible for the patients to change the idea controlling them; this preferred idea deals with their imaginary misfortune (*monideism*). The patients are frequently aware of their poverty of ideas and perceive it as dreary and monotonous. Ideas which are incompatible with the depressive thoughts can be touched upon with difficulty or not at all; so that judgment becomes considerably warped and the development of delusions is made quite easy. On superficial observation the patients sometimes even give the impression of feeble-mindedness.

Associations in Organic Psychoses

The number of individual concepts simultaneously available to patients suffering from *organic psychoses* is less than in normal; this can be most readily demonstrated when the patients attempt to do examples in arithmetic. Whereas normally the patients were able, for instance, to do mentally an addition of four-digit numbers, they can now only add one one-digit number to a two-digit number without forgetting the problem. The characteristic restrictions of organic disturbances is shown by the fact that the selection as well as the rejection of associations occurs mainly in the sense of the affective trend. Wherever it is primarily a question of affects or impulses, the associations antagonistic to the particular impulse are left out. As examples of this, one may cite the former morally senile patient, who, in a state of sexual excitement sees only the female in the child and abuses it sexually, or the paralytic who steals some tempting object under the eyes of a few dozen spectators and conceals it under his clothing, or the paretic who jumps out of an upper story window in order to pick up a fallen cigar-stump (Kraepelin). A senile patient is capable of praising his mother as a saint and immediately thereafter merge into another constellation and have nothing but evil to tell about her.

This restriction of thought for the time being to a specific cluster of ideas,—physically speaking, is like an attempt to get one's bearings through a key-hole,—exposes the patients to the danger of committing great stupidities; they enter into business undertakings without considering risks, they contract foolish marriages, or commit similar foolish acts.

When only a few ideas can be grasped simultaneously, an orderly arrangement of them becomes difficult. Thus a patient states that he was born in 1872, he knows that it is now 1917, but nevertheless thinks that he was 62 years old ten years ago. He comes to this conclusion by subtracting 10 from 72 instead of from his present age. The co-ordinating associations as such may also be affected.[9]

Furthermore, a restriction of associations may also be due to the fact that especially senile patients, and less so paralytics and Korsakoff patients, become more and more egocentric and are particularly fond of concerning themselves with their own pleasures and woes, often in a very petty fashion. Nevertheless, they are much more capable, than, for instance, organic epileptics, of occupying themselves with other things, *in so far as they can still grasp them.* They are especially capable of showing a very affective and exaggerated interest in the affairs of their friends and enemies. In conversation the patients find it difficult to pass from one thought to another. Even in cases where primary comprehension is still quite good, they answer to a question which does not exactly belong to the particular subject, frequently they answer only after numerous repetitions, or in the sense of the former trend of thought. It thus often happens that they still continue to give information about personal matters when that topic has long been finished and when the question may refer to their education.

Besides those mentioned there are other mechanisms which often prevent the patients from leaving an idea. Thus in an association test they will repeat again and again an accidental reaction word, and in a perception test they will call a penholder a cow, if the picture of such an animal has previously been shown them (*perseveration*).

The duration of time of associations in organic patients is retarded in most cases. This is especially seen in cases of senility, where one sees additional accessory processes, which hamper and retard the psychic processes, such as cerebral pressure and other phenomena that

[9] Cf. also "Orientation," p. 32.

are not yet well understood. Retardation shows itself with especial regularity in experimental associations; but in such cases difficulty of comprehension may play a part. Here the associations are emotionally accentuated, very closely related, and contain many repetitions, partly due to perseveration of ideas, and partly to poverty of thought. The patient finds it difficult or impossible to restrict the reaction to a single word.

A diagnosis can frequently be made in a few moments from the continuous associations showing the garrulous organic type, which would have been impossible to do before, when nothing characteristic could be sufficiently emphasized in the description of the case. In most cases it is a question of a slow progress of the course of ideas with a tendency to repetitions. The utterances often express a pronounced affect in its content, which is even more marked by its emphasis. Sometimes one hears nothing but wailing or boasting, with or without a definite theme. It is through the emotional accentuation rather than through the greater mobility and better intellectual coherence, that such out-pourings are distinguished from the lamentations of depressive Schizophrenic cases, whose affective expressions, even when present, hardly ever conceal a pronounced rigidity. Typical associations may be seen in the following:

"My dearest Doctor, "I'm all wrong, O God in Heaven have pity on me, Father in Heaven be compassionate. Dear good Doctor, help me. Let me out. Heavenly father, please don't forsake me. I'm not capable of that. Why, I'm quite right in my mind. Will you please take pity. I can't do anything else, O dearest God. No, no, no, I must go away, do be merciful. Doctor, won't you be merciful? O Jesus Christ, take pity on me. There is something the matter with every inch of me. My judgment is wrong. There is nothing else that is important. Have pity on my sinful self, O Doctor, do forgive me once more."

Experimental associations [10] are very characteristic in the more pronounced cases; if there is no question of epilepsy, which exhibits similar peculiarities, the associations alone are often sufficient to make the diagnosis. All reactions are retarded. The impoverishment of ideas manifests itself very clearly in reactions that are not far removed from the test word, and in generalities, thus the stimulus word "green," gives the reaction, "It's everywhere; green—the green outside." As in oligophrenic cases, a large number of the reactions consist in tautologies, definitions, designations of places, and the like. But even

[10] *Brunnschweiler,* Ueber Assoziationen bei organisch Dementen. Züricher, Diss. 1912.

these tend readily to be blurred, thus the word "family" is reacted to with "Something in the house there." Educated patients get around their poverty of ideas by means of near-by association of words. The perseveration tendency often strongly preponderates. The affectivity shows itself in many reactions as in epileptic cases, but with a much lower valuation, sometimes it evinces itself in just bare interjections: Righto—Oho! righto; or table—what-the-deuce. Complexes show themselves directly and without repression. Egocentric reactions occur frequently, and are said to be quite banal, particularly in paralytic cases, thus, "bad,"—"I don't know of anything bad," and to consist of reminiscences of former experiences in senile cases, thus: "mountain," —"I was once at Horgen mountains, from there I had to go home from the barracks on foot." As has been mentioned, when the disease has reached a certain stage, organic cases are no longer capable of answering with a single word, they cannot isolate the concept, they must tell the whole idea, or the thing which affects them.

The associations of *states of organic confusion* have not, as yet, been the subject of sufficient research. But one can often recognize even in the confusion the described type of the actual disease.

Schizophrenic (Dreamlike) Disturbances of Association (Zerfahrenheit of **Kraepelin**)

Whereas the empirically acquired structures of associations are not loosened in flight of ideas and impediment of thought as well as in organic disturbances of associations, their effectiveness is restricted in *schizophrenia*. Neither a manic patient, nor a sound person thinks of modern Italy at the mention of the name of Brutus. But a schizophrenic, by disregarding the component of time connected with the term, can call the Roman an "Italian," or he can designate the location of Egypt as "between Assyria and the Congo State," by again ignoring the periods to which each of the states belong, and at the same time exchanging in a most bizarre manner the most immediately obvious place designation (say, "the Northeast of Africa") for one altogether peculiar.

Although the following two productions lack clear objectivity the patients nevertheless stick almost perfectly to the theme which happens to refer to ancient history narrative of the Orient. The individual associations seem accidental or stimulated through sound or other factors foreign to a normal person. They differ from flight of ideas through the fact that a normal person can understand the individual steps of the latter, whereas many steps that are made in a schizophrenic train of thought are unintelligible to the normal person, or appear to be so bizarre, that they would never have entered his mind. The following examples will serve as illustrations:

"Epaminondas was one who was powerful especially on land and sea. He was the leader of great fleet manœuvers and open sea-battles against Pelopidas, but had been struck on the head, during the second Punic war, because of the wreck of an armored frigate. He wandered with ships from Athens to Hain Mamre, took Caledonian grapes and pomegranates and overcame Bedouins. He besieged the Acropolis with gun-boats, and caused the Persian crew to be burnt as living torches. The subsequent pope Gregory VII—eh—Nero followed his example and because of him all Athenians, all Roman-Germanic-Celtic races, towards whom the priests were not favorably disposed, were burned at the hands of the Druids as an offering to the Sun-god Baal on Corpus-Christi Day. This is the period of the Stone Age. Spear-points of Bronze." (Stenographically recorded.)

The Blossom-Time for a Horticulturist

"At the time of the New-Moon Venus stands in the August heavens of Egypt and with its rays of light illuminates the harbors of commerce, Suez, Cairo, and Alexandria. In this historically famous city of the Kalifs, there is situated in the museum of Assyrian monuments from Macedonia. There plantain flourishes next to maize columns, oats, clover, and barley, also bananas, figs, lemons, oranges, and olives. Olive-oil is an Arabian liqueur-sauce, with which Afghans, Moors, and Moslemites carry on the breeding of ostriches. The Indian plantain is the whiskey of the Parsee and of the Arab. The Parsee or the Caucasian possesses exactly as much influence over his elephant as the Moor has over his dromedary. The camel is the sport of the Jew and the Indian. In India, barley, rice, and sugar-cane, that is, artichoke, flourish luxuriantly. The Brahmins live in castes on Beluchistan. The Circassian inhabit Manchuria of China. China is the Eldorado of Pawnees." ("Letter of a Schizophrenic.")

The association is sometimes formed as a result of factors from without even when there is not the slightest real connection. Thus the patient explains his violent action on the ground that "the attendant wears a white apron," only because the attendant happens to be standing near when the question is asked.

Not at all infrequently new ideas crop up which have no connection of any kind with what has gone before, sometimes the patient states that they "flashed" through his mind but at other times he does not recognize anything abnormal about them. If the last-named mechanism repeatedly recurs, the mental stream becomes "distorted" and finally coherence disappears altogether. The individual thoughts then have no connection with one another from the point of view of the observer, and in most cases also from that of the patient. Indeed, it not infrequently happens that the patient never produces any coherent thought, as the concepts are piled together without any logical connection.[11]

The separation of associations from experience naturally facilitates *dereistic* thinking in the highest degree, which is actually based on the very fact that natural connections are ignored. Without the slightest regard for real and logical possibilities, the faintest wishes and fears are endowed with the subjective reality of the delusion. The most usual secondary associations, vague analogies and accidental connections determine the train of thought. Dereistic thinking is usually quite unrestricted in dreams because the latter are actively disbarred from the outer world while in schizophrenia it proceeds at a mad rate mixed with correct and realistic directives.

In the schizophrenic course of thought one observes the most varied disturbances. Of particular importance are the *obstructions* where the mental stream suddenly ceases remaining away from seconds to days ("Thought deprivation"). When the obstruction is over, a new thought, which had no connection with the one preceding obstruction, frequently crops up.

The distinction between obstruction and inhibition is very important; the latter signifies depression, the former (with the reservation stated below) Schizophrenia; superficially, however, the two symptoms resemble very much.

In profound disturbances the reactions to both anomalies are altogether or almost completely reduced to zero. But even when impeded, patients attempt to answer, the obstructions, particularly in acute cases, in order to express themselves in motion can usually be overcome only by strong and persistent effort, and even then the patient can only produce feeble and slow motions and utter words in a low tone.[12] In most cases, however, the two kinds of disturbances can easily be differentiated, inasmuch as impeded patients can react just as quickly and strongly as sound persons, once the obstruction has been broken down, whereas inhibited patients always evince the re-

[11] Cf. below, "Confusion," also the additional details about schizophrenic thinking in the chapter on "Schizophrenia: Condensations, Displacements, and Symbols."

[12] In such cases it is probably not a question of simple obstruction, but rather of a combination with a third form of retardation of the psychic processes, which we cannot yet emphasize (swelling processes of the brain, etc.).

tarded character of their movements. (If the difference does not manifest itself in spontaneous expressions, the patients can, for instance, be asked to count to twenty as quickly as possible, or to turn their hands quickly one about the other.)

The obstruction may be compared to the closing of a valve in a piping system carrying a highly mobile fluid, while the inhibition is analogous to a slowing-up of the flow as the result of increasing viscosity of the fluid. The obstruction is a sudden stoppage of psychic processes caused by affective disturbances, and in itself is not a pathological manifestation. Some affects bring to a standstill thoughts and actions even in normal persons ("examination stupor," or "emotional stupor"). Pronounced obstructions may therefore be observed in all *nervous* and particularly in *hysterical* patients. In those cases, however, where they are not sufficiently determined psychologically, where they become generalized, or last unduly long, their presence justifies the diagnosis of schizophrenia.

In neuro-physiology, such stoppages of one function through another are designated as "inhibitions" while in psychopathology, the primary meaning of the word, as the above historical considerations have shown, is something altogether different, it signifies the general retardation of thought processes in melancholic conditions. There are, to be sure, still other general retardations of the psychic processes for which we have not yet any special designation because we have no adequate knowledge of them. Many are named in accordance with their causes, as schizophrenic swelling of the brain, brain pressure in general, toxic, epileptic disturbances, and brain-torpor. In another connection "inhibitions" are spoken of in a moral sense, thus a psychosis, or alcohol destroys the inhibitions connected with wrong actions. Here again the meaning of the expression tends towards its usual physiological significance.

In superficial contradistinction to obstruction, schizophrenics often feel a *"crowding of thoughts"*; they are forced to think. In such cases the content subjectively seems rich and varied, and gives the impression of a continuous mental stream. But if the attempt is made to penetrate a little more deeply, one regularly gets the impression that the patients are forced to think always the same thoughts. The crowding of thoughts is in most cases connected with a disagreeable feeling of exertion. The feeling of activity may, however, also be lacking; "something thinks" in the patients, or "some one makes them thoughts."

Crowding of thoughts is distinguished from obsessive ideas by the fact that in the former the obsession lies in the subject-matter, while in the latter, it is in the process. The compulsive patient cannot rid himself of an apprehension or of an impulse, but in the schizophrenic it is the thinking function itself which is perceived as an automatism or compulsion, quite independent of the content, which can be principally varied in any way.

Furthermore, the thoughts may run *too rapidly*, as in the case of flight of ideas, or they may be inhibited. Such complications naturally occur regularly whenever manic and melancholic states develop in schizophrenic soil, which happens quite frequently. In such circumstances flight of ideas or depressive inhibition is mingled with the specific disturbance of the associations. The schizophrenic lack of concern about the aim of the thought naturally shows in some cases frequent manifestations which cannot in themselves be distinguished from flight of ideas. The inhibition occasionally causes the observer to mistake it for *brevity of associations,* which in most cases belongs directly to schizophrenia and consists in the fact, that the number of available concepts diminish and consequently the mental stream is always equally ready or "brief." [13]

This is seen in important as well as in unimportant trends of ideas. When the patient is asked to relate a fable which he has read, he is unable to proceed beyond the next step in the story, unless he is given an additional prod. When asked to tell about his divorce, he at first knows nothing except: "I am divorced." "Why are you divorced?" "She ran away from me." "Why?" "We did not get along." "Why." "Because of a child," etc.

Pathological brevity of associations is to be distinguished from a similar quality in persons who, for some reason or another, are not willing to give information.

In schizophrenia we often find a special kind of *perseveration,* which, to be sure, we are not yet able to describe as regards its specific peculiarities, although we must assume that it differs from other forms. Accidental psychic processes, thoughts, and actions may become stereotyped; an idea is repeatedly thought and expressed in all variations and connections, it is "worked to death." Stereotyped habits are, above all, formed by emotionally accentuated complexes (see "stereotypes").

Schizophrenic and dream-like disturbances of association may be hypothetically traced to the same origin: As sleep and disturbances of attention deflect the associations from their customary paths, it may be assumed, that a certain force is necessary to keep associations in the track laid out by experience. Now it is possible that this force

[13] Cf. p. 85.

or "control-tension" has also been diminished or hampered in its action because of the fundamental schizophrenic process.[14]

ASSOCIATIONS OF OLIGOPHRENICS

The train of ideas of *imbeciles and idiots* is restricted. But in contrast to organic impoverishment of associations, it is not the objective idea that determines here the choice of the reduced psychic material. The ideas which are left out are those which are uncommon, and do not originate from the immediate sensory perceptions, or those which are more complicated and do not belong to every day experience. The imbecile does not forget that he can get hurt by jumping out of a high window, but he might have an accident as a result of climbing down a trellis-work whose carrying strength he overestimates. An imbecile described by *Wernicke* was driving a wagon which struck a rock and therefore could go no farther. He thereupon whipped the horses instead of driving around the rock; the act of resorting to the whip when the wagon will go no farther is really the habitual thing to do, while it happens only rarely that there is need for driving around an obstacle lying in the middle of the street. Within particularly easy reach and at the same time easily stimulated are those ideas which concern the ego. That is to say, they belong to those ideas which are most easily thought of, a' fact which gives rise, in imbeciles, to a sort of egocentricity, which is further strengthened by the lack of understanding for the matters which concern others.[15]

ASSOCIATIONS OF EPILEPTICS

For obvious reasons (concomitant congenital weakness plus cerebral atrophy) the associations of epileptics often show disturbances similar to those of imbeciles and organic cases but in addition, they present the specific epileptic signs, which are so characteristic that they furnish the material for diagnosis in cases that are more or less pronounced. Nevertheless, the line of demarcation from the organic cases is not yet sufficiently distinct. The abnormities which show themselves most clearly in the experimental associations are as follows: the answers come very slowly, the patients find it difficult to respond with a single word and they frequently employ whole sentences that are often very indistinct, containing peculiar and tortuous expressions. The content is poor in ideas showing tautologies, meaningless definitions, and the

[14] *Bleuler*, Störung der Assoziationsspannung, ein Elementarsymptom der Schizophrenien Allgem. Zeitschr. f. Psychiatrie 1918. P. 1.
[15] For more details see the chapter on oligophrenia.

like, and contains many affective designations among which one frequently finds opinions of value, such as good, beautiful, just, "one should," and moral tendencies. Another mechanism observed is that of perseveration, not so much in the sense that the patient gets stuck to a reaction, but a word, a phrase or sentence form once used easily crops up again later on. The entire circle of ideas gradually becomes more and more completely narrowed down to the patient's own ego.

Examples: Poverty of ideas manifests itself among other things in senseless associations, continued grammatical constructions, tautologies, and the like: thus, long—is not short; loved—what one likes is also loved; heart—people; beat—people; sacrifice—there are all kinds of sacrifices; wonder—to wonder. *Egocentric relations:* wish—health; naturally—one would rather be well than sick; time—I would gladly spare it, for the sake of good fortune. Examples of *emotional* emphasis and affective valuation: greenish—is a pretty color; sweet— is good; to part—is not beautiful; youth—joy; to strike—evil persons strike. *Clumsy and obscure circumstantial expressions:* luck—joyfulness or something like that.[16] Wrath—man is wrathful.[17] Flower— the flower belongs to the trimmings of the window-plants in the dwellings of people, isn't that so? [18] point—one can make a point, what one does in business, if a stone is made, or something else [19] (wishes to say something to the effect "sharp stone").

A type of *perseveration* also occurs with great frequency in ordinary conversation and shows itself in the fact that patients can hardly get away from an idea. They repeat themselves word for word or in tautologies, they use circumstantial modes of expression, they present a multitude of non-essential trifles and trivialities, but they do not lose their goal, nor can they be diverted from their snail-like paths by being requested that they come to the point. Indeed the *distractability* of epileptics is abnormally slight. The *circumstantiality* of their thinking is sometimes also reflected in their actions and their entire behavior.

Whereas a sound person will, so to speak, sit down in one continuous movement, many an epileptic finds it necessary to perform this act in the following manner: He first places the chair in a special position, then he considers his spatial relation to the chair, then he proceeds to place himself in the proper attitude towards the same, and

[16] *Fuhrmann,* Analyse des Vorstellungsmaterials usw. Diss. Giesen, 1902.
[17] *Ibid.*
[18] Holzinger, Assoz. Versuche bei Epilepsie. Diss. Erlangen, 1908.
[19] *Ibid.*

thereupon he must arrange his clothes accordingly, as for example, he must draw apart his coat-tails, and now at last he can sit down in a sprawling attitude.

In speech one is frequently struck by a momentary *hesitancy* or *stalling;* in such cases the patients often repeat a syllable several times, and then they proceed further. This symptom is obviously the expression of a hesitating train of thought; it is as though there were resin in a machine, which often brings it to rest for a few moments and then lets it move again.

The intensity of these symptoms generally runs parallel to the degree of dementia; although it varies very much even in the same patients and is especially pronounced after attacks and in twilight states.

The additional part noticed in *twilight states* has not yet been characterized. In some cases the main element shows itself in an enormous exaggeration of the described peculiarities, in other cases there seems to be added something new, which has been incorrectly designated as incoherence.

THE ASSOCIATIONS OF HYSTERIA

The associations of hysteria are under the pronounced domination of the affects. Even in the habitual states the experiment shows irregular, often very high-graded prolonged reaction-times, indeed, sometimes no answer can be elicited, in content the associations are superficial and psycho-galvanic phenomena are very high.[20] Actual affects cloud the logic in hysterical patients to a very high degree. That which was today praised to heaven may be painted with coal-black colors tomorrow for just as many opposing reasons. In the hysterical twilight state reality is systematically side-tracked and another dream-world is created to replace it; this is helped by falsifications of logic and sensory deceptions.

ASSOCIATIONS OF NEURASTHENICS

In the association test with neurasthenics it is remarkable that they often answer to the *test-word* instead of to its *meaning*, they behave just like patients who suffer from acute exhaustion. For the rest their associations have not yet been sufficiently studied and can just as little be brought into a *single* purview as the morbid pictures to which the name is applied.

[20] That is, there is a diminution of electrical skin-resistance at the appearance of affects.

Associations of Paranoiacs

These associations in so far as they are pathological, are purely katathymic,[21] that is to say, they exhibit characteristic abnormalities only in cases where emotionally accentuated complexes at the basis of the delusional system are brought into play. Many things are then brought into incorrect relationship to the delusional system. Thus one finds an association-readiness for certain definite impressions, delusions of reference, coordination of inappropriate material with the logic functions, a regardless omission of contradictory matter, and a false valuation of material used. Wherever the delusions do not interfere, the thinking process appears normal.

Other Disturbances of Association

Besides these disturbances of associations, which are characteristic for definite illnesses or states, there are many others of which we have no knowledge; they form the subsoil of delirious, soporific, and many confused twilight states in fevers, inner and outer toxemias, in different brain diseases, and the like.

Outside of schizophrenia there are also *pathological brevities of the associations:* the patient always gets through with his thoughts quickly, whether they are his own or those which have been induced from the outside by means of questions and suggestions. The patient does not think of related ideas even when they might have to follow of necessity, as in the case of wishing to give an account of something (indeed, this occurs without the existence of obstructions or melancholic inhibitions). Besides certain dulled states of schizophrenia, such associations are encountered in organic psychoses, in rare epileptic conditions, in many light forms of soporific states, and in similar conditions.

A state of *monideism* may be due to many other causes besides depressive retardation; one observes this phenomenon in all forms of twilight states, where only one idea systematically dominates the patient, as for example, to set fire to something, while he has no conceptions of the cause or consequences of the action. The same state is also seen in deliria following mild cerebral concussions, where any confused idea accidentally occurring to the patient completely absorbs him for a long time and from which he cannot be freed even by outward distraction. It is quite clear that in these states, monideism is something fundamentally different from what it is in inhibitions.

The disturbances previously referred to *under brain-pressure, toxemias,* and the like, are not yet fully known.

[21] See pp. 34-35.

"Confusion"

Confusion is not a unitary disturbance of association in the same sense as those which have been described thus far, but it is the expression of quite different anomalies of the mental stream which have attained a higher grade. It is neither a unitary symptom nor a morbid picture and can even be produced by disturbances outside of the realm of the usual concepts of associations.[22]

Of the familiar disturbances of association it is naturally the schizophrenics which most readily reach to the point of confusion, because it is in their very nature to tear thoughts apart. In the acute stages of schizophrenia it happens that not only the thoughts become confused, but the false connection of the primary associations to the sense impressions already leads to illusional disorientation. Nor do the movements correspond to the thoughts, they may even appear disturbed in their coordination. In the same way paramimic and parathymic phenomena become connected with it.

Confusions incident to delirious and twilight states are still quite insufficiently known.

Occasionally flight of ideas may become intensified to the point of *confusional flight of ideas;* it is, however, necessary to guard against mistaking it for schizophrenic disturbance of associations, complicated by flight of ideas. As every one knows, marked emotional fluctuations in normal and diseased persons lead to *affective confusion* at some time or other.

The expressions, *incoherence* and *dissociation,* which often designate confused processes of thought apply most correctly to schizophrenic disturbances of association, but signify nothing of a characteristic nature.

Diffuseness and Circumstantiality

In the discussion of the associations in *epilepsy* we have mentioned *circumstantiality* and *diffuseness.*[23] This symptom occurs also as the result of other disturbances and in any case has different origins. As long as the *flighty patient* can still come back to his main subject, he may be considered circumstantial, because he works out many details and secondary material which are not needed. Thus diffuseness is often the first striking indication of incipient mania.—An *imbecile* can be circumstantial because he is incapable of distinguishing between essentials and non-essentials and hence he must go into unimportant matters as fully as into main issues. Repetitions and tautologies,

---

[22] See below: "Hallucinatory Confusion."

[23] Two not identical concepts, which, however, coincide for the most part.

characteristic of the circumstantial *epileptic* train of thought, are usually absent in manics and imbeciles. It is well known that senile patients also become circumstantial, partly because the train of thought gets into ruts which they are no longer capable of avoiding, and partly particularly, because the substantiality of the affective tone and the narrowing of the associations making reflection difficult, makes the nonessentials appear as important as the main theme. There are perhaps still other unknown reasons for the senile circumstantiality.

Circumstantiality sometimes originates from a *feeling of uncertainty* which impels the patient to add all sorts of corrective and supplementary determinants. In this form it may appear in the most varied states. It is also utilized to put off an unwished for decision.

Overvalued Ideas, Obsessions (Obsessive Acts)

Overvalued Ideas are ideas that always obtrude themselves into the foreground, they are mostly remembrances of an affectful experience, but in contrast to *autochthonous* ideas the patients do not perceive them as strange, and contrasted with compulsive ideas are not felt as incorrect. They are completely bound up with the personality and differ from ordinary affective ideas only in the fact that eventually one does not get rid of them and that they have the tendency to associate themselves with new experiences. According to *Wernicke* they are not delusions in themselves, but through morbid relationships often give occasion for delusions. They are katathymic ideas, which according to the current conception appear as the only essential symptom in persons that would otherwise be considered sane. *Ziehen*, however, also designates as overvalued ideas, obsessions, and many obtruding delusions. In positing overvalued ideas the question of the existence of *monomanias*, which for nearly a half century appeared settled in the negative, has once more been taken up, though in a much more comprehensible form. In the case of an existing predisposition or without this, is it possible for an outer experience, intensified by an accidental cause, to provoke delusions in a psyche not really morbid? I should like to answer in the affirmative. But only when these "overvalued ideas" become an active influence does one deal with a real psychosis (compare on the one hand "belief" and on the other paranoia).[24]

Obsessions or compulsive notions are ideas which continually obtrude themselves against the patient's will with or without external

---

[24] Some designate as monomanias not delusional forms in otherwise retained lucidity, but isolated morbid impulses like kleptomania or pyromania.

cause,[25] the content of which, however, is recognized as incorrect except in states of strong affects. Nevertheless they do not appear strange to the personality as they are regarded as the product of one's own thinking. They are remarkably monotonous and may be divided into four groups: Some people feel compelled to put definite questions to themselves, many of which are foolishly banal, such as, "Why has a chair four legs?", some deal with insoluble problems about final causes, such as, "What existed before the creation of the world?", some are more or less of a religious nature, such as, "Why is God a man?", or "How is the immaculate conception possible?", and some are of a sexual content, which are often also plainly an element in those previously mentioned ("Reasoning mania"). Others have anxious ideas that the match has not been put out, or the door isn't locked. They cannot mail a letter, because in spite of repeated examinations they are not convinced that it is in the right envelope, or that there isn't a serious mistake in it. They are afraid to touch a door knob because they themselves may carry germs to others, or others to them ("délire du toucher"). If a knife is lying around, they fear they may kill some-body with it—usually one of their relatives.

Others fear their father may die if a spoon lies on the table in a particular way, or if one does this or doesn't do that, in which cases one cannot always tell whether the patients are fully convinced of the incorrectness of the "superstition." Obsessions that some horrible crime was committed may merge directly into delusions of sin, which then also appear most frequently in states of melancholia. The *phobias* are also classed with obsessions. Thus one observes an agoraphobia or fear of open places, erythrophobia or fear of blushing, and similar ideas which realize the dreaded occurrence (fear of getting diarrhœa where it is impossible to satisfy this need); this can be brought about through the activity of the smooth muscular system which is not controlled by the conscious will. Other phobias, like mysophobia, or fear of dirt and eventually infection, belong to the group of *délire du toucher*, and lead indirectly to actions.

Some of the *compulsive acts* are the result of the compulsive ideas and cannot therefore be separated from them. Thus the idea that the door is not locked compels the patient to try it over and over again or ask others to examine it. Mysophobia compels one to touch the door knob only through cloth and to wash the hands continually. The notion, "If I do not return the money, my father will die," compels one to return it even under difficult circumstances. Obscene contrast ideas

[25] They are in this way also *disturbances of the will* in so far as the patient has no power to direct his thoughts to normal thinking.

compel one to utter them (coprolalia). Often the obsession and the *compulsive impulse* are identical as in the impulse to kill one's child with the nearby knife, or the thought presents itself, like a hallucination, in imperative form, "You must kill your child."

A man who has a questionable affair must turn around and look at every "dark, tall, sturdy" woman, then also at small ones, then at all women, then also at men, and then at street cars to read their numbers.

Another kind of association between an obsession and compulsive impulse was shown by a patient, who was not melancholic; he had the obsession that he had had intercourse with his mother and the compulsive impulse to write this fact on banknotes.

Connected with the compulsion is a very painful affect; still not all patients can rouse themselves to the state of really desiring to be cured, in spite of the fact that a feeling of sickness is perhaps never lacking. The ideas themselves are either of a depressive [26] content, or anxiety appears as soon as the patient wants to resist the impulse. It is anxiety that makes it impossible for the patient to suppress the impulse in spite of the fact that he is willing and knows better. But the patient has to see repeatedly that the match is out, not so much to prevent a fire, as to rid himself of his fear, indeed the execution of a compulsive act may actually be connected with "a peculiar feeling of voluptuous satisfaction." The fear itself often seems to be (incorrectly) the result of the idea (fear of germs); at times it accompanies the idea and more rarely it appears as primary, in which case the obsession may give the impression as if it were created as an explanation for the affect. But it is probably true that obsessions most frequently develop on the basis of a timid, uncertain, but conscientiously inclined character, also in exhaustions and melancholies.

Freud has attempted to explain obsessions by assuming that any relatively innocent idea is connected with another which became repressed on account of its unbearable content. The former then receives the affective endowment of the idea, which has become unconscious, and forces itself into consciousness in place of it. Thus a girl at a concert feels the impulse to micturate in the course of sexual thoughts which she rejected as immoral; thereupon at every similar state of affairs she had a phobia that she might have to micturate. It is certain that obsessive cleanliness may frequently be traced to the need for moral purity, as in onanistic pangs of conscience.

Obsessions occur temporarily in neurasthenic and melancholic states, in schizophrenia, and also as a special, and frequently very

[26] At present I doubt whether there are obsessions of a pleasant content.

severe, disease, in people originally disposed to such abnormities (Compulsion Insanity, compulsion neurosis).

DELUSIONS

Errors originate from the facts that similar things are considered identical (camelia—rose; whale—fish), that a simple coincidence is considered a regular coincidence and consequently taken as a causal determinant (e.g. the patient became well because a charm was applied), or that something important is overlooked (the earth is a plane) or also, that one is deceived by the senses, and hence unusual relations are judged according to usual relations, e.g., the sun revolves around the stationary world. Such errors may be corrected by new experiences which are enlightening to the extent that reason is capable of evaluating these experiences correctly. Even when a person is too stupid to comprehend the sphericity of the earth, we do not call his conception a delusion. Delusions are incorrect ideas created, not by an accidental insufficiency of logic, but out of inner need ("Delusional need," *Kraepelin*). There are no other inner needs than the affective. Delusions, therefore, always follow a definite direction corresponding to the patient's affects, and in the vast majority of cases cannot be corrected by new experience or instruction, as long as the condition which gave origin to them continues.

Delusions, therefore, have their psychological analogy not in error but in belief. Accordingly the chief delusion is regularly egocentric and of essential significance for the personality of the patient himself, though, of course, the forms of explanatory and secondary delusions [27] need not directly concern the patient. Contrasted with belief the main difference lies in the fact that delusions are formed by individuals from personal need and that they may relate to matters which in sane persons are subject to correction. We see that the difference is not absolute. Ordinarily we cannot speak of delusions when a pious person forms his own opinion of religious matters; but when his innovations appear altogether too gross, we designate them as "delusions of religion," although in the forum of pure logic a new prophet might have as much reality value as the older ones.

Delusions, therefore, originate as a result of affects inasmuch as what corresponds to the affect is accepted and what is opposed to it is inhibited to the extent, that it either does not appear at all in this connection, or it is of insufficient logical force. The melancholic, when he takes account of his fortune, sees continually all his debts and difficulties but cannot balance them with his assets, partly because he

[27] See below.

considers them worthless or too uncertain, and partly because he cannot connect them in a logical procedure with the idea of his debts and therefore cannot utilize them to overcome the idea of indebtedness. Such is the origin of the delusion of poverty. Not infrequently he comes to the same conclusion *by keeping back altogether the ideas referring to exact sums,* and only in a general way considers his debts. The onanistic schizophrenic fears that his vice will become known. If he notices that some one looks at him he thinks it is because of his onanism, the self-evident fact that one is looked at a thousand times without such cause, cannot be used as a counter-argument.

The delusional affect may be of a general (depressive or manic) nature, or it may be attached only to a particular idea, to a complex such as an onanistic pang of conscience. In the latter case katathymic delusional forms originate. When a person obsessed with a complex is at the same time suffering from a general depression, a frequent occurrence in schizophrenia, the katathymic and depressive effects become connected. If the schizophrenic onanist is melancholic he thinks that he is rotting because of his vice; if he is manic, he feels that he is a savior of humanity.

Some of the delusions follow logically from those already existing and do not require this mechanism. When the patient is convinced that the physician wants to murder him and after taking medicine he feels indisposed, then it is a conclusion, based on logical probability, that the physician has prescribed poison (secondary delusion). Or the patient is the son of a count, consequently, his parents are only foster parents. Or the patient is pursued everywhere, no matter where he journeys; "therefore there exists an entire organization against him, the postal authorities open his letters and tell his address" (Explanatory Delusions).

It is said that delusions are logically deduced from the affective disturbance. Thus the patient feels unhappy, seeks a cause and finds it in his sins. I have never been able to observe this mechanism.

Other delusions are said to originate in hallucinations, deceptions of memory, and in dreams. This is undoubtedly a question of concomitant circumstances, not of real causes. It is the false idea which is directly generated by the disease; it may appear first as a thought, or hallucination, or memory deception, or as a dream conception.

Some delusions, especially in schizophrenia, suddenly appear in consciousness as finished products (*délire d'emblée,* primordial delusion); [28] others have a longer period of incubation. For instance,

---

[28] If the patient takes a critical attitude toward the content of the idea, it is called an *autochthonous* idea (*Wernicke*).

the patients feel as if they were watched, as if they had sinned, until at last it becomes a certainty. Or for years the patients make a number of remarkable observations (self-references) and it suddenly comes to them "as a revelation" that it all has this and that meaning. Perhaps most frequently the delusion connects itself with external events in such a manner that the patients at first quite correctly grasp, e.g., a sermon, but later on, following a period of incubation of from hours to years, they interpret the words heard, consciously or unconsciously, in the sense of the delusion as related to themselves, that is, to their complexes.

The following classes are differentiated according to content:

Expansive forms of delusion; "Delusions of grandeur." In the mildest cases they rather take the form of overestimation of the ego, the patient surpasses other people in health, ability, beauty to an extent greater than the corresponding reality. From this we observe all stages of real delusions, from the easily possible to what is still conceivable up to the idea that the patient is capable of the most impossible discoveries, to possess "trillions," to found new religions, to be God and Super-God. Occasionally the environment is transformed to accord with the idea. The patient's companions in the asylum are mistaken for counts and potentates.

Depressive delusions refer especially to three spheres: to conscience, as delusions of sin; to health, as delusions of disease, and to fortune, as delusions of poverty.

The patient entertaining *delusions of sin* believes without reason to have committed the worst transgressions or magnifies actual trivial deeds into unpardonable sins. For these not only the patient is punished in an appalling manner here and in the life beyond, but also all his relatives, even the whole world.

The patient having *depressive delusions of sin* [29] believes that he has definite, and always especially awful diseases. The real disease, melancholic depression, is denied. The same is sometimes designated as *hypochondriacal delusions;* but we must be able to differentiate between this delusion of general depression and the katathymic delusion that stands out in the hypochondriacal morbid picture especially in dementia praecox, but also in psychopathic patients.

Usually the difference consists also in the fact that the depressive delusion of disease postpones the worst for the future, while the katathymic hypochondriac worries about the present. The depressive patient believes he suffers from closure of the intestines and will perish

[29] Not identical with the usually katathymic *hypochondriacal delusions of disease.*

in a particularly disgusting way, while the hypochondriac asserts that he actually suffers from intestinal inactivity and demands and expects relief.

Impoverishment is often thought of in forms which cannot occur, at any rate nowadays; not only is the patient punished for his debts and must starve, but his relatives also meet with the same fate.

In demented organic patients we see a fourth group of depressive delusions which, though not very common, furnishes the diagnosis when it is present,[30] viz., *nihilism*, which roughly corresponds to the *délire de négation* emphasized by the French, or delusions of negation, which are not to be mistaken for the negativistic manifestations. In this case everything no longer exists, the institution, the world, the Almighty, and the patients themselves; they have not eaten, yet they have not fasted; they have no name, are not men, women, etc. Also in the *délire d'énormité*, which occurs under similar circumstances and is frequently connected with nihilism, the same nonsense finds expression: The patients may not use a chamber because they would flood the entire institution or the whole world; they are swollen up so big that they fill up the entire house and city, and choke everybody; they must swallow everyone in the institution and there are so many of them. In a certain sense the opposite of this is *micromania*, which also only occurs in organic depressions. It consists in the fact that the patients believe themselves to be physically very small; thus a senile scholar was afraid of chickens because he believed his head was so small that it might be pecked off.

Depressive delusion may in rare cases be combined with a kind of megalomania in melancholics, who are not satisfied to be the worst person that ever existed and ever will exist, but attain the rank of the head of the devils. This is also found in schizophrenics where different kinds of affects appear together and express these in parallel delusions, such as, they are the Mother of God and at the same time the devil, or in a condensation such as, they are Queen of the Night.

Delusions of persecution do not belong to the depressive forms of delusion. The delusion of deserved punishment must not be classed with that of the unjust persecution. The former comes from a general depression, the delusion of persecution is a katathymic symptom, which grows from a single emotionally toned idea. Every depressive delusion is a symptom of a potentially transient condition, but the delusion of persecution mostly belongs to chronic diseases. An affective, not katathymic delusion of persecution is the delusion of *anxiety* seen in hal-

[30] At the most it can be said that something similar is seen in schizophrenia but it is not identical.

lucinatory conditions such as dreams, delirium tremens, epilepsy, and schizophrenia.

The real delusion of persecution may at first be quite indefinite; the patients feel that things and people about them have become uncanny ("the walls in my own home wanted to devour me"). Then they make the discovery that certain persons make signs to them or to others which refer to them. One coughs in order to indicate that here comes the onanist, or the murderer of girls. There are articles in the papers with all too plain allusions to them; in business they are badly treated, the attempt is made to get rid of them through disgusting treatment, the most difficult work is assigned to them and they are slandered behind their backs. Finally there are entire organizations, created for this very purpose, the "Black Jews," as well as the "Free-Masons," "Jesuits" and "socialists" which everywhere pursue the patient, and make him powerless. They plague him even with voices, physical influences, and other hallucinations as well as with withdrawal of his thought, crowding of thought and other annoyances. Not so seldom the delusion of persecution is combined with grandiose ideas. A certain overestimation of self generally lies at the bottom of it, insofar as the patient makes some kind of unattainable demands and then looks for the cause of his failure in the environment. It is also said that the delusion of grandeur originates in the delusion of persecution through the fact that the patient says to himself that a person who is subjected to so much persecution must be some extraordinary person. This *transformation* of the delusion I have never plainly observed. On the other hand, we frequently see that *erotic delusions* turn into delusions of persecution or fuse with them, in that the imagined affectionate lover commits sexual and finally other atrocities on the beloved.

An erotic form of delusions of persecution is the *delusion of jealousy* which exhibits several peculiarities. There are paranoiacs who have no other delusions; in schizophrenia it is not seldom mingled with other ideas of persecution, and in alcoholism and cocainism it usually appears as a temporary result of the poison which is not yet fully explained.

The *delusion of reference,* or the morbid reference to oneself, has been distinguished as a special form of delusion. It occurs especially in paranoiacs and paranoid forms, in which it often forms the base of the other delusions. Such patients can relate to themselves absolutely indifferent observations such as coughing, newspaper advertisements, and even cosmic occurrences; they think that everything occurs on their account and interpret it in the sense of their katathymic mental trend. Something similar also occurs in general emotional depressions. Melancholics especially like to believe that any misfortune is the result of their badness.

Thus one tells improbable things, to test the patient's intelligence. In the newspaper it says that some one fell downstairs in order to make the patient understand that she doesn't clean the stairs properly Some one yawns; that is to say that she is lazy.

The delusion of reference is explained by the emotional effects without anything further.[31] Every affective idea has even in normal persons many attachments that do not correspond to reality. It is known that any one coming into a ball room or wearing a uniform for the first time, believes himself noticed, etc.

It has been maintained that delusions are a *sign of mental weakness,* since a normal intelligence would see the incongruity. But it is certain that there are very capable paranoiacs evincing a complete delusional system, who exhibit no other signs of intellectual disturbance. If one bases here the assumption of mental weakness solely on the delusions, one begs the question. The essential factor in the formation of a delusion is the disproportion between affect and logical strength which may have originated in the preponderance of a general mood, as for example in melancholia, or in an especially strong affective coloring of a single idea as, for example, in katathymic delusional formations, or in the weakness of the logical capacity as, for example, in paranoid and twilight state, or in several of these forces acting together, as, for example, in manic paresis.

This formulation naturally indicates only one comprehensible condition of delusional formations out of the others that have not yet been ascertained. There are many disproportions between intelligence and affectivity that do not lead to delusions, e.g., the oligophrenias. The type of affectivity, the transformation of the entire psyche in associating, perceiving, and feeling, as is shown by the schizophrenic process, and in strongly exaggerated form by conditions of clouded consciousness, are other important foundations of delusions.

A connection between intelligence and delusions exists in so far that in mentally clear patients the *quality of the delusion* depends on the grade of intelligence. Intelligent paranoiacs "systematize" their delusions, mixed with real facts they bring them into a system that is usually logically connected, but which has a flaw especially in the assumptions based on false references to themselves, and on memory illusions—and here and there in its causal connection. The content in itself is usually conceivable to others, so that paranoiacs sometimes infect even intelligent, healthy persons.

[31] Cf. association readiness, p. 40, and attention, p. 41.

Similarly formed ideas in schizophrenia have a far weaker or no logical connection and in themselves readily merge into the absurd. Thus the patient was present at Christ's crucifixion; he has made all inventions, even those used before his birth, the bones are taken from his body, several times he has been killed and restored to life, and similar absurdities.

The disturbance of intelligence and unclear thinking express themselves in senseless delusions in manic and depressive conditions of organic patients.

The grandiose ideas of the manic depressive patient are usually only overestimations. He is cleverer than all those that lock him up, he strikes down a dozen keepers, he will expand his business, he will yet become a member of the cabinet. In manic forms of paresis the delusion usually merges at once into the absurd; the patient has large armies at his disposal which will destroy·the institution and the country in which he is; he is a general although he has never been in service; he has invented a bicycle with which you can go around the world, over seas and mountains in three minutes; he is the super-God; the female patient is the mother of everybody, every hour the Almighty takes hundreds of children from her body, etc.

The *melancholic* has committed grave sins, for which tortures will be inflicted on him as on no one else, he suffers from incurable diseases. But the depressive senile has his brain hanging down over his head, his intestines have been replaced by a snake, his head is made of wood. There develop micromania, nihilistic ideas, and the *délire d'énormité.*

In any case one must be careful in diagnosing weakness of intelligence from the senseless content of the delusions. *What has been said holds without any reservation only for conditions, in which mental clearness is not entirely absent.* In twilight states, in toxemias, in fevers absurd delusions may appear even in patients who are not demented, just as in dreams of healthy persons.

Occasionally a delusion that originated in a condition of disturbed mental capacity as in a dream or epileptic delirium and which is therefore senseless, cannot later be corrected, although the intelligence does not now appear badly impaired. Such a residual delusion may, therefore, be senseless without there being at the same time a correspondingly severe disturbance of intelligence.

The *course of delusions* is quite varied. The simple affective and delirious delusional forms fluctuate and naturally disappear with the condition which gave origin to them. The katathymic delusions which were not generated by an exceptional condition, are "fixed ideas" in paranoia and somewhat less regularly in schizophrenia, which are changed little even in decades and hardly ever disappear. Even the seemingly corrected delusions in schizophrenia should rather be considered as forgotten or pushed aside; their persistence may be shown too often, especially in corresponding affective reactions. Besides these, one observes everywhere delusions of diverse origin, which suddenly appear and rapidly disappear.

The *relation of the delusions to the ego* is usually very close. The affect upon which it is based or the ideas themselves usually compel an excessive, often quite monideistic preoccupation with it. A real attempt was made to poison a paranoiac who was always complaining in an annoying way of poisoning. The experience was not connected at all with the delusion and left him entirely indifferent. But in schizophrenics the affective disturbance and the splitting of the psyche, especially in the later stages, bring it about, as a rule, that the ideas leave the patient more or less indifferent, or that they become separated from the everyday ego, which concerns itself with the necessities of ordinary existence, and form a world of their own.

4. DISTURBANCES OF MEMORY

Hyperfunction of memory, or hypermnesia, may probably only be ascertained through the fact that occasionally recollections are much more vivid and distinct than at other times, that they deal with details that are ordinarily not noticed, and that they reach back to periods that are not otherwise remembered. Thus in a feverish disease, in deliria of senility, a memory series of early youth, even of earliest childhood may turn up. In a hypnotic state one can at times recall complicated details as distinctly as if one again saw the things in front of him. In a dream, also, details, that cannot be reproduced at all in waking state, may turn up with the clearness of a sense impression. In rare cases of schizophrenia, memory pictures obtrude themselves in the patient in a disagreeable way, in which case they are usually but slightly connected.

Much more important are the *hypofunctions*. Theoretically, one may differentiate those of formation, of retention, and those of the ekphoria of the engrams. In reality, however, the disturbances rarely concern only the one or the other function, and above all we have by no means progressed so far as to comprehend really all possible differences referring to the partial function chiefly involved. A disturbance of attention, at the time of impression, may harm the recollection in about the same way as when occurring at the time of reproduction. I can hardly conceive of a qualitative disturbance of the *engraphic* effect, and in the entire pathology I have found nothing that would indicate its existence. On the other hand, in senile atrophy of the brain the engraphic effect of the experiences on the psyche is possibly weakened, and as a result, the extensive effect must probably be reduced also, for the diffuse extension of the influence in the brain, which is to be assumed for numerous reasons, diminishes, and fewer associational connections are formed. One can also conceive that the *hypothetical elaboration* of the engrams is reduced in some way, but is not yet subject to any disturbance that would indicate the fact. From the *process of remembering* (*ekphoria*) we know that it certainly participates in many anomalies of memory, indeed there is nothing that stands in the way of assuming that disturbances of it alone can explain most memory defects. Recollection generally is disturbed, when an affect causes a diffuse blocking of thoughts as in the case of examination stupor. Individually it is difficult to remember that which is incompatible with an affect connected with self-love which strives to manifest itself. Transformations of a memory occur whenever there is an affective necessity, which also determines the direction of the falsification.[32]

To judge the unfortunate concepts "impressibility" (Merkfähigkeit) is not very easy in pathology. What is considered under this term is in reality a very complicated function which may be disturbed, without changing the engraphy or the memory functions in general. This happens when for any reason what should be noticed is not properly perceived or else not further elaborated, as in diseases of the sense organs, in all forms of disturbances of attention, and in reference to more complicated matters in various forms of dementia where things perceived are not comprehended. In the latter case there is no lack of actual engrams of the sense perceptions, but there are no associative connections to assist in bringing them to memory. As the most striking hypofunction of impressibility is that which is described in the *organic psychoses*. Thus in extreme cases every experience, even the most important, is at once forgotten; a senile woman may be told her husband has died and she will react with tears, but a moment later she knows nothing about it, and this experiment may be repeated as often as desired. To be sure, in the defective brain the formation of the engrams may be somehow impeded, but *this is certainly not the essential factor*, because the organic disturbances of memory do not confine themselves only to the period of the disease and are in no way proportional to the condition at the time of impression, but much rather to the state existing at the time of the recollection. Furthermore, in not

[32] For organic disturbances of ekphoria see below.

very extreme cases most things are "noticed," notwithstanding, but only for a short time are they capable of ekphorization. One also observes in every patient memory islands, so to say, as shown in the fact that some experience is never forgotten or that a recollection, that did not seem to be there, suddenly turns up in a certain connection. Besides, the "economy" in time, which is observed in relearning of material apparently completely forgotten, proves the persistence of a mnemonic after-effect, even in severe cases of Korsakoff's disease.

Hence, in organic hypomnesias one deals with a disturbance of memory that involves the more recent experiences disproportionately stronger than those lying further back, even though what is experienced during the disease is for various reasons often particularly poorly remembered. Only this formulation covers all the facts. The main disturbance is probably in the ability to recall, although the organic reduction of the associations hinders, on the one hand, the formation of paths, along which the recollections can be afterwards ekphorized, and, on the other hand, impedes the use of these paths in the process of ekphoria. In the same way a senile disturbance of attention not only impedes the formation of engrams capable of recollection but also their revival.

Disturbances of the retention of the engrams are not significant in psychiatry. In view of the large number of chance tests which demonstrate to us not only the unlimited continuation of the engrams but their positive consolidation through age, I cannot believe that there is such a thing as a normal weakening, in the sense, that all memory pictures become "weaker" with time and finally disappear entirely, thus producing a pathological exaggeration of such a process. Nevertheless, organic disturbances of memory are considered from this viewpoint and justly so inasmuch as the general reduction of their carriers must naturally impair the engrams in some way; but the connection of these changes with the clinical manifestations is certainly very complicated. It is chiefly the ekphoria that proves disturbed, not the preservation of the engrams. The disturbance of *acute* and *chronic alcoholism* could also be connected with the change of the engrams, where the recollections are rather readily brought up but are inexact or wrong, while the patient believes he is reproducing well. But here, too, other explanations are more probable.

In coarse brain lesions it seems that definite groups of memory pictures may become affected, such as certain speech, or motor, or acoustic, or optical memory pictures. But the extraordinarily indefinite and fluctuating border of such defects makes it probable, that even psychic structures apparently so elementary, are never totally destroyed; that they are therefore localized in the entire cortex, even though their most important part, their focus, is concentrated in a definite region of the brain. If the focus is destroyed then the engrams can only be ekphorized exceptionally and imperfectly, while destruction of other parts of the cortex affects them little or in a manner hardly noticeable.

Besides the organic memory disturbances there are also various diffuse, unsystematized forms of *memory weakness*. They show nothing that is uniform and at the present have no great significance in psychopathology; the main thing is not to confuse them with other disturbances. In the anamneses of *schizophrenics* we very frequently find the remark that they have become "forgetful," that they no longer "had any memory." If such testimony of relatives were taken literally, one would have to conclude that one dealt with an organic mental disturbance because a real weakness of memory does not occur in schizophrenia. On the other hand, schizophrenics readily become indifferent, inattentive, distracted, and inhibited in their associations, all of which can bring it about that they do not recall things at the desired time. *Neurotics*, too, have a very freakish memory for similar reasons. *Onanists* often complain of a bad memory, partly as a result of suggestion through certain books, and partly perhaps as a result of lack of concentration, which is determined by the distraction caused through the complex. In *epileptics* the memory as a rule becomes weakened when they already have a marked atrophy of the brain, naturally also in the organic sense; but this peculiarity is usually concealed by a general weakness of memory which manifests itself now here and now there but in which emotionally colored events can be retained more readily and reproduced in a stereotyped way.

Circumscribed memory gaps are designated as *amnesias;* the circumscription may be confined to content (systematized) or to time. The former occurs in gross brain lesions in such a way that all optical or all acoustic memory pictures disappear, or only those of substantives or those of numerals, etc. Naturally, here, too, it is not known what part of it is due to the memory pictures and what is merely a difficulty in ekphorization; at all events, the latter plays a big part as may be seen from the reconstruction of such amnesias.

In psychoses one meets with *amnesias for definite events* (katathymic amnesias). During the experience the patient was in an ordinary condition of consciousness and reproduced in a normal way all other events that occurred about that time. Thus an hysteric suddenly forgot everything that related to her physician *Janet*, and mistook him for a new assistant physician. In schizophrenia acts of the individual and of others are "forgotten" every day, when the memory of the same does not just suit the patient. A mild schizophrenic of *Wernicke* swore in all good faith, nevertheless falsely, that he had not insulted a policeman (katathymic amnesia). In such cases one can usually easily demonstrate in a round-about way—in hysterics most readily by hypnosis—that the engrams concerned have not been destroyed, since the recollection may again appear in another connection.

In some cases the necessity exists to omit an entire period of time, as in the case of the hysterical woman who wished to forget her husband and who then recalled things only up to the time of her acquaintance with her husband. Thus originates apparently a temporal circumscription of the amnesia but in which, nevertheless, the content is the essential factor and which furthermore differs from the ordinary temporal amnesias in the fact that it relates to a period of normal experience.

The rarer *negative hallucinations of memory* are a little different. Thus a patient, like all the others, has received his cigars for Christmas; he smoked them up quickly and then began to scold because cigars were given to all patients except to him. The distinction between this and katathymic amnesia lies in the hallucinatory obtrusiveness of such manifestations. *Wernicke's* patient did not remember something that he experienced, while upon the other the recollection forces itself that something that should have happened did not happen. The latter feel the gap in what should have happened, while the others are not conscious of any gap.

The most frequent kind of amnesia is the one that follows disturbances of consciousness of all kinds, especially twilight states and deliria. A patient wakes up suddenly after some sort of behavior otherwise not in keeping with his character, he does not know at all where he is, how he got there and what has happened. He recalls things, up to a certain moment, and then recollection ceases, somewhat as in a normal person after a "dreamless" sleep. As a rule every point of contact for estimating the transpired time is lacking; if the twilight state has lasted several days, the patient usually does not feel the lack of temporal orientation at all, or perceives it insufficiently. As a rule he underestimates the duration of the condition, and thinks it is the day following the one last remembered, as after an ordinary night's rest.

Amnesias are also not uncommon after purely affective explosions in psychopathic or in really insane patients. This is seen in outbursts of prisoners, in depressive and schizophrenic excitements, and similar states.

The amnesia is not necessarily complete. There are all transitions from absolutely no memory up to complete recollection, just as in the recall of our dreams. This amnesia also resembles that following the dream, insofar as it may be variable. Frequently, immediately after waking some things can be remembered that are forgotten some time later, and, just the reverse, an initial total absence of memory may clear up in the course of the next hours or weeks, especially when the patient is reminded of his acts. As in every case where there is a certain weakness of memory, a selection of the retained memories may take place even in quite harmless cases, which is an exaggeration of normal states, inasmuch as only what is unpleasant to the patient is altogether or mostly forgotten. The knowledge of these incomplete amnesias is very important because criminal acts are not seldom committed in twilight states and in case the patient shows a wavering recollection, the judge is inclined to take simulation for granted.

Also the exact time of the beginning and ending of the amnesia cannot always be definitely fixed, which may lead to new difficulties. In part, but not at all invariably, such a manifestation is connected with the course of the twilight state, in which clearer moments may change off with those entirely unclear.

The amnesia may also extend beyond the time of the abnormal state, taking by preference a backward direction; this is designated as *retrograde amnesia*. This is very often the case after dreamlike or unconscious states in consequence of head traumas or after attempts at hanging. The patients no longer know at all that they got into the situation that produced the trauma and how they got there. *Antero-grade amnesia* [33] occurs much more seldom and perhaps only during a gradual transition to lucidity which deceives the observer as to the severity of the condition. Here there is a prolonging of the amnesia to the time immediately following the attack, which period may last for hours or days.

During the twilight state one usually can easily ascertain that the patient can recall events experienced in the same attack. One of our epileptics, whose twilight states often lasted several weeks, pretty regularly recalled during these attacks the occurrences of the last two days; but from this period the amnesia followed continually the course of time. Moreover, the memories may turn up again in the next analogous

[33] Unfortunately this term is also used for various other disturbances of memory, as for a condition in which every experience is at once forgotten, as in our organic memory disturbance, without a consideration as to whether the disturbance of recollection also extends to former experiences. It is also used in cases like those of the epileptic, in the following paragraph, with whom the anterior border of the amnesia followed the present time by an interval of two days.

state; this is seen not only in hypnotic and hysterical twilight states, but also in epileptic and even toxic states. A drunkard, who in a drunken condition has mislaid his keys, knows the next time he is drunk where they are, etc. Also in the hypnotic as well as in epileptic states many such twilight states may be brought to light again.

In the conditions that lead to amnesias we regularly have a *markedly changed mental activity.* In the hysterical states and in attacks of rage and anxiety it is the emotional effect that produces a different relation, in alcoholic intoxication and in epileptics it is the poisoning of the brain, while in organic cases it is, doubtless, chiefly a metabolic disturbance in consequence of circulatory changes, particularly through vascular occlusions and cerebral pressure. Under such circumstances apperception is already inadequate and still more the elaboration of things perceived, that is, there is an inadequacy in the connection of normal associations with the individual's existing sum of ideas with the help of which memories are ordinarily aroused. All of these are additional impediments to the capacity to recall. Even a normal person could not recall the disorderly confusion that many states of dimmed consciousness present.

But the most important factor, which is nearly always present, is probably the entirely different state, namely, the combination of ideas changed as to content and form. Even the healthy person does not possess full control over his memory resources if he wants to make use of them under unusual circumstances or when he is preoccupied. It cannot therefore cause surprise if similar phenomena occur wherever there was a change in the usual state of the association. If one no longer remembers the events of a particular place, they often come plainly into consciousness as soon as the place is revisited; after a manic depressive attack recollections are often dimmed, but in the next attack, even if decades have since passed, they may readily obtrude themselves with most unusual clearness. We have good reason to suppose that the *amnesia for the first period of childhood* may be attributed to the powerful transformation that the personality has to undergo in this period. That the suckling has no memory is naturally a senseless assumption.

The essential factor in many hysterical amnesias is the *exclusion of an unpleasant recollection (or actual fact) from consciousness.* This necessity has usually already provoked the twilight state. To illustrate:

Through clumsy manipulation behind her husband's back, a woman has made inroads upon his fortune, on account of which her husband wanted to leave her. She now merged into a twilight state from which she had excluded a large part of time of her married existence and especially the birth of a child which occurred when her troubles began and made the situation more difficult; she could not be brought to herself through explanations.   After a while she became more lucid, but only after her husband had become reconciled to her was she able to recall her guilt and the marital difficulties; but she could not recall the twilight state.

The inability to recall frequently does not lie in the condition at the time of the experience, but in an actual resistance to the ideas about to be reproduced.   Even in the case of experiences occurring in clouded states only those that are unpleasantly accentuated are sometimes conspicuous.

Thus an epileptic teacher who had stolen during a twilight state, afterwards knew nothing either of the thefts or of the epileptic attacks, which he had while under observation in an institution, although he had not only been led over both episodes but was also convinced of them; at the same time he remembered well most of the details of his flight to a foreign country.

As disturbances of ekphoria we have still to mention the *schizophrenic states* in which obstructions, abnormal mental trends, and incoherence prevent the finding of the usual paths.   In this connection it should also be mentioned that where few associations are present, as in organic cases and in imbeciles, recollection may start from fewer points, and, therefore, under certain circumstances, proceeds less readily.

Recognition has naturally become impossible where recollection in general has ceased.   Senile patients often do not recognize their nearest relatives.   But recognition is retained much longer than simple recollection, for the association of a new impression with a memory picture of the same thing is certainly one of the strongest impressions, and very easy to find.   Thus we also see in examining the impressibility that, although the patient is unable to repeat a name just previously mentioned, he can, without difficulty, select it from a number of words presented to him.

The *alteration of the feeling tone* and other regularly occurring subjective additions of a perception which have not yet been described, can under conditions so change the latter, that the object appears strange to us and in rare cases is not recognized.   Neuropaths and melancholics very often feel that everything seems strange to them, but only seldom do they consider the things really changed, in schizophrenics, however, the reverse is often the case.

As *parafunctions of memory* (memory deceptions) we recognize, in the first place, the inaccurate recollections.   They are found, as mentioned above, in acute and in chronic alcoholism, but especially in *organic* cases and also in *epileptics*. In the latter similar memories can easily be mistaken for each other when such a patient, for example, was twice in prison, the two events merge together, especially when he is in a twilight state. He then relates about a time spent in prison which belongs to the other episode, and what is even more characteristic of epilepsy is the fact that he cannot get away from the idea of the repetition, and under conditions he will continue to relate how he was discharged from prison, then worked, then came into prison, and then he was again discharged and again locked up, etc. Indistinct and inaccurate memories are also common among those imbeciles who in their concept formations do not firmly adhere to sensory perceptions, whereas in the others we can often find a remarkably faithful reproduction of experiences.

On the whole, these inaccuracies of memory receive little attention in pathology. More important are the systematic memory falsifications which are designated as *illusions and hallucinations of memory*.

The illusions of memory (paramnesias) are exaggerations to the point of pathology, of memory disturbances which are so frequently provoked through affects in healthy persons. They play a great part in all forms of insanity, but the greatest part is played in paranoia and schizophrenia. There is no paranoiac who does not change his memories in the sense of his delusions, but just here one can sometimes verify how the original memory pictures as such have not been changed; the patient affirms, for example, "that the pastor had preached about me. He said that I am now looked upon as an insane person and I am not good for anything else." On intensive questioning one at first receives, despite all urging, the verbal quotations of the pastor's speech in the form mentioned. But if the doctor and the patient do not lose patience, one can finally show that the pastor said: "Happy are those who are poor in spirit," but that the patient referred to herself the words in the given sense and translated this sense in words which she put in the pastor's mouth without realizing it. In the delusion of princely lineage a visit paid to the parents, which in itself is perhaps insignificant, is translated by the patient as a visit from a minister. Here, too, one can often elicit through patient questioning of the patient that one does not deal with anything important.. In both these cases, however, the patients are not any more convinced by these analyses, and immediately thereafter repeat their assertions in the original form.

Melancholics entertaining delusions of sin are in the habit of investigating their whole life for faults that they may have committed.

They not only make a deadly sin out of such trivialities as stealing apples in childhood but they also often change the content of the memory in the same sense. In their excitement manic patients easily get into friction with their environment. They are regularly the aggressors and put the others on the defense. Even during the course of the illness, but more remarkably also, even after the attack, they recount these experiences for the most part in an entirely different light, they represent themselves as the ones who were maltreated, misunderstood and unjustly attacked. As they are now quite calm and, as a rule, quite sensible, it is difficult not to believe them if one is not himself well acquainted with the situation. At all events we know that patients suffering also from other mental disturbance, above all, the clearer minded and litigious schizophrenics, behave in the same manner in similar situations.

A systematic memory disturbance which is also determined by the affect is at the basis of the *alternating personality*.[34]

Memory illusions which connect the experiences of others with one's own person (as in the case of appersonation), merit special consideration. Schizophrenics sometimes aver that they experienced things which really happened, but not to them, but to their nearby patients. Whoever considers himself Christ, believes that he had been crucified, and, under certain conditions, can delude himself into remembering the details of it with perceptible acuteness; to be sure, the greatest part of such products become unclear in consequence of the imperfection of the sensible components and are thus recognized as incorrect.

Parallel with the memory illusions, we may put those memory deceptions which freely create a memory picture, which has no connection with a real experience, that is, the *memory hallucinations* which endow a phantasy with reality. The latter must be taken in the strict sense as confabulations, for they really also deserve this name. Objectively they represent ideas having a timbre of something experienced or of something remembered.

Memory hallucinations appear almost exclusively in schizophrenics. All of a sudden memories appear which have no basis in experience. The patient immediately begins to be abusive saying that last night he was taken into the tower and made to go through all sorts of gymnastic tricks, in order to throw him finally into the river. The following days the story is continued and constantly becomes more complicated but is seemingly arranged after a definite plan. He is finally made to fly (before aviation came into existence) and goes

[34] Cf. below under Disturbance of Personality.

through the whole world. At the same time it is surely not a question of verified dreams or of hallucinations of the senses, for many of these experiences are put back to a period when the patient was quite normally occupied with work or singing. In other cases the memory hallucinations are less systematized and consist only of fragmentary details. The normal person can easily read himself into this abnormity, if he thoroughly observes his dreams. A great part of the experiences which are later put into the actual dream, are in reality memory hallucinations and immediately come up in the associations as memory and not as a present experience.

Also in organic cases such real memory hallucination can occasionally appear. Thus a senile patient frequently related to us, how he was attacked in his room last night by robbers, who tied one of his arms on his back, and used his other arm with the hand as a scoop to get out the gold and silver from his own money chest. Sometimes it could be demonstrated that he neither slept nor hallucinated during the night in which he located his adventure. As a matter of fact no hallucinations of the senses have ever been confirmed in him.

In *confabulations* it is also a question of free inventions which are taken as experiences. They fill a memory gap, frequently turn out to have been produced for just this purpose, and change from moment to moment. Indeed they can be provoked and guided while memory hallucinations can no more be changed than a delusion. One asks an alcoholic Korsakoff patient where he had been yesterday, and without any reflection he recounts with great accuracy that he took a walk to the nearby mountain. If he is then asked whether he has not seen the doctor, one can expect with considerable certainty that in pronounced cases, the patient will answer in the affirmative and will describe where he had seen him and about what they talked together. Now and then such an invention adheres to memory, and what is remarkable, also when real experiences are forgotten from minute to minute.

Unfortunately the term confabulation is also used for vivid memory hallucinations and for half conscious phantasy manifestations of schizophrenia. We must, however, adhere to the concept in the above given sense of the confabulation, for thus conceived it is a sign of *organic psychoses* when observed in non-delirious states. It would be good if the name should not be applied to other anomalies.

The most vivid confabulations are seen in many alcoholic Korsakoff cases; almost their whole psychic activity often consists only of confabulations. Many paretics, especially the manic types, spontaneously confabulate in a very profuse manner. Confabulations play the smallest part in senile forms, still, even here it is in many cases quite easy to evoke the symptom if the patient is asked, for example, what he did yesterday (embarrassment confabulations).

Related to confabulations are phantasies which on occasion are formed by everybody, and are more spontaneously produced by the poets. Gottfried Keiler's Grüner Heinrich relates in an episode which is undoubtedly created from the poet's own childhood, how when in the *abc* class he was painfully taken to task for using ugly words which he accidentally absorbed, how in his embarrassment he named some place and name, following which, to further questions, a more complicated scene emerged with all possible details, which he believed was an experience from his own life.

What happened here to the future poet occurs habitually in *Pseudologia Phantastica*. Pseudologues have a vivid phantasy, they invent for themselves some fairy story about princely lineage or some other desirability and act upon it. In contradistinction to confabulations and memory hallucinations, the real worth of their phantasies becomes conscious to the pseudologues as soon as they are recalled to them by the events, and sometimes even without this; in every case a part of the fancies are just lies. Yet, for any long period the pseudologues are capable of ignoring the fact that they are living in a dream world. This circumstance, with a great talent to put a rôle into operation, which for inner reasons is regularly found at least in all cases that come for investigation, gives them the facility to deceive their environments, and if they are not very moral they are destined to become panhandlers. Pseudologia phantastica is therefore a general anomaly and not merely one of memory. The following cases will serve as illustrations: [35]

A young man of good breeding fancied so vividly that his mother died, that he rode home dressed in mourning carrying a wreath of flowers of his mother's funeral. Another young man had a quarrel with a friend. He then pictured to himself a duel with his antagonist whom he shot dead, and that he informed the latter's father of the unfortunate outcome of the duel. I found one prisoner in his cell projecting a plan for an English park. He admitted that he had already prepared in his mind the speech he was to deliver to his dinner guest on the occasion of the first hunting party.

Among the *parafunctions of memory* one may mention in the first place *the identifying memory deceptions*. Even the healthy person has sometimes the feeling, particularly when fatigued, that he had

---

[35] *Aschaffenburg*, Die pathologischen Schwindler, Allgem. Zeitschr. f. Psych. 909, Bd. 66, p. 1073.

already experienced something that happens to cross his mind at the time being. An attempt was even made to trace such deceptions to the idea of the transmigration of the soul. It occurs more frequently in neurasthenics. Now and then this manifestation is also observed in schizophrenics and epileptics, who are usually peeved over it and imagine that some comedy is performed for their benefit. A schizophrenic that I have known, believed for a long time that whatever he experienced he had already gone through in exactly the same way a year before. An epileptic who in a twilight state saw in everything that happened to him, especially visits and the doctor's words, a repetition of a few weeks before, finally remarked that everything repeated itself, and placed the actual experiences in a great number of former twilight states, a fact which at the time caused him marked excitement.

Just as the memory qualities are in this case connected with ideas to which they do not belong, so also do we find reminiscences in *cryptomnesias* which have lost the memory qualities and appear to the patient as new creations. There are learned men who at first negatively reject every new idea and then digest it consciously or unconsciously, and finally, accept it, if it suits them, but then absolutely forget that these are no discoveries of their own, and even go so far as to present them as new to the very people who discovered them. Senile patients often relate a story at a social gathering as new, which they have heard only a few minutes before from somebody else at the same gathering. Frequently, however, the cryptomnesia embraces the whole wording. In the beginning of this century an art critic was once accused of plagiarism because he reproduced word for word a criticism of somebody else. The whole state of affair points that it must have been a case of cryptomnesia. *Jung* has also demonstrated cryptomnesia in *Nietzsche* who verbally put a paragraph from the Seeress of Prevorst into his Zarathustra, and what is more, in quite a senseless connection.[36] *Helen Keller's* unconscious reproduction of the fable of the Frost King caused her a great deal of annoyance.

As *reduplicative memory deception, Pick* has described a manifestation sometimes seen in organic patients, which consists in the fact that the patients do not duplicate the actual act but double the details of it. They say that they have already been examined in the very

[36] C. G. *Jung,* Zur Psychologie und Pathologie sogenannter okkulter Phänomene, Stuttgart, Mutze 1902 Especially instructive is Flournoy's "Des Indes à la Planète Mars, Paris and Genève 1900. (Étude sur un cas de Somnambulisme avec glossolalie.)

same clinic by the very same physician, having the same name, there are therefore, two such physicians and clinics.

5. DISTURBANCES OF ORIENTATION

Wernicke divides disturbances of orientation into *autopsychic* or those referring to the individual's person, *somatopsychic* or those referring to the individual's body, and *allopsychic* or those referring to the outer world. This differentiation has a specific meaning; thus patients in alcoholic deliria are never autopsychically disoriented, that is, they can give a good account of their personal matters, their residence, occupation, and past life, whereas allopsychically they are usually deeply disoriented, especially as to time and place. However, this classification fails to give proper emphasis on the element of the situation which may form part of allopsychic as well as autopsychic orientation. Instead of somatopsychic disorientation we prefer to speak of somatic illusions and hallucinations.

In all organic mental diseases of a higher grade, the primary auxiliary functions of orientation, perception, memory, and attention are affected, and in addition there is also a disturbance of the comprehensive orientation itself. Orientation as to time and place, and later also as to the situation, are falsified. The patients are not aware that they are kept in an institution, or of the reason thereof, nor do they recognize as such the doctors who are treating them. Not infrequently one observes in the insane asylum, that orientation as to situation which is otherwise less liable to injury is falsified before orientation as to time. This is due to the fact that the patients do not wish to be in such a place.

Orientation as to time and place are always present in Schizophrenia; they are often very well preserved unless interfered with by secondary influences such as delusions and hallucinations. The patient who believes he is Christ usually considers himself **1900** years old. For affective reasons the calendar itself is often directly falsified. Places are nearly always correctly recognized by clear Schizophrenics. On the other hand, orientation as to the situation is in most cases incorrect, at least in interned Schizophrenics. The patients cannot comprehend that they are considered sick, they believe themselves unjustly confined, etc.

Furthermore, orientation can be falsified in all its relations by hallucinations and illusions. If a patient sees hell instead of the hospital ward, or a devil instead of an attendant, he cannot imagine himself in an insane asylum. The strange part of it is, that in such states of schizophrenia, hardly ever in other diseases, the correct orientation mostly accompanies the false one; one might say that there is a *double orientation*. Depending on the constellation the patient uses now one, then the other orientation, and often both together.

In all states of vivid hallucinations which conceal the real perceptions, thinking is also disturbed, often in a very profound manner, as for example in epileptic twilight states where it is sometimes more pronounced than in our dreams. In some cases the disturbance of thinking seems to be the chief cause of the disorientation, as in cases of confusion (amentia). That a schizophrenic delirium should appear to last thousands of years, and a dream of a few seconds many hours, fits in well with the absolutely changed course of the psychic mechanisms.

Disorientation as to time and place is, therefore, one of the most constant partial symptoms of all disturbances of consciousness, such as deliria, crepuscular states, confusions, amentias, and other states. Not seldom we also find here some autopsychic disturbance (referring to the person).

6. DISTURBANCES OF CONSCIOUSNESS

Under the expressions "Disturbance of Consciousness" and "Clouding of Consciousness," which do not fit in with the rest of our terminology, but for which we have not yet found substitutes, we conceive a number of anomalies in which the general relationship of the psychic processes, usually including orientation, is disturbed, or in which psychic processes are forcibly hindered from coming to consciousness.[37] The first type of disturbance is especially found in the states of *Confusion* mentioned above,[38] which may arise from very different fundamental disturbances. Marked confusion with numerous hallucinations was also designated as *Amentia*. *Kraepelin* uses this term for a definite morbid picture.[39] *Deliria* and *Twilight or crepuscular states* are concepts everywhere used, even though they are very differently defined by different authors, and not clearly differentiated from each other, nor definitely limited.

What one calls *Deliria* are mostly states of incoherent thinking combined with hallucinations and delusions, which show a certain activity and run a rapid course. They usually accompany other dis-

[37] The "conscience" of the French is a broader term than our modern consciousness. Even simple delusions are "troubles de la conscience."
[38] Cf. p. 86.
[39] Cf. Special part.

eases, such as infections, fevers, exhaustions, toxic states, and suddenly appear in the dark room in cases of diseases of the eye. But in a certain sense, some states of Schizophrenia and manic depressive insanity, may also be designated as deliria. Disturbances of consciousness in febrile diseases were all wont to be designated as deliria, although many of them clearly show connected ideas along the line of complexes and, therefore, rather belong to the "twilight states." In the newer German psychiatry the term "delirium" most frequently stands for "Delirium tremens." The memory of deliria is usually imperfect or totally absent.[40]

The name *Twilight State* suggests especially a *systematic* falsification of the situation. He who is familiar with these states finds sense and a more or less logical connection in the acts of the patient. The onset and termination of twilight states are most often sudden, the duration is brief, lasting from a few minutes to a few days, rarely for weeks or months.

In the (less frequent) *oriented twilight states* the associations are narrowed. There seems to be present only a single purpose striving to accomplish what is necessary, while the rest of the personality, at least to the extent that it runs counter to this purpose, does not exist. The patients act in a definite direction, they run away, take a journey, make a purchase, commit a crime which otherwise would be foreign to them; they do all that without any regard for themselves or others, even though at times, especially in the case of forbidden acts, they endeavor to protect themselves against discoveries. During this period if they can be observed they usually strike one as abnormal; at times, however, they can use correctly ordinary means of intercourse, can associate with fellow travelers, and can even visit relatives, without betraying their condition.

The ordinary *disoriented twilight states* present themselves quite differently and yet, as daily transitions show, they are only an exaggeration of the preceding. In spite of a certain coherence, which might be compared with a dream, thinking is not clear or it may even be confused. The connection with the outer world is altogether interrupted or falsified by illusions and hallucinations of the visual and auditory types, especially the former. The patients see robbers, animals, devils, or the Almighty with many saints; they actually believe themselves in a dream-like situation and act accordingly. As in the dream the content of the twilight ideas may be anxious, indifferent, or

---

[40] The French conception of delirium is much broader. They even call delusions occurring in clear consciousness delirium. *Bouffée's délirantes* are, according to *Magnan*, transitory deliria in his "degenerates."

rapturous. Anxious and hostile illusions provoke the patients to acts of violence; killing even several people is not uncommon. Sexual excitements lead to rape and murder. An epileptic set fire to his workshop in the belief that he was lighting a fire under a lime pan. States of rapture are designated as *ecstasies*. In such states association with the outer world is so completely interrupted that an absolute *analgesia* exits. The patients see the heavens open, associate with the saints, hear heavenly music, experience wonderful odors and tastes and an indescribable delight of distinct sexual coloring that pervades the entire body.

Some twilight states have a definite purpose such as to represent illnesses and the like, of which the best known type is the so-called *Ganser* state. The varieties of these forms are indicated under the Syndromes.

The *causes* of twilight states are very varied. Many have their origin in an affective necessity; hysterics and schizophrenics turn away from reality because it has become unbearable. An engagement which has been broken in reality continues in the twilight state and leads to marriage. Some hysterical twilight states repeat hallucinatorily an emotionally accentuated event, especially of an ambivalent nature, e.g. a sexual attack. Less frequently the delights of ecstasy can be conjured up. The basis of twilight states are the hysterical, epileptic or schizophrenic disposition, toxic conditions, especially pathological intoxication, also sleep, as pavor nocturnus, somnambulism and hypnogogic intoxication, less frequently it is migraine, concussion of the brain, and brain disturbances after hanging, occasionally it may also be caused by severe excitements as in the case of psychopathics. In hysteria the entire mechanism is psychogenetic; in the toxic states of epilepsy and schizophrenia, it is the brain disturbances which usually furnish the necessary factor. All these states produce clear thinking which becomes systematized as a result of affective aims, in consequence of which the disturbance assumes the form of a twilight state. The disturbance of thought then has a twofold origin, one in the toxic confusion, the other in the systematic formation with its misunderstanding of reality. It is self-evident, that in epilepsy as well as in schizophrenia the relation of the two causes may be entirely different. There are extreme cases in both directions, on the one hand conditions in which the organic completely dominates the picture, and on the other hand those which are of an entirely psychogenetic (hysterical) character and in which acute changes of the fundamental condition play no part. Where primary anxiety exists, as is often the case in epilepsy, the content of the delusion is colored in this sense.

Naturally, we often observe very mild twilight states and deliria, in which the thought process is only more or less unclear. These mild forms together with deliria and twilight states may be called provisionally *turbid states*.

There is still another gradual weakening of consciousness which is shown by the fact that external stimuli must be endowed with an abnormally great intensity in order to become conscious. Mild states of this sort are called *cloudiness,* a name that may also designate light grades of the twilight states. Similar states that are somewhat deeper and especially those in which movements are retarded are designated as *somnolence;* those in which only stronger stimuli produce reactions are called *torpor* or *sopor;* and those in which there is no longer any reaction are called *coma.* In the last condition one assumes that there is a state of actual *unconsciousness,* i.e., an absence of conscious psychisms. This is naturally something entirely different from the falsely designated unconsciousness in a twilight state.

In all these disturbances the *field of consciousness,* that is, the number of simultaneous ideas, is greatly diminished; in the twilight states this is more or less systematic, in other conditions it is diffuse.[41]

There is also a purely *functional attempt to keep occurrences out of consciousness.* When attention makes way for a certain group of ideas it blocks at the same time all others. In a cheerful mood unpleasant thoughts are automatically kept away. In melancholia cheerfulness cannot even be thought of. The katathymic exclusion of unbearable complexes from consciousness (repression) belongs to this category. In all these cases the functions which are not admitted to consciousness may be entirely impeded or they may lead an unconscious existence.[42]

Sleep is a kind of physiological disturbance of consciousness which also gives occasion for several pathological symptoms. I do not know whether or not one always dreams in sleep. In our present state of knowledge the forms of association in dreams are the same as in schizophrenia. The psychopetal functions usually are extremely restricted in sleep, partly in such a way that only strong stimuli arouse reactions, partly, and this is more important, in such a way that the main part of the stimuli is shut off regardless of its intensity, and its place is taken by a smaller group, which is generally or under certain constellations especially important. Thus a nurse sleeps through a great noise but is awakened by a slight respiratory change in her patient. The psychofugal connection with the outer world,

---

[41] For alternating consciousness Cf. Personality.
[42] Comp. the Unconscious, p. 8.

at least as far as concerns the voluntary muscular system, is usually limited to movements that make respiration easy, change uncomfortable positions, ward off stimuli from insects, etc. Movements that are not carried out are falsely conceived through kinaesthetic hallucinations, except in *nightmares*, where the paralysis is felt, and what is not quite the same thing, the interruption between volition and motility comes into consciousness.

Falling asleep is the result of an influence, or a special act, which is put in operation by the predisposition to fatigue, a feeling which is psychically determined. Perhaps the only thing of importance for psychotherapy is the psychic participation in the initiation of sleep. The essential thing is the "suggestion of sleep." To be sure, energetic mental occupation in the evening may for a time hinder the command to sleep. But ordinarily, it is the affects that exclude sleep. For example, one is particularly apt to remain awake when one is pleasantly or unpleasantly excited, when one is afraid of not being able to sleep, or when one "imagines" himself disturbed by a definite sensory impression. Here the sensory impression has really no significance, compared with the psychic attitude. *The psychotherapist must firmly maintain that when some one cannot sleep, let us say, because his neighbor snores, that it is his own attitude and not the neighbor's snoring that is the cause to be considered.* One can sleep in the worst noise if one is able to assume a proper attitude, and at the same time one can be awakened by the slightest sensory impression for which there is an association readiness. Millions sleep through the street noises of the metropolis. One of the most important neurotic disturbances of sleep is undoubtedly based on the fact that emotionally accentuated complexes, which are more or less repressed by the day's work, make themselves felt as soon as purposive thinking ceases.

What the *recuperative function* of sleep is, we do not know. At all events it is under a special influence, because, in states of depression, for example, one can dispense for many months with sleep, in the sense of disturbance of consciousness and association, without apparent results, while an artificial insomnia of only eight days is certainly fatal. Moreover a partial insomnia has few or no immediate ill effects, if one succeeds in lying quiet and not exhausting oneself in the "struggle for sleep."

The *dream* is classed with the twilight states because ordinarily it does not influence conduct. Nevertheless in the sleep of no person are the connections with the outer world maintained only through the merely necessary centrifugal and centripetal impulses. Through groaning, twisting, and through many somewhat uncoordinated movements and similar expressions one satisfies even in sleep some internal or external requirements. A slight increase of these normally existing motor commands permits the release of any acts corresponding to dream images, and leads to twilight states of somnabulism, hypnogogic intoxication, and pavor nocturnus.

Somnambulism occurs in nervous persons of all types, in epileptics, and to a mild degree, at times in people who must be considered healthy; this is especially the case in youth. There are all sorts of transitions from simple movements and mumbling in sleep to more complex acts as well as walking which sometimes takes place on the roof. Most frequently such little acts are performed that correspond to the daily occupation; these are sometimes senseful and sometimes senseless. Complexes may also find expression in somnambulism (Lady Macbeth).

Hypnogogic intoxication (Schlaftrunkenheit) may occur during spontaneous awakening in people who seem perfectly well, but more frequently it follows a rough waking, which generates a dream, and induces motility before the dream disappears. In rare cases something clumsy is then performed, indeed, under the influence of terrifying ideas an attack or murder may be perpetrated. A variety of sleep intoxication which is especially frequent in children is *pavor nocturnus*. It usually manifests itself in the beginning of the night when the little ones start with an anxious cry and despite all attempts to wake or quiet them, become mentally clear only after several minutes or even a longer time. The syndrome is often altogether psychically determined, in other cases it is favored or absolutely induced by respiratory difficulties. The twilight states of sleep are also regularly followed by amnesias.

"Clear Mindedness" ("Besonnenheit")

In contrast with disturbance of consciousness there is *"clear mindedness,"* a concept that is plain to all, although it cannot be quite defined. In states of clear mindedness every disturbance of consciousness is lacking, orientation is good, the affects produce neither unconsidered acts nor stupor. The most inhibited melancholic can think normally within the range of ideas accessible to him, and can orient himself, he is so to speak, clear minded. The most chronic states of schizophrenia do not lack clearmindedness, although, under certain circumstances, the patients act in an entirely senseless way. The major part of the thinking function runs along smoothly; orientation especially is good, and there is always a possibility of discussing many things sensibly with the patient. The outward indications of

clear mindedness, according to *Jasper*, are orientation, and the ability
to reflect on questions and to take some notice of them.

The concept is important because in clearmindedness identical
symptoms have an entirely different significance than in states of
disturbance of consciousness. In twilight states the most confused
delusions indicate nothing concerning the prognosis, somatic hallucinations indicate almost as little. In clear mindedness both symptoms
point to a grave condition, the latter especially to a schizophrenic
condition.

7. DISTURBANCES OF AFFECTIVITY

Since the affective dispositions fluctuate greatly in different people,
they also most readily cross the borderline of the "normal." The
so-called psychopaths are really nearly all exclusively or mainly
thymopaths. Furthermore, since affectivity dominates all other functions, it assumes a prominent rôle in psychopathology generally, even
in slight deviations, not only on account of its own morbid manifestations, but even more because in disturbances in any sphere, it
is the affective mechanisms that first create the manifest symptoms.
What we call psychogenic is mostly thymogenic. The influence of the
affects on the associations produces delusions, systematic splittings of
personality, and hysteroid twilight states; repressed pain is the source
of most neurotic symptoms, while displacements and irradiations
produce compulsive ideas, obsessive acts, and similar mechanisms.
Ambivalent feeling complexes, that is, viewed from the active side,—
inner conflicts, which the individual cannot settle but must repress,
prove especially pathogenic. To avoid repetitions the causal significance of the affects will here be passed over, and only the etiology
of certain symptoms will be briefly considered. Only the phenome-
nology of the affective disturbances will follow here.

Many affective disturbances come, as it were, from within, from
the physiology of the brain and from the general chemism. Here one
is perfectly right in thinking of the "inner secretions" in the widest
sense, without knowing anything definite about them. To this one
may add the affective bases of melancholia and mania, the euphoria
of chronic alcoholics, and most of the moody states of epileptics and
imbeciles, and naturally also the congenital abnormal emotional states.
The last may have a significance of their own, as in the case of "chronic
moods," or may be the foundation on which other diseases originate.
To become an hysteric or paranoiac one needs a distinct affective constitution which is usually congenital. Such morbid constitutions are

almost always exaggerations of the character variations of the normal type or "temperaments."

Other affective disturbances are qualitatively correct but quantitatively exaggerated reactions to an experience, which usually have their origin in the constitution. Thus a mother loses her child, and does not recover from the blow for years, remaining in mourning all the time. She shows a *morbid protraction of the affect*. Or she reacts so strongly to her misfortune that she can no longer work or eat, is entirely absorbed in the anguish and can in no way be distinguished from a melancholic. Here one sees a *morbid intensity of the affect*. In this way certain anxiety affects may lead to affective stupor [43] and confusion,—manifestations that make the examination of children and oligophrenics particularly difficult, and often lead into entirely false trails.

Reactions in themselves normal may appear morbid because the intellectual process on which they are based is abnormal. A paranoiac believes that he has made a revolutionary discovery which makes him emotionally exalted, or he considers himself persecuted and becomes irritated. In both cases the affects are normal reactions to a morbid idea; in itself the formation of the affect is normal. In the same way there is, for example, a secondary apathy in organic cases, who do not understand many experiences and, therefore, naturally cannot react to them. As soon as they grasp the true significance of anything the same patients react to it in a very active manner.

Morbid irradiations and *affective displacements* are secondary disturbances in an entirely different sense. This is shown in the following examples:

The patient feels disgust and anxiety at hornlike soup ingredients and other things shaped like horns because she was once frightened by a bull whose genitals and horns particularly impressed her. A schizophrenic woman, a patient of v. *Speyer* hated her landlord because he had cheated her husband. When she was taken with labor pains in an isolated country place, instead of a mid-wife the wife of the landlord had to assist her. The hate was transferred from the landlord to his wife, and from the latter to her own child which she tortured to death.

Most affective disturbances are transient episodes. Those which continue are usually congenital, less frequently acquired, as the chronic euphoria of alcoholics, the lability and some persisting euphoria or depressive states in organic cases, as well as the perseverance and intensity of the affects in epileptics.

[43] Cf. p. 80.

Morbid Depression

In general depression, all experiences, inner and outer, are toned with psychic pain of various kinds. The milder cases resemble normal "downheartedness." It is not so easy, however, to read oneself into the affective situation of the profound melancholic. He has lost everything that was of value to him, and nevertheless he expects still worse for himself and those he loves, the worst that one can think of. Through "diversion," i.e. an increase of sense impressions, which are really only unpleasantly toned, the pain is usually increased, except in those cases where the feeling that the patient does not feel well anywhere, leads to a continuous change of environment. In many cases perceptions take on the character of strangeness, of uncanniness, and monotony; optical impressions are double dyed gray, things seem to stand crooked, and foods lack their peculiar flavor. Thinking, in itself, is not only colored by unpleasant feelings, but proceeds with difficulty, and only ideas of a painful content can be thought out. Thoughts of a pleasant content are flighty and transient, leaving no influence on deliberation and the general condition. Only with great difficulty can the patient resolve to act, and when he succeeds in making a movement, it is with great effort.

The *mental stream* is inhibited,[44] it runs more slowly and the patient must exert effort to think out anything; a change of the ideas requires exertion or is even impossible. The patients always fall back on the same ideas of a sad content or they never get rid of them and always carry with them the same desperate thoughts (*Monideism*).

Among the varieties of depression, of which we mention only grief, desperation, and remorse, *anxiety* occupies a particular place. To be sure, it is often combined with the common forms of depression so that it merely complicates the latter. Anxiety may also appear in isolated form, which accounts for the fact that starting from different viewpoints some authors wish to differentiate an absolute anxiety psychosis and an anxiety neurosis as special forms of disease. Anxiety undoubtedly has different sources. In many cases it is plainly connected with respiratory difficulties as seen in diseases of the heart, in the respiratory organs, and in the blood. Furthermore, anxiety is undoubtedly connected in some way with sexuality, a fact which we knew for a long time but which *Freud* first made clearer. Stimulated but unsatisfied sexuality leads to various forms of anxiety. *Freud's* conception is that the sexual tension, or the sexual

[44] Cf. p. 74.

affect, is converted into anxiety, which may not be right, although sexual satisfaction may under certain circumstances remove anxiety, and although anxiety appearing in attacks, as is more generally assumed, may be converted into other syndromes, such as inordinate hunger, attacks of perspiration, asthmatic attacks, diarrhœa, dizziness and similar symptoms. We also know that normal sexuality has an anxiety component and that not seldom orgasms are generated by anxious situations such as hurrying to catch a train, scolding from a teacher in school, and difficult tasks. In many cases of psychoses connected with anxiety we see an irresistible impulse toward onanism that disappears with the affect. But there must be other pathologic sources of anxiety Wherever depression in general originates from physical processes, which we do not as yet know, anxiety too, may be generated, at least as far as we can judge at present; in other words, in all states of melancholia of the most diverse diseases.

In a more striking manner than the other affects, anxiety may exist without any association with ideas: The patient may feel anxiety without knowing why, and be absolutely certain that there is no ground for it ("free floating anxiety"). In many cases anxiety itself creates the ideas to which it becomes attached and which it apparently conditions. In most cases, however, one can easily demonstrate that such ideas are secondary; the anxious patient seizes on something that might produce anxiety such as, an uncertain financial condition, an insignificant symptom of a bodily disturbance in himself or others, or on any mistake that he made in the past; and even when circumstances can convince him that the ideas were wrong the anxiety does not improve in consequence but it attaches itself to a new idea. Often it creates one as an anxiety delusion from pure fancy without any external connection.

Katathymic anxiety referring to a particular member of the family, present in normal and abnormal individuals, is as a rule the expression of a repressed wish that this member should be dead. A latent schizophrenic woman had a child by her husband whom she did not love. Her anxiety was soon noticed even by the midwife when she expressed the idea: "I should only wish that nothing happen to the child!" A few months later she poisoned it. A young woman shows her illness through excessive anxiety for her mother. As soon as her mother has gone out, she has to stand at the window to see that nothing has happened to her, or to see if she is coming back. She is strongly attached to her father and unconsciously jealous of her mother.

Anxiety is more frequently and more visibly accompanied by physical symptoms than most of the other affects. It is especially often associated with an increased cardiac tone which is felt in the chest as something heavy, pressing and often also something painful; these feelings may be present even when the by no means uncommon palpitation is absent. As in angina pectoris the pain may even irradiate into the left arm. In the abdomen, too, a rolling or pulsing, or a hot stream may be felt, or the latter may appear to rise to the head, where other bad feelings, such as knocking, pressing, and fullness may exist. "The Anxiety" is often localized in the place where one has the greatest sensation; thus one speaks of *praecordial anxiety,* which is the most frequent concomitant of all depressions, or of *head anxiety,* etc.

Depression in general usually evinces distinct *physical symptoms.* The entire *turgor vitalis* is diminished, the patients appear older than before, and the metabolism and appetite become decreased. The muscular tone, especially of the extensors and abductors, is decreased, the latter move with greater effort than their opponents, and all show as little activity and are as slow as possible. As a result, the patient's posture becomes uniform, languid, and bowed, and manifests a tendency to draw in the limbs. The handwriting usually shows a tendency to slant the letters downwards.

In some cases, especially those showing anxiety, instead of motor retardation there is a desire to express or get rid of the inner tension through movements (*Melancholia agitata*). In contrast with the common cases of melancholia some patients have no feeling of fatigue and run around continuously and when permitted take tireless walks. In contradistinction to the normal we see more rarely, that morbid anxiety retards movement and the psychic processes generally.

Respiration is easily disturbed, in that inspiration becomes less free, and connected with this are the frequent *feelings of oppression.* The *pulse* is mostly full and small, and the artery contracted. Anxiety increases the blood pressure.

An increased tone of the *throat muscles* very often causes an annoying feeling of strangulation causing the patient to refuse nourishment; it also produces pressure in the chest. In addition all other possible dysaesthesias may accompany depression.

Depressions occur in the most varied psychoses. The tendency to it increases with age, and with increasing vascular disturbances there is more anxious excitation. Depression is the essential symptom in all states of melancholia, and above all in those of manic depressive insanity. Besides these, there are certainly depressions of other kinds which we cannot as yet characterize. Anxiety is an important concomitant of phobias, obsessive ideas and obsessive acts.

THE PATHOLOGICAL ELATED MOOD (EXALTATION, EUPHORIA)

We can differentiate two kinds of exaltation that are, however, connected by all the intermediate stages. In simple euphoria one enjoys the world and one's own existence in a particularly lively way; sensations and thoughts are pleasantly accentuated. Among the healthy of this type we have the sunny dispositions, while among the sick we see some paretics not really of the manic type, less often cases of senility, and at times, also epileptics in a euphoric mood (*morbid euphoria*). In the second form, which deserves more the name of exaltation in a narrower sense, we also see self-consciousness and with it an enormous enhancement of desires and claims. This naturally results in conflicts and leads regularly to severe outbursts of anger. The conditions therefore, in which one sees this symptom together with flight of ideas and pressure activity, are designated as mania and the affective state as *manic depression*. In a somewhat milder form and without the flight of ideas we see this exaltation in the common alcoholic euphoria.

Naturally, the pleasant accentuation may here, too, evince various shades such as cheerfulness, lack of restraint, æsthetic enjoyment, and a general ineffable feeling of delight; the last is especially observed in paresis. The blissful feeling accompanying the *ecstasy* is principally something quite different than manic euphoria, both in the quality of feeling as well as in relation to the mechanism of its origin, which in hysteria is regularly katathymic, in epilepsy usually autotoxic, while in schizophrenia sometimes more of the one, then again the other.

Corresponding to the nature of the positive affects in the normal, the mood of these patients is much more changeable than in depressed cases. They follow the different topics of conversation with their affective fluctuations, but generally do not abandon the euphoric state. In a few cases, however, such fluctuations may go as far as depressions in which the patients may be moved to tears by a sad performance.

Just as we have retardation in depression, so in exaltation we often have a fluent course of ideas up to flight of ideas; the ready translation of thoughts into acts is regularly observed. Manic patients look younger, the *turgor vitalis* is increased, the posture is the direct opposite of that of depression. The other physical symptoms are less marked than in depression, even though the pulse has a tendency to be full and soft.

Exaltation, like depression, may appear intercurrently in every mental disease; in manic states it forms part of the picture and in manic depressive insanity it is a component of the disease itself. As a chronic state it occurs in alcoholics, also as a partial symptom in psychopathic constitutions.

Morbid Irritability

A uniformly overstrong activity of all affects may be the foundation of an abnormal character as well as of hysterical and similar morbid pictures. Furthermore, such an anomaly occurs in the organic psychoses and in epilepsy, and temporarily, also, in simple exhaustion where one may see all kinds of "affective crises," not only of the endogenous but of the reactive depressive type. However, what one understands as morbid irritation is a *special tendency to ill-temper, anger, and rage*.[45] It occurs even in neurasthenics, who can become exceedingly angry over all stronger sense impressions and every disturbance. In the really insane we see it, as was mentioned, as one of 'the manifestations of exaltation, then again it may accompany, as a more independent affective disturbance, all forms of dementia. This is, in part, founded on the fact that rage is the normal reaction to a dangerous situation that one does not understand; under such circumstances reflection is useless, on the other hand, a blind effort to strike at random or tear away without consideration for the environment and the integrity of one's own body, may at times save one's life.

On the contrary, in other irritable characters we perceive the intellectual disturbance, the false conceptions of the surroundings with morbid self-reference, as a result of the affect of irritability, and even though these people always appear somewhat onesided or "narrowed" they sometimes retain an intelligence which is, on the whole, good.

Imbeciles manifest in addition moodiness which comes from within, and easily assumes the form of irritated cloudiness of thought. Here we see most frequently a peculiar symptom of rage, that actually turns the action against themselves, which rarely occurs in other patients. The patients tear their hair, scratch their face or destroy other things so that they perforce hurt themselves. Often they only tear their clothing. Such damaging of the environments, including their own clothing, are very common in schizophrenics, at times it is the result of excitations coming from within, then again it is a

[45] The disposition to anger is not always identical with rage.

reaction to outer harmless experiences. In severe cases of schizophrenia outbursts of rage and anger are often the only remaining signs of affects, while in the milder cases less severe irritability is the only indication of the disease that impresses the environment. In epileptics we often see a chronic irritability as a partial manifestation of the general increase in intensity of the affects, and further, as a passing state of depression in quite the same way as in imbeciles.

APATHY

Apathy in the sense that the affects are destroyed probably does not occur in the psychoses; as a matter of fact we see all affects retained in the brain in the most severe organic destructions. Nevertheless there are many cases of *schizophrenia* which for years show no impulses or affects. In senile patients who no longer show a proper understanding of this world we sometimes see a total lack of interest in everything that occurs about them, which is much less frequently the case in matters of personal contact with them. Melancholics, who are so immersed in their misery that everything else appears insignificant, are sometimes mistaken as apathetic. Many of them maintain that they no longer have feelings, that they are apathetic, because in the face of the great agony entailed in the disease, they can no longer discern any feelings for their own family. In contrast to neurasthenic irritability there is a *neurasthenic indifference* which no longer bothers with anything. Even more frequently do hysterics shut off their affects altogether for a shorter time, so that they appear apathetic. The chronic and totally apathetic "psychasthenics" whom the French describe, we undoubtedly would include with the schizophrenics.

VARIABLE DURATION OF THE AFFECTS

An *abnormally long duration* of the affects occurs in many people not mentally deranged, who cannot get over an ill humor and must always carry with them, for instance, a hatred. In epilepsy, the affects, once aroused, also persist an abnormally long time, even when other experiences intervene. A slight annoyance may also excite a congenital feeble-minded person for days. Such patients possess *too slight an affective distractability.*

More important and better known is the *excessive lability* of the affects, their abnormally brief duration and their increased affective distractability. Children are normally labile; they are rightly compared with seniles; except that all organic cases should in this respect be mentioned together. The affects are very easily aroused in them, but have a short duration; they are especially capable of being too easily diverted. Lability of the affects is very common also in the intervals of more advanced manic-depressive insanity. Imbeciles, too, may suffer from the same defect.

EMOTIONAL INCONTINENCE

Most patients with too great a lability of feelings display less control than the normal. They must give in to every affect, whether they express it or act in accordance with it. Yet lability and incontinence do not always run parallel. There are people without noticeable lability who cannot control their feelings. One of our imbeciles, who was none the less a pretty good workingman, could not, to his sorrow, play cards, because a smiling or a sad countenance always betrayed to the other players whether he held good or bad cards so that they could act accordingly. As far as action is concerned one can say that a real control of pathological affects is not common in the different mental diseases. When an affect is present, the patient usually acts accordingly. The best dissimulators are melancholics, and they resort to it especially for the purpose of getting an opportunity to commit suicide.

AFFECTIVE AMBIVALENCE

Even the normal individual feels, as it were, two souls in his breast, he fears an event and wishes it to come, as in the case of an operation, or the acceptance of a new position. Such a double feeling tone exists most frequently and is particularly drastic when it concerns persons, whom one hates or fears and at the same time loves. This is especially the case when sex is involved which in itself contains a powerful positive and almost equally powerful negative factor; the latter conditions among other things, the feeling of shame and all sexual inhibitions as well as the negative valuation of sexual activity as sin, and the evaluation of chastity as a cardinal virtue.[46]

But such *ambivalent* feeling tones are the exception with the normal person. On the whole he makes a decision from the contradictory values; he loves less because of accompanying bad qualities, and hates less because of accompanying good qualities. But the abnormal person often cannot bring together these two tendencies; the hate and love manifest themselves side by side without the two affects weakening or even influencing each other in any way. He wishes

[46] *Bleuler,* Der Sexualwiderstand, Jahrbuch f. Psychoanalytische Forschungen, Bd. V. 1913.

his wife's death and when hallucinations picture it for him, he is desperate, but even then, besides crying he can at the same time laugh over it.

It is chiefly ambivalent complexes that influence pathology and many expressions of the normal psyche, such as dreams, poetry, etc. In schizophrenia they come to light quite openly. There we often see directly the ambivalent feeling tones, while in the neuroses they are concealed behind a large part of the symptoms.

Congenital Deficiency and Perversions of Particular Affective Groups

Congenital deficiency is almost always described as a defect of the ethical feelings; there is, besides, though very seldom, a defect of the sexuality with all its affects.

False affective accentuations in the sense of perversions, in which the instinctive side stands in the foreground (sex impulse, hunger impulse) are described in the chapter on impulses.[47]

Exaggerations and Onesidedness of the Affective Causes, Morbid Reactions

These disturbances are of fundamental importance for the neuroses, for the understanding and treatment of abnormal characters, and for pedagogics, but of lesser importance for special psychiatry, hence we shall give here only a few suggestions.

Strong affects may lead to disturbances of consciousness in psychopathic persons. The blind rage of prisoners (prison outbreak) and oligophrenics, which may last from a few minutes to many hours, is well known. It is often followed by amnesia. Exaggerated physical symptoms such as fainting, or vomiting, may accompany the attack or represent it alone.

The characteristic factor may here show itself in the force of the momentary affect or in a lack of inhibitions, the latter occurs in definite dispositions such as manic depressions, alcoholic effects, etc. When the effect is more chronic in psychopathic individuals delusions are easily formed, which disappear with a change of the situation. A part of the prison psychoses [48] belong here.

Instead of acting forcibly, the affect can inhibit itself and then leads to *stupor* wherein thoughts and outer reactions are shut off;

[47] For Affective Disturbances of the Individual Morbid Groups see Symptomatology of the Diseases in special part.
[48] Cf. especially *Birnbaum:* Psychosen mit Wahnbildung und Wahnhaften Einbildungen bei Degenerativen. Marhold, Halle a. S. 1908.

or the affect alone is suppressed, so that a particularly terrifying experience is calmly considered and observed but no affect is felt, as in the cases of Livingstone when he was attacked by a lion and Bälzy's behavior during an earthquake. In a lesser degree we observe a kind of indifference in children and psychopaths (belle indifférence des hystériques). The mental stream may become *confused* as in making a speech.

Not quite identical with the affective stupor is the *embarrassment* which is to be conceived in the broadest sense. It is often only a question of a different attitude, as where it is impossible to do something consciously which can otherwise be done well more or less automatically, as opening certain locks and similar acts. If an affect is added, the effect is naturally still stronger. What is known in one situation is not at one's disposal in the other (Examination stupor and stairway wit). If a special effort is made to accomplish something, or when one fears lest he make a failure of it, he is then sure not to succeed, a mechanism seen in stuttering, bladder control, impotence, and erythrophobia. As a matter of fact every act which is more or less automatic, be it psychic or physical, is disturbed through the interference of the conscious will. As examples we may mention the common chronic constipation as a result of a psychic habit to drugs or occupation with the bowels, the complaints of menstruation, and the difficulties of childbirth.

Stuporous states can become chronic in connection with definite situations or a definite morbid symptom, also in the face of a certain teacher or subject where something awkward had occurred. And yet a pupil who reacts in this manner may appear normal. The most stupid way to correct it is to bully the patient. On the contrary, one must make the effort to remove the affect by kindly ignoring it; or in the more intelligent patients one can establish a different mental attitude through enlightenment. Inner complexes also act in the same way. The onanism complex, and not the onanism, continually prevents the patient from concentrating on other things, so that he gives the impression of having a poor memory. Depressive and exalted *moods* emanate from such complexes. Thus a man is more homosexually than heterosexually predisposed and becomes dissatisfied with his married life, but he cannot grasp the situation in view of his love for his wife with whom he apparently lives happily. He finally becomes depressed but improves as soon as everything becomes clear to him and he adjusts himself to it.

Continuous false attitudes result particularly from an injury to one's personality through acts which are considered "unjust." Young

people, and even children in the first years can in this way acquire
and forever continue a false attitude towards life.

*Thus develops functionally an entirely different type of character,
usually unsocial, who can be differentiated from the congenital type
only through close observation, but who can be changed back.* Of
diagnostic significance is the existence in many cases of moral
feelings from which one must naturally exclude the mere "weaknesses
of will" resulting from flighty affects.   Parents and teachers do
not understand certain reactions of the child and punish him for them.
The child conceives that as an injustice, and assumes a rebellious
attitude.   Everything is then viewed under the guise of this complex
and *a moral attitude is formed which particularly fits this purpose*
and runs something like the following: "My father has been unfair
to me, he is to blame for everything.   It is only just that I disgrace
him through stealing."   Such reflections assume so exclusive an importance that a regard for one's own welfare entirely disappears:
"It serves you right that my hands are frost bitten, it is just
what you wanted" becomes a maxim and cannot be corrected by
ordinary reflection, simply because all the associations become
only half conscious, if at all.   It is only by correct treatment,
especially by analysis that such a stubborn individual can be
saved from lasting criminality.   A young woman merges into an
"expectation neurosis" to spite her husband, who treated her dis-
gustingly, and throughout her whole life cannot extricate herself
from the disease even after her husband died.   To be sure there
were also other important factors which determined the origin
and particularly the special kind of the disease.   Little children
often cannot emerge from their spiteful attitude although they are
seemingly willing—and the same is true of argumentative adults;
that accounts for the favorable results that are often brought about
by outsiders.

Similar attitudes, though of lesser degree, result in young people
who possess special talents in manual skill, art, or in any other
sphere, but who are forced to learn to occupy themselves with something else.   They are dissatisfied with themselves and the world,
they are incapable of accomplishing things, they show a tendency
for all kinds of neuroses, *and are forced to assume a dereistic or
negativistic attitude to the world.*   The same is the case in people
who wish to go too high.   Many dissatisfactions, neuroses and some
psychoses (paranoias) result from a *disproportion between aim and
ability.*   *Bumke* tells what is quite characteristic, namely, that a
striking number of students who appeal to him for treatment be-

cause they are no longer capable of mental work think seriously of qualifying for academic positions.

An *unsuccessful separation* from the parents has similar results.

Also a *former disagreeable* experience can result in false attitudes or a tendency to certain neurotic diseases.

Affects and impulses that cannot be gratified often find spontaneously a harmless discharge, or under conscious guidance the affects and impulses may be utilized for similar activities. Thus sexual love and the childish impulse associate themselves with ordinary love for mankind and occupy themselves with charity and nursing the sick (*Freud's* sublimation). Sometimes they change into childish exaggerations as seen in the love evinced by old maids for cats and pups; frequently, however, this does not gratify the original impulse, especially when the latter is repressed. The sublimation then manifests itself only in repeated flare-ups of straw fire which can never cook the soup.

Under other circumstances the affects become stirred up in the unconscious. Every new similar experience increases the tension; thus there is on the one hand, an *explosion-readiness* to certain experiences, and on the other hand, an unconscious affective search for such processes. A child that has once experienced great anxiety without understanding it correctly, or when the experience becomes repressed by the anxiety, becomes more and more timid; it becomes sensitized to anxious experiences and peculiarly enough it repeatedly meets with accidents which stimulate anxiety. Later such a child becomes neurotic.

The *hunger for excitement* of some people comes about in this manner. There are people who must always be doing something, it matters little whether the situation is of a pleasurable or painful nature. Sometimes a decided preference is shown for the latter, they experience "ecstatic pain," martyrlike pleasure, and forever consider themselves unfairly treated. Every occasion is skilfully elaborated into a "scene;" and their own misfortunes are not only relished but decidedly more or less instigated and brought to a point. (The normal prototype is seen in the enjoyment of a tragedy.) The elaboration is often an inner one; thus any kind of experiences are misinterpreted in the sense of martyrdom and by some patients also in the sense of self-aggrandizement. Many of these patients seem abnormal only *under definite conditions* or to *certain* persons, otherwise their reactions are normal.

Complex ideas are sometimes mightier than the repressing forces. One is then pursued by a memory throughout life; any similar ex-

periences cause them to reappear with their entire affective load, or
they are even more or less constantly present in consciousness, dominating the mood and the inner and outer reactions (the dysamnesia
of Cécile Vogt).

Partly congenital and partly determined by complexes is the *exaggerated need for change*, or *the impossibility to tolerate long any
kind of situation*. No matter where the person is he is either
"homesick" or in some "mix-up." After a little while every occupation has something wrong about it. On the one side the normal need
for change is exaggerated, on the other there is a lack of love for
the customary.

A familiar feeling is the *impossibility of getting out of one's shell*,
or the *inability to express oneself*, observed in many persons who have
to endure much injustice without being able to defend themselves.
They conceal their feelings, are inclined to secretiveness, and easily
become untruthful despite their good character.

As everywhere else it is especially *ambivalent* complexes which
become pathogenic in this manner, also situations which render
prominent the negative side of a suggestion or of a tendency. If
one offers sweets to a little child and indicates by tone of voice
or in any other way that it is expected to react to it with pleasure and special thanks, he can be quite certàin that the child will
not accept it. It is really only a matter of accident whether the
machine moves backward or forward. He who reacts to a complex
with stealing is ofteñ hardly worse than another who responds to
the situation with self-sacrifice.

The difficulty lies less frequently in the events than in the
incompatibility of the characters living together. Let us say that
the husband is a very easy going person while the wife is active and
hungry for excitement. No matter how slight the difficulty is, she
finds the need for making a scene; the more extreme her expressions,
the less the husband is able to get out of himself, which thus only
enhances her affect. This continues until the vicious circle is broken
by some small or big catastrophe.

Both under occasional as well as under repeated or chronic influences there result false attitudes which not only impede the adjustment but *under certain discomforts make it more and more
sensitive*. A stimulus accepted as a matter of course causes no
disturbance. Thus if we should be disturbed at home by a person
making a big noise and shaking the chair we are sitting in, any
intellectual work would be impossible, but in similar conditions of
noise and motion in a moving train we might be able to concentrate

on any intellectual work even better than at our writing table. The baby who cannot yet think that people should be quiet for his sake adapts himself to any noise, the wife doesn't hear the snoring of the husband *she loves,* and the exertions in games of sport are perceived as enjoyment and recreation despite the fact that it exceeds by far the "tiring" resulting from work. A great part of the so-called neurasthenic symptoms and the whole "expectation neurosis" are based on such attitudes. *Depending on the attitude assumed, one becomes particularly sensitive to events which repeat themselves or particularly insensitive, a fact which holds true also for material or moral filth.*

A very useful, though, to be sure, as little exhaustive as a sharply defined classification of reaction types to difficulties, is given by *Kretschmer.* The hysteric evades the struggle, the erethic takes it up and magnifies it, the sensitive individual takes refuge in his inner self and builds up various forms of delusions and obsessions, and the asthenic person sinks into an inactive depression.

Other details concerning morbid affective reactions will be given later under "Psychopathic Forms of Reactions."

<h2 style="text-align:center">PATHOLOGY OF AFFECTIVE DISTURBANCES</h2>

The affective anomalies are in the first place a function of the disposition. The latter is acted upon, on the one hand, by various reactions which can become distorted into morbid states, and on the other hand, there are endogenous surface reactions of which the *emotional disturbances* of manic depressive insanity are the most striking examples.

These disturbances seem to correspond to physiological (chemical) attitudes. It is nevertheless remarkable that many manic depressive patients react with abnormal force to psychic stimuli during their healthy interval, which leads one to believe that the attacks of the disease may be put side by side with these psychogenic fluctuations. Moreover, a small portion of the actual manic depressive manifestations is dissipated by psychic reasons, and it is known that there are similar emotional disturbances which do not belong to this disease and which are put in operation by psychic factors. The difficulty is undoubtedly solved in the following manner: The affects like other psychisms reenforce one another; a depression, for example, unites the depressive associations and inhibits those of a euphoric tendency; in this way the affect is strengthened and maintained. In the same manner it inhibits in the physical sphere, for example, respiration and digestion, it affects the pulse more unfavorably, and lets loose the inner secretory processes corresponding to it, which can again reenforce the affect. The disease causing agent can attack in any preferred place of these two circular connecting causes. Let us assume that in the manic depressive patient there exists a special lability in the functions of the endocrine glands. The fluctuations of the glandular activities may be conditioned by causes existing outside of them; but, as probably happens in the periodicity, this function can also become too easily exhausted and then again functionate too strongly. In both cases we have the usual manic depressive attack which is conditioned "from inside to outside" —but similarly an attack results when the glands react too strongly to an exogenously (psychic) determined depression.

Most of the *emotional disturbances of epileptics and of some oligophrenics* are also conditioned by some chemism. It is nevertheless a striking fact that precisely the oligophrenics with brain lesions and particularly patients suffering brain injuries, show a tendency to produce endogenous emotional disturbances which are mostly, though not exclusively, of an irritable nature. The continuous irritability seen in those who have *brain lesions* is also anatomically determined. It is not absolutely certain, but according to many observations it is probable that there are also *periodic emotional disturbances of a psychogenic nature* analogous to the lasting attitudes mentioned above. Any kind of complex, let us say, dissatisfaction with parents, becomes half or completely repressed so that the child cannot fully account to himself for his actions. But the need for *abreaction* finds some vent through excitements or emotional disturbances and is then followed by a calm period. By and by, however, the tension accumulates again only to express itself in the same manner without any new cause, or through some ordinary occasion.

The lability of *organic patients* is but a secondary manifestation of the general cerebral disturbance. For we note a slight perseverance of the psychisms even in the spheres of memory, and the limitation of the associations is undoubtedly responsible for the fact that only actual situations are reacted to. In *epilepsy*, on the contrary, all the other psychisms run a slow course; the getting away from an idea is just as difficult as the alteration of an affect.

The *tendency to depression in senile patients* is not adequately explained by the suggestion that depressions increase with age and especially with general circulatory disturbances. Also the *euphoria of paresis* is as little explained as the rare paretic depressions.

The *morbid reactions* require no special explanation, as they spring from normal mechanisms, and act in an exaggerated and one-sided manner only in consequence of extraordinary occasions or of a disposition deviating from the normal.

8. DISTURBANCES OF ATTENTION

The pathology of attention is very complicated because its effects are strongly influenced by the other functions. Exhaustion and many morbid states weaken the faculty of concentration. The scope of attention is determined by the amount of associations that may occur at the same time; it is consequently lowered in organic patients. The exaggerated readiness of psychic processes in manic cases weakens the inhibiting effect of the effort of tenacity upon distracting influences. The lack of tenacity in organic cases is sometimes irregularly over-compensated by torpid retardation of the psychic processes, so that secondary hypo-vigility goes hand in hand with lack of tenacity. In twilight states, toxemias and similar states, where the mental trend becomes quite unintelligible, one can hardly still speak of attention, even where distinct affects are present, because the inner and outer strivings may become disconnected. The following remarks, therefore, emphasize only the most important facts in a somewhat schematical and simpler manner.

Ceteris paribus attention varies with the affects. When the latter are labile, or when the same interest is given to the most dissimilar ideas,—as raising all ideas upwards in the manic states, and lowering them to zero in cases of indifference and lack of comprehension, the vigility and the distractibility of attention naturally are quite marked. Tenacity need not here be diminished, because even without distractibility the subject may be adhered to; to be sure, there are few situations in which outer and inner distractibilities are absent for any length of time.

If the affects are stable, the *tenacity* also runs high.

In Schizophrenia and exceptional states of epilepsy, more seldom in neurasthenia and other affections, we sometimes find a strange mixture of exaggerated and slight distractibility. The patients react with difficulty to questions and other stimuli, but they react to many accidental sensory impressions such as the striking of the clock, the entrance of a person, a word not addressed to them, or to any object which happens to strike their eyes. But the epileptics and some schizophrenics will then regularly return to their former themes.

The *concentration* depends mainly upon the strength of the affectivity, yet in labile affects it is usually insufficient.

Whether tenacity is good or not in weak affects and corresponding slight concentration depends upon the accompanying circumstances. An apathetic schizophrenic can concentrate for half a day all his small strength on a little thread which he holds in his hand. On the other hand, he may be diverted by every trifle, because no interest to speak of restrains him. Hypotenacity, combined with hypovigility, is a usual manifestation where affects and intelligence are low, as in clouded states, apathetic imbecility, and other cases.

Hypotenacity, without real hypovigility, is found in *Aprosexia;* there is an inability to concentrate one's thoughts in reading, for instance, even for a short time. This symptom, which is not found very frequently, occurs in neurasthenia, and in impeded nasal breathing as a result of adenoids.

Vigility and tenacity are lowered in *Chorea Minor,* also in some cases of torpid imbecility, although here the genetic factors are quite different.

A rapid "exhaustion" of attention can be observed in many organic cases, especially in those with coarse brain lesions, also sometimes in schizophrenics during the acute stages. On the other hand, it often takes organic patients a longer time to concentrate their attention on the very subject desired. It is for this reason that perception experiments with such cases turn out very badly at first, but after some time the results are better, until the exhaustion reappears and the patients again do badly.

The *scope* of attention is diminished in organic cases and in oligophrenics because of a restriction of associations, and in melancholic and paranoid patients as a result of one-sided interest, and in epileptics as a result of both factors. In all forms of paranoia or paranoid states we also have as an important symptom the systematized vigility, the *morbid association readiness* for those events which might be connected with their delusions.[49]

In organic patients, the *habitual attention* is earlier and more strongly disturbed than the maximal attention. The patients, for instance, may seem completely normal as to attention during a clinical demonstration, but at the same time they are disoriented in the ward where they have been for weeks, they cannot locate their bedroom or their bed, because they do not register anything that happens about, and even to them, if they have no special reason for being attentive. And what is more, the memory and the comprehensive functions of orientation may still be adequate in these cases, so that the mistake can safely be ascribed to the faculty of attention.

[49] Cf. Delusions of reference, p. 94.

The patients observe, as it were, nothing, unless attention is forced upon them through some circumstance, then they behave, however, in quite a normal way. This teaches us that *intensity*, at least, of maximal attention can be good, in spite of the markedly diminished field of associations.

Tenacity of attention in organic cases is mostly lowered; the patients cannot continuously occupy themselves with one thing; they digress and *tire* simultaneously, very quickly. But the same patients find it also difficult to transfer their thoughts to another subject offered to them. They evince at the same time hypotenacity and (secondary) hypovigility of attention. In the manic stages of paresis, hypovigility may be hidden by the distractibility of the flight of ideas, yet it can usually be demonstrated through examination, for the patients after discussing their personal affairs cannot quickly answer a question about their school-knowledge, nor are they even able to understand it correctly, and this happens even where the psychic processes in general function very quickly. The excited states of presbyophrenia can also cause an over-compensation of hypovigility.

In the *schizophrenics,* the relation of active and passive attention is the reverse to that of the organics. They register excellently what is going on around them, even if they do not pay any special attention to it; but if they should have to concentrate their attention, they could not succeed, sometimes they are hindered by blockings and at the same time they often cannot hold a subject.

In some cases of schizophrenias, especially in crowding of thought, in fatigue, in hallucinations and delusions, in phobias and other obsessions, and in the pathological readiness for association, the direction of attention is obsessive.

In ordinary *fatigue,* the power of concentration and tenacity are usually very much diminished, whereas the distractibility seems to be enhanced in varying ways.

There is a tendency to explain many other manifestations on the basis of disturbances of attention, and as a deficiency of attention may be responsible for all sorts of stupidities, such deductions can be easily constructed, but just for these reasons most of these explanations have no scientific value.

9. MORBID SUGGESTIBILITY

A total lack of *suggestibility* does not perhaps occur except in such patients who evince an utter lack of comprehension and who no longer react to stimuli. A marked diminution of suggestibility we observe occasionally in imbeciles, who are then naturally incapable of any training. Schizophrenic patients are often little or not at all responsive to *direct* suggestions, but in most cases they still react very slightly to the general attitude of their environment. Wherever individual groups of affects are lacking, suggestion in the corresponding sense is naturally impossible. Moral idiots cannot be influenced in a moral sense, or irreligious people in a religious sense. Paretic patients in a manic state who look at the good side of everything and accentuate it with a feeling of happiness can hardly be brought to accept a sad situation.

The *exaggerations* of suggestibility are more important. We can produce it experimentally in a state of hypnosis. Many people are by nature as susceptible to all influences as a soft piece of dough. Fatigue and emotional experiences show a temporary disposition for suggestibility. Patients in manic states or those suffering from organic disturbances as well as alcoholics are easily influenced by suggestions.

Just as suggestibility is enhanced by the lability or resonance of the affects so it is heightened also through any decrease in the critical faculty which normally counteracts suggestions. All things being equal, the more thoughtless a person, the more suggestible he is.

Morbid suggestibility may lead to induced insanity, also to psychic and neurotic epidemics, to participations in crimes, and similar acts.

Hand in hand with positive suggestibility, there is in most cases also an increase in the *negative suggestibility*. Like children, senile patients are now wilful, and now open to the most stupid promptings. Paranoid patients allow themselves to be easily fooled by people who have their confidence, whereas they are absolutely inaccessible to other persons. In schizophrenic cases we often find command automatism and echopraxia, that is, high degrees of suggestibility combined with a pronounced negativism.

The so-called auto-suggestion is an important source of morbid states. No neuroses are possible without its cooperation ("Imaginary" diseases). Thus a girl in a street car sees an eczematous eruption on the hand of another passenger and becomes very excited because it unconsciously touched her "complex" referring to her paretic or luetic father; she then develops an eczema-like eruption in the same place as the passenger.[50] A traumatic patient *fears* that he can no longer support his family and *hopes* to assure his existence through

---

[50] *Friedman u. Kohnstamm*, Zur Pathogenese u. Psychotherapie bei Basedowscher Krankheit, Zeitschrift f. d. ges. Neur. u. Psych. Or. 23, 1914.

a pension. He observes himself anxiously and by this very means creates the necessary morbid symptoms. A girl fears lest her menstrual period fail to appear, and thus causes a temporary amenorrhœa. To be sure, auto-suggestion may have the opposite favorable effect which is curative in nature. These examples show that positive and negative suggestions are really not true opposites, and that both together are nothing but emotional effects.

10. DISTURBANCES OF PERSONALITY

Every mental disorder changes the personality in some sense if not altogether. The manic patients become reckless and actively exaggerated, the paranoid and in most cases also the paranoiac patients lose their general interests in life and live only in their delusions, the epileptic concentrates on his physical well-being and his petty affairs, the intelligent person becomes stupid and thoughtless as a result of a dementing process, and so on.

The inner disturbances of personality are not as comprehensible. Thus an ordinary citizen imagines himself an emperor. What he knows of the Emperor, he feels as part of his person: *appersonation.* Even hypochondriacal ideas can be acquired in this way; thus, the medical student in his first term of clinical experience, hearing a vivid description of some disease of the heart and seeing it demonstrated in one or several patients, becomes so deeply impressed that under certain conditions he feels that he has the same heart trouble (Morbus Medicorum).

Less frequently the personality loses some of its component parts. It naturally happens that certain events of one's life are forgotten; this is especially true in schizophrenic patients who forget a part of their disagreeable experiences, and often deny *bona fide* actions, the commitment of which they later regret. This does not, however, concern things that belong to the essence of the personality. On the other hand, the most important components are often replaced by others; thus John Smith becomes President Harding, or Christ (see below).

A special type of disturbance of personality is the *alternating personality,* also known as *dual consciousness.* Let us consider a hysterical woman who until now has lived a mediocre existence. For some known or unknown reason she falls into a hysterical sleep, and on awakening she has forgotten her entire previous existence; she does not know who she is, where she has lived until now, and who the persons are whom she sees around her. Notwithstanding this change, the ordinary faculties of walking, speaking, eating, the use of clothes and other things are usually transferred to the new state ("état second"). Whatever the patient needs for her intercourse with other people she learns very quickly. Her character, too, undergoes a change; formerly a serious-minded girl, she now becomes frivolous and pleasure-seeking. After some time, she again merges into a state of sleep, and on awakening the patient is back in her first state. She has no realization of the intervening time; all that she remembers is that she went to sleep, and has now awakened as usual. Such changed states may appear alternately for years. While in the first state the patient only remembers the former first states and when in the second she always recalls only those of the second series. More frequently, however, it seems that in the second state the patient can recall the first (normal) series, but while in the first state she cannot recall the second (morbid) series. It may also happen that eventually the second state will become permanent, and this way cause a *transformation of the personality*. In quite rare cases there may be an alternation of many such states, each with its very definite character and special memory group (personality); as many as twelve have been observed. As a matter of fact, cases of pure dual personalities are very rare. Yet their theoretical significance is very great, for they show what marked changes can be brought about by a systematic elimination or intercalation of association paths. It is not alone in hysteria that one finds an arrangement of different personalities one *succeeding* the other; through similar mechanisms schizophrenia produces different personalities existing *side by side*. As a matter of fact, there is no need of delving into those rare though most demonstrable hysterical cases; we can produce the very same phenomena, experimentally, through hypnotic suggestion, and we also know that in the ordinary hysterical twilight states the memory of former attacks, concerning which the patient shows an amnesia in her normal state, can be retained or can be aroused by suggestion.

The splitting off of parts of a personality in *transitivism* proceeds in a different manner; here the patient's own experiences become detached from him, and are ascribed to another person. A patient; for example, sees a terrifying image and screams aloud; but he then imagines that the apparition did the screaming. A woman has an operation on her toe, during the long drawn out delirium of the narcosis she continually asks the nurse to look after her bed-neighbor, because the latter is having bad pains in her toe. A person dreams during the night before he has diarrhœa that pamphlets which he has to send out suffer from diarrhœa. It is quite common to displace feeling which we have ourselves in our dreams to other persons. Transitivism is an almost common occurrence in schizophrenia; the patients are convinced that the voices which they hear are also heard by others in the same way; they frequently ascribe their own actions to others; thus, if they read something, it is really done by others; their thoughts are thought by others, and so on.

A strange disturbance of personality is *de-personalization,* in which the patients have lost the definite idea of their ego. They seem quite different to themselves, and feel that they must look in the mirror to see if they are still themselves, and even then their own images appear strange. This disturbance manifests itself especially through the fact that the patients do not feel their own will power and strivings, they feel like automatons; sometimes they are indifferent to it, but in most cases they perceive this state as extremely unpleasant. This syndrome appears in schizophrenia, perhaps also in neurasthenic-like states of psychopathic patients, and in a less pronounced degree it is also observed transitionally in epileptic twilight states. It is often connected with the analogous feelings of strangeness in regard to the outside world.

In schizophrenia one sees a great many forms of *transformations of personality* of which I only want to mention a few types. The patients suddenly imagine that they are Napoleon, and some entertain the idea without giving up their past life; it is merely an addition to their past life. In other cases they shut off at least everything incompatible with the delusion; thus, those who have grandiose ideas state they were not born in the locality in question, they did not go to school there, but in some mysterious way circumstances forced them to play the part of John Smith for some time, but now they want to re-establish their sovereign authority over Europe. In other cases, the former personality ceases to exist; sometimes, but by no means always, they have interwoven the past of Napoleon with the present of their momentary delusional personality. Others have become Christ, or even God. The latter mechanism is not a rare occurrence in paretic patients, but in most cases it exerts no influence whatever on their actions, whereas schizophrenic patients sometimes may act in accordance with the change of personality. When I expressed astonishment that he knew the whole Bible by heart, such a god said to me that there was nothing unusual about it, as he had written it himself; and to my remark that it was strange that we perceived nothing of his omniscient spirit, he answered that he had sent out his spirit among mankind, and now so little was left for him that he had come into the asylum, but that he could recall his spirit at any moment, only he would not do so out of compassion for poor mankind. Other patients imagine themselves transformed into animals and even into things, and yet they usually do not adhere to *one* idea. Just as a patient can be the Pope, the Emperor, the Sultan, and eventually God in one person, he can also be a pig and a horse. Nevertheless the patients rarely follow up the logic to act accordingly, as, for instance, to bark like a dog when they profess to be a dog. Although they refuse to admit the truth, they behave as if the expression is only to be taken symbolically, in the same way perhaps as when a man is insultingly called a pig.

It is quite an ordinary occurrence to see schizophrenic patients *identify* themselves in the most illogical way with people whom they love or admire. Under certain conditions, and in a certain sense, they *are* their beloved, they had the same experience as they, and they play their beloved's part. A non-schizophrenic patient of v. *Krafft-Ebing*, who loved only limping women, could not resist the impulse to imitate such a limping woman.

Some schizophrenics have altogether lost their personality. Formerly they have been so-and-so, but now they are somebody else, and their former personality may be in some other person. Under such circumstances it may happen that they speak of themselves in the third person, for they have the feeling that they are no longer the person whom they have designated as "I."

Temporary transformations of the person into another, as, for example, into potentates or saints, occur occasionally in the different twilight states.

Nowadays there is much talk about the *preservation* or *annihilation* of the personality. *Kraepelin's* paraphrenics are supposed to differ from schizophrenia, the arteriosclerotic and luetic psychoses from simple senile dementia, and the latter from the most disturbed paretics, in the fact that the personality is fairly well, or better preserved. By that we understand the active continuation of the hitherto existing strivings and aims of action, as well as of the more important characteristics in general. In organic diseases, where the personality is not much injured, which is especially the case in arteriosclerotic insanity, there is surely no lack of affective changes in the sense of lability, or irritability, but the patient knows something about it, and he even often endeavors to combat his faults. Having been an honest man he does not now turn into a scoundrel; when he is no longer able to support his family he perceives it painfully, and his external appearance remains relatively good, in so far as his mental clearness is not disturbed. That accounts for the fact that these people are in no immediate need of asylum treatment, and when they are sent there it is frequently only in consequence of a single special circumstance, such as a danger of suicide, or confusion.

The schizophrenic disturbance of personality is much deeper and more far reaching. Even when the organic patient changes into a different person and his strivings often change only too much, yet what he feels and strives for in a single moment is the expression of his whole actual psyche. On the other hand, the schizophrenic may at the same time strive for something contradictory, and do something that he has not desired and even despised. His personality can divide itself; now he acts and thinks like a great man, now like a scholar, or in another manner, and his hallucinations and delusions then also correspond to it. There are forever different strivings, which embody themselves in such personalities.[51] Very frequently the direction from and to a person is no longer distinguished. A paranoid patient fears in her depression that she is being harmed; she is then commanded by the voices to help others instead of that help should be given to her as might have been expected. Everyday experience shows that both ideas are identical to the patient and that it is not necessary to add a logical connecting link. A persecuted patient wants to become a professor, but he complains that people want to force him to be a professor.

In severe cases of schizophrenia, a high degree of *disintegration of personality* results because the uniform striving and the uniform memory complex become destroyed; the patients babble and show no coherence in thoughts and wishes, indeed the borderline between their own person and the environment is blurred. As in appersonation and in transitivism concepts which do not belong to the person become connected with him, and vice versa. Thus the strongest associations may finally detach themselves, while any other ideas may become associated with the person, if in such cases one can still speak of a person at all.

In general, the schizophrenic personality suffers in the following different ways: Through dementia, the restrictions or perversities of the instinctive life, through the disturbance of the uniform direction of the striving and acting, and the disturbances of will which force schizophrenics into actions that they do not strive for at all.

In most of the disturbances of personality one deals with a splitting in the direction of the affective needs, that is to say, with simple emotional effects which in themselves are very violent, or become

[51] Cf. Complexes, pp. 35-36.

overpowering in a morbid soil; this is seen, for instance, in paresis, where, owing to the restriction of associations, the wish to be God Almighty is put into reality without any further ado, also in schizophrenia particularly after the structure of associations has already become loosened; in the latter cases the complexes can actually acquire sub-personalities with some sort of independence within the psyche. Depending on the circumstances the patient is this or that personality, or, what is still more frequent, he hears in the voices, now the expression of this complex (the wish to be a Prince), and at another time that of another complex (to be condemned as an onanist).

I am not sufficiently clear about *depersonalization*, because cases giving reliable information are not very common. In part we probably have to deal with the same process which we see in the melancholic patients, to whom external things appear strange, perhaps because the feeling components are so strongly falsified. But if the patients are not conscious of their own volition-impulse it must be due to the blocking of an inner feeling, the mechanism and causes of which is not just clear.

11. DISTURBANCES OF CENTRIFUGAL FUNCTIONS

Actions as the final link in the chain of psychic processes are naturally inadequate to the situations if the sensations, deliberations or feelings upon which they depend are inadequate. He who is controlled by false perceptions, and imagines that robbers are breaking in when his nurses are coming, will defend himself. Some hallucinations influence the patient directly, and often in a forceful way; he has to act in the sense of the hallucinations even if he realizes that he does thereby something detrimental to himself and to others. This mode of action does not always need the form of commands. Thus, a periodic patient named Mantel, who was locked in his room, repeatedly heard the words: "Mantel, thou strong hero." Whereupon he reacted by demolishing his room, to show his annoyers that he was really so strong. To be sure, the hallucinations instigate only those actions for which a tendency already exists; but this does not need to be the tendency of the conscious personality; indeed, it may even be incompatible with it. At the same time there are hallucinations for the obedience of which there is little or hardly any impulse, and in later stages of schizophrenia the patients regularly refuse to obey their hallucinations, in spite of the fact that they believe in them as strongly as ever.

The so-called *hallucinatory excitements* in schizophrenia are also worthy of mention; here, under the impression of false perceptions, the patients suddenly become abusive, strike blindly, or commit any other acts of violence. To be sure, in most cases one does not know to what extent the hallucinations are only a part of the symptoms of the whole excitable action, and to what extent they are the cause of the violent outburst.

If *thinking* is disturbed so that it sets incorrect aims toward action, then the acts also are false. He who entertains the delusion that people want to poison him will in most cases react to it, which is quite correct from his viewpoint, but pathological from the observer's. An aimless or feeble-minded thinking will condition aimless or feeble-minded actions. If the thinking of the psychopathic and insane deviates from the average thinking, it means in most cases a deterioration of quality; the actions of the real insane persons are nearly always of inferior quality or of negative value. In exceptional cases, however, and especially in mere psychopaths the anomaly leads to new values.[52]

Action is for the most part influenced by *affectivity*, if one at least agrees with us when we designate the force and direction of the impulses, or of the "will," as partial manifestations of the affects. He who is happy, sad or furious, will react accordingly. Fear can make a person motionless and rigid or limp, it can urge him to aimless flight, or merely to a restless manifestation of the affect, such as restlessly walking to and fro, or to brutal acts of violence. The last named are especially striking when motility is otherwise practically absent and the anxious or depressed patient suddenly gives vent to his feeling by destroying some object or even by committing a murder. Such reactions to unbearable tension are designated as *raptus*.[53] The absence of ethical feelings brings to the surface anti-social actions. Lability of feelings and emotivity make the actions unsteady and capricious. Absence of feelings in general or weakness of the same diminishes the impulses, and makes them weak. The expression *"Weakness of Will"* designates three totally different things: (1) A lack of will impulses due to a weakness of the affects, or a lack of steam pressure in the engine, *abulia* as a result of apathy. (2) Inconsistency of the aims in the face of very vivid, but too labile affects, which make its bearer dependent on outer influences; a slight push causes the engine to run backwards too easily, when it should go forward, which is due to the fact that the direction-switch is too easily movable. Frivolous people and those who are unable to act in

[52] Comp. remarks on Genius, p. 171.
[53] There is also a raptus in schizophrenic patients which is merely an execution of sudden impulses without affective tension.

accordance with their own resolutions are congenitally weak-willed in this sense; manic and organic patients become so through their illness. This kind of weakness of will can also be ascribed to an exaggerated suggestibility, which only partly coincides with the lability of affects. (3) Incapacity to make decisions through counter reflections and impulses in persons who are too conscientious and too deliberate in everything, and in those who are in a depressed state.

Wherever one does not observe any, or very slight expressions of will, one speaks of *stupor*; in such cases thinking is usually at a low ebb; indeed, in some states the disturbance of thought as such may be in the foreground as in the emotional stupor of imbeciles. *Stupor is no uniform syndrome, but an outer form of manifestation of the following different states:* maximal apathy, inhibitions, obstructions, overpowering through fright or anxiety, and cerebral torpor of any kind. Thus we find stupor, especially in schizophrenia where apathy, blockings, inhibitions, and sometimes cerebral torpor appear together, furthermore in epilepsy, in organic diseases, and in manic-depressive inhibitions. Nevertheless, in regard to the latter, it must be observed that one does not like to call melancholic inhibitions stupor, if, as is usual, they are distinctly connected with signs of severe physical pain. Melancholia *attonita,* as it was formerly called, is usually a catatonia, with or without depression. Stupor resulting from strong affects (emotional stupor) we find in its highest development especially in hysteria, and to a lesser degree very frequently in forms of congenital feeble-mindedness.

A *hyper-function of the will* in the sense of special strength is naturally difficult to establish, because a person seems to us the healthier, the stronger his will is. Yet, in hysterical and other psychopathic cases we sometimes see a force of impulse, of endurance, and capacity to bear pain, which far exceeds the normal. Also schizophrenic patients sometimes develop a special energy or will, as, for instance, when they pull out their own teeth, squeeze out one of their eyes, or do something similar without being analgesic. The dissimulation of symptoms of disease, especially in melancholics, points to an enormous force of will. The occupation urge of manic patients who constantly want to do all sorts of things and accomplish much has also been regarded as a hyperfunction of will. We also mention here the hyperkineses of many catatonic patients (see below) which in everything else are principally separated from them.

A morbid facility of the *capacity to make decisions* is observed in manic patients and under mild alcoholic stimulation. Also in affects which compel actions such as fury, or fear, but here it is naturally one-sided, acting only in the direction of the affect; every idea which has a centrifugal component leads straight to action. The possibility of an accurate reflection is hereby always diminished; the actions become precipitated. If reflection is primarily inhibited the reverse is the case, all things being equal; any kind of stimulus leads to action more easily and more quickly.

The ability to make decisions is primarily badly impaired in melancholic states, secondarily it is still more diminished through the feeling of insufficient reflection and especially through the general unpleasant accentuation of all the possible objective ideas. If the patient is inclined to go in the open air he feels it as something too terrible; if he thinks of remaining in the room, that too, seems just as unbearable. In apathy no decision can be taken, because the impulse is lacking; the same is the case in torpor, where all psychic processes are low. In states of obstruction, as long as it exists, the physical processes are interrupted either altogether or especially in the direction of the decision, and nothing happens. But there can also be too much thinking. Whoever inclines to take into account every imaginable possibility can hardly arrive at a conclusion. A certain onesidedness is necessary in action; one must give up advantages in big or small matters and must be able to risk something, if one wants to act at the right time and with the necessary force. The ambivalence of the feeling tone [54] is an obstacle to the decision. If one loves and hates at the same time without summing up the positive and negative feelings into a unified difference, one is torn to both sides and does not get any results even in deciding. The so-called *psychomotor excitements and inhibitions* naturally concern the whole psyche; in any case they are not strictly confined to motility, but distinctly influence also the need for action, the ability to make decisions, and the facility of the transition of the excitement over the true centrifugal paths. The *manic pressure activity* (the urge to occupy oneself) expresses itself in the fact that the patients can never permit themselves to rest; something has to happen all the time. In milder cases it is merely a quantitative increase of action that is observed, which can also be accomplished by a normal person, such as an increase of business activity or similar acts; in more severe cases it comes to excesses; thus one notes a thoughtlessness in all spheres of action, and finally there is a destruction of objects and a building up of new combinations from the material acquired; there is a constant smearing, screaming, jumping and similar acts. Taken singly, the aims usually change very quickly under these conditions; nothing is finished, and

[54] Cf. p. 125.

even in mild cases one notes a lack of perseverance in the business enterprises of manic patients. The pressure activity is naturally also disburdened through talking. The patients are very talkative and they can not really get away from their talking which becomes more and more incoherent (*Logorrhœa*).

The *depressive inhibition of action* causes actions to be avoided as far as possible, in more severe cases altogether, or if motions and actions still exist, they represent the monotonous discharge of the dominating affect, especially that of anxiety.

The highest degree of inhibition of motion is designated as *attonity*. For long periods the patients really make no active movement. They have to be dressed and undressed like puppets, they have to be fed with a spoon or even with the tube, their saliva is not swallowed, but drools from the corners of their mouths, and even the movements of the eyelids can stop. Such states nearly always belong to the schizophrenic stupor, especially of the depressive type.

There exists also a simple schizophrenic *akinesis*, which we cannot at present very well refer to other disturbances because the accompanying symptoms seem insufficiently developed. In contrast to this we have the schizophrenic *hyperkinesis* where the patients are in constant motion, but yet do not seem to "act." Without any apparent reason, as far as we can learn, without any motive known to themselves, they are actively violent, they are destructive, they throw themselves or only their limbs in the air, they play tricks, etc. Nevertheless, both subjectively and objectively the action appears to be intended: it is a psychic motion impulse without motive, one might say, a kind of convulsion of psychomotility (but not at all a motor spasm in the usual sense). *The mere pressure motion should be distinctly differentiated from the pressure occupation of the manic patients which always has a meaning.* The attempt has been made to classify also *verbigeration* as an analogous "cramp of the speech centre," but it is not particularly often combined with hyperkinesis.

The concept of *jactation* refers more to the outward appearance. Here also we deal with mere motions, which are especially weak; at most they represent rudiments of actions and have quite different causes. Under certain conditions hyperkinetic states in the sense just now described may be called jactations; the term may also be applied to agitation caused by fear or other uncomfortable feelings, or the tossing about in pain; but the concept corresponds best to the movements in cerebral irritations, as seen in meningitis or acute delirium.

In schizophrenia there is sometimes a motor parafunction which actually calls to mind *apraxia,* but at all events it is not genetically analogous to the organic syndrome of this name; it resembles more the opposite actions produced during shock or distraction: Thus, the patient wants to put the spoon into the place, but with uncertain movements he takes it in a strange way first in one hand, then in the other, where he turns it around, until at last he places it on his knee; or instead of the spoon he grasps anything else which happens to be at hand. When walking, his legs move in an uncertain way, in various long steps, not exactly towards the goal. *Kraepelin* grouped analogous disturbances of a lighter grade under the term: "loss of gracefulness." As the patient is simultaneously moved by different feelings, and as they are badly suited to the ideas, all actions often appear unreal, artificial, and affected, and as the associations of ideas also in regard to the carrying out of the movements do not proceed in usual paths, they acquire something of the bizarre.[55]

Sometimes movements, that is, actions, become *stereotyped*, in which case quite different mechanisms may come into play. Catatonic patients sometimes cannot get through with a movement manifoldly repeated, such as wiping the face, or scooping up their soup, or they do not think of stopping even after they have finished these acts. A strong accompanying affect can easily stereotype an action which then continues to repeat itself without any voluntary effort on the part of the patients. In the course of time, it generally becomes more or less shortened in form, or it changes in regard to place. Thus an original onanistic movement of the pelvis may finally change into a shaking of the head. In this, and in still other ways stereotyped movements originate in catatonic patients, which often last for decades and seem absurd to the patient as well as to the observer. Customary acts may undergo changes which then become stereotyped. For example, the patient taps seven times on his coat at every button he is about to close; he shakes hands in quite a strange way (*Variation stereotypes, mannerisms*).

There are still other mannerisms besides the variation stereotypes of which the following may be mentioned: independent clownish gestures, spreading out of fingers, also bizarre expressions of every description, exaggerated style of dress and hair, caricatured elegance and finally morbid expressions of affects, exaggerated pathos, and self-satisfied attitude; in short, the patient evinces all the faults of a bad actor. As many show an indication of these changes at puberty, an attempt was made to regard them as symptoms of puberty, which were fixed and exaggerated by the disease.

When language becomes stereotyped it is called *verbigeration*.

[55] Cf. below, "mannerisms."

Here quite senseless words and sentences, at least for the actual situation, are constantly repeated, often in a striking tone which is also stereotyped.

Besides the *stereotypes of motion* there are those *of posture,* the patients always assuming exactly the same position,—and *of place;* they want to sit, or stand, or walk always in the same place.[56]

The stereotypes, in the sense amplified so far, belong to the *catatonic* symptoms, and outside of schizophrenia occur perhaps also in organic patients; but it is not at all certain that they are then genetically of the same value. In any case the *perseveration* in the organic patients, which we see most typically in coarse brain lesions, especially in aphasic patients, is something quite different from stereotypes. The patients cannot rid themselves of a word which they have just heard, or which they have just said, and repeat it constantly when they wish to say something else. And even when the patients execute a simple action, such as wishing merely to think of something, this impulse may under certain conditions proceed against their will in the path of the preceding action, or in the one thought of immediately before.

Other stereotype-like manifestations are the homogeneous actions, which some epileptic patients perform in post-epileptic twilight states, the repetitions of terrifying experiences through hallucinations, and (mostly abbreviated) actions in the twilight states of the hysterical patients. The manifestation of a lasting strong affect, like the stereotyped screaming or wailing of depressed organic patients, the tics, some actions which have become automatic, and the movements of idiots,—all these movements which outwardly resemble the schizophrenic stereotypes have quite a different genesis and meaning.

Parafunctions of the will attach themselves mainly to the so-called *impulses.* The *nutrition-impulse* has been stunted in the cultural being who rarely feels real hunger, and when he wants to starve himself to death he is forcibly fed. This impulse is also very indirectly satisfied, in so far as one learns to write at the age of six, in order to earn his living from ten to twenty years later. Even the *impulse of self-preservation* in general is no longer at its height with us, either with regard to the individual, or his family, or his race. The suicide-impulse, which under simpler circumstances very rarely occurs even in pathological conditions, has become a calamity in our asylums. The *sex impulse* has been preserved only in some measure of its original form, and is pushed back by culture in different ways, such as through chastity, monogamy, asceticism, and birth control. But this impulse breaks through with elemental force and creates in the individual those

[56] For more details Cf. chapter on Schizophrenia.

inner conflicts which mostly become pathogenic. Preserved is the *ethical* or the altruistic impulse, although just now it is being subjected to a certain transvaluation. In place of the primary impulses there are others, which are particularly active, such as the impulse for knowledge, and tend more towards the preservation of civilization than life.

The morbid disturbances of the nutrition-impulse are not so important in psychiatry. Beside excessive gluttony of the paretic and idiots, we find in depressions and in catatonics a peculiar lack of appetite; indeed there is an aversion to eating and drinking resulting in a total abstinence for any length of time. Besides these, nervous patients evince peculiar cravings (*picae*), and schizophrenics a tendency to swallow all kinds of things, even their own excrement (*coprophagia*), which is sometimes accompanied by gustatory enjoyment and sometimes not.

The *sex-impulse* has a special pathology, which will be dealt with in the special psychiatry. The *ethical impulse* varies constitutionally from the "genius of altruism" to the moral idiot, who is devoid of all altruistic feelings.

The expression "impulse" has quite a different meaning, if one speaks of *"morbid impulses."* In most cases this word refers to the impulses for actions, which are accomplished unexpectedly, without real reflection or with inconsistent reflection, or without the assent of the whole personality. Such actions are often distinguished by violence, hastiness, skill, and regardlessness of the interests of others, as well as of their own. But even under the name of impulsive actions, one includes chiefly different symptoms of various grades. Thus one speaks of the morbid impulse to set fire to places (*Pyromania*), of the stealing impulse (*Kleptomania*), the murder impulse and similar pathological states. These disturbances will be described later on under the heading of "Impulsive Insanity."

All impulsive actions have one thing in common, namely, they are carried out without the cooperation of reflection and aimful willing.

The expression *"Impulsive Actions"* expresses only a part of the same thing, that is, it refers to various indefinable kinds of actions carried out suddenly and without proper deliberation. This may be in the form of incomprehensible "affective-actions" in emotional persons, or actions which are conditioned by inner motives of which the subject himself is not sufficiently conscious, and this is especially the case in schizophrenics. Some sudden obsessive actions are also often inaptly called impulsive, and of course also the raptus observed in melancholics.

Certain pathological actions, like *obsessive* and *automatic actions* are abnormally related to consciousness or to the will.

Obsessive actions are conscious actions running counter to one's own will, and proceed from an inner impulse which the personality cannot resist. In most cases the resistance is connected with fear or some other vague uneasiness, to the influence of which the personality finally yields, in the same way as a physical pain forces a person to do something which he does not wish to do.

Impulses towards indifferent actions, to the extent of compulsive-like exclamations of indecent or sacrilegious words (*Coprolalia*), occur frequently in different states. In so far as they refer to serious crimes, like murder of relatives, they are rarely irresistible outside of schizophrenia. Indeed, one deals most frequently with *apprehensions* lest one might do something, rather than with real impulses.[57] To be sure, those apprehensions are nothing but effects of impulses repressed into the unconscious.

Automatic Actions are not directly noticed by the patient himself: he neither feels that he wishes to accomplish the action, nor that he executes it. If the action lasts for some time, he takes notice of it like a third person, by observing and listening. This occurs in schizophrenia, where in this way windowpanes are frequently broken, clothes torn, and beating administered, but automatic actions may also be present in an especially clear formation, in forms of hysteria and in artificial trance-states, where they may appear in complicated and senseful actions. Here the mouth speaks, reproduces apparently the thoughts of the spirit, preaches, and the hand writes. Most people can apparently be quickly educated to automatic writing by skilful suggestors; I know of a quack who made all his patients automatically write out their diagnosis and the remedies to be applied. Every "medium" in spiritistic circles does automatic speaking, and in religious epidemics (preachers in the Cevennes and others) automatism draws quite a large circle of followers. It is easy to understand that such people acquire the idea that they are possessed of a spirit (*Demonism*). If the latter expresses what they consciously think or wish, then it is a good spirit, otherwise it is a bad one; it is not at all unusual to observe that the patients frequently have to do exactly just what they do not want to do as, for instance, to utter ugly or sinful words (*Automatic Coprolalia*).

A very good description of a schizophrenic patient is the following:

"Suddenly Dolinin (the writer himself) felt, that not only without his wish, but even against his will, his tongue begins to express loudly

[57] Cf. obsessive ideas, and Compulsion Neurosis, p. 87.

and at the same time most rapidly that which in no case should have been uttered. At the first moment the patient was perplexed and frightened by the very fact of this unusual occurrence, because to be suddenly and obviously aware of a wound up automaton in oneself is *per se* disagreeable, but when he began to grasp the meaning of what *his tongue* chattered, the horror of the patient increased, because it showed that he, D., openly confesses his guilt to a serious political crime, sometimes ascribing such plans to himself which he had never entertained. Notwithstanding this fact, *his will did not have the power to restrain his tongue, which had suddenly become automatic.*[58]

Within the automatic actions there are different mechanisms. It may happen that something is executed which the patient wishes to do, but he does not feel the will impulse nor its accomplishment. When he wants to eat, to give his hand, to walk, or when he merely would be ready to do so, his limbs carry out the action, and yet he has not the feeling that it has been accomplished at his instigation (in schizophrenia). His limb can also carry out something, his mouth can say something, which the patient might not wish. He feels the impulse, wants to resist, but has no power; the innervation of his muscles is directed by another will. From this there are all transitions to the obsessive actions, and the other will is naturally not a strange one, but a repression of the patient's own striving (in Hysterics, Schizophrenia). Not a few automatic actions remain also unconscious in execution, for instance, when a hysterical woman crushes rose leaves against her temple during conversation as a symbol of the thought of her lover's death, who shot himself through his temple. Such automatisms may also be the prototype of many schizophrenic stereotypes.

Automatic actions which are formed by *practice* evidently have quite different mechanisms. In walking, riding, cycling, piano playing and indeed in all our occupations we carry out a number of simple actions which we neither start consciously nor direct consciously. As a rule, these are willed actions, but not always; somebody may do something which he would not carry out consciously, as to pick his nose in company, to show a sign of disdain, and similar acts.

Similar to such actions are some of the apparent *stereotypes of organic patients* which evidently pass off automatically in most cases, but represent actions which already have been practised before the disease, like the incessant twirling of the moustache, etc.

The list can still be completed by some types which although

---

[58] *Kandinsky* in *Jaspers*, Allgemeine Psychopathologie, p. 121. Julius Springer, Berlin, 1913.

markedly differing from each other, however, have these in common: sometimes they are carried out quite consciously, sometimes quite automatically, sometimes they are done only in partial consciousness; and sometimes they are only the expression of a mood. The twirling of thumbs, scratching of the head in healthy people, and the swaying of idiots represent some examples.

Just as in outer actions, *thinking* also may proceed compulsively or automatically, without and against the will of the patient. If an idea continually keeps on obtruding itself against the will, we deal with an *obsessive idea*. But beside this form of obsessive thinking there is another quite different form of *compulsive thinking*, which only occurs in schizophrenic patients, and rarely in epileptic equivalents where the patients feel that "it" thinks in them often the same thoughts that they themselves think spontaneously, but often the thoughts are quite different; sometimes there is a confused crowding as in the "thought crowding" of schizophrenic patients. Hence in such cases the thought process as well as its contents are withdrawn from the will.

The *theory of the automatic actions* can easily be understood from our conception of psychic processes. The associative connection between the conscious ego-complex and the functions of acting is lacking. The impulses to action are direct effects from the unconscious acting upon the motor functions. The complexes from which they logically originate can be demonstrated by the analyses of accessible patients. Automatic actions of various kinds can be experimentally produced in hypnosis.

Half automatic, though to a certain insufficient extent accessible to the will, are the *tics*, which according to *Oppenheim* are movements of a reflex, defensive, or expressive nature, which have deteriorated into compulsive acts; among these we have the displaying of the teeth, clenching of fists, and closing of eyelids. They are morbid because they are repeated again and again without apparent motive. The patient can resist the impulse for a short time, but not for very long. Tics are naturally quite stereotyped.

The impulse for an action carried out sometimes consciously, and sometimes compulsively, can also come from without, as, for instance, in *automatic obedience*, that is, the compulsive-like or also automatic obedience to requests for simple actions of all kinds. The patients carry out any commands whatsoever, even also if it is against their will, as, for example, putting out their tongue when they know that a pin will be stuck into it (Schizophrenia). The impulse for such an action can also be given by means of example alone, as in *echopraxia* and *echolalia*. Although this symptom is so closely related to automatic obedience that *Kraepelin* makes it a part of it, I have never seen the two peculiarities run parallel in development. The echopractic patients imitate whatever strikes them in the actions or words of their surroundings. As far as we know, it is partly a question of hysteria-like mechanisms, as seen in the echopraxia of primitive people,[59] and certainly in most cases of schizophrenia, and partly a matter of an incapacity to get away from a conceived idea, so that instead of giving an answer the question is repeated, or instead of a new action the preceding act is imitated (organic echolalias and echopraxias). In the latter case the patients usually *wish* to do or to say something quite different, but the impulse turns into a wrong path. In hysteriform, or schizophrenic echopraxias, the person does not "wish" to do something different; it is not a question of a derailment of an impulse actually desired, but of an influence of the conscious or unconscious wish itself.

According to *Kraepelin,* the phenomenon of *flexibilitas cerea* (wax-like flexibility), also commonly called *catalepsy,* also belongs to automatic obedience. The patients make no movement of their own volition; but if they are placed in no matter how uncomfortable an attitude they maintain it for a very long time. Thus, the patient can hold his limbs in an extended posture for a much longer time than a normal person could do voluntarily; usually they gradually sink without trembling, and without any evident exertion on the part of the patient. Some patients offer a certain resistance to the passive moving of their limbs, which gives the impression as if a wax statue was modelled. Most patients, however, move their limbs at a slight push, as they guess what is wanted of them.

Much more frequently one finds in patients whose movements are obviously quite normal, that if, for instance, an arm is somewhat brusquely raised upwards, it remains so for a long time (*Pseudoflexibilitas*).

The schizophrenic and hysterical catalepsy can be psychically influenced to a high degree, which makes it probable that it is essentially a psychic symptom; still there is a probability of its being based on a peripheral tendency to tonic muscular disturbances. The other forms are too little known.

Besides the flexible, there exists also a *rigid catalepsy.* Patients evincing a stereotyped attitude must naturally keep the corresponding muscles in constant tone, and every passive change of the same is often energetically resisted, giving the appearance of a wooden statue.

---

[59] In the Malays the compulsory imitation of simple actions is described as Latah, in S'berian tribes as Miryachit.

The apparent counterpart of automatic obedience is *negativism*, which, however, frequently appears with symptoms of automatic obedience. Negativistic patients refuse to do exactly what is requested or expected of them (Passive negativism), or they do the opposite (Active negativism), so that in pronounced cases it is possible to direct them by requesting the opposite of what is wanted of them. Negativism is often, but not always connected with an irritated response to all influences from without, and consequently with a tendency to anger and violence. Not infrequently negativism expresses itself in the fact that the patients make an effort to start an action, when a counter-impulse, or only a mere blocking appears and hinders them in its execution. It is also probable that quite different impulses (cross-impulses) interfere. In this way, negativism can also express itself against its own impulses (Inner-negativism).[64]

Centrifugal disturbances have especially many relations to schizophrenia while they recede in other diseases, or only appear as a natural consequence of other disturbances. The schizophrenic morbid pictures in which they appear in the foreground are called catatonias, and the symptoms, which associate here particularly often in various combinations, are called *catatonic symptoms*. But the latter partly in other genesis, and partly in a somewhat different form, may also occur now and then in other diseases. Catatonic symptoms are: stereotypes (of action, of attitude, of space, and verbigeration), mannerisms, automatic commands with waxlike and rigid catalepsy, echokinesis and echolalia, mutism (see below), negativism, impulsive raptus, the catatonic form of stupor, and the disturbances of the will in the stricter sense.

In general the will is indirectly influenced by the disturbances of perceptions and thinking, and more directly by disturbances of the affects. In catatonia there are disturbances of the will in a different sense. What we call will seems to merge independently into wrong paths. The patients cannot do what the conscious part of their ego would wish, they cannot will what they recognize as good; yet these actions are not automatic, but conscious, and in a certain respect they are also willed by a split off part of the will. The following disturbances have here been particularly emphasized: Hyperkinesis and akinesis, impulsive actions, automatisms, negativism, and obsessive actions.

The *affective manifestations inadequate* to the feeling belong almost entirely to schizophrenia. What impresses us in the affective conduct of the patient outside of schizophrenia is conditioned by the

[60] For further details about negativism Cf. Schizophrenia.

abnormity of the affect itself; an exaggerated manifestation is based on an exaggerated affect. In schizophrenia one cannot so easily judge from without to within: behind a tragic pathos there may be a very light or even no affect at all. At the same time the manifestations easily strike a false note which is often sensed with true instinct by naïve persons, and by very small children. Very frequently one observes an unmotivated laughter, which sounds artificial, and from which we can easily recognize that it is not the expression of a real gaiety. It can also be easily distinguished from the convulsive laughter of hysterical patients. In lesions of the thalamic regions one finds occasionally obsessive laughter or crying in consequence of any psychic stimuli with, or particularly without, a corresponding affect.

The abnormities of the mental trend are naturally expressed in the content of speech. It is noteworthy, however, that not only in aphasic, but also in schizophrenic patients, the speech utterances may be quite incomprehensible (*confusion of speech, "word salad," schizophasia*), while the corresponding thoughts remain clear as shown by the orderly behavior and work of the patients.

Formally, the vivid speech of the manic patient expresses his euphoric excitement, the retarded and low speech of the melancholic his depressive inhibitions, the babbling and stammering speech of the idiot his sensory and motor awkwardness, the inarticulate, syllable stumbling speech of the paretic, his disturbances of coordination, and the hesitating, singing speech of the epileptic, the dullness of his affect and mental stream. The different dysarthrias in apoplexy and other organic disturbances of the brain do not directly belong to our field of research, as they are only accidental complications of the psychoses.

A persistent not speaking is called *mutism;* it is variously determined by negativism, delusions, and by hallucinatory prohibitions to speak, but mainly by the fact that schizophrenic patients have nothing to communicate to their environment, and that they do not even take notice of questions put to them.

The handwriting shows quite analogous disturbances. Orthographic and grammatical mistakes, wrong corrections, and blots, give evidence of the patient's psychic defects. Imbecilic awkwardness and paretic disturbances of coordination impress on the handwriting a mark which is easily recognizable; the same is true of the manic mobility and excitability as well as of the melancholic inhibition. Some schizophrenic handwritings contain all kinds of strange letters and flourishes, orthographic peculiarities, abnormal formations of lines mixed with unintelligible signs, and similar peculiarities. The content of the writings gives us just as important enlightenment as regards the psychic life of the patient as the spoken utterances; often it is even more important, because in writing the patients are by themselves and are more free in expression. A skilfully dissimulating paranoiac used to confide his delusions only on toilet paper; and as his wife, who suffered severely in consequence of his disease, collected these documents she obtained the necessary material for divorce and guardianship.

CHAPTER III

PHYSICAL SYMPTOMS

Among the physical symptoms those of a neurological nature are especially important, because on the one hand many psychoses are partial manifestations of an organic affection of the central nervous system, and on the other hand the functional neuroses are mental diseases. Although it is a matter for the neurological clinic to deal with the semeiology, we shall mention here some of the most important symptoms for orientation.

Paralyses occur in the organic brain diseases, especially in idiocy, paresis, and in Korsakoff's disease. In the latter case paralyses are, of course, mostly peripheral. Psychic paralyses occur less frequently and are of hysterical genesis, even if found in cases other than hysteria. Many paralyses result in *contractures*. There are also primary (hysterical) contractures.

Real *convulsions* occur in epileptiform, paretic, catatonic, and hysterical attacks. Huntington's disease is always accompanied by *choreic* movements. In ordinary chorea the psychic disturbances sometimes rise to the height of a psychosis. The slow *athetoid* movements which ordinarily confine themselves to a limb or to half of the body are manifestations of brain lesions in postencephalitic idiocies or apoplectic dementia, and other similar cases. Other convulsive manifestations are chewing motions and grinding of teeth in idiots, in organic patients, and in acute delirium. The European sleeping sickness (Encephalitis lethargica) shows all sorts of hyperkinesias, particularly a stiffness of the muscles of mimicry which is not the same as the schizophrenic "rigidity" but as it is often associated with indifference and lack of energy, it cannot in itself be differentiated from schizophrenia.

Disturbances of coördination of a very definite form belong to the picture of paralysis, while bad coordination of motion in general, to the middle and higher grades of oligophrenias.

Tremors very frequently accompany the psychoses. Thus we have the fine, even tremor in uncomplicated chronic alcoholism and in some cases of schizophrenia, the various kinds of coarse tremors in all organic diseases, such as the severe forms of alcoholism and delirium

157

tremens, the febrile toxæmias and some cases of exhaustion. A form of organic tremor is especially seen in simple senile dementia and quite regularly accompanies this disease. Irregular tremors are often only a sign of some form of excitement.

With the exception of the *Babinski*, the cutaneous *reflexes* are practically of no significance in psychiatry. More important are the tendon or deep reflexes, the latter are increased wherever control by the cerebrum is disturbed, as in idiocy, in hysteria, also in dementia præcox; this phenomenon is naturally most pronounced in the organic psychoses. The crossing over of the *patellar-reflex* to the other leg most frequently to the adductors (contra-lateral movement), if the reflex can be elicited through the tibia or patella, indicates with reasonable probability an organic disturbance. Through affections of the peripheral nerve and the cord the exaggeration can be overcompensated even to the total disappearance of the reflexes (Alcoholic Korsakoff, tabo-paresis).

In the diagnosis of hysteria some people attach importance to the absence of the *pharyngeal-reflex*. This reflex is also absent in bromism and in many normal persons, depending entirely on the examination.

The disturbances of the *pupilary-reflexes* depend on the organic affection. In paresis, one usually finds rigidity to light (Argyll-Robertson's phenomenon), but it is also an important sign of other syphilitic affection of the nervous system; it may also occur transiently in organic forms of alcoholism and also in sleeping sickness. Catatonia seems to favor functional pupilary disturbances which are as yet incomprehensible.

Anesthesias and *analgesias* have already been mentioned, also *hyperesthesias* (p. 55). *Paresthesias* can have an organic origin in degenerations of the central or peripheral nervous system, or they can be psychically determined. Slight degenerative and toxic processes seem to produce changes in the physical sensations in cases of schizophrenia, which in turn give cause for hypochondriacal delusions and interpretations in the form of physical hallucinations.

The *remaining physical functions* are effected in some cases by the psychic alterations (loss of appetite in depression), in others they are organically determined by the underlying disease, such as paresis, and in still others they are the cause of the psychic alteration (Basedow psychoses, athyroidism, cases of amentia). The insomnias which regularly accompany the acute states have very divergent connections.

Menstruation often stays away for some time in acute psychoses; at least the subjective sensations of menstruation such as pain, etc., are very uncommon in chronic diseases where the patients no longer think of the function this is particularly the case in schizophrenia. In cases of debility where, on the contrary, such things are very important, one finds many menstrual difficulties. *Childbirth* proceeds very smoothly when the disease absorbs the patient to such an extent that the physiological act is not disturbed by the psyche. This shows that it is essentially the interference of the psyche which makes the function of childbirth so remarkably burdensome. Even women who at former confinements needed artificial assistance are wont to go through easy births in the psychoses, unless serious anatomical hindrances are in the way. The *potency* with the *libido* is diminished in some depressions, in morphinism, in many schizophrenics, in the excited initial stages of organic psychoses, especially in paresis; but in senile cases whose sexual impulse seems almost extinguished the potency and libido are sometimes increased. In chronic alcoholism, only the libido is enhanced while the potency is diminished in most cases.

At the height of the depression there is an absence of tears. In schizophrenia all *secretions* may be disturbed quite capriciously in the most varied ways. In cases of refusal of nourishment and naturally also in diabetic psychoses, one often finds acetone in the urine. *Metabolism* is markedly influenced in a most incomprehensible manner, especially in paresis and dementia præcox where one frequently notes fluctuations from extreme marasmus to excessive obesity and the reverse. In acute diseases the *bodily weight* usually diminishes, and increases during convalescence.

For the rest one knows a *lot of details* about disturbances of *digestion*, of *metabolism*, and of the *blood picture*, but as yet very little that is constant, that is sufficiently comprehensible, or that would contribute to the understanding. The *temperature* is normal in almost all psychoses, but one also observes febrile attacks, particularly in paresis, where it is cerebrally conditioned, and in hysteria where it is psychogenetically induced. Subnormal temperatures are sometimes encountered in marasmic conditions, in cerebral affections, and also without any explanation in schizophrenia.

The *heart* and *vasomotor* system remain uninfluenced in no psychoses, except perhaps in paranoia.

In paresis, perhaps also in senile processes, and in schizophrenia, one sees tabetic and other *rarefications* of the bones. Other *trophic disturbances* such as the tendency to otohaematoma and decubitus are variously determined in organic diseases.

With the aberration of the cerebral predisposition which is at the basis of many mental diseases, the *physical development*, too, merges into false paths. A great number of patients carry with them many malformations, or surely more than the average of those mentally normal, from a subnormal bodily height, deformed skull, badly formed ears and palates, irregular position of the teeth or insufficiently developed teeth, to the abnormal length of the vermiform appendix. For a long time great stress was laid on these "degenerative signs"; in individual cases it is hardly permitted to draw any conclusion about the psyche from either their presence or absence. On the other hand, they predominate as a whole in oligophrenics, in epileptics, and criminals, and less in other mental diseases. They have apparently something to do with injuries of the germ and point to a teratologic origin of the disease. The diseases which are sometimes described as "degenerative psychoses," namely, paranoia and manic depressive insanity are very frequently found in persons of particularly good physical development.

CHAPTER IV

THE MANIFESTATIONS OF MENTAL DISEASES

A psychosis is generally a complicated structure which may manifest itself in very different ways, not only from one patient to another, but in the same patient at different times. The manifestations were formerly taken for the diseases themselves,[1] and even yet it is of practical value to emphasize them as *pictures of morbid states and as syndromes.*

MORBID STATES

The manic state: On the affective side one observes an exalted and very changeable mood which is especially easily transformed into anger; in thought, there is flight of ideas, centrifugal pressure activity; as accessory symptoms one not seldom sees overestimated and grandiose ideas.

The expressions "mania" now usually means the manic state of manic depressive insanity. In countries speaking the Romance languages or English it still designates generally any excitement especially when it evinces itself in motor expression.

When the euphoric excitement gives a feeble and stupid impression, some still speak of it as *Moria.* Distinct flight of ideas need not be present. Moria occurs especially when manic attacks are subsiding, and in lesions of the frontal lobe. To be sure, exalted moods in dementing psychoses of any kind frequently also manifest a similar appearance.

Depression or *Melancholic states* with a painful accentuation of all experiences, retardation of thought and of the centrifugal functions. As accessory symptoms: depressive delusions.

The expression *"Melancholia"* designated for a long time the form of melancholia of the "involutional period," especially emphasized by *Kraepelin,* and is now also used to designate the depression of manic depressive insanity by those who have fused the two morbid pictures into one.

---

[1] *Kahlbaum* deserves the credit for having made a deliberate and sharp differentiation between "conditions" and "diseases," even though in his time the position of science had not yet made it possible to circumscribe natural morbid pictures more exactly.

The manic and the melancholic (depressive) states we see almost in pure form in the common cases of manic depressive insanity, also accidentally more or less frequently in most other mental diseases.

Delusional insanity refers to acute conditions in which delusions and hallucinations or even only one of the two symptoms dominate the picture to such an extent that the patient loses his pose, and frequently also his orientation.

The expression is now rarely applied to chronic conditions. When a distinct emotional fluctuation is combined with it, or, what is usually the same thing, when one deals with an onset of manic depressive insanity, one also speaks of *manic* or *melancholic insanity*.

What for a time was called delusional insanity ("Wahnsinn") were mostly hallucinatory excitements of schizophrenia. We still use the name only for the forms of manic depressive onsets, which cannot be otherwise classified, in which hallucinations and illusions more or less conceal the fundamental complex; we use it at times for similar schizophrenic pictures.

Meynert once believed that under this name ("Wahnsinn") he described a particular disease. He later substituted for it the term *amentia*.

The term *Confusion* is ambiguous; in the first place it designates the thought disturbances described above [2] that have no limits as to incoherence and dissociation. But more complicated conditions of very different origin are also designated in this way, being conceived at times as syndromes, at times as pictures of conditions and at times as diseases. According to *Ziehen*, confusion is a symptom complex, consisting of disorientation, incoherence of the course of ideation and motor incoherence. The "diseases" designated as confusion corresponded approximately to the newer amentia of average degree. Here we use the expression only for the above named mental disturbances.

"Hallucinatory Confusion" is symptomologically about the same as the broader amentia; therefore, what is still so called belongs nearly altogether, in part to our amentia, and in part to schizophrenia.

Only conditions that last for a long time and that are conceived as an entire disease are called *amentia*. Like *confusion*, it cannot be sharply defined symptomatically from twilight states and the deliria,[3] concepts, that we cannot as yet dispense with entirely. Transient confusion, twilight states and deliria, be they pronounced or merely indicated, we called "clouded states."

[2] Cf. p. 86.
[3] Cf. p. 111.

Acute delirium is now a rare brain disease. It is evidently based on different infections or on schizophrenic processes, and shows itself in deliria, convulsive manifestations, and in most cases in a rapidly ending death.

Hallucinosis is Wernicke's designation for acute hallucinatory conditions in which, in contrast with the deliria and the greater part of the twilight states, orientation and, in part, clearness, are retained (alcoholic hallucinosis).

Dreamy state is nothing but another name for twilight state.

Transitory psychoses [4] are attacks which appear and disappear suddenly, with disturbances of consciousness of brief duration. They occur in the manifold psychopathic states (Magnan's bouffées délirantes) with or without affective or toxic cause, then too, in latent and manifest forms of real psychoses, especially in schizophrenia and epilepsy. Many may be included in the concepts of twilight states. At times they are the cause of crimes.

Stupor [5] is a state of various origins that occurs especially in schizophrenia, then in hysteria, epilepsy and also in auto-intoxication, etc., rarely in manic depressive insanity. *Emotional stupor* is a syndrome seen in different conditions, especially in the different kinds of "nervosities," in the widest sense, and in the oligophrenias.

Stuporous forms with almost complete immotility are designated as *Attonity*. This is usually a catatonic condition; but a *melancholia attonita* has also been distinguished; whether the latter exists, i.e., whether the retardation of merely depressive conditions may rise to a continuous immotility, is questionable.

Under *cloudiness* we understand different conditions of narrowed, unclear, slowly performed thinking, in which stimuli are lacking or at any rate merge into the background. Such conditions are seen in slumber, in fever, in epilepsy, in schizophrenia, and in organic states of all kinds. A part of these pictures naturally may just as well be called stupor.

The picture of the condition of *hypochondria* consists in continuous attention to one's own state of health with the tendency to ascribe a disease to oneself from insignificant signs or also without such. It occurs in dementia præcox, in depressive and neurasthenic conditions, in initial stages of organic psychoses (arteriosclerosis, paresis), and in psychopathic states of all kinds. We no longer recognize *hypochondria as a disease*.

Catatonia as such is a manifestation of schizophrenia. But cata-

[4] Formerly in their excited forms also called transitory manias.
[5] Cf. pp. 143-144.

tonic symptoms also occur in organic mental diseases, in epilepsy and in fever psychoses.

Paranoid symptoms is the designation for hallucinations and delusions when they appear in a state of mental clearness and without (primary) fluctuations of the affects.

"Acute (hallucinatory) *Paranoia"* was conceived by *Ziehen* and others as a disease. The majority of these so called conditions belongs, in our opinion, to the acute manifestations of schizophrenia.

Religious mania, or *mania religiosa,* is any mental disease with religious delusions; it is thus mainly a question of dementia præcox. Nevertheless some observers still designate a melancholia with pronounced delusions of sin as religious mania.

Dementia (feeble mindedness) is not a uniform condition. One deals here with a purely practical conception. Whoever fails in life because of intellectual insufficiency is demented. In a scientific sense there is no uniform dementia, but only an oligophrenic, epileptic, organic dementia, i.e., forms which in their entire character are very different from one another. The diagnosis "dementia" is scientifically never sufficient; one can diagnose only a particular kind of dementia.

As *psychopathies* we designate the mass of congenital or at any rate permanent psychic deviations from the normal which have not yet been included into any other class, and which exist chiefly in the borderline between health and disease. Among these one naturally finds many undeveloped real mental diseases, especially latent schizophrenia. Many believe that they connect a well defined conception with this expression, but they are certainly mistaken.

Degeneration.[6] "Degenerates" are usually about the same type as psychopathics, namely, individuals who intellectually and especially affectively react differently from the average. "Degénérés supérieurs" (superior degenerates) are psychopaths who stand above the average in some line and can maintain themselves in the world. It is only just to state that famous men belong to this class.[7]

SYNDROMES

Syndromes are complexes of symptoms that belong together genetically. A part of such pictures as manic depressive insanity, eventually with their corresponding delusions, represent at the same time such syndromes. One speaks, furthermore, of an *"organic symptom complex,"* also called the *Korsakoff syndrome* and understands by

---

[6] Cf. p. 201.
[7] For some etiological designations see end of the chapter on Causation.

this term the sum of the psychical fundamental symptoms of a diffuse atrophy of the cortex, or of a general lowering of the function of the cortex through shock or injury of the brain.[8]

The *Katathymic delusional formation,* i.e., a delusional formation with clearness in other respects, which is not due to a general moodiness but to a definite "complex," or a particular experience, is a syndrome in itself. It alone or combined with hallucinations forms the *paranoid syndrome,* which is to be distinguished from the *paranoid constitution.* The latter type of personality readily refers the actions of others to himself, or interprets them in the sense of a definite attitude (suspicion, persecution, grandeur) without progressing to the distinct formation of a real delusion. We can also mention here the *hysterical* and *neurasthenic symptom complex,*[9] the *compulsive symptoms,* the *anxiety psychosis* and *anxiety neurosis,* also the *fright neurosis,* the *expectation neurosis* and the *twilight states,* because they are all produced by definite mechanisms on different foundations such as the psychopathic, hysteric, and epileptic. Under the twilight states several types are to be distinguished, which permit of fairly good differentiation on the basis of their psychic genesis: thus we have the *Ganser Syndrome,* which represents a "mental disease," in the form of acting and thinking in a manner which is the reverse of the normal; the *buffoonery syndrome* in which the patient plays the fool in the "vulgar" sense;[10] puerilism,[11] when the patient behaves like a little child and the *pseudo-dementia* in which the patient "knows nothing." Moreover, wishes are not only realized *through* the twilight states but also hallucinatorily *in* the twilight states, inasmuch as the patients dream themselves into the desired situation. The wish to be insane and to appear irresponsible is fulfilled *through* the Ganser state which *is* a mental disease, or the wish to be innocent and pardoned is realized in the prison delirium which *deludes* the patients with the fact that they are innocent or forgiven. The maximum of wish fulfilment is achieved by the ecstasies.[12] These syndromes are also called *Purpose psychoses.*

Among the twilight states the *wandering mania* (poriomania, fugues) deserves special consideration. It manifests itself in a running away that is completely aimless, or dominated by a single confused and uncontrollable idea; at times it is merely motor without

---

[8] Cf. p. 230.

[9] For the kinds of manifestations see the corresponding diseases.

[10] As in spoiled children, the buffoonery observed in schizophrenia may exceptionally be used as a means to hide the despair.

[11] Not to be confused with infantilism.

[12] Cf. p. 113.

any consideration for the outer world except what is necessary for running; at times it is externally inconspicuous, the act seems planned with correct use of transportation and with the possibility of contact with other people; at other times it is done in a way that it can be placed between these two extremes. The milder forms are rather psychogenic and may therefore occur everywhere, even in hysterics and ordinary psychopaths, especially in those who are young, as a result of an exciting experience, a temptation, or an unbearable situation. The severer forms belong chiefly to epilepsy, while those who are midway between the two classes belong in the main to schizophrenia.

Querulousness is generated by an exalted self-consciousness where there is activity and lack of understanding for the rights of others; this occurs in schizophrenia, paranoia, manic depressions of long duration, traumatic neurosis, and prison confinements. Aside from the affective explosions of rage (prison outburst), confinement produces conditions in which on the one hand the patient imagines himself pardoned, acquitted, or innocent, on the other hand persecuted by those about him. Syndromes that are put in motion by a definite situation, as prison psychoses, Ganser, etc., transitory affect psychoses, and eventually also querulousness, are also comprehended under the name of *situation psychoses.*

Further syndromes are "attacks," such as the epileptiform in the narrower sense with petit mal, Jacksonian epilepsy, paretic, and catatonic attacks.

Hoche wanted to supplant the pictures of diseases that are still too fluctuating by the theory of the syndrome, urging that one should be satisfied with a diagnosis of the latter. But even the syndrome theory is by no means complete; the identical syndrome has an entirely different significance for therapy and especially for practice, according to whether it occurs in an hysteria, or epilepsy, or schizophrenia; besides we now know altogether too much about the "diseases" in the ordinary sense to be able to disregard these conceptions without a severe loss to science. *On the other hand, it would be an advantage to carry out a syndromistic treatment of those symptom complexes that are only deviations from the normal average either in predisposition, as in psychopathic conditions, or in reaction as in neuroses, purpose and situation psychoses, and paranoias.*

CHAPTER V

THE COURSE OF MENTAL DISEASES

Few generalizations can be made concerning the course of mental diseases. The congenital mental diseases run a "course" only to the extent that at times they show acute syndromes or sometimes progress as in puberty, or that they combine with a new disease such as epilepsy, schizophrenia, alcoholism, or atrophy of the brain.

In acquired psychoses one frequently speaks of *prodromal stages*, but here as in most cases they represent nothing but such mild morbid symptoms, that a diagnosis is impossible. The most frequent of these are: depression, exaltation, eccentricities, nervous symptoms or changes of character, in which the new attitude may resemble the character of many healthy people, and in itself, therefore, does not necessarily seem morbid. To be sure, all the real signs of mental diseases in a less marked form may also have the significance of prodromes.

The *"beginning of the actual disease"* is usually furtive if one does not designate acute episodes in chronic pictures as "the" disease, as frequently used to happen and even now occurs in the onsets of manic depressive insanity. At all events certain deliria, hysterical twilight states, and similar processes are in the real sense acute.

The entire course is mostly chronic, even in the sense of psychiatry, which also designates as acute diseases depressions extending over a period of years, provided they regain normal balance. Here the term "acute" has come to mean approximately something transitory while the term "chronic" something incurable. In organic psychoses, which after a long while end in death, one usually avoids the division of acute and chronic, as far as the disease is concerned.

During the course one encounters *acute shifts, acute onsets, exacerbations* and *remissions*. *Shifts* are rapidly appearing aggravations of the disease; the concept usually indicates that the given aggravation does not usually equalize itself. Shifts are often connected with some form of excitement and other accessory symptoms, which except for the given lasting injury may recede to former states. Paresis and schizophrenia are usually first recognized as diseases during such

167

"shifts" after they have furtively transformed the patient for some time. In dementia præcox many of these shifts assume the form of schizophrenic manias and melancholias, of catatonias, and other syndromes that were formerly considered special psychoses. *Exacerbations* are aggravations in general, especially such as readjust themselves. Among them one observes many psychically determined excitements, or twilight states (e.g. in schizophrenia), that are not directly connected with the process of the disease, but are only transient reactions of the diseased psyche to certain stimuli. To be sure they generally disappear, leaving no trace of themselves. The term, exacerbation, does not usually designate the acute attacks that belong to the morbid picture, such as the moodiness and twilight states of epilepsy or the manias and melancholias of manic depressive insanity. All the mentioned transient states of chronic diseases, taken together, may be designated as *acute onsets*. Between the aggravations there are *remissions;* whether one may also assume *intermissions* in forms like manic depressive insanity depends on the conception. With *Kraepelin, Magnan* and others, we designate the whole permanent state of manic depressive insanity as the disease, and the acute appearances may also alternate with one another in regular sequence so that mania follows melancholia and the latter follows mania, etc., eventually with normal intervals after the mania or after the melancholia or after both. Such formations are called *circular* or *cyclic* forms. Outside of manic depressive insanity they occur occasionally in schizophrenia and also in paresis.

How many insane patients are *cured* depends in institutional statistics very much on the quality of the cases received into the hospital, otherwise primarily on the physician's conception of cure. Whether a schizophrenic patient who is perfectly competent socially, and in whom some remnants of the disease can only be demonstrated after a minute examination, may be considered as cured or not, is a matter of taste. I would rather not call him cured, in view of new aggravations that usually appear later, such as the question of marriage, and similar consequences, although I am aware that the disease may also "definitively remain quiescent." Delirium tremens, which in hospital statistics often shows a large percentage of cures, is, to be sure, as a rule totally gone at the discharge, but not the alcoholism that lies at its basis, i.e., the disease is cured but the patient is not. In residual schizophrenic states "cures" sometimes take place even many years after the patient has long been given up; this occurs in some without any visible reason, in some as a result of a febrile disease, or a change of environments, and similar things.

Cure with a defect is also spoken of by formulating the conception, suitable only to few cases, that the acute disease has left a defect just as a healed wound leaves a scar. A "psychic scar" may be formed by definite "residual symptoms," as in the case of a delusion which in spite of returned clearness following a delirium is no longer corrected. If the psychic scar is so severe and multiform that it may be considered as a disease in itself, the morbid picture was formerly designated as *secondary* to distinguish it from the *primary disease* that formed it ("secondary dementia," "secondary paranoia"). The conception must now be given up as in such cases it is nearly always a question of dementia præcox, which does not change its nature.

Nearly all organic mental diseases and some severe cases of other forms, e.g., of catatonia end in *death*. Of the remaining a small part indirectly ends fatally through suicide, unhygienic living, refusal of nourishment, exhaustion from restlessness and insomnia, injuries, and infection.

In making the *prognosis* we have to differentiate the "direction prognosis" and in chronic diseases, in addition, the "extent prognosis." Organic mental diseases run in the direction of a definite dementia and end in death; the epileptic and schizophrenic follow the direction of other kinds of dementia and usually do not end in death. Within the realm of schizophrenia there are again different directions such as the paranoid, catatonic dementia, etc., that have to be considered in the prognosis. Not less important is often the "extent prognosis," i.e., the prediction how far the disease will progress within a conceivable period. Will the disease soon come to a stop, or will there be some improvement? Will the patient become socially incompetent through dementia? Or will he be able to maintain himself in spite of the disease? And under what circumstances? In dementia praecox, epilepsy and the severe forms of manic depressive insanity these questions must often be put and sometimes their answer is possible with considerable probability.

CHAPTER VI

THE BORDERLINES OF INSANITY

Nowhere is the question: "sick or not sick?" put so often, in such an inexorable manner and with such heavy consequences as in the judgment of mental conditions. But the given question is false. *There are no borderlines of insanity*, no more than for any other disease. In every person a tubercular bacillus occasionally takes hold; one or the other of the microbes may even divide once or twice. How many bacteria must be present, how much living tissue must have been destroyed before the individual should be called tubercular? Or beginning with what degree of susceptibility is the "predisposition to tuberculosis" morbid? No one will want to answer such a question. Still more senseless is the question about well and sick where it is not a case of something added but of a plain deviation from the normal. Where is the borderline between healthy stupidity and morbid feeble-mindedness? Where is the boundary between normal and supernormal size of body? If the boundary line is lacking here, then there are extensive fields in which the conceptions "sick" and "healthy" are not at all applicable, as little as the various shades of light in a photograph can be divided into black and white; most of them are gray as a matter of fact.

That the people and jurisprudence repeatedly demand an answer to such senseless questions from the psychiatrist is due to the consequences. They really do not want to know whether a person is healthy or sick, but they want to know whether he is to be taken seriously, whether he is to be committed to a hospital, whether he is responsible and capable of acting, etc., and all that they want to infer from the confirmation "sick or not sick?" This method of inference is in itself wrong, not only because in a very wide zone the conceptions sane and insane cannot be applied at all, but also because there are patients that need not be committed, that may have good ideas, that are not incapacitated, that are not irresponsible. Today Schizophrenia and paresis may frequently be diagnosed before one would care to act upon the social consequences of such a confirmation, and with the refinement of our diagnostic resources such cases will always increase. On the other hand, under certain circumstances a

170

psychopath, who is not insane, may for a definite period have lost his ability to reflect, to such an extent, that he is neither responsible nor capable of action. And one will often have to decide within the border zone according to external circumstances, since the same degree of feeblemindedness, that does not harm the day laborer, at all, incapacitates the man who has inherited a large business.

The whole difficulty lies in the fact that there is no definition of "disease" and there cannot be any. The fruitless controversies can only cease when the ambiguous and indefinite concept is entirely excluded. *It is easy enough* to examine how a person is and reacts, and draw conclusions *from the facts*, instead of from a concept, and then determine our actions accordingly.

Where chapters of the code contain more detailed descriptions of the concept of disease, they vary greatly according to the context. *As far as the concept of insanity has become at all practical, it rests not on medical or psychopathological criteria, but on the idea of social incapacity.* That is why, from practical points of view, the *neuroses* which are purely psychic diseases, are not included in insanity, when they do not lead to severe syndromes like clouded states. All the more they belong to theoretical psychiatry because they are comprehensible only psychopathologically and have to be accurately known to differentiate them from the other mental diseases. But much more severe mental disturbances, as those in coarse brain diseases and in infections, are usually not classed with the psychoses. From a medical point of view the basic disease is taken as the only thing important; socially, these disturbances have no significance especially because of their brief duration, unless an important legal transaction happens at this time.

Hence we shall use the expressions sane and insane only in very pronounced cases and otherwise, in so far as we are compelled to. At the same time, in the aberrations like mental debility, or psychopathy, we shall take the capacity required under the given conditions as a criterion to determine the boundary of disease. But as soon as an acquired disease is definitely proven, even though by few and relatively mild symptoms, we shall speak of "disease in the medical sense" and shall then have to put the questions, whether any conclusions and which ones are to be drawn from this finding after a consideration of all the circumstances.

A question which touches many people deeply is this, "Whether *genius* is a disease or not?" Lombroso asserted that it was a disease, while others have indignantly rejected this view. Now here, too, we do not know all we should like to know. But matters stand about like this: 1. Genius is an aberration like any other; that it is much less common than undesirable deviations is self-evident, because few defects in disposition can make a man useless.   One only becomes a genius when a large number of attributes are simultaneously very highly developed.   Genius may therefore run just as little true to strain as a particularly fine variety of peach which as a single aberration was accidentally cultivated by the gardener. 2. The tendency to aberration usually involves the entire organism.   Every domestic animal and every plant, which can be cultivated along a definite characteristic, deviates more readily in another direction.   Those who are psychically abnormal have (in the average) many physical "stigmata of degeneration" and those who are physically abnormal have (in the average) many psychic defects.   In the aberration of genius we therefore, as a rule, also find relatively frequently other abnormal qualities, which we must usually give a negative value (sensitiveness, nervousness, etc.). 3. Besides, there is a connection between genius and mental abnormality: The normal philistine is adjusted to the conditions in which he was born, and balances with their little changes without thinking or noticing much in the process.   The psychopathic individual cannot adapt himself so well, or not at all; he reacts to difficulties resulting therefrom either by evasion,—he may take refuge from the demands, in hysteria or neurasthenia,—or he may create an imaginary world for himself through grandiose and persecutory delusion,—or aggressively by attempts to adapt the external world to his necessities, or by both together.   Whoever would like the outer world different in large or small matters is compelled to ponder over it and strive for inventions, social betterments, etc.   If he is also sufficiently intelligent, the facility of avoiding the usual paths may be directly conducive to finding something new.   Often the lack of adaptability lies rather in inner difficulties, because the different tendencies do not equalize themselves but lead to a lasting inner schism.   Such people may combine the contrasts in dereistic thinking or obtain satisfaction from without; if they have the other necessary qualifications, they become poets or artists.   It is, therefore, not chance that famous men are so frequently the offspring of unlike parents, whose tendencies do not fuse into a unified whole in the psyche of their descendants, but throughout their lives strive in different directions.   Poets and musicians must also be more sensitive than other people, a quality which is a hindrance to the daily tasks of life and often attains the significance of a disease.

CHAPTER VII

CLASSIFICATION OF MENTAL DISEASES

One class of the psychoses shows itself as a morbid reaction to an affective experience, as a prison psychosis to a confinement, and an hysterical twilight state to a jilting on the part of the beloved (*reactive psychoses, situation psychoses*). In the other class there is a morbid process in the brain, that conditions the psychosis (process pychosis, progressive psychosis).[1] But no division can be based on these classes because the two symptomologies intermingle.

The terms "organic"[2] and "psychogenic" indicate similar differences. With the organic one naturally also classed the toxic psychoses resulting from changes of metabolism, hormones, and from infections and poisoning in the narrower sense. The idea of the Psychogenic is not clear to many. It is said that psychogenic manifestations, too, must "naturally" have an anatomical substratum; indeed, an anatomical change has even been postulated for things like hysterical paralysis of the arm. That is wrong. An hysterical paralysis as such has only substrata, which in themselves are not pathologic; but as the foundation of the hysterical *disposition* there is a nervous system anatomically —chemically somehow differently formed from that of the normal disposition. In a house there are doors and windows so that at times they may be opened, at other times closed. If they are open or closed, it is in itself no derangement of the structure; but if they close or open too slowly or too easily, or if there is a rogue who brings it about that they move too slowly or too easily, or who breaks them or opens them when they should be closed, and closes them when they should be opened, those are changes that may be compared with the anatomical.

Endogenous and *exogenous* psychoses cannot be sharply differentiated, not only because the two factors mingle or combine in their effects but because the two concepts in themselves have no definite

---

[1] For details see *Jaspers*, Schicksal und Psychose bei der Dementia Præcox, Ztschr. f. d. ges. Neur. u. Psych. Orig. XIV, S. 158.

[2] The word "organic" designates here a much broader conception than in the expression "organic psychoses" which—in order not to have to coin a new name—I use for those psychoses that are based on a different reduction of brain elements.

limits. Idiocy, whether stationary or progressive, may be endogenous in relation to the patient but may be the result of an exogenous influence on a parent. If schizophrenias are based on autointoxications, they are exogenous in relation to the brain but endogenous in relation to the body. Nevertheless *Bonhoeffer's* investigations of the exogenous reaction types in toxic states and infections have been very enlightening.

The attempt has also been made to classify on the basis of *causes;* for example, alcoholic, infections, and traumatic psychoses have been differentiated. But this principle cannot be carried out because some causes produce very different morbid pictures, as syphilitic paranoid states and paresis, alcoholic insanity and alcoholic Korsakoff's disease. And conversely, the same morbid pictures might be produced by different causes, thus Korsakoff's diseases may be due to alcohol or carbonic oxide gas. That the idea of causality is not clearly limited need not nowadays be explained in detail.

Under *Kraepelin's* guidance the course of diseases has been particularly emphasized, thus the same terminal state was supposed to be proof that two different groups (not diseases) were formed which are entities even in other respects, and will probably remain so for us. We refer to dementia præcox and manic depressive insanity. It is nevertheless impossible to base a classification of morbid pictures *only* on the course of the disease.

According to a more recent theory of these two groups of psychoses one observes *even in normal people* a syntonic ("cyclothymic") reaction type, in which the whole personality uniformly participates in a definite and relatively vivid affect, suitable for the situation of the moment, and the train of ideas follows substantially quite logical laws, in that the affects disturb it only by connecting and overvaluing what conforms to it, and by inhibiting and undervaluing what opposes it. If at the same time the physiologically conditioned mood remains uniform throughout life and maintains an average pace, the representatives of this type then pass as the most normal people. If it permanently deviates to euphoric or depressive paths, its carriers are then in a chronic mood; if the mood fluctuates (always for physiologic reasons), those so afflicted are cyclothymic, or in the pronounced cases, manic depressive. Studies of heredity show us, that the peculiarities mentioned, somewhere belong together, that they represent a uniform super quality, the "syntone," in which, although the individual sub groups follow by preference a similar heredity, they can nevertheless substitute one another in almost every family. *Manic-depressive insanity, Cyclothymia, chronic depressive and manic moods, appear as exaggerations or other deviations of "normal" syntonic reaction types.*

Whereas the relationship of even the uniform (most normal) syntones to the morbid fluctuations was first demonstrated by Kretschmer, the "schizoid" peculiarities of healthy persons was long known. Thus there is a lack of uniformity of the affectivity, actual coexistence of different, nay, contrasting strivings, and a slight deviation of the associations from the usual paths. Here too one must differentiate the various qualitative or quantitative sub groups, which are frequently inherited as such, but still change frequently within the main type. Among those one finds persons who are dereistic, who show an affective poverty, who are irritable, eccentric, paranoid, schizophrenic, schizoid, etc. Now, even if the schizoid reaction appears mostly abnormal following the canon which we have made for ourselves about psychic normality, that too has as much biologic significance as the syntones: Psychic new creations, inventions, political and religious revolutions almost always owe their existence to it. *Exaggerations or caricatures of this reaction type come into existence as schizophrenic manifestations.* But whereas according to our present, still very limited knowledge, the manic depressive attacks are designated as "functional," at least the more serious schizophrenias are connected with tangible cerebral changes; hence the most marked deviation from the normal seems to be here in the first place not merely a strong fluctuation but something new, still even in this relation it is nevertheless possible to form a parallel syntone, at least hypothetically, between manic-depressive and schizoid-schizophrenia.

Every man then has one syntonic and one schizoid component, and through closer observation one can determine its force and direction and can also put it in relation to his heredity, if the members of the family are known.

Either both or only one of the reactions may be morbidly exaggerated in the same individual. The extreme cases then belong to the pure manic-depressive and the pure schizophrenic diseases. Frequently, however, we find distinct mixtures; preponderating manic-depressive types with schizophrenic accessory symptoms and the reverse. These mixtures have been known to psychiatrists for a long time, but they have been guided by it only in the prognosis and treatment of the disease but not in naming it. Except in the rare extreme cases we now no longer have to ask, is it manic-depressive or schizophrenia? but *to what extent manic-depressive and to what extent schizophrenia?* Confronted with such mixed forms we can say that if the schizophrenic components, though distinct, do not definitely follow the paths of dementia, the prognosis is still good, at least as regards the present attack, otherwise it is bad; for the manic depressive part of the disease is almost always transitory.

For not only would the schizophrenic-like symptoms in all manic depressive forms owe their existence to schizophrenic components, but conversely most of the melancholic and manic states in schizophrenics would probably be an expression of the manic depressive components; they would really have no direct connection with the schizophrenic process. In many cases the latter connection could always be made with the greatest probability by studying the heredity.

The theory has also some bearing *on other diseases, namely, organic psychoses. Poisons* coming from without (alcohol, infections), as from within (uræmia), will set free more schizoid symptoms, if the schizoid factors of the individual are stronger, and more manic depressive symptoms, the more syntonically the patient is predisposed. This would thus furnish us with the explanation not only for the mixed forms of manic-depressive and schizophrenic symptoms, but also for the admixture of manic depressive or schizophrenic symptoms in quite different diseases. As far as our experience goes this theory can be fully applied to senile dementia. The preponderance of euphoric or even manic symptoms in general paresis requires a special explanation: Does the disposition to manic behavior also contain a disposition to the localization of the spirochites in the brain? Or what seems more probable, does the paralytic process or toxin produce a tendency to euphoric reaction?

That under these circumstances the paraphrenias must all be added to the schizophrenias is self-evident. One thinks less of the fact that also the essential factor in all *neuroses* rests on schizophrenic mechanisms; one may think of the splitting off, the pinching off, the arraignment of one impulse by the other, the inability to adjust to certain situations (or better the will not to adjust oneself), etc. To be sure the syntonic components play some part in the formation of even these morbid pictures. Thus to produce a hysteria in the ordinary sense there must be a tendency to a labile affectivity in order to accentuate one's own personality; a more depressive affectivity in the same schizophrenic mechanism would lead to "neurasthenic" pictures. If the affects are very constant and maintain themselves in a more central position, a paranoia will develop in a schizoid mental type as a reaction to inner and outer difficulties (Studies in heredity seem at last able to furnish the long expected proof of the relationship between forms of paranoia and schizophrenias). A simple uncontrollable affectivity which leads to all sorts of primitive reactions, such as crying, window breaking, scratching up the husband, extravagance in love and veneration, has its origin in the syntonic components.

The fragmentary theory here presented is for the present only an hypothesis; but could be demonstrated with remarkable elegance in a large amount of material of healthy and sick people; its correctness at least as far as its general features are concerned can therefore hardly be doubted. It is even more important when we find that the two psychic types also show a certain predilection for definite physical constitutions; to be sure these connections are more complicated and less definite than those based on psychic spheres; but *Kretschmer's Pyknical* physical type, e.g., must somewhere show a particular relation to the stronger syntonic reaction types.[3]

In recent years *anatomical investigations* have carried us forward very nicely, in that, for instance, a clearly circumscribed picture could be distinguished of dementia paralytica, of various forms of senility, and of several diseases that may be designated clinically as epileptic.

As in somatic pathology we are not accustomed in psychiatry to apply concurrently different principles of classification, and through the services of *Kraepelin* we have attained in barely two decades a point of view, which compared with the earlier one, is entirely satisfactory. Even though, as everywhere else, there is much we should know in order to see clearly, and though there are surely still many diseases that we do not know, nevertheless compared with the complete helplessness of previous years we have achieved a point of view from which it is possible to gain new ground steadily.

Therefore I follow, as far as possible, Kraepelin's classification which is now pretty well understood in the whole world, even if it is not everywhere accepted, while all other schematizations are usable only in certain schools.

Combinations of psychoses are still insufficintly studied. A schizophrenic or a manic depressive patient may be taken with feverdelirium, delirium tremens, paresis, or dementia senilis; alcoholism is not at all rare, especially in women where it is a symptom of schizophrenia. In such cases the symptoms of the two psychoses combine and under certain circumstances as in the interconnected hallucinations of the schizophrenic delirium tremens, they fuse into a unified and peculiar nuance. Sometimes one disease apparently forms the essential picture; there is no pronounced second disease but a mere predisposition colors the symptoms.

[3] For more information see Kretschmer Körperbau und Charakter, Springer, Berlin 1921, and Bleuler: Die Probleme der Schizoidie und der Syntonie, Zeitschr. f. d. gesam. Neurol. u. Psychiat. 1922.

Recently an attempt was made to place the classification of the psychoses on an entirely different basis by emphasizing the various factors participating in the causation, development, and course. I made the effort to initiate these viewpoints also here but had to desist from it.[4]

Even if only the most important combinations would have been presented it would have been so complicated that not alone the beginner would have had much trouble in understanding them. On the other hand if one is well acquainted with the present grouping of the symptoms, it is no longer a clever feat to recognize and sufficiently differentiate in the same patients such conditions as congenital debility, alcoholism, manic states, and perhaps even the beginning of senile dementia. If the new demands would be followed many repetitions would be unavoidable. Moreover our knowledge is by far too meagre for such description. Thus in the case of apparently catatonic symptoms in organic psychoses, we must, for example, first find out whether and to what extent they are based on the same schizoid mechanisms as in schizophrenia before we can say in a given case that the morbid picture is colored by a schizoid disposition. We do not know the somatic (toxic?) part, that probably conditions the tendency to euphoria and mania in paresis, and consequently cannot tell to what extent an induced paretic mania results from the disposition, etc.

Besides, the diagnosis in the present sense still remains the important factor. If we formulate our findings in such words as "organic disease," "epilepsy," "manic depressive insanity," or "neurosis," we have at the same time drawn from it the most important practical and theoretical consequences, which at least for the present cannot be substituted by any other theory. What would be the use of recognizing an hysterical mechanism, if we would not know whether it developed on a schizophrenic, paretic, epileptic, or on a mere nervous constitution? And if instead of calling a disease schizophrenia we would have to describe all the individual mechanisms which we see acting in unison, we would hardly ever get through, and we would then still have to keep the whole story in our heads, in order to decide upon the prognosis and treatment. Also the two latter deductions could be the same as in any other psychosis, which is composed of quite different individual syndromes, that is, it would look quite different in the description, but would become attached to the former, without anything further, through the diagnosis of schizophrenia.

The first thing to consider in the "Strata-diagnosis" ("Schichtdiag-

[4] Comp. also the end of Chapter IX on "syndromes," p. 198.

nose") of *Kretschmer* is the *constitution*, whereby there is tendency of late to understand only something acquired through heredity, although it is natural to suppose that some qualities, as e.g., the weakness of an endocrine gland, can be just as well acquired as congenital. But the constitution even in this narrow sense is by no means a factor acting only in one way. It acts *pathogenetically* when it gives direct origin to an amaurotic idiocy, to a schizophrenia, or a manic depressive insanity; it acts "pathoplastically" (*Birnbaum*) when as a schizoid disposition it determines the formation and the kind of delusions in an organic disease, or when it causes an alternation of manic and depressive moods in the same disease. In the latter case it influences besides the course of the external morbid picture, and it is assumed that it can determine the severity of the disease in its manifestation and outcome.

The concept of *disposition* includes the constitution and with it also all the not familiar factors, congenital and acquired, that may come into consideration, such as poisons, infections, traumas and physical diseases of various kinds. It acts exactly like the constitution: pathologically, pathoplastically, and determines the course and the severity of the disease.

A particularly conspicuous side of the disposition is the *character*, which acts pathoplastically; thus certain ideas of persecution and grandeur are only possible in definite strivings and in definite characterological relations to the environments; the economical person becomes miserly in senile dementia.

But indirectly the character also acts pathogenetically, not only by assisting in the acquisition of a syphilis or an alcoholism, but also probably through the fact that certain diseases, like paranoia or even paranoid conditions, i.e., diseases which are made up, as it were, of delusions, would not have broken out, if the character would not have assisted in determining the possibility of delusional formation. The neuroses too require a soil of a definite character foundation.

However, the character may also be the result of a morbid disposition, which later leads to a psychosis (schizophrenia, manic depressive insanity, epilepsy), or it may be the partial manifestation of the disease (oligophrenia, schizophrenia epilepsy), or it is the disease that first emphasizes definite features of character, exaggerates, or caricatures them (a punctual and conscientious person becomes querulous in old age, the generous becomes thoughtless, and the one who is somewhat below par morally becomes an unscrupulous criminal as a schizophrenic).

Quite independent of the disposition, as far as its psychic expression is concerned, is the part played by individual cerebral processes which change the material foundations of the psychic life. Among the first to be named is the *diffuse atrophy* of the brain, that is, its cortex, which in very different diseases is the most essential factor for the structure of the psychic picture of the symptoms; and quite independent of all other manifestations and dispositions determines what we call clinically "organic mental diseases." In reference to the psychosis the cerebral alteration acts pathogenetically, while in reference to the symptomatology pathoplastically. That the localization, and the kind of the process leading to the atrophy must exert a formative influence on the distributions of the picture, which we consider as accessory manifestations, is self-evident. But as yet we know too little about it to give these factors serious consideration. The invasion of the spirochites exerts a tendency to euphoria; certain senile processes like cerebral pressure determine a torpor of all psychic processes. Multiple sclerosis (and epilepsy) and other organic brain diseases dispose one to hysteroid symptoms, while paresis and senile dementia often cause them to recede.

Circumscribed injuries of the brain also come into consideration both in regards to causation as well as formation. Lesions in the basal ganglia diminish the energy from the impulsive life (sleeping sickness); other lesions at the base of the frontal lobe lead to moria, facetiousness, and a tendency to mischievous teasing. Other circumscribed lesions in the basal ganglia determine a labile affectivity, while all destructions of parts of the brain are likely to produce irritability and transient moodiness.

Congenital dispositions also influence the form of the symptoms in these cases, in that the force of the schizoid functions adds to the picture schizophrenic symptoms, and pronounced syntony manic depressive symptoms; the other dispositions of character also color the disease. That former experiences, e.g., delusions, can color the organic, and that poisons (alcohol) can influence the entire psychic picture even here, is well known.

More difficult is the formation of the theory in *epilepsy*. The epileptic process (chemical or anatomical) produces a marked change in the psyche, but only in the same direction as the epileptoid foundation showed itself before the appearance of the disease in the patient himself or at the same time in his blood relationship. We shall therefore do well here to reserve our theory for a while.

Still more complicated are the relations in schizophrenia. Here too there is a disposition, which psychically shows itself as an embryo of the later insanity, then there are elementary disturbances in the thought apparatus, which are still hard to understand, somewhat later or in acute shifts there are distinct organic changes in the brain and on the top of this as accessories there develops the entire polymorphous complex of the schizophrenic manifestations, as reactions of a sick organism, or as deviated functions of the psyche.

Besides the epileptoid and schizoid characteristics, which have some connection with the disease itself, other qualities of character must naturally co-determine in many directions the outward appearance of the psychosis.

Some *toxins*, like alcohol, morphine, and cocaine, act causatively and at the same time formatively, so that one can tell the cause from the picture; in their manifestations these poisons are also definite forms of psychic disturbances.

When different causes producing definite symptom complexes co-operate, for instance, a spirochite invasion and an alcohol poisoning, it is customary to view the one disease as the essential and the admixtures of the other as a "coloring" of the same. In a delirium tremens we sometimes find the signs of paresis, in senile dementia those of alcoholism. As a matter of fact, it concerns here a mixture of two diseases, of which, to be sure, the one without the other would often not come to light. Similar conditions prevail when only dispositions, and not a pronounced disease complicate the main psychosis. Febrile deliria, and delirium tremens, are influenced by schizoid factors, schizophrenia by alcoholism, in that, e.g., the hallucinations and delusions become more united. A schizoid disposition or schizophrenia and the effect of alcohol mix with a uniform picture, in acute alcoholic delusions, in so far as the two components are even much less separable than the algæ and fungi among the lichens.

The psychosis or the disposition can also counterbalance the other in individual symptoms: organic psychoses loosen the blockings and other catatonic manifestations of schizophrenia. The original character can be turned into its opposite.

There are also definite syndromes ("diseases") which are produced by definite causes or cerebral processes. On the other side it has been said that similar causes may produce different pictures of disease, depending on the reaction type of the patient. Thus a fever, an alcoholic poisoning, a delirium tremens, a paresis, even a manic depressive attack will set free schizophrenic symptoms in a schizoid individual. Depending on the disposition, psychic influences will evoke twilight states, hysterical attacks, a neurasthenia, a schizophrenic attack, or chronic delusional formations. The correct concept is that a disposition and a chance cause manifest themselves in the morbid picture in just such cases, or, what is the same, that two causes participate in the formation of the picture.

Individual diseases are direct products of the disposition: they are nothing but the expressions of the congenital disposition, which manifests itself at a certain age (amaurotic idiocy, process shifts of schizophrenia, arteriosclerosis). We assume that in accordance with fate the disease would here break out under all circumstances. Nevertheless in the individual case some still think of chance causes, which were necessary to *set free* the disease, or have at least participated in some way (reenforcing, hastening the outbreak) in the success of the disease. Precisely in arteriosclerosis one always looks for external causes.

Besides, the layman, and even now many physicians still have the same idea about the appearance of a disease, to which one is predisposed, as about the appearance of a running nose through a cold. In addition, when it is a question of the psychoses one thinks mostly of psychic injuries. But as far as temporary injuries are concerned, there is not the least basis in experience for such an assumption. People who consider it quite obvious that any unfortunate occurrence "can drive one crazy," and that confinement in the insane asylum will "surely make one crazy," mistake transient reactions for permanent maladies resulting from dispositions. Only where the harmful influence is permanent can it sustain a permanent reactive psychosis: delusion of being pardoned in life-prisoners, paranoid, or damage suit neurosis. And when we speak in such cases of a "disposition" for the concerned diseases, the expression means here something quite different than the disposition for schizophrenia or for arteriosclerosis, which in the light of hitherto conceptions is nothing but the germ of the disease, whereas in the latter examples the disease represents only an accidental special reaction to a general reactive predisposition.

As to the very different things that are understood by "occasion for something" ("Anlass"), and what causative and at the same time formative meanings it conveys, is too familiar to require here more than a few suggestions. In the vocation of the saloonkeeper there is the "occasion" for becoming an alcoholic, in the war, for dreaming or hysterical manifestation, in fever or in a nephritis, there is the occasion for a catatonically colored delirium, in alcoholism for the outbreak of epilepsy, in Bright's disease for an amentia, in a fracture of the head of the femur or in an exhaustive disease for a senile dementia, and in childbirth for a schizophrenic shift. The latter connection as well as the hysterical manifestations with their causes belong in the sphere of the psychogenetic, which are not unknown in the present time; an exaggerated or qualitatively abnormal stimulus in a corresponding disposition leads to a psychosis or neurosis; the same happens in the case of a normal stimulus, if the kind or force of the reactivity is abnormal.

Still more could be said about the "structure of the psychosis"; the material mentioned should show only about what points of view come into consideration, and how complicated are the various factors influencing one another. Analogous points of view could also be considered in the study of the *demolition*, improvement, and flattening down of the diseases.

CHAPTER VIII

THE RECOGNITION OF INSANITY

In the diagnosis of insanity in general it is hardly ever possible to obtain in *a single examination* a complete morbid picture, or to follow a general plan of examination.[1] One would never finish and would worry or irritate the patient unnecessarily. And only at exceptional times is it feasible to keep to a definite procedure in the examination. When the patient indicates a symptom to us, e.g., an hallucination, it is usually advisable to follow the trail at once. Often, too, we are forced to verify only a few cardinal symptoms and of the others as much as is still necessary and possible under the circumstances.

But in this respect one must not be too modest; the more one knows, the more certain the diagnosis and the more definite the therapeutic measures. *The human psyche is so complex that much that at first seems a sure symptom of a definite mental disease is not infrequently explained as something else when all the circumstances are known.* It frequently suffices to make only the diagnosis of the mental disease without, however, ascertaining the particular psychosis. This is the case when an excited, or violent, or fasting, or suicidal patient is to be committed to a hospital as quickly as possible. The eventual necessity of a neurological, ophthalmoscopic, and general physical examination should always be borne in mind.

Since a general examination is not possible as in somatic diseases where one begins at the head, and ends with the feet, the only thing to do is to follow up those symptoms which one was called to treat

[1] Plans for examination have been devised which naturally take into consideration everything existing and, for that reason, must give a too large number of viewpoints. It may be a good thing for a beginner to read them through carefully and note everything that might be considered. But in the examination itself one must be able to hit upon the selection necessary for the special case, not only in the interest of the patient, but especially of the physician who otherwise, as experience shows, easily neglects the important point. This important point, namely, the examination of the chief symptoms with their theoretical and practical associations, simply does not permit of schematization and, therefore, compared with the remaining trifles in the scheme, necessarily falls short.

or that immediately strike one's eye, and think of those diseases that can produce such manifestations, and then look around for other signs of the disease. If the suspicion is neither positively nor partially confirmed, then other possibilities will have to be considered. *In order to do this, it is necessary to carry in one's head the symptomatology of at least the more important individual diseases.*

The *kind of questioning* is of the greatest importance. In the first place, if it is at all possible, one must not irritate the patient until the most important information has been obtained. It is much better to gain his confidence, naturally without taking him in. An examination under false pretenses should be avoided. If a patient does not talk, a physical examination can be made, perhaps occasionally, as if by accident, a question may be put to him as "Does this hurt?" or something similar and so induce the patient to speak. One can observe much in both the mental and physical field without the patient's noticing it; thus one can become accustomed to notice the pupilary reactions in an ordinary conversation. One will always keep in mind the whole situation *as it appears to the patient.* The identical question with or without introduction may, in one situation or another, be a very good one, or such that it makes the patient unfit for a further examination. "How much is twice two?" may be a good question but under other circumstances it may suggest to the patient another question, viz., whether the physician is crazy. A test of the sense of pain with needle pricks is something entirely different if the patient is distracted or not, if one dashes at him with the instrument, or first begs him to indicate whether he notices the prick, etc. In short, in these matters one must have some practice and above all native tact and comprehension of the situation and the consequences, otherwise all special directions and details are useless.

One must never forget that the examination in the clinic, where the examiner usually knows the patient and where the entire situation facilitates many questions, is entirely different from the examination in a first consultation. The latter requires much greater care.

Naturally, whenever possible, one endeavors to obtain a good *anamnesis.* If this is possible before the examination, it can materially shorten the entire procedure, since in many cases one then needs only a confirmation of its important data by the patient to be sure of the diagnosis. But even after the examination one must not hesitate to supplement or obtain the anamnesis, because only now does one know in all respects the drift of the situation. In this matter one must not be too gullible. No anamnesis is entirely impartial; purposely or accidentally with good or bad intentions, a great deal is invented both on the good and the bad side. One should be especially careful about an anamnesis which is obtained from the patient himself. Correctly used, it frequently furnishes an absolutely clear diagnosis despite the patient's wishes.

Something entirely different from a single examination is a *complete examination or observation* which is usually necessary in giving a professional opinion. Here one must be assisted by the other departments which the clinic offers and possibly by other specialists, such as the examinations of the eyes, ears, blood, fluids, etc. This technique must be acquired in institutions or at least from textbooks. Such examinations can usually only be done in institutions.

The intelligence examination will be discussed in the chapter on Oligophrenia.

If a case is not clear without it and under all circumstances, if one must handle the patient oneself, *a minute physical* and *especially neurological examination* must not be omitted.

In patients who are inclined to assume tense attitudes or who are otherwise awkward, the *patella reflexes* are best taken not with the knees crossed but with the feet somewhat forward and the whole sole resting flat on the ground. If they are absent, they can sometimes be obtained by Buzzard's method, that is, by raising the heels in this position with the point of the foot left on the ground.

In testing the *pupillary reflexes* the beginner often makes mistakes. The directions recommended for avoiding them are contradictory; clinical experience, one's own good sense, care and adaptation to the special case must help along.

One does well to observe the pupillary reflexes while conversing with the patient. In doubtful cases the room should be darkened and lighted. Restricted sources of light, especially the pocket flash light, are likely to result in false reactions. Touching the lids is often responded to by patients with irritability or stubbornness. One should be careful not to confuse in the insane, light—and accommodation—and psychic reactions.

For examination of *cerebrospinal fluid* see the section on organic psychoses in general (p. 238).

Clinical experience alone can teach the *technique of mental* examinations. One must know from observation what a blocking or a rigid mimicry is; whoever would depend on theoretical descriptions will be helpless before the patient, or make the crassest mistakes. Most psychic symptoms are exaggerations of normal mechanisms; for that reason one must not only see them, but also evaluate them. Whether an affective stupor, a blocking, or a speech disturbance is pathological cannot be described, and still less whether these matters are pathognomonic of a particular disease. *Clinical experience, too, must teach one to understand the descriptions with the necessary grain of salt. Words cannot do more than seize upon a pronounced "typical" facies from the endless variety of psychic manifestations; only observation can decide to what extent such an example should be generalized and to what extent not.*

As far as the individual functions are concerned, attention should be called to the following

Whether the patient is *oriented,* usually shows of itself. When necessary, a few questions will make for certainty.

Even the layman can recognize *sense deceptions* usually from some contradiction with ordinary experience, although in individual cases one will have to prove the reality of the perceptions. A great many hallucinations may be recognized by the fact that they cannot be described in such detail as a perception. Like dreamers, the patients often hallucinate only what matters to them; they can see a part of a body, but then rather imagine the person to whom it belongs than perceive him. Concerning the voices, the patient at times gives only the sense; the hallucinator cannot say which of several synonymous expressions he has heard, or even when he states it positively, he frequently contradicts himself in repeated accounts. Upon exact quest oning the illusions often are differentiated from reality as "pictures," or "inner voices," or something similar. But there are many exceptions; the visual hallucinations of delirium tremens are especially distinguished for their detailed elaboration.

Direct questions concerning *hallucinations* are frequently incorrectly answered in the negative (denial, inhibition); with patients whom one does not yet know, it is advisable to inform oneself indirectly through such questions as "Do you sleep well? Does any one disturb you? Do the neighbors concern themselves with you much?" etc.

Similarly in *delusions.* Where their content does not prove incorrect from the first, one should, when possible, test their objectivity. But this is not the only criterion and, precisely considered, not at all the decisive one. A mistake involves also an incorrect judgment, and a delusion may by chance correspond with reality. It would be really futile to examine the objective foundation of a jealousy delusion; the decisive factor is the patient's subjective confirmation of it. If for his firm conviction he offers no other grounds than that his wife's bed was once particularly warm, that twice in succession the same man met her as she was leaving the house, that she looked frightened when the patient came home unexpectedly, then it is a question of delusions whether the wife is in reality faithful or not.

In many cases, *perception* is naturally tested indirectly. One can easily see whether people see and hear correctly. One will notice how quickly they comprehend questions, whether one must repeatedly explain things, and for what reasons. Optical comprehension can also be tested by reading; especially convenient for this examination are suitable pictures that are not too large, which one quickly uncovers, and then covers, but in this connection one must know what may be expected from a normal person.

In most cases the *associations* need not be specially examined; every conversation, especially when one lets the patient talk, is an association test. Milder flight of ideas becomes evident, if one stimulates the patients somewhat and lets them tell what interests them. The association experiments which are ordinarily unnecessary have to be practised somewhat if one wants to use them.

Memory is already tested in taking an *autanamnesis;* many questions can be put in such a way that they will throw light also on this function. The memory for happenings in the course of the examination (impressibility) is examined by again asking the patient after a little while what was discussed in the beginning and by having him repeat examples that have been given him. Isolated numbers of from four to six digits and rare words or whole sentences very often cannot be reproduced at once even by healthy persons when they are somewhat excited. At all events, one must make sure that the patients understood what was said to them and to a certain degree comprehended it.

Affectivity can be examined directly only in very few cases; one can always see how the patient reacts; furthermore one can give him an opportunity to show a difference in his reaction to important matters and to trifles, and to exhibit morbid lability, etc.

For anomalies of the *impulses* one must usually question, if they are not indicated in the anamnesis; but perversions like homosexuality and similar anomalies are often indicated in the whole behavior and in the dress of the patient.

If in order to test different functions one wants the patients *to read and recount a story,* the following illustrations, according to our experience, are especially well adapted for it, obviously because they contain repetitions. The first, exacts the easiest and the last, the most difficult demands:

The Donkey Loaded with Salt

A donkey, loaded with salt, had to wade a stream. He fell down and for a. few moments lay comfortably in the cool water. When he got up he felt relieved of a great part of his burden because the salt had melted in the water. Longears noted this advantage and at once applied it the following day when, loaded with sponges, he again went through the same stream.

This time he fell purposely but was grossly deceived. The sponges had soaked up the water and were considerably heavier than before. The burden was so great that he succumbed.

A remedy does not do for all cases.

Neptune and the Laborer

A day laborer worked along a stream. By accident his ax fell in and, as the stream was so deep that he could not get it out, he sat on the bank and bemoaned his fate to the river god.

Neptune took pity on the man's poverty, dived down and brought up a golden ax. "Is this yours?" he asked the laborer. The latter honestly answered "no." Suddenly Neptune dived down again and appeared before the woodcutter with a silver ax. To this one, too, the laborer made no claim. For the third time the god dived and brought up the right iron ax with the wooden handle. "Yes, that is it. That is the right one. That is the one I lost," the laborer exclaimed joyfully. "I only wanted to test you," replied Neptune; "I am glad that you are as honest as you are poor. There, take all three axes; I present them to you."

The honest man told this story to several acquaintances. One of these wanted to misuse Neptune's goodness and for this reason he purposely threw his ax into the stream. Hardly had he begun to bemoan his fate to the river god when the latter appeared with a golden ax. He asked, "Is this the one that fell into the stream?" He quickly exclaimed, "Yes, that is it," and grabbed for it. But Neptune denounced him as a shameless liar because he wanted to deceive even a god and turned his back on him. With him disappeared the golden ax and the laborer had to go home without even his own ax.

Honesty is the best policy.

A Miser Trick

The inhabitants of Cufa were considered the stingiest Arabs. Once one of them heard that in Bassora there lived a miser from whom all stingy ones might learn something. When he came to him he frankly confessed the reason for his visit. "You are welcome," said he from Bassora; "we will go to the market and shop."

They went to the baker. "Have you good bread?" "At your service, gentlemen, fresh and white as butter!"—"You see," said the man from Bassora to him from Cufa, "Butter must be better than bread because bread is compared with butter. We will, therefore, do better to buy butter."

They went to the butter dealer and asked if he had good butter. "At your service, butter as fresh and sweet as olive oil!"—"You hear," said the host, "The best butter is compared with oil, this will therefore be better."

They went to the oil merchant. "Have you good oil?" "Of the best, light and clear as water!" "Hoho," said the man from Bassora to him from Cufa, "according to that water is the best of all! I still have a whole barrel at home with which I will serve you liberally."

In fact he served his guest nothing but water since water was better than oil, oil better than butter and butter better than bread. "Good," said the miser from Cufa, "I did not come here in vain; I have learned much."

Under certain circumstances one can draw conclusions concerning attention, impressibility, registering in general, if after the patients have been some time in a room unknown to them, one has them close their eyes and then asks them to tell what objects are in the room.

One must never forget to obtain a clear idea of the *attitude of the patient toward the examination.* Some errors are not due to inability but to emotional stupor, indifference, negativism, and ill will. Characteristic of embarrassment in examinations are answers in which the given material is mixed up, as when in figuring, single figures in the problem are put into the answer, etc.

Moreover, neither in the diagnosis nor in any other examination must the totality of the objective and subjective conditions be overlooked. In the complicated psychic mechanisms the identical manifestations have under different circumstances an entirely different significance. Senseless delusions indicate in the clear average patient an existing dementia, but not in the oligophrenic, or in the delirious patient. Somatic hallucinations only when accompanied by clear mindedness are sure to demonstrate a schizophrenia. Catatonic symptoms in acute conditions becloud the prognosis little, in chronic conditions they have a bad significance. A "rigid" affect may indicate an examination stupor or schizophrenia. "Negativism" in a sensitive person may be the result of the physician's demeanor or of some other part of the situation. A delirious patient with whom it is difficult to establish a relationship is, as a rule, a schizophrenic or he has epilepti-form attacks. But in exceptional cases such behavior may be a symptom of a *light* delirium.

Such a patient who for the three days showed an otherwise typical alcoholic delirium turned his back on us, gave either no answer or short, rejecting ones. He was a vagrant of rather exaggerated joviality, who had often been locked up for trifles and considered such measures as unjustifiable, especially too, his commitment to the clinic because they had lied to him about it. In the mild development of the delirium he was conscious of these circumstances, and on account of which fact he later explained his reaction.

Some psychic symptoms also occur in diseases which we do not describe here, such as fevers, traumata, heart diseases, uremia, eclampsia, and similar diseases. What is still more important is this: *one must never expect the reverse, namely to see in a given moment all the important symptoms of a disease. One must never, for example, conclude that if there is no affective disturbance, therefore it is not a case of Schizophrenia. Indeed under certain circumstances even in a pronounced psychosis one can temporarily find nothing morbid. A negative finding without prolonged observation, therefore, never proves that the patient is normal; it only indicates an absence of proof of the disease.*

Simulation and Dissimulation. Simulation of insanity is not nearly so common as the layman supposes. *Those who simulate in-sanity with some cleverness are nearly all psychopaths and some are actually insane. Demonstration of simulation, therefore, does not at all prove that the patient is mentally sound and responsible for his actions.* The decision as to whether there is simulation must in most cases depend on the evidence of the absence or presence of inimitable symptoms. Those who have not had long experience in hospitals for the insane, and present a consistent morbid picture, rich in symptoms, are not resorting to simulation. If the deception is not readily trans-parent, observation in an asylum must be required in order to "un-mask" the person.

Simulation is, moreover, proven by inconsistencies, clumsy exag-gerations, and by a representation of a morbid picture, that exists only in the layman's imagination (Beware of *unconscious* simulation as in the Ganser and buffoonery syndromes, puerilism, etc.). A supposed insomnia can be controlled by watching the patient at night. Ex-citements that entail exertion cannot be continued very long because of fatigue; in thrashing about with or without convulsive movements the simulator plainly takes care not to hurt himself, etc. One can also suggest that this or that symptom that belongs to the disease is lacking, whereupon the simulator usually hastens to complete the picture. These are a few indications. All details cannot be described, as one would have to repeat the entire symptomology from this point of view. A very thorough uninterrupted observation, if possible both by day and night, is important. On the one hand this will tire the simulator and, on the other, it will usually produce many evidences of the attempted deception. The first glance often arouses a suspicion of simulation when one notices that the patient who has just been admitted acts in an excited and confused manner and at the same time attempts to orientate himself by glancing about and following carefully everything going on around him.

It is more difficult to judge simple exaggerations in psychopathic or even insane people. Here, too, the line of demarkation between conscious simulation and disease is as faint as in the case where the unconscious acts the part, e.g., in the Ganser syndrome. At times, therefore, one cannot decide how much of the "simulation" is conscious deception and how much emerges from the unconscious as a product of the disease.

Much more frequent than simulation one observes *dissimulation* of a mental disease. Melancholics make it appear that they are cured in order to carry out suicide; other patients, so that they will not be limited in their activities or to obtain an opportunity for carrying out their plans, etc. This dissimulation on the patient's part is, naturally, only a concealment of thoughts and symptoms which they know others regard as signs of insanity. For they themselves do not consider themselves sick.

CHAPTER IX

DIFFERENTIAL DIAGNOSIS

In differentiating the psychoses one has to keep in mind that most of the *individual pictures of conditions and syndromes may occur in different diseases;* one must therefore look in addition to these for concomitant specific symptoms and for specific shades of the syndrome. None of the diseases have specific symptoms and *except perhaps from the course they take, they should therefore be diagnosed only by the careful exclusion of other diseases* ("negative diagnosis"), such as manic depressive insanity, paranoia, hysteria, compulsion neurosis, and the psychopathic conditions. Specific symptoms of amentia, uremia, and many other rarer diseases are not yet known.

In the differential diagnosis also one cannot expect to find at any particular moment all the differentiating characteristics; and there, too, nearly all symptoms are to be valued only in connection with the psychic environment. The psyche offers so many possibilities that through a chance constellation a symptom of one disease, considered specific, may sometimes be imitated by another. Our language, even, cannot cope with the wealth of manifestations and must designate different things with identical or similar names; the pressure activity in mánia, in presbyophrenia, in paretic and several other organic deliria, and that in delirium tremens, are of entirely different varieties and cannot be differentiated by brief designations.[1] Whoever follows diagnostic catch words without paying attention to constellations and nuances will go wrong any moment.[2] Also the *diagnostic observations in the special part of this book make no claim to completeness but emphasize only that which might be insufficiently stressed in the symptomology of the disease, especially in the diagnosis. The essentials for the diagnosis must be gathered from a knowledge of the entire disease. The following remarks, too, are only to be utilized in this sense.*

[1] In many twilight states, too, and in erethic idiocy there are syndromes which could be called pressure activity.
[2] Cf. also footnote, p. 84.

COMPILATION OF THE DIFFERENTIAL DIAGNOSTIC SIGNIFICANCE OF INDIVIDUAL SYMPTOMS

DISTURBANCES OF PERCEPTION [3]

Sense perception is retarded and often falsified in the *organic psychoses,* and in a very similar but not identical sense in *epilepsy;* in *alcoholism* it becomes inexact, but no retardation is seen when tested without apparatus. In all cloudings of consciousness it can be disturbed in various ways.

In *forms of idiocy* the synthesis of combined impressions is affected; the patients see and comprehend the unit but cannot work it into a complete picture. At times the meaning of simple pictures is not recognized, even perspective is not understood.

Real *illusions* may occur everywhere, and are especially prevalent in *clouding of consciousness.*

Of the *hallucinations* those referring to sight usually preponderate in disturbances of consciousness such as delirium, twilight states, etc.; in mental clearness they are rare.

In chronic conditions of schizophrenia accompanied by clearness *auditory* and *somatic hallucinations* predominate; under these circumstances the latter are characteristic of the disease. *Hallucinations and illusions of smell and taste* occur especially in schizophrenia, but also in *delirium tremens,* and in various *twilight states.*

Characteristic of *delirium tremens* are in the first place *tactile hallucinations,* then the numerous *visual hallucinations,* which are multiple, moving, and mostly colorless, often representing particularly small or diminutive objects, especially animals. Along with visions of this sort the patients frequently feel and see threadlike objects, wires, ropes, spittle, and streams of water. Auditory hallucinations, in pure delirium tremens, have noticeably often the character of music, which is otherwise rare. If verbal auditory hallucinations are prominent, it is a question of complications, especially with schizophrenia or with alcoholic insanity.

Auditory hallucinations of a dramatically connected character that refer to the patient in the third person indicate with great certainty abuse of alcohol and occur in acute alcoholic insanity and in alcoholic schizophrenics.

Microscopically reduced hallucinations of sight and touch belong to cocainism. In sniffing cocainism, one frequently observes tangibly distinct voices, visual illusions, and vividly colored visions.

[3] Cf. also p. 56.

In *manic depressive* and in *organic psychoses, visual* and *auditory* hallucinations are most common. In organic patients they are much more frequent at night than in the daytime.

Visual and auditory hallucinations in themselves have no specific significance; they are the ones that may occur in every mental disturbance.

DISTURBANCES OF ASSOCIATION

Flight of ideas occurs in the different *manic states,* at times in *exhaustion,* otherwise hardly ever; thus in epileptic excitements it is extremely rare.

Inhibition of associations, retardation and inability to rid oneself of a sad subject which may run to monideism is a partial manifestation of the various *depressive states.* Other forms of retardation of thought may occur in various diseases such as brain pressure, organic inertia, and toxic states.

In *schizophrenia* and under certain circumstances also in *hysteria* we find blockings as an exaggeration of a mechanism that occurs in every healthy person; moreover, some or all of the influences that otherwise guide associations are often lacking, which results partly in bizarre, and partly in entirely disconnected chains of ideas.

In *epilepsy* ideation is slow and hesitating, the mental content becomes restricted to the ego, there is an inclination to affective colored associations especially to those containing judgments of value, and further to perseverations, tautologies and to circumstantiality in particular; the patients do not easily get rid of a subject without thinking it out in many directions.

In *organic* conditions, too, there is a tendency to perseveration and there is frequently a retardation of all reactions. But more important is the restriction of the number of ideas simultaneously possible. Especially readily absent are those ideas that contradict an actual purpose, whereby organic dementia is most strikingly characterized.

In *oligophrenics* the range of associations is also limited; but what is lacking belongs to the complicated associations, the attainment of which requires a higher psychic activity, and to those that are extraordinary. The patient thinks of what is plain, tangible and ordinary.

In *paranoia,* and in a certain sense in *hysteria* also, some associations are facilitated and others are inhibited, according to whether or not they harmonize with the purposes that are interwoven with the disease. Aside from this there are no anomalies of association.

DISTURBANCES OF ORIENTATION

Orientation as to place and time is disturbed in *advanced organic mental diseases,* and generally in *delirious* and *twilight states of all kinds.* In schizophrenic twilight states correct orientation often exists with the falsified. The other patients know where they are and what time it is, unless chance circumstances falsify these concepts.

Orientation as to situation is as a rule naturally also incorrect if place and time are registered incorrectly; but in addition it may be disturbed in every hindrance to judgment, or as a result of manic ideas or similar anomalies.

Autopsychic orientation, the personality with its relation to the family, occupation, dwelling place, etc., is most readily falsified in paresis and in dreamlike twilight states. It is striking the way it remains intact in the deepest delirium tremens, while an apparently sensible paretic or a schizophrenic readily declares himself to be the emperor or a particular saint.

DISTURBANCES OF MEMORY

In *chronic alcoholism* the memory becomes inexact; katathymic memory illusions, whose content apparently is not far removed from reality, are not rare. In dementia alcoholico-senilis and in Korsakoff's disease there is also an organic memory disturbance. After *delirium tremens* remembrance is incomplete and very inexact; after uncomplicated *acute alcoholic insanity* it is good. After pathologic drunkenness there is usually amnesia. The tendency to phantastic stories is heightened in delirium tremens to *confabulation-like* excuses, and to real confabulations.

The memory of the *organic* group is characterized by an especially marked, or exclusive confusion of the more recent memories. The void is often filled by provoked (perplexity), or spontaneous confabulations. Amnesias after deliria, and confusions are not rare even after mere excitements.

The schizophrenic memory retains all experiences; but blockings and other affective reactions in a given moment very often make it impossible for the patient to utilize his engrams. As there is no elaboration of perceptions in certain chronic stages, the schizophrenic memory often retains insignificant details better than does the normal memory. Memory hallucinations and katathymic illusions are frequent. In spite of the frequent occurrence of deliria and twilight states amnesias are rather rare, and still more rarely are they complete.

In *epilepsy* the memory becomes unsystematically poor. Complete or partial amnesia is an ordinary occurrence after twilight states.

Hysteria at times very markedly transforms memories in accordance with the momentary affective requirements. After twilight states amnesia is apt to be complete, but it is relatively easy to remove it by suggestive influences.

In the *paranoiac*, memory illusions, combined with the morbid self-reference, form the most important foundation of the delusions.

In *oligophrenics* memory varies greatly. All things being equal, the incomprehensible is naturally retained less readily than the comprehensible, and the patients understand poorly the very things that appear interesting to the normal; but hand in hand with this there is often a noticeably good reproduction of unelaborated material.

In *conditions of melancholia* the past life is readily explored for sins. Small errors are transformed into unpardonable crimes; if none are found, they are invented as a sort of memory hallucination or memory illusion.

Even during *manic conditions* but very noticeably after them, the morbid behavior of the patient is later readily justified through transformations in the memory and by putting the blame on the environment. During and after confusions seldom accompanied by flight of ideas, the memory is very incomplete.

Amnesias are to be expected after all disturbances of consciousness and after transitory psychoses generally, that is, after hysterical and epileptic attacks and twilight states, confusions of all kinds, toxemias, especially drunkenness. After similar conditions of schizophrenia (twilight states, hallucinatory states with dreamlike episodes), memory is not always defective and when it is, it is usually only partly so.

Amnesias as to content referring to events, the recollection of which is at the time disagreeable, are frequent in schizophrenia and hysteria.

AFFECTIVE DISTURBANCES

The affectivity is *labile* in organic patients, in alcoholism, in hysteria, and in the later intervals of many manic depressive cases.

Acute displacement of the affective attitude (moods) in the sense of manic or melancholic appearances is seen in alcoholism, in the rather uncommon alcoholic melancholia, in organic psychoses, in schizophrenia (very common), in epilepsy which is of brief duration and also shows the very common irritable depression, in manic depressive insanity, in hysteria, in all kinds of psychopathic states, especially in the cyclothymias, and in oligophrenics where it is as a rule of short duration and often manifests irritable moods.

The *organic* affective disturbances regularly show lability, accessory moods, which are preponderatingly manic in paresis and melancholia, especially in the senile forms.   In alcoholic Korsakoff's disease besides lability, there usually is also a euphoric basal mood, which is not apt to disappear until the later stages of crossness and irritation.

In *schizophrenia* the affects cease to function altogether in severe cases; in milder cases affective reactions sometimes appear and sometimes not; when they are present, they are often rigid.   At times they are absent just at the most important events, whereas trifles are normally accentuated.   In many cases irritation up to the stage of unbounded rage is the only reaction which one sees for a long time; in mild cases irritation may be the only striking symptom.   Parathymia and paramimia are not infrequent.   Ambivalence is nowhere so conspicuous as in schizophrenia.   Besides these, one also sees melancholic and manic affective fluctuations.

In the *epileptic* the affects are easily stirred, readily attain an abnormal intensity but last abnormally long.   At the same time they are massive and not finely differentiated.   Fitful moods of an irritated, depressive or euphoric character are probably never lacking.

The *manic depressive* patient in the interval between manic or depressive attacks often has lability of the affects or lasting states in the sense of milder manic or melancholic moods.

In *hysteria* one sees slight outbreaks during which there is heightening and falling off of the affects.   Reactions to similar stimuli are quantitatively and also qualitatively different, depending on chance intervention.

In *paranoia* the affective state corresponds to the content of the real or delusional experiences.   The affective anomalies that must lie at the root of the disease cannot yet be described more minutely.

Among *oligophrenics* there are excitable and torpid types; briefly all the variations occur that we see in normal and psychopathic persons, and only when possible they run within wider limits.   Besides, many cases evince the same moods as epileptics.

In all *forms of dementia* there is a tendency to outbursts of anger.

Some Special Syndromes

States of stupor occur most frequently in *schizophrenia*, next in *epilepsy, hysteria,* and besides in melancholic states, in the mixed states of manic depressive insanity, and in paresis.

Twilight states are seen in *epilepsy, hysteria* and in *schizophrenia*, occasionally perhaps in *manic depressive insanity*, then in the various *toxic states* (as in the pathologic drunkenness), in states of ordinary *sleep* (somnambulism, etc.), following *cerebral concussions* and *hanging*, in very severe *migraines,* and even as *states of excitement* of purely affective origin in psychopaths (jail outbursts, fugues, etc.).

Symptoms of the *Catatonic type.* Symptoms which from their external appearance must be designated as catatonic,[4] besides occurring in *schizophrenia* appear also in the *organic psychoses;* furthermore catalepsy is not rare in *epilepsy* and is also said to have been noticed occasionally in *hysterical twilight states,* in *oligophrenia,* and in *manic depressive insanity.* Something, that must be called echolalia in spite of an apparently very different origin, besides occurring in schizophrenia and the organic psychoses (very rarely) appears also in *epilepsy, hysteria,* and *oligophrenia.*

Epileptiform attacks, besides occurring in the epilepsies appear in schizophrenia, paresis, presbyophrenia, some forms of arteriosclerosis, alcoholism, including delirium tremens, as affective epilepsy in psychopathics, and outside of psychiatry, in all coarse cerebral diseases, in uremia and eclampsia.

Paretic-like attacks occur in all coarse brain diseases, especially when they involve the cortex.

Compulsive ideas and eventually compulsive impulses we see rather frequently besides in the independently considered compulsion neurosis and compulsion psychosis, also in schizophrenia, but pretty rarely in the various depressive states.

Uremia may also simulate the psychic symptoms as well as most physical symptoms of an organic brain disease or of epilepsy. Eclampsia, too, may for a short time act exactly like epilepsy.

[4] Cf. p. 153.

CHAPTER X

CAUSES OF MENTAL DISEASES

I. Germinal Predisposition. It was always known that mental diseases converge in one family and lack in another, and that in the families with mental diseases the members that are not really diseased very frequently show certain deviations, which often run in the direction of the disease. To be sure those families are rare which on careful search prove entirely free, and the cases with only a few diseased members are always the more common. Nevertheless the *family predisposition* is surely one of the most important determinants for the development of mental diseases.[1] To be sure a predisposition alone need not find expression in disease, even when it undoubtedly shows itself in the particular individual through minor deviations from the normal and through transference to the descendants. Either there are different grades of hereditary predisposition or the predisposition does not "develop" in all into a pronounced disease, or both cases may occur. Besides, we have to presuppose some predispositions which in themselves are not diseased but still form necessary or at least furthering determinants in the development of exogenous diseases: Not every inebriate becomes a "psychic" alcoholic and not every luetic becomes paretic; but certain psychic peculiarities that are discoverable in most candidates for alcoholism and paresis and their families indicate that inherited factors play a rôle even in exogenous diseases.

Formerly it was necessary to assume a general *neuro- and psychopathic family predisposition* that might express itself in the most variegated nervous and mental diseases and psychical peculiarities. But since *Kraepelin* taught us to recognize natural boundaries between several clinical pictures, the concept of psychotic heredity began to be more and more clearly divided into several predispositions, among which may be mentioned in the first place the big groups of schizophrenias, epilepsies and manic depressive insanity. A part of

[1] The conspicuous significance of predisposition shows itself especially in *the insanity of twins* where occasionally both members become sick at the same time and with very similar symptoms, and what is more, that may happen even when they do not live together.

the psychopathies as well as most of the neuroses proved to be the lighter and simpler forms of these hereditary groups.

Very recently the attempt was made to apply the *Mendelian laws* to the hereditary mental diseases and endeavor to make it probable that these are transmitted recessively according to the Mendelian type. But the theoretical and practical difficulties are far too great to have produced something useful so far. We are far from understanding what is involved. With the endless shades of morbid predispositions, from the slight peculiarity of character up to the most pronounced insanity, it is out of the question that the predisposition to a psychosis or even the disease itself should be a plain indication that can be present or absent only as a whole; we would rather say that at present we cannot dispense with the assumption of a mechanism, which may be provisionally designated as "intermediary heredity." [2] Furthermore the small number of children and the long duration of a generation increase the difficulties of the survey in these studies to a particularly high degree.

Besides these lasting family predispositions *"Degenerations"* are spoken of. The term designates very different but very vague ideas, and most observers are so little conscious of this that they do not at all express themselves about it, but secretly permit one meaning to pass over into the other, or suddenly substitute one for the other. These concepts may be arranged into four classes, two relating to the family, and two to the individual:

1. It is assumed that some families degenerate through the different generations, that they become more and more incapacitated and generate severer forms of mental diseases, until they die out. *Morel* even supposed that this occurs so regularly that it was possible to prognosticate definite diseases for each of the last four generations. As a matter of fact there is really no such regularity and we cannot say anything worth while either about degeneration or regeneration. Furthermore the Mendelian conceptions which are clear and hold good for certain conditions present an insurmountable opposition to such views. In more recent times morbid predispositions were progressively (not regularly) produced, throughout generations, by means of poisons.

2. It has also been customary for some time, regardless of the progressiveness of the predisposition, to designate families in which insanities are very common, as degenerate, especially if the healthy members also show striking peculiarities.

3. Depending somewhat on this concept, constitutional peculiarities

---

[2] *Bleuler*, Mendelismus b. Psychosen spez. bei der Schizophrenia. Sheweiz. Arch. f. Neurologie und Psychiatrie. Vol. I. Zürich 1917.

in the individual are designated as "degenerative," in which case usually the impression is made as if a definite concept were being used. But actually the *most different* deviations from the normal in all directions are so designated, provided they are not included in one of the familiar morbid pictures. In this sense all families burdened with heredity and their individual (abnormal) members are degenerates.[3]

4. There are also *degenerative psychoses* that are again divided into two very different classes: (a) those that show the characteristics described in classes 2 and 3, that develop, or are supposed to develop from an abnormal constitution (Paranoia, "periodic forms"), or where serious peculiarities of character are observable as causes or concomitant of the "real" morbid picture (degenerative hysteria). (b) Such diseases as have the tendency to "degenerate" i.e. they show a tendency gradually to become worse, to degenerate into dementia as seen in our schizophrenias so far as they really merge into idiocy.

One should avoid working with such an ambiguous conception as degeneration and its designation. The concept of degeneration would most readily fit blastophthoric conditions, the most marked developments of which we call teratologic, and the milder forms perhaps might include all kinds of predispositions even those of psychoses. Families with many abnormal members like those abnormal individuals mentioned in class *3* we call *psychopathic;* those with a tendency to definite mental diseases like those mentioned in class 2, or with less pronounced peculiarities in the sense of a psychosis we name accordingly manic depressive, schizoid, or epileptoid families.

Race is an important consideration for the origin as well as for the formation of the diseases, even though at present we know very little that is definite about it. The great number of insane we find in the present culture races; but whether, and to what extent, more insanity occurs, or more remain alive, and how much the damaging influence of natural selection amounts to, has not yet been investigated. Many peoples, notably North Africans, Abyssinians, South Slavs, Turks, and Australian aborigines, are entirely or to a high degree immune to paresis, although syphilis is common among them. Still our ancestors more than four generations ago were also apparently immune and, on the other hand, the Japanese who are far less closely related to us are now as subject to paresis as we. The more or less extensive use of alcohol does not explain all these differences. Dementia præcox, epilepsy and idiocies also seem to occur in lower

[3] *Magnan's* idea of degeneration is a combination of 2 and 3.

races as with us, the first, to be sure, in somewhat different forms. *Kraepelin* observed among the Malays an absence of the catatonic forms; I could ascertain the same among negroes and Indians as far as modes of appearances are concerned that could be observed as pronounced catatonias on just walking through institutions and in questioning physicians and head nurses. The same may be said here of suicide, whereas just the Germanic race and especially the Saxons are very frequently victims of suicide. It is said that *Jews* are especially predisposed to manic depressive insanity and psychoneuroses. According to a very experienced older psychiatrist they did not develop paresis until they took to "Christian customs and Christian champagne"; in general, race and manner of living, that is to say culture, are difficult to separate.[4]

II. Blastophthory. It seems that even with sound parental predisposition the germ may be so damaged in its development that the descendant becomes (mentally) diseased. Such influences are ascribed especially to debilitating diseases, poisons (alcohol!), and infections. But in the last, among which syphilis comes into prominent consideration, one cannot properly separate the transference of the disease to the child from the germinal damage. In this field many assumptions are opposed by a few definite facts.

III. Germ Fusion. There are a few cases that seem to prove that an unsuitable fusion of healthy germs ("germinal enmity") can generate diseases; thus a couple produced only microcephalics, while each of the individual parents had healthy children with another mate. Also marked differences in the character predispositions of the parents make themselves felt, according to all we know, in a certain lack of equilibrium in the descendants. To be sure, in individual cases this may become the foundation of, and the impulse to, great achievements, especially the artistic; generally it is nevertheless an unpleasant supplement to life and one that readily erupts into the neurotic. The intermingling of races, even those closely related, often has still worse results although, at least according to superficial observations of masses, the West Indian negroes in whom a white streak is easily noticed, are a tribe so capable of enjoying life and so unburdened with any sense of responsibility that one may well ask whether it is not we who constitute the unsuccessful variety of humanity.

Relationship between parents (inbreeding) is also much feared. But it turns out that, in spite of the experience of animal breeders, who have to reckon with many more generations, that under human

[4] See below, American Negroes.

conditions injury through intermarriages is not demonstrable unless there is a summation of a common predisposition to disease in the vulgar sense, or a cumulation in the Mendelian sense. In Incas, the Pharoahs, the Ptolemys, propagated themselves through numerous generations by marriages between brother and sister, and an inter-marriage within a healthy family in every event offers better chances than the intermingling of doubtful or perhaps diseased foreign blood. Nevertheless, in view of the many cases of deaf mutism and of optic atrophy observed in intermarriages as well as the experiences with animal breeding it behooves one to observe a certain caution.

IV. Fœtal Diseases. The embryo, too, may be harmed by diseases of the mother, lack of room in the pelvis, by traumatic occurrences, as well as by intrauterine diseases, so that it comes into the world as an idiot or psychopath. To what extent psychical influences on the mother harm the fœtus, has not been scientifically determined. Undoubtedly sorrow and other chronic depressions may disturb nutrition; and a psychic shock—perhaps through a spasm of the uterine vessels—may be noticed by the foetus to such an extent that it may find a vent in wild movements with change of position whereby injuries of various kinds are conceivable.

The categories I to IV are often designated as *"endogenous causes."* But only I, the pathological germ predisposition, is really endogenous; the remaining, at least in relation to the family, are exogenous, and in relation to the individual they may be called what one pleases. In studies of heredity all four categories were hitherto usually thrown together. It is very important for future research that this should no longer be done.

If all people were designated as "burdened" who have among their blood relations (parents, grand-parents, children, brothers and sisters, aunts and uncles) members who suffer from mental or nervous diseases, alcoholism, apoplexy, abnormal character or have committed suicide, then according to *Diem* [5] 67% of the healthy and 78% of the insane who are admitted to institutions are burdened. But the difference becomes greater, if one counts only those burdened with insanity (7: 38%) or with abnormal characters (10: 15%) and still greater, if these categories are supplied merely to the direct burdening (through the parents), since only 2% of the healthy have insane parents as against 18% of those who are mentally diseased, and 6% abnormal characters against 13%. Apoplexies and nervous diseases are observed

[5] Die psycho-neurotische Belastung der Geistesgesunden und der Geistes-kranken, Archiv. für Rassen-und Gesellschaftsbiologie 1905.

less frequently in the families of the insane than in those who are healthy.

Nowadays heredity is talked about too much, although in practical affairs it is not often considered. Many people actually make life hard for themselves because on account of a hereditary burden they are afraid of getting sick or being sick. As a matter of fact, families in which the majority of the members are sick are rare. Furthermore a sort of regeneration is possible, even though we do not feel at all clear about this term, and above all the difference between those considered burdened and those considered healthy is not so great, because on careful examination abnormalities are generally to be found also in the latter. It should not be forgotten, also, that many diseases have no hereditary significance, as for instance most acquired forms of idiocy and paresis. Furthermore, a sick member of an otherwise healthy family is usually less dangerous even as a patient than a relatively sound member of an otherwise heavily afflicted family. In the former case the exception may be determined by an acquired disease, in the latter it may represent a chance aberration upwards; both variations are not true to kind. For questions of eugenics *Forel* described the risk as follows: that a family in which insanities occur, but which in spite of this maintains itself, is not to be feared; while members of a declining family should not marry or be married.

V. The exogenous causes affecting the individual sometimes create disposition, sometimes they precipitate the disease either as a necessary consequence (carbon monoxide) or as the cause (psychic reasons), or as one of the various necessary conditions of the disease (syphilis in paresis). It is furthermore to be kept in mind that while individual causes frequently produce definite morbid pictures, (e.g. traumatic neuroses; alcoholism, paresis) nevertheless, depending on the disposition and the constellation of other contributing conditions, the identical (major) causes may generate and occasion different morbid pictures, such as different traumatic neuroses, hysteria and neurasthenia in certain conflicts, and various alcoholic forms. The same psychic influence may release a schizophrenic attack in one person, a neurosis in another, a manic attack in a third. Furthermore, depending on the disposition the cause may be indifferent, thus a woman predisposed to cyclothymia can become manic through a psychic influence or through a childbirth, and the epileptic disposition can probably be developed into pronounced epilepsy just as well by a trauma as by alcoholic poisoning. It can be seen from the illustrations that no decided distinction is to be made between causative and merely precipitating conditions; but we must understand that it is a different matter when a fright neurosis or carbonic oxide poisoning develops in a healthy person than when the disease becomes "manifest" through a psychic influence, in a latent schizophrenic or manic depressive patient. But intermediate cases make it impossible to carry out a sharp separation.

Among the exogenous causes discontinuation of *soothing with the natural nourishment* is to be mentioned also,[6] although here, too, we should like to know something more definite.

Moreover all diseases are to be considered that *directly affect the brain,* such as traumata, and in childhood above all polioencephalitis and meningitis, which create oligophrenias, psychopathies, epilepsies, and organic diseases. Scleroses, tumors, and other brain diseases cause different pictures. *Infectious diseases* may change the anatomical consistency of the brain, as cerebral lues, paresis, encephalitides, and lyssa, or they may affect its function through poisoning as in fever psychoses, and in the forms of "delirium acutum," or they may indirectly disturb its nutrition as in syphilitic diseases of the blood vessels. Besides the fever psychoses, infectious diseases can probably precipitate schizophrenic "shifts."

Other physical diseases which in respect to the brain may be called exogenous not seldom cause mental diseases; carcinomatous dyscrasia and perhaps stomach and bowel disturbances can also produce states of confusion; diabetes seems to favor depressions; through the neuritic processes in the brain it can bring about Korsakoff's syndrome, and through acetone poisoning delirious conditions. Of course, diabetes is also frequently only a parallel manifestation of the mental disease, e.g. in organic brain diseases. Hypo-function of the thyroid gland causes myxedema and cretinism; a certain complicated hyper-function causes Basedow's psychoses. The other glands are also connected with the psychic, but they are very far from being sufficiently understood.

Of the external *poisons* alcohol is to be particularly mentioned. It is responsible for 20 to 35% of the male admissions to the hospitals, and probably makes alcoholics of 10% of the men outside,[7] but it also complicates, co-determines, or aggravates other psychoses, especially epilepsy, traumatic neuroses, and paresis.[8] A similar even though numerically a vastly minor rôle is played by ether, opium, morphine,

[6] Bunge, Die zunehmende Unfähigkeit der Frauen, ihre Kinder zu stillen. 7. Aufl. Rheinhard, München 1914.

[7] Schweizerische Statistiks. Sanitarisch-demographisches Wochenbulletin, 1903, und Internationale Monatschrift zur Bekaempfung der Trinksitten, 1904, p. 183.

[8] The influence on posterity was discussed in Part II.

and cocaine.[9] Other poisons that enter into consideration here are lead, carbon monoxide, pellagra and ergotine. Some also wish to blame here tobacco, which is probably an unjust view. Lack of *vitamines* acts like the poisons, as in the case of Beri-beri.

Among other diseases those of the sense organs, especially that of hearing, are to be mentioned; the latter do harm rather through their psychic influence. Thus paranoid distrust and irritability result from defective hearing, heart and vascular diseases occasion anxiety states and atrophies of the brain, while kidney diseases are often at the foundation of amentia.

Exhaustion[10] also is said to produce insanities; there is no doubt that hunger in its last stages causes deliria. That *over-work*, which is frequently mentioned may bring on mental diseases, is not to be assumed; it usually conceals politely our ignorance of the causes,— a good physician works much more than most of the patients that come to him because of over-work. It is more proper to assume that the congenital "morbid exhaustiblity" expresses the predisposition to psychoses. But usually it is emotional difficulties that "exhaust the nervous energies," or the slowly advancing schizophrenia deludes the patient with a feeling of exertion and over-exertion. Among ten thousand Serbs captured in the late war, who were all subjected to the most miserable state of maximum over-exertion and severe undernourishment, only five became insane. Therefore, acute physical exhaustion, at least, may be crossed off the list of the causes of psychoses. Weakness from *acute loss of blood* is also not a cause of psychoses, according to statements that I have received from surgeons.

Among *living conditions* climate should be mentioned; but as yet we do not know its influences. Concerning the so-called *Tropical mania* which is naturally a collective term for different things, it is not even certain to what extent it is really brought on merely by the heat, and to what extent by the use of alcohol and by other diseases, and by the feeling of being absolute master of life and death among savages (a sort of Cæsar mania).

Occupation may cause poisoning, thus employees of the alcohol industry readily become alcoholics, and persons occupied with the healing art become morphine addicts. In the army many psychopaths succumb to disease less from exertion than from psychic causes. Some occupations, such as school teaching and acting, are said to dispose

[9] Most recently the use of cocaine in the form of snuff powders is very rapidly gaining the ascendency with the demi-monde and its associates.

[10] According to *Kraepelin* exhaustion is the excessive consumption or insufficient replacement of the active substances, while fatigue is the accumulation of waste matter that has a paralyzing effect.

people to mental diseases. But what is more likely to be the case is, that affected or rather psychopathic people show a preference for certain callings, just as no occupation or tramping is selected only by morbid or insane individuals.

According to the classification of *civil conditions* there are a great many single persons among the insane, and it is plausible that the more regular life of the married, in sexual and other respects, is a slight protection against disease. But it should be remembered that half of all the patients, the oligophrenics, cannot marry because of their disease; and the same is true of those schizophrenics who are afflicted when young. Other abnormal individuals do not marry because of various psychic reasons, and people who are divorced are very often not normal. Thus there remain only the widows and widowers that could demonstrate the danger of being single and it is really said that the latter become sick more frequently than the married.

According to experience *civilization,* so called, is one of the most important breeding places of mental diseases. The "higher" the scale of civilization the more insane are noted. Of course, this is in part misleading because the care of the helpless that civilization demands simply does not permit them to perish as they do under natural conditions. Nevertheless there is no doubt that our *kind* of civilization does favor the disease causing agencies, of alcohol and lues, and in America it was discovered that the negroes, who as slaves had no percentage of insanity worth mentioning, become insane in greater numbers the more they approach the manner of living of the whites, and that in the northern states where they are quite acclimated they also attain the same morbidity. Furthermore, it cannot very well be otherwise than that the elimination of natural selection gradually increases the number of abnormals. As far as the neuroses and obvious psychopathies are concerned, it goes without saying, that under complicated living conditions, where a conscience and feeling of responsibility exist and are continually needed, they must more frequently—let us say come to light than in carefree and unconcerned people. That those who lead the parvenu life of a metropolis commit race suicide in doing so, has been known for a long time, but the path from the normal to extinction probably traverses in part mental degeneration. Furthermore, just as in domestication of animals the artificial construction of human relationships will produce all sorts of deviations from the normal. Though difficult to evaluate, it is an important circumstance that education is now fraught with infinitely more dangers than in primitive times when the little ones did not soil the curtains and could not break the statuary.

Naturally this is not the place to go into the details of the complicated conditions of the artificial deterioration of race hygiene in a big city; it is sufficient to know that insanity increases with the density of population.

Great significance has always been ascribed to *sexual* conditions, and it is not to be denied that at times a case of gonorrhœa in a college boy who still has a sense of decency may release a depression that must be designated as morbid. Diseases of the feminine genitals are still more frequently blamed and for that reason operated upon— but without valid proof. The most severe blame is attached to onanism, which is supposed to cause all neuroses and some of the more serious mental diseases, and the patients themselves like to support this view. But we see that it is carried on to an incredible high degree by care-free insane patients and moral defectives without visible harm. Direct bodily injury can hardly be proven unless one wishes to regard here the more or less painful feeling of weakness in the back that suggests similar menstrual complaints and not seldom seems to follow excesses. The real conditions are about as follows: Onanism is an unnatural gratification of the most important instinctive impulse of mankind which can be carried on very easily and consequently leads not only to over-indulgence but would endanger the existence of the race if there were no inhibitions against it. It is therefore comprehensible that our instincts are so ordered that our feeling revolts against it. This feeling is supported by social and religious command and, perhaps, most strongly, even though in a harmful way, by a literature that pictures for the adolescent in the most horrible colors the consequences of the evil, in order to extort money from him for cures. Thus where anxiety states and ideas of sin appear, we usually also find accentuated ideas of self-accusations concerning onanism which is thought at least, even if not always expressed. Onanism then becomes the unpardonable sin, and we see, moreover, that the fear of having harmed oneself becomes the cause of many neurotic conditions, which can improve as soon as this fear is removed.[11] Naturally the useless struggle against the bad habit and the resulting loss of self-respect result in very harmful factors. However, onanism is often a *symptom* of disease, especially when it is overdone or carried on in early childhood; or *as a result* of schizophrenic shamelessness it becomes apparent not only because

[11] *Bleuler:* Der Sexualwiderstand. Jahrbuch f. Psychoanalyt. Forschungen Bd. V, 1913.

it is more frequent but also because it is practiced without fear before others.

With a certain emphasis some nowadays also include sexual *abstinence* among the causes of neuroses and even of mental diseases —but again without any proof. The daughters of certain classes, catholic priests, as well as other chaste people, really offer sufficient refutation; but it must be admitted that the general attitude has become so frivolous that in many places, at least among the males, almost only psychopaths remain chaste. If then many of these become sick, it is surely wrong to blame their continence.

Among the sexual functions *menstruation* has a certain causal significance for the psychoses. It rarely happens that the beginning of maturity is marked by conditions similar to twilight or schizophrenic states, which recur a few times at intervals corresponding to the menstrual period but disappear with the regular setting in of the menses, without leaving any psychopathic traces. Later the menstrual moodiness which is not uncommon in "normal women" might be heightened to a degree that may be designated as melancholic depression; at all events suicides among women occur noticeably often at this time. States of confusion also are said to occur with or without impulsive acts. In addition the menstrual period can set free fairly regular attacks of manic depressive insanity, while existing psychoses are very often temporarily exacerbated at this time. But it is a plain confusion of cause and effect, if the cessation of the flow, so common at the beginning of an acute psychosis, is represented as the cause of the insanity. A "menstrual insanity" in any definite sense has not been demonstrated in spite of different attempts.

The name *puerperal psychoses,* those psychoses that appear during delivery and up to about four or six weeks after it, are contrasted on the one hand with pregnancy and lactation psychoses, and on the other hand the term is used to designate all of the three forms. But there are no special puerperal psychoses either in the wider or narrower sense of the term. Nevertheless *pregnancy* in psychopathic women, aside from the most different neurotic symptoms, may obviously also condition melancholic depressions in both psychic and somatic ways, or in both together. The delusions of such a psychosis usually refer to the pregnancy and future of the child and disappear after delivery without leaving any traces. It rarely causes the exacerbation of a schizophrenia, otherwise it is probably a case of chance coincidence of pregnancy and insanity. Cases of amentia resulting from exhaustion, hemorrhage, or infection are said to appear in *child bed.* According to my experience it is nearly always a case of schizophrenia which becomes manifest or a schizophrenic exacerbation, the release of which is to be explained mostly along psychic lines. Even a manic depressive attack may sometimes be precipitated by parturition. The *lactation psychoses* have little practical significance.

At the time of the female *climacterium* a slight accumulation of exacerbations of different psychoses shows itself; it also brings with it a particular tendency to depressions. About a decade later we also see in men mild but long lasting curable depressions that belong to the period of involution (climacterium virile). Real *climacteric psychoses* in women, which formerly were not uncommon, have disappeared from the literature of the last few years.

For the remainder, the sexual life has much to do with the causation of mental diseases, especially of the psychoneuroses by way of psychic influences; but we are far from being clear concerning the degree and kind of its effects.[12]

Among the other psychic causes an unsuitable *education* is certainly to be mentioned; as a matter of fact it is always being discussed although to be sure very little is known about it. We have good reasons, however, for the assumption that many neuroses originate through the aid of poor educational influences.

In later life it is only affective influences stirring the mind deeply or for a long time that enter into consideration as causes of neuroses and psychoses. To what extent care and sorrow produce real psychoses is not yet known; no doubt the importance of their rôle is exaggerated by the layman, whereas dissatisfaction, the feeling that life has been a failure and, above all, erotic difficulties (in the wider sense) causes flare-ups of neuroses and exacerbations of the psychoses. In psychopathic persons terror, anger, or despair can produce excitements of blind rage with subsequent amnesia or stuporous states (*emotional psychoses, anxiety deliria*), which quickly pass away. Imprisonment precipitates different psychopathic conditions, also such resembling paranoia; it is also said that *operations* produce mental diseases. This is undoubtedly very rare.

Modern accident laws arouse imaginative desires and have consequently become the most important causes of traumatic neuroses in the wider sense. Other transient mental and nervous disturbances originate in great catastrophes, as in earthquakes.[13]

The public often fears *infection* from the insane. It does not

[12] Concerning the Freudian viewpoint Cf. some observations in the chapter on neuroses.
[13] Cf. Fright neuroses.

exist in this form. On the other hand energetic patients can impart their mania to the apparently healthy who live with them (*induced insanity*). To be sure, occasionally even the entirely healthy are dragged along by insane litigants or reformers. Thus from induced insanity there are all the intermediate stages to psychic and nervous epidemics, such as chorea major, tic epidemics in schools, and religious epidemics, that certainly¹ may attack even well balanced natures.

Childhood disposes to brain diseases, and above all to polioencephalitis. "*Child psychoses*" *sui generis* are not known, unless one so designates oligophrenias which are to be attributed to diseases of infancy, paresis which comes from hereditary syphilis, and the epilepsies that break out at this age. Schizophrenia also, and more rarely manic depressive insanity, at times begin in early childhood. Deliria in childhood are comparatively frequent in cases of intoxication and infection; occasionally they show at these times catatonic symptoms, (e.g. catalepsy), which have no deleterious significance under these circumstances. Hysterias in childhood are frequently monosymptomatic and have less the character of a psychic general disease than those of adults.

The disposition to mental disease increases explosively with *puberty;* and where neither alcoholism nor paresis constitutes an essential part of the disease, the disposition decreases slowly from the twenty-fifth year and quickly between thirty-five and forty.

A "puberty psychosis" peculiar to the period of development is not yet known, unless the above mentioned coincidences previous to the inception of menstruation are to be called so. What used to be so designated were usually schizophrenias.

During *manhood* the alcoholics, paretics and paranoiacs become manifest, then, also the traumatic cases from comprehensible external causes.

The *period of involution* brings with it a small increase of schizophrenic conditions, a more considerable increase of depressions, and then a number of less common diseases, some of which were described by *Kraepelin. But the period of involution is to be sharply differentiated in this respect, as well as in general, from senile degeneration,* even if the two processes may touch each other. Like puberty, it is a *re*-formation for another stage of life; the normal matron for more than two decades is still a capable person.

Senility, on the contrary, is a *retro*-formation, a dying out. If the retro-formation of the brain precedes the retro-formation of the other organs, it shows itself clinically in the pure form of dementia senilis. Moreover, arteriosclerosis and presbyophrenia, while not entirely peculiar to senility, are still most commonly met with it.

The male *sex* is disposed more than the female to idiocy and epilepsy, and less to neuroses and manic depressive insanity. If alcoholism and paresis primarily affect men, this is due to their manner of living; that they prefer this manner of living, is again based on sex. On the whole more men are taken into the insane asylum; but their numbers are generally less than those of women, because the alcoholics are usually quickly discharged and the paretics die. Among the older insane patients there are more women because of the greater longevity of the sex.

CHAPTER XI

THE TREATMENT OF MENTAL DISEASES IN GENERAL

The treatment will here only be considered as far as it concerns the requirements of the practicing physician—and as far as its discussion, independent of clinical demonstration, may be of some use. *Concerning the neuroses reference must be made to textbooks on neurology.*[1]

As yet very little is done for *prophylaxis,* and without a change of the general attitude and legislation very little can be done. The more severely burdened should not propagate themselves. Some have recommended "social sterilization"; others have challenged "the infringement upon human rights" and found it useless. Many diseased and degenerates are themselves quite willing to undergo the operation, and though the opportunity may not be very frequent, it may be of use in individual cases. Moreover the idea is capable of expansion, and that is just what is feared. I do not fear it: because as long as the now current attitude is not completely changed, the danger of overdoing exists almost only in so far as the practice would get ahead of the development of the ideas and consequently might for a long time discredit these measures. I would begin with compulsion in the case of incurable criminals and on the basis of consent in the case of other more serious psychopathics, and then gradually alter the general attitude and legislation in accordance with experience. But if we do nothing but make mental and physical cripples capable of propagating themselves, and the healthy stocks have to limit the number of their children because so much has to be done for the maintenance of the others, if natural selection is generally suppressed, then unless we will get new measures our race must rapidly deteriorate.

Also the *deleterious influences* that act on the germ, among which I class the living conditions in large cities, should be seriously attacked. To quote *Kraepelin:* "It must also be the sacred duty of physicians

[1] Comp. especially the chapter on Psychotherapy by Mohr in *Lewandowsky,* Handbuch der Neurologie, Julius Springer, Berlin. And *Schultz,* Die Seelische Krankenbehandlung (Psychotherapie). Fischer, Jena 1920.

to increase gradually the pressure of public opinion in such a way that the resolution will be formed to take up the battle against alcohol and syphilis with the same emphasis and the same resort to remedies as in the battle against tuberculosis." All "Back to nature" move- ments also are to be supported much more energetically than here- tofore, but not to the bogey that is called nature. Even in our in- dustrial age the race sustaining power of agriculture could be utilized for prophylactic measures.

A purposeful *bringing up* might perhaps prevent many a neurosis. We see, at least, nervousness and morbid characteristics grow directly from an inadequate training and must therefore conclude that proper influences with training of the will and particularly of the character to become habituated to tolerate the disagreeable, including pain, and hardened within sensible limits—all that could preserve from sickness many who are not too severely burdened. A careful *selection of vocation* will also furnish a certain protection. It is also conceivable that the timely solution of inner conflicts in the milder schizophrenic process could postpone the breaking out of secondary symptoms, i.e. of the manifest insanity.

In pronounced disease the chronic cases should be differentiated from the acute. The chronic cases, for the great part, are to be *trained* to normal conduct and work; but since besides physicians few people understand such a training, its direction is still the task for medical men. The layman, even when he is ever so well mean- ing and intelligent, still forgets too easily the difference between sick and well, and thinks he can work with logic and indignation and kindliness, as is properly the case with the healthy. But just in those things that matter, the sick frequently have a false logic and still less do they understand indignation at their acts, which they con- sider proper. Or can gratitude be expected when they do not at all value our sacrifice or only negatively, i.e., when they take them as chicaneries? Here it is a question of carefully ascertaining the patient's general modes of reaction and especially those toward par- ticular individuals, and then act as seems best in the particular situa- tion, and not from a sense of justice, or anger, or sentimental sympathy.

An indispensable means of training is *work*, which also renders incalcuable services against many symptoms. Whoever considers him- self too good for this or whatever kind of work he could still accom- plish is not good enough for it. But also in the beginning of mental diseases, especially of schizophrenias, one should not permit work to be dropped at once without some definite reason. When *adapted to the ability* of the patient, it usually does more good than so-called rest and recuperation, and this is particularly the case in many light melancholias such as the physician will most probably have to treat in his private practice. Mental work, also, is not to be excluded on principle, even though it is frequently not applicable, more because of practical than inner reasons. But the worst is "the poison of laziness" (*Rieger*).

Milder chronic cases can be sent with very good results to a *Psychiatric clinic* where the patient is braced up from time to time, where he receives the necessary remedies, and where a special effort is made to make the external conditions bearable.

In acute diseases the object of obtaining a *cure* is of uppermost consideration, but unfortunately we cannot do as much as we should like. In individual cases special psychiatry has to lay down the necessary rules.

An important question is "Which patients are to be committed to a *hospital for the insane?*" Naturally, all those who cannot be kept outside because they are too dangerous to themselves, to others, or too disturbing. Some can be properly treated only in an institution because they themselves or sometimes their relatives oppose a proper management of the case. Where the danger to the patient's fortune is the chief indication, a legal *guardianship* can at times take the place of an institution or shorten the stay. Not seldom patients must be interned, not because their conditions directly require it, but because their relatives are worn out by taking care of them. It is also not unusual that the family exerts a directly harmful influence on the patient, hence the indication for institutional care lies in the existing conditions.

To intern an insane patient compliance with a number of formalities is necessary, which unfortunately vary in different states. *Every physician who settles down to practice should inform himself about these local formalities;* if he waits until the occasion arises he is apt to encounter many difficulties. In almost every state a physician's certificate is required. In the state of New York it is a legal act and must therefore be carefully filled out with the required data. Besides the petition to the court, signed if possible by the nearest relative, it must also contain a physician's certificate signed by two qualified examiners in lunacy who must examine the patient conjointly within five days of the presentation of the petition. Such a certificate must contain information about the patient's legal standing whether he is charged with a criminal act or not, his financial standing whether he has relatives who are able to pay for his maintenance in the hospital (if not committed to a private institution) and the physical and mental states of the patient, whether he is dangerous to himself and others, whether he shows hallucinations, delusions, depression, exaltation or other abnormal signs. It is often not possible to make a definite diagnosis after one examination but for purposes of commitment this is not essential. It is merely a question whether the patient is insane and unmanageable at home. The necessity for institutional care must in every case be specified. (Is the patient dangerous to the community, does he refuse nourishment, has he suicidal tendencies, etc.?)

Without the legal commitment no insane patient will be admitted to a state institution, so that it is advisable to inquire first of the hospital superintendent whether the patient can be received. Not all hospitals are in position to receive patients at all times.[2]

So much for the administrative details. In addition the physician at the institution should receive all the data required for the treatment of the patient, his outward behavior, presence or absence of particular inclinations or impulses, so that a harmless patient does not have to be sent at once to the observation ward. He should also obtain the anamnesis, information concerning the patient's past treatment and its success; whether the patient was given narcotics on the trip to the hospital, which kind, and in what doses? Hyoscine can give the appearance of a pupillary disturbance and lead to a wrong diagnosis. It is best not to give narcotics on the first day if one does not know whether the patient has already been given the same. Sometimes the physician has no time to ascertain all this and make a note of it. Then he sends with the patient a preliminary certificate with the necessary data and states that the detailed report will be sent on the following day.

Moreover the hospital physician will be grateful to get not only the practically necessary information but also that which may be scientifically interesting.

In bringing a patient to an institution one should not resort to lies and false pretenses; that would make a beneficial treatment impossible and especially in the case of patients who have some self-respect, it would permanently disturb the entire relationship with their relatives. In an emergency it is better to use force or a hypnotic, which is more readily forgiven by the patient. But force is very rarely necessary when the proper procedure has been followed. A large part of the patients can be persuaded, if, without losing one's own

[2] This is not necessary in most of our big cities where psychopathic hospitals or pavilions are maintained for observation, treatment and commitment when necessary.

self-possession, one explains the decision for a hospital on grounds of necessity; but it must be told so decisively that they feel that any discussion whatsoever is useless, and that there are enough people present who would be capable of putting the thing in operation in the face of resistance. It should not be forgotten that it is only in the rarest case that logic itself makes the patient yield; it is the personality of the individual who applies the logic.

When the patient is in a hospital, the family physician frequently has to continue his function as advisor of the family. The questions about private or public institutions, about visiting the patient and taking him home must all be advised by him. In this matter it is difficult to give general rules. One must guard against giving advice without knowing exactly the actual state of the case. It is best to get in touch with the hospital physician; moreover, in such cases professional courtesy is of greater value to the patient and his family than to the professional relationship. At all events the physician should know that manic depressive patients are frequently taken out too soon, and schizophrenics very rarely, unless other considerations than the patient's condition come into account. Only in exceptional cases is home-sickness an indication for taking the patient home; usually what the patient and relatives take as such is not home-sickness at all. The patient does not feel at ease anywhere and then the cause is sought in the separation from home. Patients who are cured hardly ever urge to be sent home. The dreaded "living with other markedly insane patients" is sometimes an unpleasant experience but it is not a hindrance to the cure. It is very harmful if visiting relatives give the patient hopes of coming home or of anything else that cannot be fulfilled later. Moreover, *visits* are sometimes harmful; they frequently disturb an acute patient, especially in the beginning when he has to get used to the institution. I should like to call attention to the younger children who almost without exception overcome home-sickness after a few days, but on condition that they are not visited. But even in the case of chronic patients visits interfere with the adjustment to the new home even where they are carefully and tactfully carried out.

The selection of an institution is frequently not easy. Where overcrowding has not become excessive, public institutions are generally the ones that accomplish most for the least money. This is naturally counterbalanced by the fact that there is frequently less comfort and less consideration for the wishes and moods of the individual. *The latter may also be an advantage.* All private sanatoria are far from being well equipped for restless patients. Sometimes because of the "odium," or from false pride relatives want to avoid public institutions and sacrifice money to this idea that would be better applied in other ways, e.g. during the period of recuperation.[3] But it is self-evident that good private institutions can offer much, especially to spoiled patients, that they are deprived of in a public institution. But it is more difficult to carry out a rigid training there than under the inexorable rules of a general institution (care should be taken especially in deprivation cures, see morphinism).

Some patients, e.g. oligophrenics and cases of schizophrenia that have run their course, can often be trained with success or also kept for a long time in a private family, with a doctor, teacher, or minister. In some places private *family* care is publicly organized also for the poorer classes and has proved to be very successful. The guardians are preferably farmers or former nurses and attendants from hospitals.

The *disease itself* can only be attacked directly in a few cases such as cerebral lues and epilepsy. On the basis of chance experience with dementia præcox, an artificial fever has been produced by the injection of bacterial toxins (*Wagner von Jauregg*). The toxins, however, can be advantageously replaced by somnifen. Tertian plasmodia seem to neutralize the spirochites in paresis.

In despair the family often assumes expensive treatments in cases of incurable patients that set the family back financially and thereby make a later proper treatment of the patients impossible. This is a grave wrong. It should not be forgotten that curable cases are usually cured for the most part by time.

Against emotional fluctuations, distraction sometimes has an effect only in milder cases. To argue with the patient about his delusions is nearly always useless or harmful. One should not conceal his own viewpoint from the patient but at the most,—it should be left to the future to prove who is right.

With the exception of the psychoneuroses, mental diseases offer

---

[3] Such an odium is especially entertained in reference to our State Hospitals, thus furnishing no little problem for the consulting psychiatrist. It is easy enough to dispose of the wealthy patients, they are invariably sent to private sanatoriums, and of the greater part of the poor, who go to state institutions, but one is often at his wits' end to know what to do with middle class patients who cannot afford a first class sanatorium and would under no circumstances go to a State Hospital. I have known families who actually became ruined financially in their zeal of maintaining a præcox in a third rate private sanatorium. The State Hospital could have offered them just as good,—in my opinion much better—service, but owing to the mediæval prejudices which our newspapers continually change into modern garb, the average person is still horrified when a public institution is suggested. (*Editor.*)

no fertile field for *psychotherapy* in the narrower sense.[4] Manic depressives, and similar cases recover from the attack, organic cases perish, while schizophrenics live on uncured. But just in the case of the latter it is of especial importance, whether one understands them, and can think oneself into their condition, only an extensive occupation with psychopathology, delusional and symptomatic formations, blockings and inhibitions, can assist in this. *Suggestion*, whether direct or concealed, will always be carried on, just as in medical practice and in life generally. In some cases *hypnosis* may make many things easier, e.g. in residual conditions like insomnia following melancholia. On the whole, its significance in real psychoses[5] is not great, because as *Forel* expressed it, in hypnosis one works with the patient's brain, which in the case of mental diseases is an inefficient instrument. One of the most important psychical means of therapy is patience, calm, and inner good will for the patient, three things that must be absolutely inexhaustible.

From definite "procedures" in the case of psychoses in the narrower sense, very little is to be expected even though milder cases at times are favorably influenced in hydrotherapeutic institutions where one exercises care. A careless application of cold water may do decided harm. On the other hand baths of normal or near normal bodily temperature are an important help in the treatment of restless and sometimes also of depressed patients. Excitements are often reduced by a bath; a feeling of tiredness without a real reduction of psychical and physical capacities makes the patient more accessible. But even in those cases where this result is not visible the tepid bath (35 to 36° C.) is an excellent resort for the patients who can constantly occupy themselves with the water and thus remain harmless to themselves, to others and to the objects about them. The introduction of the *continuous baths*, used also in some institutions throughout the night, and the use of wards for sleepless patients, has given the modern insane asylum a much better appearance. The depressed patients also are frequently better off in the bath; a warm bath, taken at night, is especially conducive to sleep.

Cold packs are also frequently applied, and the patient is kept in them for about twenty minutes until he gets warm or even for many hours. The latter is only resorted to in the case of good con-

---

[4] That is, psychotherapy according to definite methods, such as that of *Freud, Dubois*, hypnotism, etc. It is self-evident that "psychotherapy" in a wider sense is practiced by every psychiatrist,—I should almost like to say, not as such.

[5] In contradistinction with the neuroses. Even those who are not very skilled in hypnosis will find that such cases as monosymptomatic hysteria or enuresis are frequently readily susceptible of this treatment.

trol of temperature, appearance, and psychical condition. Occasionally they also have a soothing effect. But if the arms are not wrapped up, they are not tolerated for long, just by those patients who need packs most; and if they are put under the blanket this procedure, according to my way of thinking and that of my patients, becomes, under the guise of medicine, the worst means of restraint that exists. I therefore avoid packs as much as possible.

Very many patients, especially the depressed, also schizophrenics who do not occupy themselves, and mild manics are best off *in bed;* if they want to occupy themselves, there is no objection to reading, writing, and feminine handwork. Every modern institution has a number of wards where the patients remain in bed day and night under constant surveillance, but there must be a definite indication for this; one should not merely feel that "patients should be in bed." In chronic cases work is to be preferred if it is possible.

If patients are very excited or annoy and injure others, they are under certain circumstances *isolated.* Nowadays there are physicians, and there were even more ten or twenty years ago, who regard isolation as an atrocity. With discrimination, properly applied, I consider it a blessing for all concerned. In the case of manics who do not necessarily soil everything it is the preferred therapy. And at night probably every healthy person would prefer to be alone in a room, even if it is called a cell, rather than in the company of many lunatics.

Other means of restraint are to be applied most rarely; but when there is a special indication, as in the treatment of a fracture, I consider it wrong to let the patient become a cripple because of consideration of principle.

Where *artificial feeding* is necessary, the patient can only rarely be kept in a private house. A well nourished person, if he remains in bed, can go without food from five to seven days without harmful effects, unless he has previously put himself on half rations. One should not bother with rectal feeding and similar emergency measures. On the other hand there are sometimes roundabout ways by which nourishment may be given the patient; thus some will eat secretly, if food is left within their reach as if by accident. If tube feeding is necessary, it is best done through the nose. The patient is held in a reclining or sitting position firmly enough to preclude a struggle during the process. Then a well lubricated soft tube is inserted into the wider nostril, so thick that it just goes through. The bending at the posterior wall of the throat is forced by a little push. From here on the insertion should be made somewhat quickly, so that the patient has not time to guide the tube into the mouth.

In any case, it is often well to wait for the pharyngeal reflex and as soon as it begins, to shove the tube into the œsophagus. It is then inserted into the stomach, and through the auscultation of a little air, blown in by balloon or mouth, one makes sure of the correct position of the tube. *Lack of reaction by the patient, especially in the case of catatonics, is no guarantee that the tube is not in the trachea.* When the tube is withdrawn the tube should be pinched shut so that nothing flows into the larynx. The simplest thing to inject is milk and half as many eggs as a deciliter of milk. After a prolonged fast one may pour in five deciliters at the most the first time, later one liter of milk and five eggs at a time. Two daily feedings will then usually suffice. The state of nourishment, digestion, vomiting, are naturally always to be watched carefully. Medicines may also be mixed with the food and in case of a longer period of illness a different food, in fluid or semifluid condition, will probably be given in place of, or in addition to, milk.

If the patient causes special trouble, he should be committed to an institution. In case of narrow nostrils the insertion of the tube through the mouth may sometimes become necessary, also to wash out the stomach after poisoning. In the case of patients who offer resistance one must use a gag and be sure to protect one's fingers; then insert tenderly but without fussiness the left index and middle fingers until reaching the back of the epiglottis which is pressed forward a little. Guide the tube between the two fingers directly to the entrance of the œsophagus, which can only be forced in this way by a soft tube against the patient's will.

Electricity, massage, climatic influences cannot be used as yet. Nor can hardly anything be gained by a definite *manner* of *nourishment;* special additional indications naturally excepted (compare also therapy of epilepsy). On the other hand strong nerve stimulants such as coffee and tea should be avoided, and above all alcohol has so many disadvantages that the little benefit which here and there is sometimes claimed for it does not enter into consideration.

Hypnotics can never be dispensed with entirely; in institutions they must often be given because of the other patients whom an excited patient keeps awake. Certainly the less one uses, the better; but if one is careful, *that is, if one never gives it daily for any length of time and changes the drugs, one will* not have any unpleasant experiences. To be sure one must watch the urine for the effect on the blood when administering Sulfonal and Trional. Chloral Hydrate is still one of the best drugs when given in doses of 2-3 Gm. (Blood pressure!) and eventually in smaller doses together with morphine. Of the newer drugs Veronal (0.5 to 1.5; care nephritis!) and Veronal of Soda (0.5 to 1.0) are particularly useful. The latter may also be given in enemas. Trional and Sulfonal are also given; the former acts quickly but not continuously, the latter slowly but effectively and very readily shows a cumulative effect. Hence 1.0 Trional can sometimes be combined with 2.0 Sulfonal to obtain an immediate and, at the same time, a more lasting effect. In the case of excitations of not too long duration a certain calming effect can be attained with Sulfonal, if it is frequently given (the cumulative effects manifest themselves by disturbances of coordination). The specified doses, with the exception of those of Sulfonal and Trional, may be exceeded without danger with patients whose reaction is known. In real excitations energetic doses should be administered or none at all; one should be glad if anything at all produces results. Paraldehyde (5.0 per dose and more, always through the mouth) would be one of the best hypnotics if it did not have such a bad taste and odor. In single doses it is entirely harmless, but it cannot be given for a long period. Amylene hydrate (2.0 to 5.0) is well adapted for rectal administration and is sometimes successfully used especially in status epilepticus; but it must be well diluted with starch or something similar when given as an enema, otherwise it attacks the mucous membrane of the intestines.

Many recommend *alcohol* as a hypnotic. It is the pleasantest, but as it may become a habit it is the most dangerous and least effective. I do not think it worthy of physicians to prescribe a drug which is most pleasant but most dangerous and ineffective.[6]

In nervous excitements resulting from fatiguing work *bromide* in smaller doses is excellent (1 to 3 grammes to be taken evenings all at once, or perhaps still better in two doses, but it must be thoroughly diluted). In milder depressions it is more rarely effective, in severer ones not at all (comp. Melancholia).

Opium and *opiates* are not hypnotics. But indirectly by removing fear and psychic pain they can have a calming or even hypnotic effect. In psychoses, however, they do not achieve by far what their effects on the healthy would lead one to expect. With the exception of a few cases, their use can be dispensed with, and because the danger of habituation to opiates is very great, especially with psychopaths, there is good reason to avoid them as much as possible. To give opiates

---

[6] If it is supposedly necessary for any other reason to prescribe alcohol as a medicine, it should be prescribed like any other remedy in definite doses and—for self-evident reasons—without the patient knowing it, as: Spir. Vin. 30.0, Aqua 130.0, Syr. Liquir. 40.0.

to an excited patient to facilitate the transfer to an institution is hardly ever of any use but it constantly occurs nevertheless.

Hyoscine (Scopolamin, Euscopol) hypodermatically in doses of 0.8 to 1 mg. (above the maximum dose!) is best in such cases; if the patient's reaction is known and the drug is fresh, more may be given, up to 1.5 mg. It has a decidedly better effect in combination with morphine—ten times the dose of hyoscine—and in frequent use this addition overcomes the harmful influence of hyoscine on the digestion. If one gives smaller doses of hyoscine (about 0.3 mg.) as some recommend, one can add more morphine, e.g. 0.015 g. per dose. Within more recent times *somnifen* has been used both as a hypnotic and sedative (40-50 minims internally; some give bigger doses). The more exact medications are still to be determined.[7]

Among particular symptoms which the practicing physician has to deal with, *uncleanliness* should be mentioned. Many mechanical arrangements have been constructed, particularly for the unclean bed cases, and all have been given up. The best thing is immediate cleaning, day and night, after every evacuation. In many patients, especially those not paralyzed, smearing of feces can be done away with, if every evening, if possible at exactly the same time, they are given an enema and urged to move their bowels.

Formerly it was thought necessary to do much to prevent *masturbation*.[8] This struggle, which is not only useless but which also keeps the attention of the inmates of the institution directed to the evil, I gave up long ago and am glad of it. But at all events care must be taken that onanistic acts are not carried on openly and do not anger the others or infect them. In cases where the patients themselves are struggling against the impulse, medium doses of bromide (2.0 to 4.2 per day) are sometimes effective. Epiglandol, which to be sure is better, can also diminish the impulse.

For a treatment of the danger of *suicide* see manic-depressive insanity.

If *operations on the insane* are to be undertaken, unless it is a question of life and death which makes immediate action necessary, one should obtain the consent of the relatives or of the guardian, perhaps of a counsel named for the purpose. The practice in this case is pretty well free from trouble; the theoretical difficulties, however, are numerous; there are foolish people who do not wish to deprive a person incapable of action of "the disposition of his own body" and would rather deprive him of life or limb than amputate

[7] See also Treatment of Schizophrenia.
[8] Comp. p. 209.

a couple of gangrenous toes against his will. The reduction of a dislocation, the proper treatment of a fracture naturally do not belong to the "operations" in the specified sense; this is not true, however, of lumbar punctures which require considerable skill. Every beginner does well in these matters to ascertain exactly the customs or requirements valid in his district.

The *interruption of pregnancy* [9] requires special indications. In depressions of pregnancy [10] the intervention frequently only causes the patients severe reproach and the condition is aggravated, while by mere waiting with sufficient oversight the psychosis is regularly cured, not seldom even before the delivery. However, the psychogenic depressions or situation melancholias of girls and women for whom the child will make difficulties are theoretically to be judged differently. Such diseases can naturally be cured by the removal of the cause; but with our present views and laws this cannot be a sufficient indication for abortion. Even in the case of schizophrenia and oligophrenia in spite of all the valid reasons that may be advanced, the sacrifice of the child is only decided on in exceptional cases. It is quite different in the case of early and severe eclamptic or choreatic psychoses. In Germany and in Catholic districts, according to the weight of opinion, a special indication (danger of a diseased progeny in the case of the insane and idiots; reaction of nursing difficulties on the condition of the mother) does not properly exist. In the Protestant part of Switzerland the sensibilities of the people demand an attitude that is more favorable to abortion and I should let social considerations count with the legal. Plain legal determinations exist nowhere; one has to fall back on local and customary interpretations. *At all events, it is wise not only to weigh carefully all the circumstances that enter into consideration, but to consult an experienced colleague.* Psychiatric indications of premature birth are more rare and simpler.

[9] Comp. E. *Meyer*, Künstliche Unterbrechung der Schwangerschaft bei Psychosen (mit Einschluss der Hysterie und Neurasthenie). Med. Klinik 1918. No. 7 u. 8.

[10] Cf. pp. 210-211.

CHAPTER XII

THE SIGNIFICANCE OF PSYCHIATRY

The frequency of psychical diseases is fairly great. Some are of the opinion that about two per thousand of the population is pronouncedly insane; but this does not include those "who were insane," the mental defectives, who are more than again as numerous as the manifestly insane, and most epileptics. And it is not to be doubted that the facts exceed by far the estimate. The most exact enumerations give about one percent of the population as insane and oligophrenics. From an investigation of conscripts *Maier* goes so far as to raise it to two percent. In its insane asylums alone Germany has to care for more than one hundred thousand insane. According to statistics obtained by the National Committee for Mental Hygiene there are about two hundred and fifty thousand patients in the hospitals for the insane in the United States. New York State supports about forty-three thousand patients in its State Hospitals.

But the estimated pecuniary loss to the individual is not less than the loss to the people generally. The paretic who has made a position for himself and has a family and then permits both to go to pieces is a frequent occurrence, the same is seen in the case of the hebephrenic, who for a half century has to be maintained at the expense of the family and the state and who retards the former economically.

Added to this, is the peculiar significance of insanity. The psyche is the essential element in man, not only from a religious but also from the viewpoint of natural science. Strong muscles and solid bones are still agreeable attributes for those who have them, but one can direct a world without even having arms and legs, while a slight disturbance in the psychic mechanism can change the strongest man into a pitiable object of care or into a dangerous enemy of society. It is for this reason that the psychoses attain their social importance much more than other diseases; they spread their harm to wider circles and they rob the patient himself of his independence in all his relations to his fellow men. They falsify or destroy his social position. He can no longer maintain himself, and he loses his qualifications as a legal subject. What was said applies only to the recognized insane, but if the insane person is not recognized, the consequences are often more serious for him, above all for the family, and sometimes for society. In many cases unbearable conditions improve as soon as the diagnosis is made.

Hence the great and sometimes dreaded import of psychiatric expert opinion.

And the significance of psychological and psychopathological considerations is always becoming greater. The *penal code* whose old standards are no longer adequate for modern viewpoints and conditions, is about to forge new weapons for itself in the battle against the enemies of society. This can only be accomplished with success if the conclusions drawn about criminals are based on studies and application of psychiatric methods of investigation and psychiatric prognostication. In *civil jurisprudence* psychical conditions are ever becoming more important; the psychological problems, which the antiquated insanity code presents to the judge and the expert, are already so large and so numerous that the profession will have trouble to meet them. A jurisprudence without a thorough psychological training is becoming more and more insufficient.

The same is true in other sciences. Our *ethical instincts* are no longer equal to the modern conditions of life and like the other instincts become inadequate with a progressive civilization; indeed, under certain conditions they even become harmful, (e.g. the instinct of revenge). Religions which since Buddha have regarded ethics as their domain, no longer have the general influence that they had in the last two thousand years. A conscious ethics can naturally spring only from the intimate study of the social psychology of man.

History is at last beginning to become psychological and consequently a comprehending science, because it is the product of the human psyche.

Pedagogy is getting ready to derive benefit from a penetrating study of the soul of the child.

In the last half century our *literature* has become immeasurably more psychological, even though in this respect it has not yet caught up with the French and Russian. Poetic compositions and especially their creators, themselves, can only be properly understood by an extensive psychological study.

A particularly fertile field scientifically and practically is the borderland between the normal and disease. The normal and average man is the product of adaptation to conditions and must consequently always hobble along somewhat behind the requirements. He dare not conspicuously develop a single characteristic at the expense of others, because he is above all the physical forebear of the future generations and as such must be able to bequeath in proper proportion all psychical gifts needed by society. But civilization is furthered by those who are developed in a one-sided manner, who inwardly and outwardly specialize themselves, who carry out the division of labor, and by those who are not sufficiently adapted to be satisfied with everything that exists.

But while the lines of deviation are countless, the useful possibilities are naturally few. Thus the bad prophets, the clumsy world reformers, the fanatic partisans who are inspired by all sorts of unrealizable dreams, and those who are really regarded as sick are and will continue to be the majority of the abnormal. To recognize them in the morbidity of their inner life is a problem that is practically important, that could contribute materially to the improvement of our public affairs.

The study of *race and mass psychology,* which is dominated by such people, should complete this knowledge. Psychopaths and insane, such as Mohammed, Luther, Loyola, Rousseau, Pestalozzi, Napoleon, and Robert Meyer, have influenced the course of our civilization in a fateful or beneficent way. The psychic epidemics from the crusades and the dances of St. Vitus to the twitchings of modern school children, and the numerous sectarian and party movements in religion, politics, and art, all represent the readily discernible peaks of the fluctuations of ideas, in which the psychic life of races expresses itself and from which the achievements of individual leading spirits grow as advanced pathfinders, as complements or as negatives to the general current.

For the *physician* a psychological training is nowadays particularly necessary. While the naïve practice of medicine was always in great part psychic, and the quack even yet partly heals and partly shears his patients by following psychic lines, the development of the exact methods of modern times has diverted the physician from psychical conceptions; indeed, as *Adolph Meyer* expresses it it has engendered an actual "Psychophobia." But theory and practice are suffering severely from this, when one side of a man is neglected and to be sure it is the one which through ideas and affects is the chief regulator of all bodily functions, and which alone decides the relation between physician and patient. The good practitioner is still preponderately the good, though usually instinctive, psychologist. The origin and disappearance of "Neuroses" goes by way of the psyche. The control of diseases of accidental origin, which cost the exchequer millions, and which make permanent cripples of many people, is only possible since their psychic origin has been grasped, and the manifestations of a good many other diseases in the single individual are modified and modifiable by the psyche. The usual digestive and menstrual difficulties are in large part entirely psychogenic diseases. Mental hygiene in the family is not less necessary to the happiness of mankind than physical hygiene; in short, a complete physician must understand the complete individual.

Now experience has shown here as everywhere, that it is difficult, yes, impossible to obtain insight, if only the commonplace, the normal is considered. *That accounts for the fact that psychology in the past could not only not contribute anything to all these purposes, but was positively a hindrance to better insight.* Only the newer schools such as those of *Marbe* and *Stern* tend in this direction. Hence what is important we shall only recognize from the study of the growing psyche of the child and, above all, from the aberrations of those already developed in psychopathology. At this time one of the most important, if not the most important path to a knowledge of the human soul is by way of psychopathology.

CHAPTER XIII

THE INDIVIDUAL MENTAL DISEASES

I.—V. THE ACQUIRED PSYCHOSES WITH COARSE BRAIN DISTURBANCES. THE ORGANIC SYNDROME

Kraepelin has here differentiated injuries and diseases of the brain and for practical reasons syphilitic diseases are separated from the latter. Among the syphilitic conditions again the most important, paresis, has been emphasized because of its historic, symptomatic, and practical individuality. With the senile forms and the real Korsakoff disease resulting from intoxication (alcohol, CO, lead, bacteria toxins, etc.), it has in common the diffuse reduction of the brain and with this, a large part of the symptomatology. These three forms are thought of first when the **organic psychoses** are mentioned. But they include also the various forms of degenerations of the nervous system, such as the glioses, multiple sclerosis, cerebral changes in tabes, tumors, etc. They alone have in common the "organic syndrome," which with a one-sided emphasis of the memory defect was also designated as the *Korsakoff symptom complex*.[1] Naturally it can also be found in other brain diseases, as soon as they result in a diffuse cortical lesion. If the cortex as a whole is only functionally damaged by a trauma, these symptoms may again disappear—"curable Korsakoff"—the same is true in an intoxication with adjustable anatomic disturbances (delirium tremens).

Only *diffuse* disturbances of the cortex cause a real weakening of intelligence, whereas certain affective disturbances can already manifest themselves in cortical brain lesions, most frequently when it affects the thalamic region. Irritability and a tendency to all sorts of temporary moodiness, again in the direction of anger and rage, are the most common persistent manifestations in most focal lesions of the brain, but in diffuse disturbances as well as in lesions in the thalamic region, the general affective lability would seem to be more marked.

[1] Korsakoff's disease is really a toxic neuritis of the peripheral and central nervous system. The name was then incorrectly transferred to other diseases showing similar memory disturbances.

THE ORGANIC SYNDROME

The diffuse reduction of the functions of the cortex results in definite symptoms, which only vary in detail according to the circumstances and the diseases.

Memory: [2] All things being equal, the fresher an engram, the worse is recollection ranging up to complete absence of impressibility,—the older it is, the less the memory is disturbed. Patients who evince a greater poverty of thoughts often fill their memory gaps with (real) *despairing confabulations,* while the more productive ones, going beyond this, revel in spontaneous pseudo-recollections. Transitory confusions or other disturbances of consciousness (attacks of all kinds) are frequently followed by amnesias.

The extent of *associations* simultaneously possible is restricted. [3] The choice of the latter is chiefly decided by the affects, that is, by the momentary strivings. One of the first results of this is *an absence of the critical faculty and a disturbance of judgment.* Recall the paretic who jumps from a high window to get a cigar butt, and the one who steals an object when everyone is looking and then carefully conceals it. Another paretic stole a barrel of wine from in front of a wine shop in bright daylight, and rolled it homewards; when he became tired, he begged two policemen to help him, and they went so far in their good nature as to give him his way. A paretic physician threatened to run away from us; he said that he could accomplish this very easily in the following way: he would go walking with us, and then he would step aside for a moment and not return. When the organic patient in a state of euphoria comes to an institution and finds a nice room and a friendly attitude, he very frequently overlooks the entire internment with its element of force, and declares that he will remain there for such and such a time. A paretic finds an old bag, cuts up several new ones to mend it, then gets the idea to make it big enough to reach the ceiling. Patients at the height of their disease only exceptionally acquire wisdom through experience. In every institution one is well acquainted with the variations of the paretic, who for several years has greeted the physician at every visit with the words: "Next Tuesday my wife will come and take me away."

Complicated *pictures* can sometimes no longer be grasped in their context; the patient counts up details and in this respect then reminds one of imbeciles.

[2] Cf. p. 100 and following.
[3] Cf. p. 74.

The various intellectual abilities do not disappear uniformly, but at present no other rule can be stated except that especially developed and practiced abilities escape the general deterioration the longest. The senile bookkeeper can be markedly demented in all other directions and yet surpass many a healthy person in addition. A paretic physician, who had previously made quite a name for himself as a chess player, when in all other respects he seemed completely childish, could still announce to a less skilled player at the opportune moment: "In ten moves I will checkmate you on this particular square," and he was nearly always right.

The psychic processes are usually more or less retarded, even aside from the torpid conditions evidently directly based on the disease process. But the retardation can, in certain respects, be over-compensated by manic moods with their rapid succession of ideas. Sometimes the patients evince distinct difficulty in passing from one topic to another. In the later stages the tendency to *perseveration* exists, in severe cases so strongly, that a patient, for example, answers the most varied questions about his personal details with "61," after he has given the year of his birth with this number. Intercurrent stronger associative disturbances are the bases of the deliria and states of confusion.

Of the disturbances of euphoria those individual concepts are naturally most strongly affected which are in themselves difficult of access, indefinite, and hard to determine. In place of them the patients reproduce simple, vague and general ideas such as: "building" for summer house, "man" for carpenter. Their answers to questions are also characteristically indefinite as shown by the following: "Where do you come from now?" "I have come forward from in back there." "Where is our institution?" "Why, it is in this city." Such answers are not given in the manner of intentional evasion but with a good natured sincerity. The patients are evidently satisfied with them and expect the questioner to feel the same about them. Very often the form of the answer is influenced by the mood: "In what ward are we now?" "In a nice one." "What sort of people are they?" "The right sort of people." In other cases a more or less conscious embarrassment is shown, which, however, does not really change the character of the answer: in the case of questions concerning the date, the patients have not seen the newspaper or the calendar just of today, or refusing to recognize the significance of the question, they turn to a companion and ask him to give the answer, etc. This symptom also is especially marked in cases of senility.

The *affectivity* is labile; it manifests itself more strongly and quickly than normal (emotional incontinence): but emotional excitements peter out more readily, either spontaneously or because the patient is led to think of something else. In the latter case, too, a lively mood may be supplanted by another without leaving any trace, often in a few seconds; the actual emotion dominates the patient absolutely. Trifles make him happy or desperate. A paretic woman seriously attempted suicide because her husband was late for a meal. To the extent that the insight for complicated relations is absent, these, naturally, can no longer become accentuated with feeling. The feeling reaction is easily restricted to certain fields also by the decrease of associations, and the *patients appear indifferent, although the defect is not really in the affective element.* A general brain torpor naturally expresses itself also in the affectivity; on the other hand, other patients have an exaggerated general excitability, and consequently also an affective excitability. The egotistic interests are naturally among those most difficult to suppress. As these patients cannot easily or at all think of other corrective ideas, especially contrast ideas in conjunction with their egotistic ones, many appear egotistic in their thoughts, feelings and acts. This is particularly evident in the simple senile forms; while in erethic and manic conditions, which occur especially in paresis, the more varied change in thinking over-compensates this tendency.

It is usually said that the *ethical feelings* of the organic patients deteriorate early and very markedly. I believe this is wrong. Some of these patients, no doubt, commit all sorts of crimes, but—to the extent that they were previously decent—according to my experience they commit them because they no longer have an insight into the entire situation and its consequences. If they can be made to comprehend what they have done, they regret it in the normal way. If they previously had anti-social tendencies, the disappearance of inhibitions naturally permits these to become more easily dangerous.

The cooperation of this labile affectivity with the restricted reflective ability makes purposeful action impossible. Tenderness, consideration, tact, piety, æsthetic sensibility, sense of duty, sense of right, feeling of sexual shame—all these may fail at any moment, even when they are present. Any sort of impulses from within and without are translated into action without any restraint.

Acute manic and *melancholic moods,* lasting for months and sometimes longer, appear frequently. The *mood,* chronic throughout the entire course, may also be a morbidly euphoric or depressive.

Corresponding to this condition of affectivity and the restriction of associations, the positive as well as negative *suggestibility* is heightened; on the one hand such people are easily influenced and, on the other hand, they are stubborn.

Apperception is retarded and unclear. The patients require more time to recognize pictures and often deceive themselves anyway; failures to recognize are sometimes caused by perseverations. Things read are easily perceived imperfectly and incorrectly. Questions to the patient often must be repeated and are sometimes answered in the sense of the previous trend of thought.

Orientation as to time and space often also, the autopsychic, is disturbed. The patients lack the "inner clock." Many of these patients no longer differentiate whether they or others are being spoken to, which is also a part of disturbed orientation. When presented at the clinic, for example, many, like patients in alcoholic delirium, answer regularly, when one speaks to the audience.

Attention,[4] aside from the restricted extent, is made difficult; this is seen more in the habitual and the passive than in the maximal and the active attention. The *intensity* of the latter may be normal, even if the *extensity* has already suffered severely. Sometimes *vigility* is reduced at the same time with *tenacity*.

If *Delusions* are present, they obtain as a rule the character of senselessness in the severe cases. Among the depressive delusions one observes commonly exaggerated ideas referring to diseases; the délire d'énormité and nihilism when present are especially characteristic.

Hallucinations usually affect sight and hearing. Corresponding to the brain process other kinds of parasthesias also occur, which, under certain circumstances, attain a similarity with real (body-) hallucinations. This is usually brought about through misinterpretation in a state of delirium. Many of our patients are excited and hallucinate *at night*, while during the day they are quiet or actually sleep.

With depressive patients, screaming throughout the night, lasting for months, is not rare, and generally, stereotyped whining and complaining are nowhere more pronounced than here.

Severe *anxiety attacks* with senseless or confused reactions, pushing away, clinging, brutal, and often clumsy attempts at suicide, hiding away, hitting at random, etc., are in part results of the brain disease, and in part probably results of disturbances of the circulatory apparatus; at all events they are most frequently seen in sufferers from arteriosclerosis.

Besides, various kinds of *delirious*, perhaps also of *twilight states* occur, which under no circumstances manifest the same genesis. We

[4] Cf. p. 134.

find them as intercurrent symptoms of paresis; in arteriosclerotic psychosis especially after the inception of diffuse softening, etc.

The organic psychoses are usually accompanied by *physical symptoms*, which are, in part, the result of the brain affection (paralyses, trophic disturbances), in part concomitant manifestations (senile marasmus, neuritis). An irregular coarse tremor, especially of the hands and the organs of speech, is most constant.

As physical symptoms one often designated also the "nervous" manifestations which can mark the beginning of every organic insanity. Among these we have: pressure in the head, headache, parasthesias, flickering of the eyes, buzzing in the ears, etc. Later they are in part concealed by the deeper psychotic symptoms or in delirious conditions they are misinterpreted as illusions and delusions referring to the body.

The *disturbance of memory* is most often characteristic of the simple forms of dementia senilis. Here one sees cases in which the limits of absence of memory may be determined to some extent. For instance, the patient does not remember anything that occurred in this century. After a while the memory gap extends back to the nineties of the last century, then to the eighties, etc. If only memories of youth are present, they often have a greater freshness than under normal conditions; they may even attain an hallucinatory vividness so that the patients believe they live over scenes which in reality took place seventy years ago. In arteriosclerotic forms irregular fluctuations of memory disturbance, both as regards content and time, readily occur. In paresis the difference in the ability to recall earlier and fresher experiences is sometimes not so striking as in the senile forms, but it can be invariably demonstrated, even though sometimes it first appears only when the dementia becomes deeper. Alcoholic Korsakoff's disease when it is acute usually shows at first a well defined limit of the ability to recall at the beginning of the disease; the patients have at their disposal nothing that occurred since; what occurred previously they recall pretty completely. However, this demarkation becomes blurred rather quickly, in that earlier experiences also are not remembered at all or incorrectly. In the magic form of paresis and alcoholic Korsakoff, confabulations often appear altogether without any restrictions. In many torpid forms of the senile psychoses confabulations are almost absent. Other things being equal it increases and decreases with excitement and activity.

The *absence of the critical faculty* appears to be, on the whole, more pronounced in paresis than in the senile forms, where the personality with its strivings in relation to the elementary disturbance is often better preserved, to the extent that a miserly old man, for example, is not easily talked into making gifts, etc. The uncertain answers, which are to disguise the dearth of ideas, are found most frequently and in a most pronounced form in the simple senile dements. Coarse brain lesions lead most readily to marked perseverations.

The *productivity* of the delusions in manic paresis is enormous but in the other forms it is very limited. Moreover the *phantasy forma-tion* in paresis and in alcoholic Korsakoff is usually very vivid, else-where it is rather reduced.

The *lability of the affects* also occurs frequently as the result of a hemorrhage in the thalamic region; it may then remain as an isolated symptom, in that the intelligence is not affected at all or only after months and years. In paresis there is a marked tendency to euphoric moods, and in the senile forms to *depressive* moods. Alcoholic Korsa-koff cases are usually very euphoric for a long period.

Apperception is often preserved much longer in the simple senile forms than in paresis.

Certain variations of the organic forms are often determined by congenital predisposition of the brain; thus emotional people, especially members of families with manic depressive tendencies, more readily have affective forms of paresis and of the senile psychoses; indeed, even the depressive or manic dispositions become particularly marked by the addition of the brain disease; paranoid forms occur in patients who have always been distrustful and inclined to false interpretations, while schizophrenic forms in those who originally belong to the schizoid type, etc. Nevertheless the kind of process has its influence also; thus paresis inclines to euphoric states, arteriosclerosis to depressive and anxiety states; delusions of stealing is an organic-senile mani-festation, not a constitutional symptom, etc.

Corresponding to the underlying brain disease the *outcome* of organic psychoses is usually fatal. Intoxication psychoses, like Korsa-koff, can improve more or less, or after a slight improvement remain essentially stationary. In spite of a course which is progressive on the whole, remissions in paresis and in the arteriosclerotic forms may go very far; in the latter the particular improvements can also last only a few days or hours; but then they are usually more frequent and constitute an important element of the entire picture; this is probably the only occasion on which one can properly speak of "Lucid intervals." The prognosis of particular senile diseases will be discussed later.

A *differential diagnosis* of the organic psychoses is not easy in the beginning. The disease must already have attained a certain height before a large part of the disturbances mentioned become evident. Orientation, for example, in patients whose sensorium is clear is only falsified in the more advanced stages of dementia. But it may also happen that intelligent witnesses in court pronounce a man entirely capable of action who, literally, mistakes night and day and wants to go to his office at eleven o'clock at night and closes his office in the forenoon. On the other hand in senile dementia the difficulty lies in the fact that normal senility indicates similar symptoms: One does not know at what stage of memory disturbance or of affective lability one should count the beginning of the disease. In these cases practical reasons must sometimes serve as criteria.

If a pronounced melancholic condition exists, then a petty reaction to minor affairs like a belated meal, or a striking affective distraction, perhaps by a joke, point to organic lability.

More important still is the *nonsense* of the *delusions* and here especially the form of nihilism and of the Délire d'énormité. Disturbances of orientation may naturally only be evaluated in cases where it occurs in a clear sensorium. Nocturnal excitements with sleeping by day must be weighed carefully because they also occur elsewhere, e.g. sometimes in schizophrenia. Slow functioning of the psychic processes, even though of a somewhat different kind, occurs in epilepsy, where one also sees blurred perception and perseveration.

States of *organic unclearness* can be recognized most conspicuously by a good affective rapport with a declining intellectual rapport; this is differentiated from epilepsy by the fact that fluctuations of emotional reaction readily occur. Usually the patient is eagerly occupied with any obviously foolish action, which is to be designated as imaginary, since it is not based on hallucinations. The patient endeavors, for example, to fold the comforter, if he succeeds, which he rarely does, or if we fold it for him, he nevertheless continues in exactly the same way to fuss around with it.[5]

Frequently while the diagnosis of the organic disease is not yet possible, the specific manifestations, especially physical symptoms like neuritis, pupillary and speech disturbances (Korsakoff, paresis) permit a definite diagnosis of the special psychosis. More frequently the reverse holds true; that is, the "organic psychosis" can be generally recognized while the specific symptoms of a definite form are still lacking. The latter is especially true in view of the fact that there are also organic psychoses resulting from brain diseases which are not yet known.

An important means of recognizing and differentiating organic dis-

[5] Comp. presbyophrenic delirium, pages 290 and 294.

turbances of the central nervous system is the examination of the cerebrospinal fluid. The lumbar puncture also has therapeutic significance in various diseases. But one must be cautious, especially in brain tumors, because of the danger that the medulla oblongata may be pressed into the occipital foramen, and in traumatic neuroses, in which new complaints may be attached to the operation.

The technique of puncturing should, in the interest of the patient, be learned by practical demonstration and initial practice under supervision. To refresh the memory the following points are mentioned here: If a line is drawn on the patient's back connecting the two crests of the ileum, then directly over and under this line one finds the space between the third and fourth and the fourth and fifth lumbar vertebræ, respectively, one of which is selected for the puncture. This is the region of the cauda equina, so that injury of the cord is impossible. Disinfection of the region must be most carefully done. The puncture needle should be at least ten cm. long and as thin as possible; the elastic instruments of platiniridium are the best. In the insane it is often an advantage to puncture them while in a sitting position, because it is easier to hold them, and because they are usually less excited than when they are put in a reclining position; in both cases the most important item is the very decided flexion of the spinal column ("hump back") because then the inter-vertebral spaces open; but the spinal column must not be turned laterally because the location of the spinal canal is then more difficult to find. The sitting patient is best placed so that he sits backwards on a chair and throws his arms around its back; an attendant kneels in front of him and holds his legs symmetrically upwards. The puncture is made either in the middle line directly under the third or fourth lumbar spinous process which is located with the finger of the free hand. The direction of the puncture should be slightly oblique tending upwards; the lateral method penetrates a little deeper, one cm. beside the middle line. In the first case one has the great advantage that one must puncture directly in the middle line without a lateral deviation, while in the lateral puncture the correct estimate of the angle requires more practice; on the other hand, in the median puncture one must go through the hardest part of the ligaments which occasionally may deceive with a resistance equal to that of bone. Frequently the puncture is made too deep; then a slow withdrawal of the needle suffices to permit the outflow of the liquor which had apparently not been reached.

For purely diagnostic purposes six to ten ccm. should be withdrawn; in cases of paresis one can usually go a little higher without disagreeable consequences. Rapid decline of high pressure even after a slight emptying indicates danger because of defective communication between the cerebral fluid and spinal canal.

If one wants to measure the *pressure of the liquor*, one must naturally do that first and with the patient lying on his side. One attaches to the needle a sterile tube of small calibre with a glass attachment, lifts it as long as the fluid in the glass attachment rises, then one measures the height from the point of puncture with a scale held alongside. The normal height varies between 90 and 140 mm. H_2O. In case of very high pressure the withdrawal should be retarded and ended before it has come to the normal height. After the puncture the patient should lie in bed for 24 hours in about a horizontal position. If there is slight temperature or headache or heaviness in the head, as occasionally happens, he should remain in bed two or more days and take, perhaps, some pyramidon (0.2 to 0.3 per dose).

In the normal person the fluid is clear and colorless; intermixtures of blood resulting from the puncture settle quickly when permitted to stand. (Sera containing blood are naturally useless for the Wassermann reaction.) In yellowish discolorations that do not come from bleeding of the puncture, bleeding of the brain should be thought of especially, then of cerebral inflammation and pachymeningitis. *Counting* the cellular elements of the fluid must be done as soon as possible, as otherwise they turn to sediment; it is best done with the blood cell chamber as modified by Fuchs-Rosenthal, which has a depth of 0.2 mm. instead of 0.1 mm.; as a stain, for example, one can use Methylviolet 0.2, Acid. acet. glac. 1.0, Aq. dest. 50.0. The normal number is 0 to 5 cells in the cubic millimeter; 6 to 10 is suspicious; what exceeds this number may be considered pathological. A psychosis with an increase of the cells is generally paresis.—If one wants to differentiate the individual cell forms, one had better stain according to well known methods after the fluid is centrifuged. Plasma cells found in a psychosis usually indicate paresis.—Still more important is the Wassermann reaction of the serum, in which the evaluation with different doses of liquor is frequently necessary. In paresis the reaction is usually strong; in lues of the central nervous system it is frequently weaker.[6] Chemically, *Nonne's* "Phase I" is significant: About 1 to 2 ccm. of the fluid are mixed with an equal amount of a saturated aqueous solution of ammonium sulphate, not warmed: In central syphilogenous diseases a discoloration or at least an opalescence appears, which proves the increased presence of globulin and nuclein. If it is then boiled the remaining albuminous elements precipitate (Nonne's "Phase II"), but the latter examination is better made with

[6] See page 248.

Nissl's graduated tube, in which 2 ccm. of the fresh fluid is replaced by 1 ccm. of the common Esbach reagent and then centrifuged for one half to three quarters of an hour; the precipitate gathers at the bottom of the tube and can be removed; the normal liquor hardly contains more than 0.2 to 0.35% of albumin; in pathological conditions a twofold or greater increase frequently occurs.

Phase I is regularly positive (opalescence) in paresis, congenital syphilis, in extra medullary tumors, a little rarer in tabes and other luetic forms of the central nervous system, only in some cases of brain abscess and other diseases of the brain, spinal cord, and its meninges.

According to *Kafka* [7] the chemical diagnosis may be carried further. The Globulines, which already separate when a 28% saturated solution of ammonium sulphate is added, indicate acute meningeal inflammation but do not exclude tubercular or luetic processes. The euglobulins (fibrinogen, fibrinoglobulin), whose presence proves paresis, still separate with reagents saturated to 33%. The pseudoglobulins only occur in chronic lues cerebri and only become visible with the application of a solution saturated to 40%.

I. INSANITY IN INJURIES TO THE BRAIN [8]

In the confusing mass of external pictures resulting from brain injuries one still misses a systematic viewpoint. A few types that I mention, following *Kraepelin*, may give an indication of what occurs in this connection.

Concussion of the brain with its symptoms of unconsciousness, collapse, vomiting, etc., is familiar to physicians from the study of surgery.

Traumatic delirium or commotion psychosis. A delirious state sometimes follows directly after the accident or brain concussion in which disturbance of memory of the organic type, or *traumatic* in uninjured brains of curable Korsakoff, is usually plainly recognizable; sometimes it is connected with nervous symptoms like headache, dizziness and with focal symptoms that do not always indicate a tangible anatomic brain injury. The state of affectivity varies. The disease usually lasts only a few hours or days, occasionally several weeks, the last especially when it has developed only after days or weeks after the trauma. Later one observes usually a lack of memory with a tendency to *retroactive amnesia*.

[7] Münch. Med. W. S. 1915, p. 105.
[8] Besides *Kraepelin*, comp. *Schröder*, Geistesstörungen nach Kopfverletzungen, Enke, Stuttgart 1915.

As transitional states during improvements, and more frequently as a chronic state, that can attach itself to the trauma immediately or after a longer latent period even without a commotion psychosis, we notice different pictures of *traumatic* states of *weakness.* Common to most of them are rapid exhaustion,[9] irritability, tendency to spontaneous and reactive moods, up to the most intense anger, which is in part labile and in part of a more torpid persistent affect; more rarely we notice a stupid euphoria with a mania for joking (Moria). Not rarely epileptic attacks appear in which the typical *epileptic dementia* may occur (traumatic epilepsy).[10] Pictures similar to Catatonia can last for a long time. Even after a long time subdural or cerebral bleedings with the consequent manifestations can occur.

Not very rarely milder injuries to the brain cause indefinite symptoms that give the appearance of a *neurosis.*

In children injuries to the brain readily lead to idiocy, especially to the irritable forms with moods.

Berger [11] differentiates (1) commotion psychosis, (2) traumatic dementia, and (3) traumatic twilight state. He divides commotion psychosis into (1) hallucinatory confusion, (2) those with the Korsakoff (=organic) symptom, (3) those with a manic tinge, (4) those with catatonic symptoms.

The *treatment* of these conditions unfortunately is not very successful. In the delirious forms the only thing that can be done is to await recovery and protect the patient from himself. In the chronic forms it is important to abstain from *alcohol* which enhances the symptoms and causes excitement. It should also be kept in mind not to give such people cocaine injections (dentist!) because permanent epilepsies may be released as a result. The excision of a scar from the brain (more frequently from the meninges), leaving perhaps an opening as a pressure vent, is said sometimes to effect a cure especially in the epileptic forms; perhaps more frequently the same may be

---

[9] Under certain conditions, e.g. in continuing to add numbers, many of these patients seem to tire less than the normal, apparently because they do not concentrate.

[10] The numerous "war epilepsies" do not confirm these peace epilepsies. However, on the one hand, the time since the war is still somewhat short; on the other hand, the various brain attacks which do not belong to our concept of epilepsy are here included—for the present, because it is not quite possible to differentiate them, as the different kinds of attacks frequently change from case to case and even in the same patient (comp. e.g. *Jacksonian* Epilep. p. 342). Cf. also *Forster* on later clinical experiences with bullet injuries of the brain in the Handbuch der ärztlichen Erfahrung im Weltkrieg, Barth, Leipzig, 1922, IV, p. 198.

[11] Trauma und Psychose. Springer, Berlin, 1915.

effected by a removal of a bone splinter irritating the brain. Bromide is sometimes effective against irritability. It is still more important to be extremely considerate of the patient and to avoid every irritating circumstance. Headache and similar symptoms frequently only become worse through treatment, while ignoring it may make the condition more bearable. In addition a suitable selection and education of those persons who are wont to come in contact with the patient is necessary. It is taken for granted that the patient is trained and practiced in a line of work carefully adapted to his abilities.

II. INSANITY IN BRAIN DISEASES

These psychoses also have little significance for psychiatry. The thing that is essential from a practical viewpoint is usually the basic disease; but the psychosis must not be overlooked because of the possibility of its being mistaken for other mental diseases and neuroses. *Diffuse nutritional disturbances of the cortex in every case result in the organic syndrome.*

In connection with the psychical disturbances in the various forms of *meningitis, Kraepelin* discusses the insanity in cases of *brain tumors.* Here too the most different disturbances have been described, and the connections between the tumor and the psychosis are not often clear. Large tumors may remain with hardly any psychic symptoms or at any rate may run a course without any severe manifestations. Brain pressure retards all reactions, but need not disturb them in any other way. I have seen a case in which it might take five minutes before the patient answered a simple question; but the answers were appropriate. Of theoretic interest, even though still incomprehensible, is the frequent occurrence here of the "facetiousness," which perhaps appears as a local symptom of the base of the frontal lobe. It is interesting also that, according to *Schuster,* tumors of the corpus collosum are regularly connected with psychic disturbances.

Where pronounced psychical morbid pictures are found in tumors, it is usually a case of the organic symptom complex (lability of the feelings, Korsakoff memory disturbances, etc.)—for comprehensible reasons, because the nutrition of the brain is easily disturbed in toto. Under circumstances still unknown, catatonic symptoms may also be connected with brain diseases, especially with tumors.

The disturbances of the psyche in *multiple sclerosis* are mainly those of the organic psychoses. In the field of affectivity, irritability is often in the foreground; in other cases it is euphoria, or the reverse, depression. *In most cases the diseased is animated by psychogenic neurotic symptoms;* since these are amenable to the right psycho-therapy it is very important, and usually very easy, to recognize them. In later stages delusions and delirious conditions may also be seen. The diagnosis is based on the neurological signs of multiple sclerosis.

Huntington's chorea, which is almost always hereditary, is more important. I knew a family in which four generations were so afflicted. The transmission is usually of the same variety. But not seldom other severe cerebral disturbances such as epilepsy, idiocy, etc., are also found among the relatives. The psychic and motor manifestations, as a rule long unrecognized, appear stealthily mostly in the second to the fourth decade, occasionally still later, and rarely earlier. Such persons are often considered inattentive and careless and are blamed for their clumsiness, in the appearance of which the motor-choreatic disturbances participate just as well as the psychical. The chorea in itself, when it is once pronounced, looks exactly like Sydenham's disease, only the movements are mostly less brusque. In the psychic sphere one observes an organic dementia. Often, however, there is a marked indifference to the disease and about their own affairs which is generally noticeable. When the patients are no longer capable of speaking and writing they usually take no pains at all to make themselves otherwise understood. Changes of mood are not so rare but they probably never attain the degree of a melancholia or a mania.

Death results in the course of a few decades during which the severe mental affliction either progresses steadily or shows minor fluctuations.

The brain shows markedly diffuse changes of the nervous elements, which as yet have not been sufficiently investigated to permit of an anatomical diagnosis.

Kraepelin includes in here the *amaurotic idiocy* of *Tay* and *Sachs,* which affects mainly Jewish children in their first year. It is not a form of idiocy but a peculiar brain degeneration involving the visual apparatus including the retina and ends in death in several months or years.

An organic brain disease, which affects the cortex relatively little and for that reason lacks the organic syndrome, is *Encephalitis lethargica,* the European sleeping sickness, which has no connection whatever with the African sleeping sickness. Anatomically it is a *poliencephalitis* in which there is a round cell proliferation of the vessels and in which more rarely there are also slight hemorrhages. Its favorite location is around the Aqueduct of Sylvius but it also spreads to the canal root ganglia and their surroundings and invariably descends into the spinal cord but it probably does not leave any part of the gray matter entirely free. The physical symptoms are paralysis of internal and external eye muscles, sometimes also paralysis of the facial nerve, parasthesias not only in the form of itching, etc., but also pains and burning, paralyses in general, and mild muscular rigidity. The development of the disease is from several days to weeks; fever appears mostly at the height of the disease; it is frequently not particularly high and may disappear after a few weeks.

Psychotic symptoms of a toxic rather than organic character appear chiefly in the initial stage. Thus one observes: motor restlessness, which sometimes lends a choreic character to the movements. This is frequently accompanied by deliria, which resemble the ordinary fever psychoses, but because of their complex character they may be readily taken as hysterical, especially before the temperature rises. In severe cases they increase to the point of apparent confusion. Somewhat later the clouded state often assumes the character of occupation deliria, which alternate with the ever-increasing lethargic state. In milder cases one sees at least occupation dreams. Except in the most severe cases the patients can be roused from their sleep and, after the disappearance of the initial deliria, evince their mental clearness, even though strikingly uninterested in their own condition as well as in the environment. Left to themselves at the height of the disease they invariably go to sleep again. The hyperkinetic deliria of the beginning are easily mistaken for catatonic especially because, in spite of existing affects, the facial expression regularly has something rather stiff about it, and because the torpor may assume a real cataleptic appearance. The occupation deliria may occasion its being mistaken for delirium tremens. The disease' often results in death in the early weeks, in many other cases later, even after more than two years. About two thirds recover almost entirely in the course of a greater number of weeks or months. But the rigidity of the pupils is often said to remain permanently. The differential diagnosis is based mainly on the proof of the following encephalitic symptoms: parasthesias, hyperkinesis with chorea-like movements and above all disturbances of the eye muscle and eventually of the optic nerve; also then the mania for sleep with the possibility of being aroused to an intellectually clear condition.

What excites the disease and the manner of infection are unknown; the treatment is symptomatic.

III. SYPHILITIC PSYCHOSES

Among the infectious diseases of the brain and its meninges syphilis is the most important. To be sure even without the confirmation of a luetic process in the central organs there are already disturbances at the beginning of the secondary stages of lues, which are designated as "neurasthenic." The latter are due in part to the psychic effects of the infection, which nowadays is no longer taken so light heartedly, and in part probably to the direct weakening or poisoning influence of the virus, which to be sure we cannot as yet define more exactly. Manifold signs of milder disturbances of the nervous system, such as dizziness, headache, diminished pupillary reaction to light, an increase in the cells and albumin in the spinal fluid, which are frequently a result of an antiluetic treatment, lead to the supposition that as a third factor some unknown early alteration of the brain or of the meninges can produce or condition symptoms resembling those of neurasthenia.

Sometimes the thought of being infected and the fear of the consequences of lues form the conspicuous part of the picture. There develops a *hypochondriacal neurasthenia,* altogether or mainly psychogenetic, with an eager searching for morbid symptoms that might be ascribed to syphilis. According to some, hysterical pictures are also said to be produced by the infection.

In other cases, according to *Kraepelin,* one deals with a *general nervous uneasiness,* increased difficulty in thinking, irritability, disturbance of sleep, pressure in the head, vague and alternating feelings and pains, later on anxiety feelings, pronounced depressions, dizziness, clouding, difficulty in finding words, transitory paralyses, disturbances of perception, nausea, and a rise in temperature. The latter group of manifestations might perhaps be ascribed to the third cause, or to some direct anatomical or chemical disturbance in the cranial content.

For a second group of syphilitic psychoses which are about equally frequent in men and women we have an anatomical basis; among those one observes *gummata, slowly progressing meningitis,* and *luetic vascular diseases.* In most cases one of these processes predominates, but the disturbance is rarely limited entirely to one of them. The vascular alteration is most often found alone but it frequently accompanies meningitis and both together are often found in an affection which is primarily gummatous. The combinations and the changing intensity and location of the processes produce a great variety of the clinical pictures, but the anatomical findings are as yet only roughly paralleled with the clinical.

The *Gummata* in themselves naturally produce the identical symptoms as other brain tumors of equally rapid growth and similar localization. Luetic *meningitis* is mostly localized at the base, especially in the region where the various optic nerves have their exit, it moves rarely; also affects the convexity and then usually to a lesser extent. The variety of symptoms caused by meningitis naturally depends on the increase of the pressure and the luetic process, or on whether the disturbances of nutrition extend to the cortex or not. The diseased pia is usually thickened, clouded, infiltrated with round cells, and shows an increase in connective tissue.

The *vascular changes* in themselves produce symptoms similar to the non-luetic arterioscleroses. They can affect more extensively either the large or the small vessels. The syphilitic vascular disease shows itself in the larger arteries in an exuberance of the cells of the intima and adventitia, in the former to the extent of occluding the lumen. The elastica becomes split apart. The process has a certain tendency towards regeneration, but when the arteries of the brain are involved, the region they supply is usually permanently injured in the way of a simple gradual destruction of the nervous elements with an infiltration of the glia to the extent of softenings and hemorrhages. The process is most marked in the pia and seems to extend from it to the cortex.

In contradistinction to paresis one notes here a massive infiltration of the entire vessel with round cells, among which the plasma cells constitute a small minority or are absent, while in paresis the marked infiltration of the vessels with plasma cells is particularly characteristic, and the extensive exuberance of the intima is foreign to this disease. What is also characteristic is the more circumscribed dissemination in contradistinction to the diffuse disturbances of paresis.

The luetic arteritis of the smaller vessel often consists in an enlargement and proliferation of the cells in the adventitia and intima but without an infiltration of round cells. Side by side with the destructive processes one also finds newly formed vessels in the pia and in the brain.

The brain substance is naturally injured in the most varied ways both qualitatively and quantitatively by the alteration of the vessels and the meninges.

The *organic-nervous symptoms* can assume pretty nearly all forms that are produced by the contents of the cranium and the spinal canal. The most frequent symptoms encountered are reflex disturbances of the pupils, pressure symptoms with clouding of sensorium, desire for sleep, etc., and apoplectiform and epileptiform attacks as well as attacks showing a Jacksonian character. The psychic symptoms are those of the organic psychoses. The specific peculiarities are similar to those of arteriosclerotic insanity—for the self-evident reason that in both diseases the cortex needs not be affected in toto. The personality is retained for a long time.[12]   The patients maintain their outward demeanor and take part in external events.   Judgment is not so much disturbed; thus a far-reaching insight into the disease exists, in quiet times even considerable clearness.   As in arteriosclerotic insanity, here, too, the psychic symptoms, both as to time and number, are lacunary: many good individual functions cause surprise when found where others have been lost; moody fluctuations can appear temporarily, regardless of the general course toward improvement or aggravation.

After all this, no sharply distinguishable morbid pictures can be expected.   It also happens that a genuine brain syphilis can be followed later by a real paresis.   *Kraepelin* makes the following distinctions: *Forms with brain pressure,* mostly based on gummatous growths, clinically not essentially differentiated from diseases resulting from other brain tumors, and the *syphilitic pseudoparesis* (corresponding approximately to the *post syphilitic* dementia of *Binswanger*).

In the latter it is most frequently a case of a morbid picture very similar to the simple demented form of paresis; in the physical spheres besides the rigidity of the pupils to light, the frequency of irregular paralyses of the ocular muscles, and disturbances of vision are the most important to be mentioned.   Disturbances of speech and writing may be present but they then are of a different type from that of paresis.

Much rarer is the *delirious confusion* of *Marcus* which is to be classed with syphilitic pseudoparesis.   It manifests itself in rather sudden organic deliria with symptoms of insomnia, confusion, anxiety, mistaking the environment, hallucinations of hearing and sight, mostly of a terrifying content, active excitement, and acts of violence against one's own person and others.   Besides these one also finds organic nervous symptoms.

Other forms resemble expansive paresis.   The prominent feature of the fourth group is an organic memory disturbance ("Korsakoff").

Syphilitic pseudoparesis takes an entirely irregular course; it can be stationary for years.   The outcome in all cases, when no antiluetic treatment intervenes or when this is not effective, is an organic dementia combined with paralysis.   The patients die of intercurrent diseases, or from weakness, or cerebral attacks, or marasmic pneumonias, etc.

The *differential diagnosis* between *pseudoparesis* and paresis cannot be made at once in individual cases with absolute certainty.   Improvement in the course of antiluetic treatment does not exclude the

[12] Cf. pp. 139-282.

element of coincidence. The probability favoring cerebral syphilis is the lighter intensity and extent of the psychical disturbances. It may also be worth noting that in paresis milder psychic symptoms of "the neurasthenic" type have in most cases preceded the physical symptoms, while here both groups usually appear together.

According to *Plaut* the following should be especially considered: Wassermann in the blood proves lues; its absence permits the exclusion of the possibility of cerebral lues with a probability of 80%. A pronounced pleocytosis of the spinal fluid in the advanced stage of lues (not in the initial stage) proves an organic (meningitic) process in the central nervous system; the same holds in Nonne's Phase I. Wassermann in the spinal fluid proves the luetic affection of the central nervous system; contrasted with the invariably strong reaction in paresis (already plain in 0.2 ccm. of the liquor) it is here weak; the fluid must be tested up to 1.0 ccm. Lues cerebri may be excluded with great probability when there is no Wassermann in tested fluid, an absence of Wassermann in the blood, an absence of pleocytosis, and, with least certainty, when there is a failure of the globulin reaction.

Apoplectic cerebral lues is supposed to be the commonest of the syphilitic psychoses. It presents about the same pictures as the common post apoplectic dementia, but it appears most often at an earlier time of life, shows a greater desultoriness and regenerative possibilities of the symptoms, and then again as a sign of brain lues it shows frequent paralysis of the eye muscles as well as pupillary disturbances.

Furthermore there is a *luetic epilepsy* which differs from the other forms by the existence of lues, its appearance late in life, occasional (not invariable) cure through antisyphilitic treatment, and finally by disturbances of the eye muscles.

An entirely divergent form without plain psychic organic symptoms has been described in detail chiefly by *Plaut*, as *hallucinosis of syphilitics*, but he did not establish with entire certainty the conception of a particular disease. It is a question of cases which as yet are not to be differentiated clinically from mild paranoid types with senseless delusions, voices, very rarely other hallucinations. Hallucinations referring to the body probably also occur; the patients sometimes feel as if they were hypnotized. However, pronounced specific schizophrenic symptoms, especially actual dementia, are absent. Depressions with ideas of sin and, more rarely, exaltation of a minor degree, but still with grandiose ideas, are also met. Usually there is a certain feeling of sickness. The course is similar to many cases of schizophrenic paranoid types and shows irregular fluctuations up to hallucinatory excitations, which, however, remain without disorientation. Cures do not seem to occur in spite of antisyphilitic treatment. Sometimes one also notes paralytic manifestations, pupillary disturbances, bladder weakness, disturbances of speech and writing, dizziness and other cerebral attacks. The disease usually breaks out more than ten years after the infection.

Plaut also described similar *acute cases* with symptoms of anxious excitation, with voices and delusions of persecution without disorientation, which lasted from 18 days to 10 months and usually recovered.

The most important syphilitic affection of the central nervous system is *Dementia paralytica*. Contrasted with the other luetic diseases it has some peculiarities in common with tabes and is not seldom associated with this disease as taboparesis. But besides this there are *"Tabes psychoses"* which neither clinically nor anatomically belong to paresis. They mostly show mild indications of organic symptoms, especially lability, but also disturbances of memory, attention, etc. In all other respects they take very different forms. Following *Kraepelin* affective and paranoid forms are mostly differentiated, of which the latter are the more frequent.

The *affective pictures* manifest themselves in persistent moods, in the form of depression, irritability, or abnormal euphoria. The *paranoid forms* develop vague delusions, usually of persecution, intermingled at times with delusions of grandeur; they also have hallucinations of hearing and occasionally of sight, more rarely of smell and taste and of body sensations.[13]

Even in the chronic course, these conditions show a rather marked fluctuation; on the other hand cases are not rare in which the disease manifests itself only in acute shifts of such hallucinations and delusions mostly with anxious excitements extending to the point of delirium. Between these forms there are all combinations and transitions, i.e. cases in which the delusions continue more or less in the clear state and now and then one also observes deliria. In clear mental states all these patients are usually allopsychically oriented.

The much more frequent occurrence of disturbances of the visual nerves in tabes with psychoses than in mere symptoms of the spinal cord makes it probable that the tabes psychoses also are based on a variety of cerebral lues.

Hereditary syphilis also generates numerous brain diseases, which are associated with psychic symptoms, they range from simple nervousness up to idiocy, epilepsy, infantile paralysis, and other progressive forms of dementia which have not been properly described as yet.

[13] Cf. pp. 64-65.

According to *Kraepelin* a part of the luetic idiocies already originated within the uterus, chiefly through meningo-encephalitis; others develop later, some suddenly, others gradually; later they may again become stationary. Local disturbances of the brain texture, e.g. through arterial occlusion, naturally leave pictures similar to those of acute encephalitis. According to some about 10% of idiocies are conditioned by syphilis. In some, besides severe or very slight intellectual disturbances, one finds chiefly anomalies of character, vehemence, maliciousness, cruelty, and uneducability in general. Under certain circumstances paranoid pictures also appear. In all these forms the entire constitution is mostly impaired; the children develop late, remain weak, small, or deformed. The luetic cerebral symptoms may appear at any time, but most frequently in the first years. But *infantile paresis* may first begin in the second decade; in very rare cases the outbreak is said to have been delayed to the fourth or fifth decade.

The *diagnosis* of paresis in children rests on the same principles as in adults. The other hereditary syphilitic forms are first proven as definitely syphilitic by the success of therapy or by the anatomical examination. At all events the specific origin is indicated with great probability by the demonstration of syphilis, such as direct luetic manifestations, positive Wassermann, Hutchinson's triad, namely, semicircular lower edges of the middle upper incisors, keratitis parenchymatosa, and sudden deafness in childhood, further by the eye symptoms and by the fluctuating progressive course.

IV. DEMENTIA PARALYTICA

Dementia paralytica, which is commonly incorrectly called softening of the brain and in science briefly, paresis, is a peculiar syphilitic brain disease with the general symptoms of the organic psychoses and peculiar physical manifestations. It mostly runs a course of a few years and ends in death.

Besides the above mentioned [14] psychical peculiarities which differentiate paresis from the other organic psychoses, there are still others, but as yet it has not been possible to isolate them clearly, and still less to formulate them.

On the other hand the *physical symptoms* of paresis are plain specific signs. Just as in tabes we find reflex rigidity of the pupils (Argyll-Robertson); that is, the pupils react to light slowly or sluggishly or not at all, while reaction to accommodation is usually longer or better preserved. The pupils are frequently unequal, abnormally

[14] Cf. pp. 235-236.

dilated or abnormally contracted, and not seldom changed in form. Psychical pupillary reaction (to pain, mental exertion) is also impaired, but not to the extent that these disturbances would show a proportionate relation to the reflex rigidity of the pupil or to the stage of the disease.

The remaining *reflexes* have nothing characteristic about them; the tendon reflexes in simple paresis are naturally exaggerated because their control through the cerebrum is diminished; when complicated with tabes, that is, when there is an interruption of the peripheral spinal reflex arc, they are absent at least in the lower extremities.

The *coordination of muscular action* suffers in a striking manner which is most pronounced in the delicate adjustments of the movements of speech. Individual sounds are badly formed, successive sounds are "run together," the patient prolongs the semi - vowels, sounds and syllables are omitted, repeated, or misplaced (stuttering of syllables), and occasionally the sound components of a word are changed.[15] The psychic disturbances are naturally also present, since inattention and weakness of impressibility or amnestic difficulties, make repetition as well as spontaneous speech more difficult.

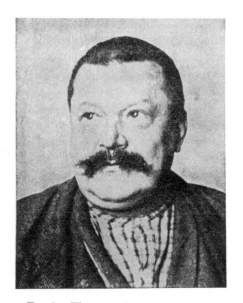

Fig. 1.—The typical flabby paretic expression. It looks as if the mimetic modelling had been erased by excessive retouching, while the eyes betray an affective life. If the eyes are covered, the face looks like that of a sleeper. Asymmetrical noso-labial folds.

Especially in the later stages, the voice easily becomes trembling, monotonous, and towards the last speech is usually slow, babbling, and hardly comprehensible.

In many cases the tone of the mimetic muscles decreases, the nasolabial folds seem wiped out (often more so on one side), the finer

[15] *Ziehen* speaks of "hesitating speech." It is, of course, correct to say that paretics speak slowly as soon as coordination becomes seriously difficult; but the term should be limited to the entirely different *epileptic* speech disturbance to which it is better suited.

mimetic movements are lost. As a result the *face* assumes a flabby and stupid expression, which often enables one to recognize the paretic immediately. Even earlier tremors of individual groups of the facial muscles are sometimes seen ("Heat lightning").

The *tongue* is often put out hesitatingly and shows tremors of individual muscle groups.

The *handwriting* is changed in an analogous manner to speech. Aside from the frequent coarse and irregular tremors of the organic brain affection the lines do not go where they should; the letters become abnormally large and long and unequal; curves are made with corners, etc.; pressure is irregular. The psychical difficulties are as follows: omissions, repetitions, interchange of letters, syllables and words, blotting, wrong corrections, incorrect syntax, the end does not fit the beginning of the sentence and, finally, only an illegible scribbling is produced.

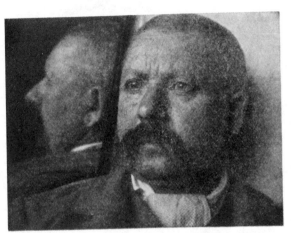

Fig. 2.—Paretic. In spite of a strained pose, expressed in the frown and eyes, the part of the face below the eyes remains flabby.

Disturbance of the *gait* usually becomes plain somewhat later, unless tabes with its characteristic signs of the psychosis precedes. The foot misses its mark, deviating now to the front, now to the rear or side ways. Thus the walk becomes irregular, swaying, with legs spread apart, and at the same time weak, and in certain respects spastic (but not in the sense of spastic spinal paralysis with its difficulty of freeing the tip of the foot from the ground). Inequality of the two sides, "hanging" of the entire body to the left or right is not rare. In the last stages walking is generally impossible.

Gradually the entire *muscular system* attains a condition of extreme spastic paralysis; the patient becomes entirely helpless. The involuntary muscular system is also affected: swallowing becomes difficult and impossible; the intestines no longer advance their content; more frequently *incontinentia alvi et urinae* exists, the latter often together with paralysis of the bladder.

A

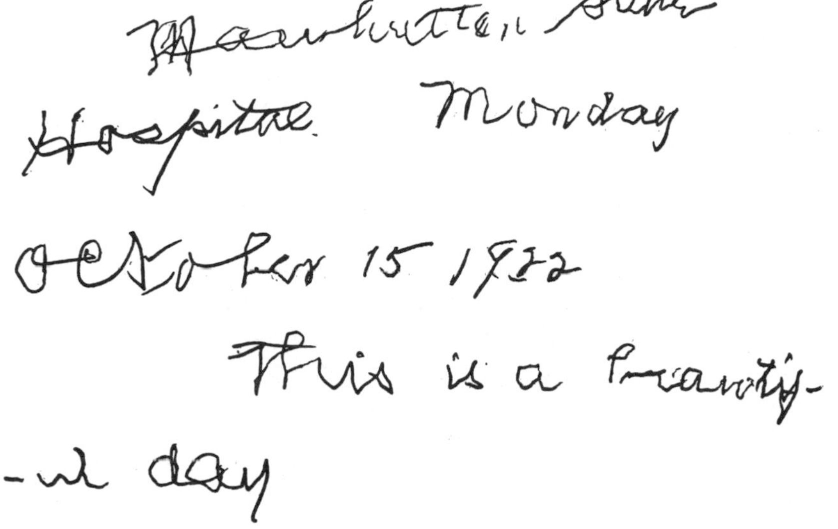

Manhattan State

Hospital.   Monday

October 15 1922

This is a beautif-

-ul day

B

Manhattan State Hospital

This is a beautiful day in April

Around the ragged rock the ragged urchen ran

Benjamin Becker

April 7, 1908.

1919.

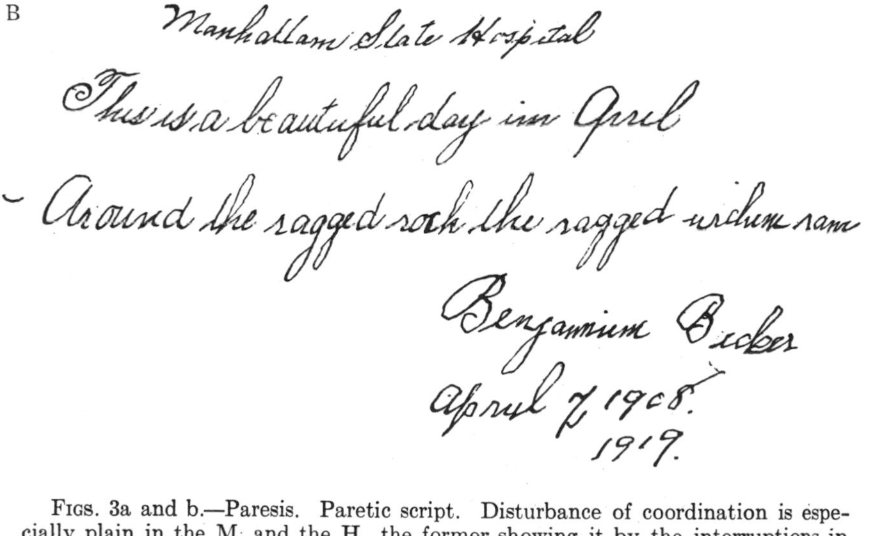

FIGS. 3a and b.—Paresis. Paretic script. Disturbance of coordination is especially plain in the M: and the H., the former showing it by the interruptions in the lines, numerous but vain efforts to continue the strokes. This is particularly seen in the letters r and in the word *beautiful,* which is hardly legible. In example (b) one sees besides some reduplications of strokes and letters and a fusion of letters, etc.

The *blood* in most cases shows a positive Wassermann, the *liquor cerebro spinalis* nearly always. The latter [16] is mostly under increased pressure and because it contains globulin it is clouded by the addition of an equal amount of saturated solution of ammonium sulphate (Nonne, Phase I) ; it also contains an abnormal amount of albumin (Nissl reaction with the Esbach reagent), and shows always a hyper-lymphocytosis, in which the presence of plasma-cells especially (and eventually broken-down cells) is said to be important for the special diagnosis. The number of cellular elements may rise in paresis to several hundred in the cubic millimeter.

The above mentioned physical symptoms must be classed with the fundamental symptoms of paresis, even though in very rare cases they may be only indistinctly evidenced throughout the entire course. Neither in the time of appearance nor in regard to their intensity is there a definite correlation with the psychic defects, and they may appear earlier or later than these. Disturbance of coordination is not seldom found afterwards in earlier specimens of the patient's hand-writing, and the pupillary disturbances especially may manifest them-selves years before the outbreak but may be lacking in a pronounced psychosis.

Among the *accessory physical symptoms* the paretic attacks are most frequent. They resemble those of other severe brain diseases. Mostly, but not always, they appear suddenly; consciousness is usually lost and then convulsions appear, in part general, in part somehow localized, sometimes also they are of the Jacksonian type. There is no "striking blindly" as is so common in epileptiform attacks. They may last for seconds or for days, and consciousness often returns before the convulsions cease.

Besides these attacks, which are characteristic of gross brain lesions in general, mere fainting spells, epileptiform and apoplectiform attacks occur. The latter may leave half sided or monoplegic paralyses, which mostly have a spastic character and need not be based on ascer-tainable anatomic lesions, even when they no longer disappear, which is the exception. Attacks of fever lasting for hours or days may be based on abnormal conditions of the heat centers or on a sudden in-crease of the spirilli.

Aside from *decalcification of the bones various kinds of trophic disturbances occur.* Decubitus cannot sometimes be avoided in the final stage, not only because of the paralyses and uncleanliness but because of trophic changes. *Othaematoma* may also appear without the application of violence.

[16] Comp. pp. 238, etc.

The *weight of the body* is strongly influenced by the disease; the euphoric forms are mostly well nourished, sometimes till death; but usually marasmus appears in the final stage of the disease. Other cases are marasmic from the beginning.

The *appetite* is at times excessive, at times lacking, as a rule fluctuating with the prevalent mood; exaggerated gorging often exists, especially in the demented stage of the manic form.

Sleep is very variable; in all excited states it is naturally brief; in the quiet stages preceding the deep dementia it is mostly normal; in the last stage the nights easily become restless. Pathological sleepiness is much rare.

The *sexuality* is usually changed; in the beginning of the manic forms the libido is mostly increased, later potency disappears first, then, also, the desire.

Like tabes, paresis also is sometimes accompanied by optic atrophy which, however, may fluctuate strongly in a striking manner, that is, vision, in the course of months becomes worse and better; total blindness is an exception. Paralyses, mostly transient, of individual eye muscles are not so rare (especially in the incipient stages) ; definite degenerations of individual nerve roots may occur.

Sensory symptoms in the form of headache, ordinary and "ophthalmic" migrain, and other parasthesias are not rare and are prominent, especially in the preparatory stage, where they are taken for neuritis and rheumatisms. The very frequent hypalgesia or analgesia which mostly affects only the skin, is diagnostically important.

Among the *psychic accessory symptoms* endogenous affective fluctuations of the manic or melancholic type dominate the external picture so frequently that they have been used as characteristic of sub-groups.

Hallucinations (almost entirely of sight and hearing) do not play a large part; most cases run their course without them. Only rarely are illusions prominent for any length of time.

On the other hand *delusions* are frequent and are mostly connected with the emotional shiftings. They are not nearly so fixed as in the paranoid conditions, and especially in the manic forms they change in extent and intensity with the strength of the affective fluctuations and the weakness of judgment; they also increase through preoccupation with them. The patient has the idea that he owns twenty horses; as soon as he has imagined this, it is not enough and he owns one hundred, then two hundred, etc. Delusions may also be provoked or modified by remarks: The patient is asked whether he did not have a rank in the army and he readily becomes a general. They are senseless, partly because of the enormous exaggeration, partly qualitatively: A paretic wants to become rich by purchasing a house with a mortgage of $70,000, that pays $1600 interest; he wants to earn a million with a toboggan slide: "Admission with a bottle of fine wine two dollars." Another buys for his own use one hundred cases of macaroni and all sorts of perishable things in similar quantity, he orders "a boat load of champaign."

In some cases severe focal symptoms are noticed, indefinitely circumscribed paralyses of the cerebral type (*facial nerve inequality* especially of the lower branch is very frequent), aphasic and apractic disturbances, etc. In the later stages manifestations of irritation as smacking the lips, grinding the teeth and other spasmodic, more or less coordinated movements sometimes appear.

Especially in the final stage, symptoms also occur that externally look the same as those of catatonia and cannot as yet be properly differentiated from them; they show themselves in manifestations which one is inclined to designate as verbigerations, stereotypes, and echopraxias.

Course. As a rule paresis results in death within a few years. The few so-called cures, which are mentioned in the literature of the subject, are doubtful (wrong diagnoses? long remissions?). In rare exceptional cases a remission may last a decade or even longer and even without a plain remission a case may be drawn out for many years. That is so rare, however, that it should not be considered. The galloping form may result in death after an excitement lasting eight days.

The *onset* is probably always gradual, even in the case where an acute attack first makes the disease manifest to those around it. Pupillary disturbances as well as transformations of character in many cases can be shown to have taken place a decade before the actual outbreak and symptoms like those of neurasthenia may for a few years exclusively announce the severe disease.

But when the paresis is once noticeable, extensive remissions may simulate a cure. This hardly ever occurs in the simple demented form.

The different manifestations may appear in an entirely irregular sequence. In the prodromal stage, i.e. before the disease is recognized, pupillary disturbances and those of writing, and transformations of character, are most frequent. A neurasthenic symptom, a paralytic attack, or another physical sign may begin the action just as well as a pronounced psychic syndrome, e.g. a senseless or criminal act. For the later stages, too, no rules can be set up, except perhaps that the excitements in severe dementia naturally readily assume the character of confusion.

As the most frequent premonitory symptoms should be mentioned the *pupillary disturbances* and in complication with *tabes* the *absence of the patella* reflex, then irritability, anxiety, excessive ambitions or, the reverse, unusual weakness of will, twilight states lasting for minutes or hours, very similar in appearance to the epileptic, often with some incorrect act, attacks of dizziness, fainting spells, transient double vision, temporary failure of speech, sleep disturbances and especially the neurasthenic syndrome.

The *last stage* is essentially the same in the different forms; nonessential differences are brought about by the affectivity (euphoric in most cases, depressive or indifferent in others), and by the existence or absence of erethic conditions. The individual morbid pictures will be discussed below.

Death results in the uncomplicated cases from marasmus with or without pneumonia. Paralysis of the bladder and decubitus give occasion for infections of all sorts. Paralysis of the muscles of swallowing and respiration may produce pneumonia and choking. Paralytic attacks may also prove fatal. Many patients come to grief because of their motor or psychic deficiencies; suicides occur in the depressive, more rarely in the simple forms.

The *duration of paresis* is difficult to determine. The better the anamnesis the further it can be dated back, not so seldom to a decade before the manifest outbreak. From this period on the disease lasts, on the average, about three years; the shortest course runs in the agitated forms. In all forms, except the agitated, single cases may be protracted over a very long period; the maximum noted so far in one case is thirty-two years.

Grouping. To present the different clinical pictures of paresis, four main types have been differentiated into which most cases can be classed. But there are continuous transitions from one form to another. The individual case, however, remains usually, not unexceptionally, within the type of the form it has once assumed.

1. In the *simple demented form*, stronger exaltations and depressions, delusions, and confused states are lacking. On the other hand besides the typical organic dementia it exhibits as a rule the different physical symptoms, especially attacks. For self-evident reasons it is usually recognized rather late. At first not much else is noticed than that the patients very gradually decline in their occupation—the simpler this is the later it is seen,—then they become more and more demented, awkward, and weaker.

2. The *manic or expansive form,* also called the classical form, because it was the first type recognized, often becomes manifest through a very acute manic attack with a feeling of intense joy and power, flight of ideas, enormous impulse to activity in which the most senseless delusions of grandeur betray the deep seated disturbance of intelligence. The patient is not only God, but possibly a super God, he possesses trillions, and with millions of ships as large as Lake Superior, he constantly brings home diamonds from India, hunts on the moon, has invented a bicycle, with which in three minutes one can ride over land and sea around the earth, etc. He is a general, salutes everybody at the railway station and whoever does not respond to the salute he wants to have shot. Paretic women are the most beautiful that were ever on earth, all human beings are their own children whom God brings forth every second from their womb. The imagination does not always reach so far, and in the later stages of dementia the evaluation of the possession sometimes takes the place of its magnitude: The patient boasts that every month he kills five or six pigs; he can lift a half a hundred weight; he tells that he has inherited a dollar or that he has a fine hat at home, with the same satisfaction as if he owned the earth.

Delusions of grandeur, pressure activity, and lack of critical attitude are often expressed in *inventions* which are usually colossal nonsense. At times, however, something less stupid may result. Thus a man suffering from paresis invented a mixture to freshen up high hats temporarily and supported himself with it for two years after he had become useless for other work. Another speculated on the rise of cotton prices while a fall was generally expected and won nearly half a million francs.

3. The *melancholic* or *depressive form* usually begins less acutely; the fluctuations also are rarely so great. The patients usually never come out of their depression. The delusions are just as senseless but take the form of ideas of impoverishment, of sin, and especially of the hypochondriacal and nihilistic types.

4. The rather rare *agitated form* is defined in various ways. I should like to include here only those cases in which one sees violent motor excitements with confusion and failure to recognize the environment, *without a manic condition;* in addition hallucinations and illusions of hearing and vision invariably occur. Furthermore one also finds coarse cerebral irritating manifestations such as gnashing of teeth, convulsive movements, later carphologia. The disease thus runs a course resembling the picture of the old "acute delirium"; the patients exhaust themselves after a week or more and therefore usually

succumb during the first attack. In milder cases the disease drags along for months and in very mild cases remissions may even occur.

Other observers designate also as agitated those cases of manic paresis which show marked excitement and rapidly succumb to exhaustion, cases which, corresponding with the virulence of the morbid process, show more confusion and agitation than mania and pressure activity. From the two forms described those that run a rapid fatal course, from one to a few weeks, are distinguished as *galloping paresis*.

In the common classification one does not find *euphoric paresis* which, though showing a persistently exalted mood with some grandiose ideas, never reaches to the height of a manic condition. To be sure, it may be regarded as an intermediate form between simple and manic paresis into both of which it extends without limits but because it is the most frequent form, at least with us, I should like to emphasize it particularly.

Of the *related forms* one should mention the *cyclic*, in which manic and melancholy states alternate for a time with or without intervals of an indifferent mood. It is very rare.

Many cases, which later are to be classed mostly with the depressive, somewhat less often with the simple form, are conspicuous because of an extended incipient stage, closely resembling neurasthenia and frequently mistaken for it. If the nervous symptoms are permanently prominent, it is sometimes called *neurasthenic paresis*.

A *paranoid form* is rarely met which for several years impresses one as paranoia and only then takes the usual course. The picture may also be complicated by depressive moods and corresponding delusions.

Tabo-paresis is the designation for the rather frequent association of paresis with tabes; it is supposed to be peculiar also in the entire combination of the paretic symptoms, in so far as it runs a slow course with less pronounced real paretic manifestations.

A *catatonic variety* has also been distinguished but it is still an open question on what the addition of catatonic or apparently catatonic symptoms is based (the occurrence of paresis in a case of schizophrenia or in a schizophrenic disposition?).

Some cases, which in other respects are different, incline to *stupor* lasting for weeks or years. Here it is possible occasionally, but not always, to prove a complication with a previously existing schizophrenia.

Morbid Picture of the Manic Form. In individual but rare cases, occulo-motor paralyses, pupillary rigidity to light, diminution of the tendon reflexes precede the acute outbreak several years. The ocular paralysis can usually be cured by antisyphilitic treatment; but the other symptoms improve less often. These cases then have a pause of several years after which the real onset does not differ from the usual outline that follows.

A man, mentally and physically robust, begins now and then to complain of "nervous" symptoms; a little headache or head pressure or fatigue, either general or localized, e.g. in the eyes; his sleep becomes irregular. This is considered natural and is ascribed to overwork. Treatments at times seem to bring about a temporary improvement, sometimes none; a review of the history extending over longer periods would show that the uncomfortable condition gets rather worse and the ability to work decreases. Topalgias or any other pains, which are interpreted and treated as nervous or rheumatic, are sometimes quite prominent.

At the same time, or even a few years earlier there begins in many cases a very gradual transformation of character that is so stealthy that it is usually overlooked. The careful head of a family now and then seems selfish or careless in a particular act, perhaps, contrary to his previous disposition, he engages in a careless business transaction or without sufficient reason he at times does not feel like going to work.

An able country doctor gives up his practice; he wants to be a surgeon and enters a clinic as an assistant but fails in spite of other good qualities because he does not learn to control asepsis sufficiently. Then he buys a second house and arranges it as a sanitarium that prospers for a few years. Another physician begins enthusiastically and with great success to carry on abstinence propaganda, but then leaves everything to become the head of a cooperative private institution with a doubtful future. Both physicians after a few years are stricken with pronounced manic paresis.

Later in the disease intellectual disturbances become plainer, even though in the incipient stage they are rarely noticed and still less considered morbid. The physician who took over the new institution once figured in all seriousness that he need only prescribe double the length of stay in the sanatorium to his patients, then he would have twice as many inmates, and this he did several years before the disease became manifest; later he was still capable of picking up in a clinic a considerable knowledge of psychiatry and of establishing a thriving city practice.

Intelligent relatives are first conscious of the increasing lability of the feelings, at times in the sense of irritability, at times rather in the sense of sanguine temperament with emotional flights, up and down.

Shortly before the outbreak one notices trespasses against good morals; the patient begins to cheat at cards or he becomes sexually offensive or commits crimes.

There is reason to suppose that such prodromal symptoms are not lacking in any case; but they are not always noticed. *In most cases the acute manifestation usually surprises the family.*

Within a few weeks, often even within a few days, a manic condition attains its highest point with flight of ideas, exalted mood, tireless pressure activity, and flourishing delusions of grandeur. The patient feels capable of anything, undertakes senseless transactions, makes inventions, becomes engaged to three women at the same time, for whom he bought three identical brooches with stones made, in order to send them to all three on the same day. Whoever hinders him is brutally treated as an enemy; it comes to noisy scenes, peace and decency are violated, and then the patient is quickly taken to an institution. Here right at the beginning one often finds, in mild or pronounced form, the symptoms referring to speech, pupils, and hypalgesia of the skin. The absence of critical faculty usually increases very quickly, the patient is God, the President, or Pope; he throws millions around. Thus a chemist discovered the fourth dimension: "right—left, two dimensions, front—rear, two more, equals four, strange that the world had to wait for me to find this egg of Columbus."

Such patients are restless day and night; they tear up things, rattle, sing, and scold.

After a few months the manic condition usually dies down and gives way to a quiet euphoria. The physical symptoms also may subside, in rare cases to complete disappearance. The patient now considers himself cured, he has a certain insight concerning his excitement, and corrects the worst delusions but considers the attack not so severe, or as the self-evident result of confinement, etc. In some cases, which are described as rareties, he may for a few years regain complete capacity for work. Usually, however, he is more or less markedly reduced, affectively too labile and uncritical, but, in spite of this, he may be considered healthy by his relatives. And herein lies a great danger. If he has not ruined his fortune at the beginning of the attack, he is now in danger of doing so. Moreover it is sometimes noticeable that he does not observe the rules of social intercourse; he may go to sleep at a gathering and pass the matter by with indifference.

The remission usually lasts a greater number of months; then there sometimes follows a manic condition similar to the first, more frequently a milder excitement with increased dementia. This game may be repeated several times. A number of delusions are retained and

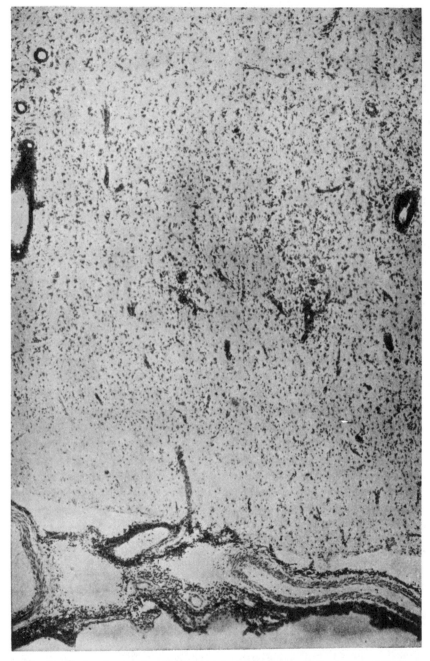

FIG. 4.—Cortex in paresis. Cells stained. Disturbance of the layers. Thickening of the pia. Enlargement of many vessels. Infiltration of small cells into the pia and walls of blood vessels.

produced at every opportunity, even during the remission: "Tomorrow I dine with the President." In many cases such ideas are produced in ever increasing numbers and in even more senseless quality, and are mingled with the products of confabulation. Educated patients endeavor at the same time to retain their bearing; but they do not succeed in every respect; they easily become filthy, and lose their self-control. With or without external causes excitements arise; if the physician, as is often the case, must refuse the patient something, the latter promises to have his head cut off; he summons a regiment, a billion soldiers, who will shoot down the physician and the institution and the entire city. But very soon he is friendly and happy again. Excitements from within usually last longer, sometimes weeks or months.

In the meantime paretic attacks may occur from which the patient mostly recovers very well.

As times goes on, the weakness of judgment and lack of critical faculty becomes more marked, new material is less and less produced; the patient still repeats in a stereotype fashion his old ideas; he industriously gathers all sorts of refuse, and becomes unclear in all respects. He becomes entirely incapable of comprehending the environment; he does not know where he is, and what happens about him. Even without aphasic disturbances it ultimately becomes impossible for him to comprehend even the simplest requests, let alone comply with them. The physical symptoms take the upper hand, his speech becomes a hardly comprehensible babble, his helplessness in all respects becomes worse, the patient has to be kept in bed more and more, he cannot attend to any of his needs himself, he becomes unclean, partly from psychical indifference, in part from paralysis of the sphincter muscles or from *incontinentia paradoxa*. He chokes easily, or in great gluttony he shoves in so much food that the mouth cavity and throat are completely stuffed.

The state of nutrition is mostly noticeably good for a long time, often until death. In some cases marasmus occurs during the final stage; and in rare cases it is followed by marked obesity. The end finally results from an attack, a simple cortical paralysis, a terminal pneumonia, decubitus with infection, or a fracture resulting from the osteoporotic bones; in the majority of cases death comes without the patient being conscious of his misery and without the disappearance of his euphoria.

Morbid Picture of the Depressive Form. Many of these patients, simply because they are timid, exhibit the "nervous symptoms" at an early stage and to a marked degree. Such patients are frequently

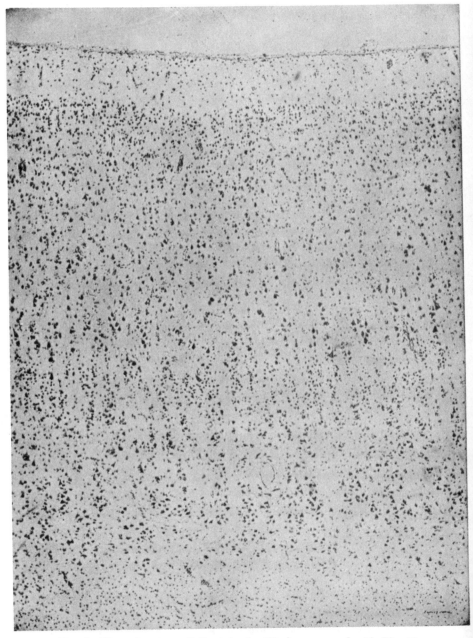

FIG. 5.—Normal cortex. Cells stained. (To be compared with Fig. 4.)

treated for several years as neurasthenics. Ultimately, however, one notices the decline of the ordinary psychic functions, or the paretic physical symptoms. The depression becomes worse, coming either in attacks or progressing gradually; it is usually connected with anxiety. An attempt at suicide often brings the patient into the institution. There he is terribly unhappy, he feels that he has committed every sin, he is punished in an appalling manner here on earth as well as in the hereafter, the world has come to an end or has never existed, his entrails have been consumed, and his limbs are wooden; "I have large legs, I no longer have any legs, I do not exist." Some

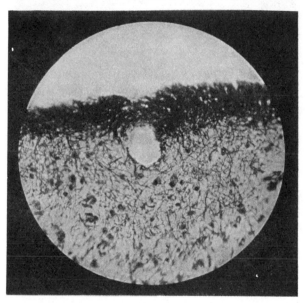

FIG. 6.—Paresis. Gliosis at the cortical edge and around a smaller blood vessel.

bear their fate with a certain outward calm and remain in bed, others run about, cling to everything, push away, scream incessantly, until death relieves them.

The picture of *simple paresis* is more monotonous. With or without nervous symptoms, often slowly in the course of several years, often more rapidly in a few weeks, the patient fails in his work and in his social conduct. He becomes flighty and careless, forgets to pay his club bills or gets served without having any money. He becomes selfish, dissatisfied with his clothes, although he neglects himself, scolds if everything is not according to his wishes, buys four umbrellas at once without knowing why, or cannot find his way in the city. The cook puts too much salt into the food or none at all, or pours petroleum on the salad and puts sugar into the soup; later she throws into one pan "everything that is in the larder." The wife knits stockings of senseless shape and size. A woman patient brought into the institution five pounds of cigar butts in her coat pockets. Aside from this, the mental and physical basic symptoms gradually become plain; the latter often follow paralytic attacks which seem to be here particularly frequent. The patient mistakes places, calls a seal a sleigh ride, etc.

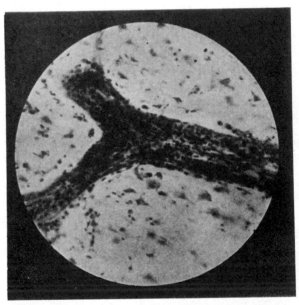

FIG. 7.—Paresis: Infiltration of round cells into a cortical blood vessel.

Mild excitations are sometimes observed. The patients change their vocation several times, they are little concerned with time and custom, e.g. they get up in the middle of the night to take senseless walks. Frequently they indulge in drinking and sexual excesses.

The simple demented paretics usually come to the institution in a seriously reduced state. As there is nothing acute that can become regenerated, extensive remissions are very rare in these cases. Usually they are entirely lacking and the mental and physical decline begins pretty quickly.

The *euphoric* form most closely resembles the manic, only the fluctuations in a good and a bad direction are lacking, or they are slighter, and especially never attain the height of a manic state. The delusional productions are also less and invariably have the identical character as those in classic paresis.

Morbid picture of agitated paresis. The course of this form may be illustrated by the following specific case.

A substantial baker has become less reliable in the last twelve years; with unfortunate inventions and speculations he has squandered a neat little fortune. Suddenly he becomes more restless, stays away from home very often, though to be sure he gives definite excuses, he no longer wants to tend his oven himself, etc. Several months later a hallucinatory delirium breaks out very suddenly, voices command him to undress completely, to partake of only three mouthfuls of food at each meal, and to cut off three of his fingers. Brought into the institution, he throws together everything he lays hands on, pours the soup into the plate and back into the bowl and then again into the plate until everything is on the floor; day and night he pounds on the doors, tears things up, jumps around, attacks the attendants in a brutal way, fails to recognize his surroundings, and does not permit his attention to be held in any way. His talks appear entirely incoherent. Besides he has the physical signs of paresis. After about a week he is completely exhausted, permits himself to be kept in bed, at first with the aid of hypnotics, but he is still in incessant motion, which in the meantime quickly appears weaker and less systematic and after another week he dies from exhaustion.

Anatomical Findings. In paresis the *nervous elements* of the brain, and often those of the spinal cord also gradually disintegrate, and to be sure in different ways, without anything in common to the destructive processes being known. The arrangement of the ganglia cells in rows and layers seems disturbed. The glia grows profusely in the cells and fibres and in such a manner that these elements seem to be increased and enlarged, that is to say thickened. This increase can readily be differentiated, even on superficial examination, from the increase of the glia in senile forms, by the degree of the increase, and specially by the marked thickening of the elements. Mitoses of the glia cells are not rare. The sheaths of the smaller vessels of the cortex and pia (and even of other organs) are infiltrated with round cells, which usually show the *character of plasma cells.* This latter finding is said to be characteristic of paresis, as it only is met elsewhere in the African sleeping sickness and, according to *v. Monakow*, in multiple sclerosis. Other frequent alterations of the vessels of an atheromatous or other degenerative character are probably complications. The formation of new capillaries is often plainly observed. In the tissues are sometimes found the red cells described by *Nissl*, "very elongated, uncommonly narrow formations, at times curved, which consist almost only of a single bright nucleus with several nucleolar bodies, beyond which the body of the cell extends at both ends, sometimes more and sometimes less." Their significance is not yet evident. Lately spirochites have been demonstrated in the central organs by *Noguchi* and others.

Macroscopically the brain is diminished,—in very old cases to less than 1000 g., the surface has frequently lost its smoothness as a result of an atrophying process; the convolutions are narrowed, and the fissures widened. The white substance is of a dirty discoloration and often contracts in the plane of incision, if its severer atrophy is not concealed by *œdema* of the brain. It is striking that for the clinical focal manifestations an anatomical substratum is not always found. But sometimes it is a case of *Lissauer's* paresis, in which very acute shifts with violent cerebral manifestations have affected circumscribed regions, especially in the occipital region.

The *findings in the pia* do not stand in a definite relation to those of the brain. But the usual findings are as follows: The pia is thickened and opaque; it often shows adhesions, sometimes to the cortex, so that in peeling it, parts of the upper cortical layers come off (decortication), and sometimes to the adjacent folds so that one can only go through the median fissure or the fossa Sylvii with the help of a knife. Microscopically one observes an increase of the pia tissues, round cell infiltration (especially plasma cells) and the identical changes in the small vessels as in the cortex.

Nowhere is *Pachymeningitis hœmorrhagica* found so frequently as in paresis, and often the dura adheres to the skull. A certain weight has been attached to the fact that the diplöe is frequently lacking.

Naturally the *spinal cord* shows secondary degenerations as a result of the changes in the brain, but very often there are primary alterations similar to those in the brain.

The *peripheral nervous system* sometimes shows chronic degenerations. The aorta is mostly luetically altered. The other organs also, above all, the liver, are usually not normal; but more definite characteristics are still lacking. The ordinary manifestations of lues and their remnants are remarkably rare (except in the vessels) in paretics.

Causes. The disease which is now differentiated from the other organic psychoses as paresis is in the same sense as tabes, a "metasyphilitic" disease, i.e. at the present time it is a late manifestation of lues, hardly ever associated with ordinary luetic symptoms, and uninfluenced by antiluetic treatment. According to statistics of army officers about 4 percent of syphilitics are afflicted later with paresis.

Severe or mild, thoroughly or superficially treated syphilis may be followed by paresis. It is not, however, without reason that some speak of a special "lues nervosa" which is said to run an easy course and to dispose one to tabes or paresis. It is supposed to be transmitted as such with its peculiarity. However, paresis in married couples is not so frequent that the element of chance be excluded; it is more likely that cases of paresis with a common source of infection favor this conception. Since tertiary manifestations are practically never found in people having paresis, and as secondary symptoms of lues, also, are infrequently noticed in the anamneses, it may be assumed that the mild forms of lues are especially predisposed to paresis. But it may be that the tertiary and the metasyphilitic symptoms are mutually exclusive. At all events it is striking that in marital infection from

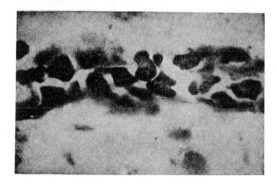

Fig. 8.—Paresis. Plasma cells on the wall of a capillary.

a paretic the lues is latent much more frequently than is otherwise the case. What the personal predisposition to this kind of brain lues is, no one knows; that paresis is the psychosis of the healthy brain has been supposed with just as little reason as that it appears only in cases of psychopathic heredity. However, in the previous history of many paretics a very unsteady manner of living is found, and *Savage* once called attention to the fact that they have mostly taken wives of a markedly sexual type. Where this type is the exception as in Switzerland, this can be confirmed. *Reichardt* claims to have demonstrated a small cranial capacity as very frequent in paresis.

That mental exertion is an important factor has not been proven. But it is probable that alcoholism plays an important part among those predisposed, because paresis is extremely rare among those who have been total abstainers from youth. On the other hand there is a racial predisposition which we do not as yet understand. Among the natives of the Balkan States it is rare; among African Arabs, Abyssinians and Australian negroes it seems practically never to occur; with the Japanese it is said to have become more frequent only in the last decades; with the negroes of North America it was formerly rarer, now it is especially frequent. It is much rarer in rural districts than in cities. The deciding factor, therefore, is probably not the race as such, but the manner of living or some added determining cause, e.g. a second infection of a different sort.

As precipitating or secondary causes one names mental exertions, heat, traumata, and other influences, but none of these assumptions have even been confirmed. The various injurious consequences of the war have, as far as known, conditioned no noticeable increase of paresis. Nevertheless injury in the service, be it in the sense of causation (precipitation) or in the sense of merely aggravating the disease, was assumed after over-exertions, head trauma, infectious diseases, etc. Scientific proofs of such connections are still lacking.[17]

Paresis appears most frequently from about eight to twenty years after the syphilitic infection; but there are also belated cases and those that become manifest after a fewer number of years (up to two years). The disease, therefore, occurs in the period of most active endeavor, after the man has established a family (maximum between 35 and 45) and thereby attains an especially great social significance. To be sure there are cases of *infantile paresis,* that are based on hereditary lues and that mostly run a course following the type of the simple demented form. In contradistinction to many other manifestations of hereditary lues they break out mostly after the sixth year, indeed in some cases not until around the age of twenty.

In accordance with its nature the male sex is much more frequently afflicted than the female, but the morbidity of the latter is rapidly increasing, especially in the large cities, where the proportion is one to two, while the average proportion may be still about one to four. Men are afflicted relatively more in the upper classes, while women in the lower. Cases of infantile paresis are naturally equally divided between two sexes.

Pathology. The finding of spirochites in the brain tissues and of plasma cells in the walls of the vessels shows that it is a question of a direct manifestation of lues in the brain. Whether it is a particular species of spirochites, an inherited predisposition of the patient,

---

[17] Compare especially Bonnhöffer, Die Dienstbeschädigungsfrage in der Psychopathologie. Die Militarärztliche Sachverständigentätigkeit auf dem Gebiet des Ersatzwesens. Vorträge . . . redigiert von Adam. Vol. 1. Fischer, Jena 1917, p. 86.

or later additional influences that make a case of paresis out of a case of lues is not known. Racial dispositions may be variously interpreted; that paretics are somewhat more burdened with psychoses and neuroses than the normal, even though less burdened than the insane, and that they themselves, for the most part, had something psychopathic about them even before, seems to point to endogenous influences; on the other hand, the additional effects of alcohol point to exogenous. It is interesting that cases of paresis from manic depressive families have a particular inclination to the affective forms, while those with schizophrenic relatives get, by preference, paresis colored in the sense of schizophrenia. Besides alcohol we do not know any contributing causes that are favoring or necessary to the origin of the disease.

Diagnosis. In the prodromal stage it is necessary to seek the premonitory symptoms enumerated above,[18] among which migrain with or without scintillating scotoma may be mentioned when it has rather suddenly appeared in the critical age, and is not inherited; furthermore all premonitory symptoms of tabes, such as the crisis and above all pains of uncertain origin falsely interpreted as rheumatic.

The organic disease is confirmed by the affective state and the associations, the dementia by the lack of critical faculty and the kind of delusions, and the paresis in particular by the somatic symptoms.

The diagnostic significance of the individual psychic symptoms may be inferred from what has been said. Prodromal violations of ethical principles by people formerly decent are perhaps the only ones that should be particularly mentioned here.

The physical symptoms without certain proof of an existing mental disease can in themselves be generally decisive. Paresis has the characteristic pupillary disturbance in common with the other luetic psychoses and tabes; encephalitis lethargica also at times leaves pupils that are irresponsive to light. Unequal pupils occur persistently in normal people, then also in catatonia, but they usually change quickly, while in paresis they change at the most in the course of weeks and months. Sluggishly reacting, or rigid *pupils* are often found in the alcoholic psychoses with an organic element, very rarely in the hysteric with contraction of sphincters, then in the epileptic in the course of the attack, etc. One must hear the paretic *speech disturbance* but after that, one very rarely mistakes it. The stuttering of imbeciles is something entirely different; here the sounds may be inexact but they are not misplaced and are not run together; on the contrary they are

[18] Cf. p. 257.

combined less than in skilled speech. The dysarthritic disturbances of other organic brain diseases have not yet been sufficiently described, even though they are in most cases easily differentiated from those of paresis. One has to think only of the hesitating and singing of epileptic speech to recognize it when it is developed. Yet slightly developed speech disturbances in paresis and epilepsy can have a certain similarity.

The speech disturbance must often be looked for. For this purpose one finds useful some test words which make a great demand on co-ordination: Above all "Third riding artillery brigade," or "Electricity," or "Methodist Episcopal Church," where the patient usually gets stuck on the *p* and *s* sounds, or "Around the rugged rock the ragged rascal ran." Such long test words as "Constantinopolitan ladies" are not as good as those cited, and test more the psychic qualities like attention and correct reproduction, than coordination. One must particularly learn to distinguish between psychic and speech errors. He who instead of "Third riding artillery brigade" repeats without coordinating disturbances "third artillery brigade" is, to be sure, usually an organic case but seldom a paretic. Furthermore, it must be considered that many patients by strained attention succeed even with difficult words, while in ordinary conversation they fall down on more simple ones; or the paretic, who has been examined by several physicians in succession, is specially practiced in the test words and, therefore, reproduces them particularly well. On the other hand anxious attention may in itself cause the downfall even of those not suffering from paresis in the speech stunts of the tests. In many cases this danger may be circumvented by permitting the patient to read something aloud, and this can be done with better results when the patient is not aware that his speech is tested.

The *handwriting* cannot always be evaluated because it is changed in a similar manner by other diseases, and the results of severe trembling are sometimes difficult to distinguish from those of disturbances of coordination. But the examination of the handwriting need not be dispensed with, and in cases where the diagnosis is definite the examination of previous handwritings is sometimes the safest means of determining how long ago the disease began. Moreover, in an existing psychosis it can at least present evidence of a cerebral affection, which in most cases indirectly assures the existence of paresis. Neurasthenics and other excited people, also, sometimes make mistakes in handwriting both as to quality and quantity that are difficult to understand. But they can easily correct them; on the other hand the person afflicted with paresis leaves most of his errors uncorrected, he also cannot readily find them and when he does make corrections they are very often wrong.

Paralyses are also significant when it is certain that they have been acquired which, e.g. in the case of facial inequalities, is not always easily determined.

Paralytic attacks are often mistaken for apoplectic attacks but in the latter the protracted twitchings are rare. Apparently severe attacks with consequent paralyses and very rapid complete recovery point to paresis.

To be sure the easiest way to make the diagnosis at present is through an examination of the *cerebro spinal fluid*. If pleocytoses, Nonne and Wassermann, are found in an existing psychosis, the diagnosis is as good as settled. To be sure tabes can produce the identical manifestation; but their existence only increases the probability of paresis because with the rarity of "tabes psychoses" in the narrower sense, a mental disease combined with tabes, is very probably paresis. In some exceptional cases of paresis the Wassermann findings may at times be negative for a shorter or longer period; this is mostly the case in stealthy or stationary stages or in very slowly progressing varieties. *Cave:* In the secondary stage of syphilis one sometimes observes in the cerebro spinal fluid the same findings as in paresis, but its only significance is that it is a transient mild cooperation in the infection on the part of the central nervous system and its integuments. Paresis at this period is extremely rare.

The *differential diagnosis of manic paresis from the manic attack of manic depressive insanity* rests on the demonstration of the physical symptoms, also on a thoughtlessness and lack of regard in all actions which are exaggeratedly out of proportion to the excitement, and above all on the foolishness of the delusions. Mistaking individuals is rather a trick with manic depressives; whereas paretics believe in their fictions. But particular care must be taken in the case of initial outbreaks during manhood, because paretic symptoms that are lacking today may appear tomorrow. At any rate in a pronounced manic state of paresis the delusions are nearly always present.

The differentiation from *states of melancholia* rests on the same principles.

As against *schizophrenia* the diagnosis is often not easy, when we have mere conditions of excitements with a senseless and confusional trend of ideas which do not assume a distinct and specific form. Individual catatonic signs, which under such circumstances usually cannot be anaylzed, are not yet evidence of catatonia, but affective stiffness and lack of intellectual and affective rapport furnish such proof. Since so many paretics were always pronounced psychopaths, the anamnesis may often only confuse instead of enlighten. Here, as in all psycho-pathies, it is often of decisive importance, if from a definite time a change of the psychic attributes in the sense of paresis can be ascer-tained or excluded.

As against *epilepsy*, only the specific signs of the two psychoses can be decisive; when epileptic attacks appear in middle age, they are mostly not pronounced in any direction, and therefore there are cases where for a time one wavers.

Because of the tendency of paretics to excesses the *alcoholic forms* frequently give occasion for doubt. Korsakoff's disease as an organic psychosis has the most important psychical symptoms in common with paresis, but the neuritis and the lack of the specific paretic signs (pupillary disturbances also occur there!) usually remove the diffi-culties; sometimes the mode of onset of the disease also helps the diagnosis. But the peripheral neuritis is not always present. *Alcoholic pseudo paresis* causes still greater difficulties. I have never seen pro-nounced delusions of grandeur accompany it, but it is said to occur in rare cases. Progression during abstinence instead of gradual, and at least partial, regression decides in time for paresis. To be sure the examination of the spinal fluid is a quicker way.

Not at all seldom it is a *delirium tremens* that first brings the real case of paresis into the institution. The former passes away, the latter progresses.

The *paranoid forms* of dementia paralytica are very rare, so that here I would like only to call attention to them; if the symptoms are still barely pronounced, then for a time the differentiation from paranoia or paranoid states can only be made by lumbar puncture.

The differential diagnosis from *brain tumors* is self-evident, only it must be mentioned that there are slowly growing, infiltrating gliomas which may run their course entirely under the picture of a simple paresis with indicated local symptoms. Without a lumbar puncture one can miss the diagnosis up to death, and it is just in the case of suspected tumor that the puncture is dangerous.

From the remaining *organic psychoses* paresis can be certainly differentiated only by the physical symptoms (including the fluid), even though pronounced paretic grandiose delusions alone permit the diagnosis without too great a risk.

To draw the boundary line between *neurasthenia* and paresis is one of the most important problems. The complaints are frequently the same for a long time. The neurasthenic supposes, e.g. that he is suffer-ing from weakness of memory; but when he is examined for it nothing is found, or instead one sees affective memory difficulties; he fears he is suffering from "softening of the brain" and thinks he has a speech disturbance, but the latter shows itself, when it is present at all, to be graduated not according to the articulatory difficulties of the words, but according to the momentary degree of anxiety. Especially important is the *attitude* of the patient toward these symptoms. The neurasthenic pictures everything as more difficult than it is; he likes to hear himself consoled but is not quieted immediately, or at all. The paretic usually does not take matters so seriously; he very readily offers excuses: Just at present he is somewhat tired or frightened by the examination or he is chilly or anything similar. And when, in depressive cases he really is anxious, he remains inconsistent and readily neglects the physician's directions which the real neurasthenic does only when he is bothered by several "Systems of Treatment." Above all the neurasthenic shows an exaggerated self-observation and is accustomed to attribute an exaggerated importance to the symptoms while the paretic usually appears indifferent and exhibits a striking incapacity for self-observation. This difference is also seen in the depressive conditions with retained intelligence (e.g. in the manic depressive states).

Treatment. Prophylaxis consists in the avoidance of, or combatting syphilis and alcohol, the latter, because on the one hand it increases the chances of infection, on the other hand because it helps lues to develop into paresis. It has not been proven that the energetic treatment of erupted syphilis betters the chances against later affliction with paresis. It is not a rare technical blunder to prophesy the approaching paresis (or tabes) to patients with pupillary rigidity or absent patellar reflexes. If later difficulties are to be anticipated, a responsible person should always be informed of the *possibility* of the future outbreak of such a disease; the patient himself, who breaks down anyway at the critical moment, should be spared and, when possible, his wife also.

The treatment of pronounced paresis as a disease has so far been hopeless. Antisyphilitic treatment as well as salvarsan are ineffective. Very recently successes have been reported from the infection of patients with *tertian plasmodium* (Wagner v. Jauregg).

An early diagnosis is most important, in part to save the expense of ruinous and useless treatments, in part to secure the existing estate. When cases of paresis come into hospitals, they have, in great part, impaired their estate severely as a result of their grandiose delusions or of the dementia. It is the duty of the family physician to instigate the necessary steps in time. Above all there is danger in the long remissions upon which judges and relatives like to look as a cure, whereas the existing feeble-mindedness and the euphoric mood as well as new shifts impair the patient's capacity for independent action.

The obvious general rules of treatment should be followed in the excitements as well as in the stage of helplessness. In anxiety states opiates often render good service. Careful oversight of the bladder is essential, as otherwise paradoxical incontinences remain concealed and may lead to paralysis or rupture of the bladder. Many patients can under favorable circumstances be treated at home as soon as it is certain that they will permit themselves to be managed, and will not endanger their estate or compromise themselves by sexual excesses or criminal acts.

In paralytic attacks a simple conservative attitude is best; the patients are protected from harm through collision and rubbing, but above all against uncleanliness. Artificial feeding is resorted to only in cases of necessity; the patient will not die at once from inanition but with these helpless patients the danger is especially great that some of the liquid food is inhaled into the lungs when the tube is taken out or when they gag. Nutritive enemas are often not retained. When necessary an infusion of a physiological salt solution beneath the skin can at least maintain the supply of water at the proper level. If the relatives demand "that something be done," ice-packs applied to the head are advisable, and amylenehydrate or paraldehyde or chloralamide are said to reduce sometimes the violence of the convulsion. The first two drugs can also be given as an enema in a vehicle that protects the bowel (chloralamide 4.0 to 6.0 (!), Amyli 4.0, Ap. dest. 150.0; or Amylenehydrate 4.0 to 6.0 Aq. dest. 60.0, Mucil Gummi arab. 30.0 for enema). Heart stimulants are also given, when a collapse is threatened.—But I do not have the impression that the attack runs its course the worse in any respect whatever, if the patient is not bothered at all.

V. SENILE AND PRESENILE INSANITY (SENILE PSYCHOSES)

Under the name of senile psychoses *Kraepelin* includes the *presenile and senile mental disturbances*, among the latter separating *arteriosclerotic insanity* from *senile dementia* with which he also classes *presbyophrenia*.

The presenile forms are as yet symptomologically as well as systematically entirely obscure. It has not even been definitely proven that there are such forms. No doubt certain forms are favored at the period of involution since, e.g. depressions and anxiety states increase greatly from this time on and it is possible that certain psychoses still occur in this period. The morbid pictures here considered as presenile are with difficulty separated from the senile forms, in part because a few of them also evince an organic character, in part because naturally in case of a protracted duration a senile brain alteration may very easily be added to the presenile, in which case the furtive development of the organic symptom for a long time easily conceals the fact that something new has stepped in.

The conception of "Involution" which is infused with the idea of "presenility," is sometimes conceived in the sense of a regression that ends with death, sometimes in the sense of transition to a new age, similar to the "climacterium": The designation "Involutionary Psychoses" is based on the latter conception, directing attention to a difference as opposed to the senile psychoses.

The *actual senile psychoses*, that we know, all have a definite tendency to progress, or expressed anatomically, to the gradual destruction of the brain. That there are not also curable psychoses belonging to senility, is naturally not excluded as yet. But with these I should not like to class "senile melancholias" with mild organic features or organic confusions and deliria, because on closer examination it is always found that after the disappearance of the striking symptoms the patient is, in the sense of dementia senilis, a weakened individual. Therefore, I conceive such storms as intercurrent manifestations of a senile brain degeneration, just as in pronounced senile dementia and analogous to the acute appearances in paresis and schizophrenia, and theoretically I place the major disease in the foreground, even though there are cases where the restoration of equilibrium has practically the significance of a cure. On the other hand *Kraepelin* usually places the practical result in the foreground and designates many senile melancholias with nihilistic delusions or other organic manifestations as curable, as long as the psyche is not as yet materially damaged otherwise.

Furthermore other psychoses, like manic depressive shifts, which also occur at this age, naturally do not belong to the senile; here the disposition lies in the native constitution and not in the age.

The senile psychoses offer three different classes of anatomical findings: arteriosclerosis with its effects on the nervous system (*arteriosclerotic insanity*), simple atrophy of the brain (*dementia senilis in the narrower sense*) and spherotrichia (*Verdrusung*) with or without alteration of the neuro-fibrils (*presbyophrenia*). *With the first and last alteration there naturally also appears regularly sooner or later a nutritive disturbance of the entire brain and besides, the three processes can, from the beginning, be combined in all possible combinations.* We rarely have pure forms in practice.

The essential thing is above all anatomically the diffuse reduction of the brain substance and symptomatologically the complex of the "organic psychic" symptoms. The latter alone are present in the simple senile forms. In arteriosclerotic insanity there are also neurological cerebral manifestations and the psychical defects for a long time have something lacunar about them. In the presbyophrenic forms the picture is complicated by excitation and some other symptoms.

The three senile forms have within the organic group a *common differential diagnosis*, which, as against paresis, is decided chiefly by the absence of the paretic signs (speech, pupils, fluid, blood Wassermann). As against alcoholic Korsakoff the decisive points are the lack of the signs of alcoholism and, up to a certain degree, neuritis. The remaining organic diseases (brain tumor, multiple sclerosis, etc.) carry their particular neurological signs which are wanting in the psychoses previously mentioned.

The alcoholic Korsakoff patient is as a rule euphoric in the beginning but not manic as in classic paresis. The deeper moods of the senile patients are in the great majority of a depressive type.

Organic depressions, especially senile, externally often closely resemble late catatonias since they are rebuffing (like negativism), mutistic, and have moods and fits (like the stereotype forms). The general specific signs, especially memory defects, may still be absent in the beginning. For purposes of recognition the good affective reactions are especially of service, which, to be sure, may manifest themselves only in little noticeable movements of the corners of the mouth; then also the accumulation of organic delusions:—a million years in purgatory, the abdomen is a sewer, it is blown up like a baloon (while in reality it is entirely empty and contracted). Such ideas are not excluded in dementia præcox but are very rare.

A number of *therapeutic* viewpoints also are common to the group. Like paresis they jeopardize the fortune and the legal relations generally. Therefore in every individual case the question arises whether a legal guardianship should be instituted.

Beware of the advice that the patient should give up the accustomed occupation without, a substitute, unless it is absolutely necessary. *Senility often becomes a disease only as a result of the sudden cessation of the ordinary attractions of life.*

Interning in an institution should be much less frequently recommended and should be less often permitted to become protracted than in a case of paresis. If a senile patient has a home, under ordinary circumstances he should be able to remain there. Only when accessory symptoms (restlessness, confusion) or danger for himself and those about him appear, when he is melancholic, when he handles light and fire carelessly, leaves the gas jet open, is inclined to sexual attacks, threatens his wife and children,—then only should he be placed in an institution. If the danger is past, it should be seen to it that he is again brought into normal condition.

The nightly deliria which are very annoying to all concerned may sometimes be overcome by hypnotics but not nearly in all cases. Besides the ordinary remedies bromidia may be recommended here which contains a happy combination of narcotics precisely for just such cases. Its formula is a secret; how to compound it is stated below.[19] But the remedy can be compounded in every drug store. Only the preparation then looks cloudy and must be shaken. *Ris* recommends for the "reversed daily program" (restlessness at night, sleep during the day) that 0.03 opium be given evenings around eight o'clock; after one or two weeks, sleep would occur at night, when the remedy can be omitted until further needed. In severe cases two doses (6 and 8 o'clock) should be given; a triple dose daily (4, 6 and 8 o'clock) should rarely be necessary.

PRESENILE INSANITY

Under this name are described entirely different, insufficiently classified and characterized pictures: 1. rare *subacute cerebral degenerations* which result in death or dementia often after a few months of senseless delusions, delirium, usually anxiety conditions, and which are to be classed with diseases of the brain. 2. more frequent *melancholy conditions* of varying appearance, usually improving (see manic-depressive insanity and climacterium virile): 3. pretty frequent paranoid and catatonia-like forms, the former passing more chronically, the latter rather in shifts, but on the whole with a bad prognosis. A part but not all of the third category are belated schizophrenias. According to my experience, *Kraepelin's presenile delusions* especially belong to dementia præcox.

ARTERIOSCLEROTIC INSANITY

Arteriosclerotic insanity has very manifold ways of manifesting itself. Usually arteriosclerosis of the brain with different symptoms

[19] Ext. Cannab. Ind. Ext. Hyoscyami fluid. āā 0.5. Kal. bromat. Chloralhydrati āā 50.0. Aq. dest. ad 250.0.

is present before a psychosis can be mentioned. Very few cases generally reach the psychiatrist. Arteriosclerosis in itself does not condition a psychosis; this only happens when there is a diffuse reduction of the brain substance (aside from transient delirious conditions and the emotional disturbances from large brain lesions).

The neurologic cerebral symptoms consist of head pressure, headache with marked fluctuations, dizziness, fainting spells, buzzing in the ears, scintillating before the eyes, eventually paralyses and all possible focal symptoms such as hemiplegia, hemianopsia, and aphasic and apractic disturbances etc. The latter manifestations of organic deterioration are in the beginning usually unstable and can regenerate very decidedly (i.e. they need not be based on hemorrhage and softenings).

In very many cases other symptoms also appear as a result of arteriosclerotic changes in other organs, especially the kidneys and the heart.

As long as the psychic symptoms do not dominate the picture, the disease is also designated as *"the nervous form of arteriosclerosis of the brain."*

The psychic symptoms like the physical begin very insidiously and come and go in the beginning. The patients often feel something like a void in their mind, their initiative weakens, it becomes difficult for them to rouse themselves to action. Their endurance is diminished, the accustomed attention is trying to them, they tire much more readily than they used to. *These symptoms invariably have a painful effect whereby* the morbid picture is again made more serious. But undoubtedly there also exists a primary tendency to depression and to an anxious conception of experiences, often even to severe anxiety conditions, which evidently are frequently the direct result of circulatory disturbances of the brain.

This stage may last for years without material aggravation. Nevertheless the affectivity usually becomes more labile in a certain sense; emotional incontinence is plainly developed. The patient's interest becomes narrowed and the tendency to depression inhibits somewhat the emotional fluctuations; nevertheless it is evident how they can react in all directions in the sense of irritability and psychic pain, and in periods of improvement also in the sense of joy and longing, and what is characteristic is the fact that they react even to trifles.

Gradually disturbances of *memory*, especially for recent experiences, become more pronounced, at first only on certain occasions, as on seeking a name, etc.; later it is more generally noticeable, but always oscillating up and down. Confabulations may appear but are rarely numerous.

As a result of many fluctuations in the course of many years the picture may become more and more serious. *Anxiety states* lasting for minutes or weeks can assume a delirious character with failure to recognize the environment, dreadful delusions of being cut up, burnt, buried alive, usually as punishment for sins. The patients struggle for breath, yell, accuse themselves, strive to get away, and make brutal attempts at suicide. In the intervals also there is a tendency to real melancholia. The patients become less courageous, they are timid, conceive everything as painful, and form depressive delusions, especially also of a hypochrondriacal type.

Other *delirious* states are rather rare in the simple forms, but they are all the more frequent in the apoplectic types.

Apperceptive ability and *attention* are only gradually changed in the sense of the organic syndrome.

Orientation at first suffers only spasmodically and finally it is entirely destroyed, the physical strength is impaired, the patients finally remain bedridden and die of marasmus or of *apoplectiform* attacks.

Apoplectic Forms. Very often the entire disease has its origin in the attacks or these chiefly determine its course. Here one deals with hemorrhages as well as softenings. The first attack occurs after arteriosclerotic prodromal stages of varying intensity and varying duration, or also in people who were still entirely well, with the usual symptoms of headache, irritabilities, dizziness, fainting, and consequent general symptoms and focal manifestations, the latter remaining or regenerating according to their location. Depending on the general nutritive condition of the brain and perhaps also on the localization of the focus, the psychical signs of diffuse brain atrophy can sooner or later supervene. According to my experience, lesions especially in the region of the pons seem to be deleterious, although at first they produce the least change in the psyche (circulatory disturbances starting from the vascular centre?). On many cases, however, the psyche remains for years disturbed so little that the patients are properly regarded as mentally sound. Only the affectivity is often plainly changed in these cases also, and this change is in the direction of lability. Often immediately after the stroke the patients can be made to cry and even to laugh much more readily than before. In many cases they feel this as positively unpleasant; real compulsive laughing and compulsive crying, i.e. mimetic expressions to which no real felt affect corresponds qualitatively and quantitatively, is a rare local symptom emanating from the thalamic region.

Otherwise *dementia apoplectica* is not materially different from simple arteriosclerotic dementia without apoplectic strokes with which it is connected by transitional forms with rare or frequent minor attacks.

Both forms may be complicated by moods (nearly always depressive), and especially by irregular, fluctuating anxiety-melancholic states.

Invariably the personality with its strivings is maintained for a relatively long period; even when the patients already appear decidedly demented they are not much changed in the fundamental aims of their will, only they no longer understand everything and they permit themselves to be dominated more by their affects. The symptoms of deterioration also are "lacunary," i.e. as to time and in respect to special functions they are entirely irregular, present or absent in part; thus good memory may be surprisingly present in complete helplessness of the ability to recall, and correct judgments may be evinced side by side with completely narrowed ones. While in paresis, dementia senilis and presbyophrenia, one can infer with great probability from the general condition as to individual abilities, in this case it would be very deceptive.

Individually the pictures are naturally very different according to the location and diffusion of the lesion on the one side and according to the intensity of the general cerebral atrophy on the other.

Concerning the *course* of all forms *Kraepelin* emphasizes the fact that first, the decrease in the elasticity of the vessels produces troubles in the adjustment of the blood apparatus to the momentary needs; this adjustment is particularly infinitely graduated in the brain. This naturally also impairs the capacity for functional adjustments and consequently produces the exhaustion, the difficulties in doing things and perhaps, also a part of the early affective disturbance. It finally produces wrong reactions of the vessels, sometimes surely local paralyses of the vessels, which causes the transient local troubles and many fluctuating general symptoms Later one observes an insufficient blood supply of circumscribed regions which are ever increasing in numbers, sometimes even embracing the entire brain (e.g. in sclerosis the entire circulus Willisii) with the various consequent manifestations, and in the third place the hemorrhages and softenings resulting from the breaking of the arterial walls and the blocking of the lumina.

The outcome is death following organic dementia. The latter may not occur when the course is shortened by apoplexies and other attacks. The duration of the disease may vary from a few weeks to two decades.

Age. Arteriosclerotic insanity appears most frequently between the ages of 55 and 65 years. But cases occur even in the forties; they are mostly conditioned by a family predisposition.

Both sexes are about equally represented in the apoplectic disturbances, in the other forms, according to Kraepelin, 71.5% affect men.

A functionally limited morbid picture is *arteriosclerotic epilepsy*, which usualy appears very early in the various localizations of arteriosclerosis and sooner or later leads to dementia. It is said to occur mainly in alcoholics.

Concerning the *anatomy* of arteriosclerotic insanity nothing can really be added to what has been said. Most of the varieties of arteriosclerotic thickening through proliferation of the vascular cells, hyaline degeneration, etc. are found in the most different distributions, and as a result of these there is local destruction of the nerve tissue through degeneration and a filling in of glia ("perivascular gliosis"), through capillary and large hemorrhages, through softenings, and besides in most cases there is a diffuse reduction of the brain substance as the expression of a *general* metabolic disturbance. The sum of countless small lesions can perhaps also have the same effect as a complete diffuse disturbance. The entire brain is invariably atrophied; at death it is reduced on an average by about 150 g. The pia is often thickened with connective tissue, but hardly infiltrated or adherent.

The *etiology* of arteriosclerosis is for the most part still obscure; it is not only a disease of civilization; its traces are said to have been found in prehistoric races. At all events the family disposition is of importance. On the basis of experimental facts, tobacco has been blamed very recently; alcohol for a long time. Furthermore the attempt has been made to include among the causes of arteriosclerosis a number of circumstances such as conscientiousness and dissipation, overexertion and laziness, and many other things, but as yet without sufficient proof. In the ordinary cases, where the Wassermann is negative lues probably plays no part; as yet we do not possess sufficient knowledge to differentiate anatomically the ordinary arteriosclerosis from the specific in all cases.

As *precipitating causes* debilitating diseases are to be mentioned, as in simple dementia senilis; the brain, the blood supply of which might just suffice under ordinary circumstances; can then no longer obtain nourishment and atrophies *in toto* or in certain places to such an extent that the psychic symptoms break out. Stronger affects, especially depressive ones, often induce the rapid appearance of the arteriosclerotic syndrome; the connecting link is probably the inadequate regulation and adaptive insufficiency of the vessels.

Naturally in pronounced cases the *diagnosis* is relatively easy.

In the beginning it is based on the different neurological symptoms with their characteristic change.

The hardening of the cerebral vessels is not always easy to diagnose. More severe sclerosis of the arteries of the body offers a certain probability of similar changes in the brain; but the latter can just as well be free in the case of pronounced hardening in other organs, just as the reverse occurs. Importance is properly attached to increase of blood pressure, slow pulse, to its abnormal increase after slight exertions (climbing on a chair or bending ten times), then especially to the marked differences between systolic and diastolic pressure. The normal figures (measured according to *Recklinghausen*) are minimum pressure to 100 mm. Hg., maximum pressure 160 mm. Hg., resp. 140 and 220 cm. H_2O.

From paresis which is sometimes combined with arteriosclerosis, it can be differentiated by the absence of the physical signs of paresis, especially pupillary rigidity which is never found here, negative Wassermann in the blood and fluid, absence of pleocytosis and globulin reaction in the fluid,[20] absence of expansive delusions and excessive euphoria. Manic states hardly occur in arteriosclerotic insanity. Anatomically there need not be in paresis a thickening of the vessel walls, while the infiltration with plasma cells is foreign to arteriosclerosis.

From *dementia senilis* and *presbyophrenia* it is differentiated particularly by the fluctuations in the course and by the presence of the signs of arteriosclerosis. Heredity also sometimes offers differential points. When there are no circumstances that favor cerebral atrophy such as a manic-depressive constitution, congenital weakness of the brain, alcoholism, and heart troubles, an age of less than sixty-five years speaks against mere dementia senilis. *But it is self-evident that the various senile processes frequently take place together.*

Senile dementia and, to a still higher degree, paresis alter the personality much earlier and fundamentally than arteriosclerosis; the entire functions of memory, of the critical faculty, etc. are damaged in senile dementia and paresis while arteriosclerosis at least for a long time manifests itself in a "Mosaic of individual symptoms."

From *brain syphilis* arteriosclerotic insanity is differentiated by the absence of the neurological signs (eye troubles, etc.) and by the serological signs of lues.

Treatment. Because of our ignorance of the etiology we cannot carry on much *prophylaxis* against arteriosclerosis. It is undoubtedly good to avoid tobacco and alcohol. Still, pronounced arteriosclerotic

[20] Increase of albumin occurs, as it seems, but no globulin reaction.

insanity is in many cases a grateful object of treatment. Mild, slowly progressing disturbances are often markedly improved and there is also occasion to prove that this is not chance but really the result of treatment.

It is very often possible to free the patients from all the psychic and physical exertions that they cannot bear, that is, from those burdens which according to experience aggravate their condition. If it is not known what the patients can stand, it is necessary to try them out carefully. Neither the psyche nor the heart should be overtaxed. As far as possible the patients should be protected against affective disturbances. If the heart does not respond it should be treated but not without care (digitalin; once in a while perhaps strophantus, etc.: sensible treatment with digitalis hardly increases the danger of apoplexy). We also have had good results with *diuretin* in small doses, e.g. 0.5 three times a day. Anxiety states can also be combatted from the psychical side with opiates or at the same time with heart remedies. Very often, too, a bromide preparation, especially sedobrol, produces calm; it can be combined very well with small doses of iodide. Iodide is generally given and under certain circumstances it probably has a certain effect on the arterial walls or, at any rate, on their regulation and, as has been lately supposed, on the viscosity of blood also. At present many are afraid of such big doses as 3.0 per day, and prefer smaller doses, e.g. up to 0.5 per day. All drugs should be stopped after a few weeks or months until there is a new indication for their reapplication. For example, an iodide cure can perhaps be given once every year.

Proof is lacking that any of the usually recommended diets are useful; excessive meat diet is said to be injurious. *Lewandowsky* claims to have observed benefits from a diet with little salt. At all events the patient should guard against overfilling his stomach either with solid or liquid food. Stimulating substances as well as alcohol [21] should be avoided on principle.

The *psychic treatment*, which should calm the anxious patient with consolations, is especially important.

But under all circumstances, as soon as the condition permits, the attempt should be made to keep the patient busy. In the beginning of the disease before employment has been given up, this usually succeeds without much difficulty by having the patient do a smaller amount of his ordinary work. If this is not possible, other work must be sought for him that holds his interest. Exercise in the open, adapted

[21] Total abstinence from alcohol is a *condition sine qua non* in any treatment. (Pilz, Wiener med. W.S. 1910, p. 626.)

to the strength of the heart, is naturally to be recommended. In this way fairly tolerable conditions are often obtained for many years. Naturally this is also the case when the arteriosclerosis has been complicated by an involutionary depression independent of it, which heals in time of its own accord, after it has made the picture appear too serious.

Strenuous measures, like hydrotherapeutic treatments, especially thermal cures, are naturally to be avoided. To prevent apoplexy in pronounced arteriosclerosis, everything is to be excluded that increases the blood pressure or leads to a rush of blood to the head, especially hot baths, excessive eating and drinking, etc. Experience shows that a cerebral hemorrhage is occasionally connected with such influences; but too much cannot be expected from these regulations.

In arteriosclerotic *epilepsy* besides bromides, iodide may also be given. But it is usually an incurable disease.

In accidents following sudden cerebral diseases the family physician's most important psychiatric problem often is to obtain a clear idea of the patient's mental condition; because he sometimes has to decide his testimentary ability either for present purposes or later in court as expert or witness. Care must be taken not to mistake aphasic or paraphasic symptoms (including paragraphia) for confusion and dementia. In all cases where it would be a question as to the patient's responsibility for his actions pains should be taken to get in contact with the patient through the most various means of understanding. Since wills frequently are attacked only after years have elapsed, pains must not be spared to make exact notes of the case.

Senile Dementia (Simple Dementia Senilis)

Even though the normal regression of the brain begins in the early fifties, it does not usually become plainly noticeable until the last decade of the normal span of life. The earliest sign we meet with in most cases—in many people even before the end of the sixth decade—is a certain inability to assimilate the new ideas of others. Such persons become passively neophobic even though they are still capable themselves of creating new combinations of ideas to a limited extent. But after a while the entire ability to assimilate is weakened; the old man is less and less interested in what goes on in the world; his thoughts, now egocentric, are withdrawn to the more personal necessities, both in emotional and intellectual relations. The feelings become more labile, and react to trifles; more protracted moods readily occur. In social intercourse some cases show a tendency to empty chatter, others to torpid monosyllabism. Besides excessive suggestibility one is struck by a stubborn intractableness. Not only the impressibility but the entire memory becomes poorer, at first for names and similar efforts which are otherwise also particularly difficult. The inability to understand and recall new experiences, the relatively or absolutely easier reproduction of the old memory material in connection with the general trait that memory pictures of a pleasant character can be more readily revived than the unpleasant, makes them into *laudatores temporis acti.* All psychic processes become more trying and slower, particularly in proportion to their complexity. That the capacity for practical work declines under these conditions is self-evident.

Simple senile dementia is said to be a simple exaggeration of these symptoms which in a mildly indicated or pronounced form are found in nearly every person who attains his normal end through "weakness of old age."

As the first morbid symptom there is often noticed a *change of character,* sometimes at first in the sense of caricaturing personal peculiarities; a sense of order develops into picayune pedantry, firmness into stupid stubbornness, care into distrust, economy into filthy stinginess. Then as in paresis there comes the falsely so-called *ethical obtuseness* which here also is a combined product of imperfect conception and elaboration of experiences and ideas; and perhaps at the same time there appears the lability of the affectivity with its heightened negative and positive suggestibility: "The old man is a child." The beginning of the disease is sometimes marked by sexual excitation. Men, who have long been impotent, "feel young again" and under certain conditions actually perpetrate excesses. Others remain more or less impotent but the libido is enhanced.

Then the *memory* fails more and more and just in simple senile dementia this often occurs in an entirely systematic manner; the more recent an experience, the sooner it is forgotten; (usually it is still "noticed"; but is capable of being recalled only for a short time). At first single experiences of the immediate past, which naturally is also the period of disease, are irregularly forgotten; these gaps increase slowly and with fluctuations; they coalesce until the last years disappear from the memory at first in part, then entirely. Then in the course of years the limits of recollection are pushed back farther and farther and at last the patients live only in their childhood. An old woman, who in the ninety years of her life had changed her residence several times, at first believed herself in her last residence, then in the next to last, etc., until at last she returned to her birthplace. Another patient was just coming from school. It is very common for senile women to give their maiden names, to believe that they have just recently been confirmed and to have no recollection of their marriage and their entire adult life. The most important events, such as the husband's death, etc., can be told to the patient in this stage several times within a few minutes and they always conceive the information as something new with the corresponding emotional reaction; they themselves are untiring in recounting the same news; in severe cases they not only do not know what they experienced the day before, but under certain circumstances forget everything from one minute to another. Sometimes, however, experiences that intimately concern the personal complexes are retained like memory isles; it may be an unjust accusation or an attempt to obtain money from a stingy old man, etc. As in paresis practiced streams of thoughts also are sometimes still capable of relatively good reproductions.

Lively natures fill up the memory gap with spontaneous *confabulations,* they tell fantastic stories of what they have accomplished and experienced; in torpid natures the symptom has to be provoked by questions. Many of these people do not like to say "I do not know" and produce an answer invented for the occasion which they themselves believe.

The range of ideas is markedly restricted, even though the lack of critical ability rarely, and then much later reaches the high degree as in paresis.

In the first years the patients usually try to act as usual; only torpid and depressive cases give up the active relations with the environment. But then actions become clumsy, unsteady and finally entirely senseless. Because of their lack of thoughtfulness they permit themselves to be misled into stupid financial transactions and uncalled for gifts and bequests. Seniles are favorable material for legacy hunters not only because they will die soon but especially because they are helpless against clever external influences. The attempt to obtain the fortune is frequently made by way of marriage in which case the heightened sexuality in many patients offers a good opportunity. In a great many cases the external forms are retained for a long time. A woman entirely unknown to me, about whom I was consulted, received me as a female acquaintance (although she could see very well); she entered into a conversation with me in the usual social phrases without making a single slip, aside from the fundamental fiction, she asked what my children were doing, said that it pleased her that I had at last come again, and remarked that it was cold but pleasant weather, etc.

Some do not feel comfortable anywhere, especially at night. Without purpose, or with unclear ideas, or to look after their things, they wander about the house spook-like with a light and consequently often become dangerous. In the last stage real deliria are usually added, especially those occurring at night; the patients then live in hallucinations of experiences of youth but also in other adventurous and, usually in emotionally accentuated phantasies.

Perception and *attention* are gradually changed in the sense of the organic disturbance.

Orientation is disturbed rather late, often at first transiently at night, then also during the day. The patients no longer know what year it is, often not even the century, and when the year has been told them they are not capable of reckoning their age, usually state it incorrectly, even when they know the year of their birth, as they often do. They can mistake day and night though in the nightly excitations they want to go to their customary daily occupation more frequently than they mistake the day for the night. Sometimes they themselves feel that they are in a confused condition; one of our patients has maintained for two years that she is at home and sleeping, and that her being here and everything she experiences here is only a dream.

In the last stage disorientation also affects the simplest situation. Then it is particularly characteristic that anxious senile patients, when they have to be lifted or carried, grab hold everywhere of people and doors and every object that they can reach, whereby they naturally increase the danger of falling.

The large majority of seniles have only these basic symptoms; it is a case of *simple senile dementia* analogous to simple paresis and simple demented schizophrenia. But these people rarely come to the insane asylums; their death is awaited in their families and in the poorhouses.

But various accessory symptoms can change the picture and often make institutional care necessary. Even among the simple senile cases some are more torpid, others more lively. The torpidity can increase to stupor, the liveliness to an erethism in which the patients who are in continuous activity combined with a talking mania can hardly be made to rest. The mild affective displacements which are frequent in old age can rise to melancholic and manic conditions, of which the first are very frequent, the second rather rare (*senile melancholia and mania*). The depression is frequently accompanied by anxiety though perhaps less often than in the arteriosclerotic forms.

In such affective conditions *delusions* are invariably formed, and depending on the mental state they are either delusions of insignificance or greatness. The latter is always very weak and does not attain the multi-colored and fantastic magnitude of the paretic delusion. In the depressive delusional forms the delusion of poverty usually recedes before the horribly developed delusions of sin and hypochondriasis. These are often accompanied by nihilistic ideas and ideas of enormity, which are specific in organic diseases, and occasionally also by micromanic ideas, the patients believing themselves or some parts of their bodies to be very small, which gives them occasion for anxiety and justification of the anxiety. The mere poverty of ideas is shown in the following complaint; "I must make so much water; the nurse will not empty the chamber; what will happen? I have such parched feeling and what if the nurse will not give me any water? And when this jacket is dirty, then they will send me one that is too thin."

Very often these affective delusions are mingled with delusions of suspicion, self-reference and of persecution; the *delusion of being robbed* is something quite common in senile diseases.

Even in otherwise simple forms delirious conditions with *hallucinations* occur in the final stage. Individual hallucinations may now and then be noticed earlier; it is generally a case of auditory and also visual hallucinations. Hallucinations of smell and taste are rare. The patients see and hear dreamlike transactions; for instance, they live in a previous activity, or like presbyophrenics, they busy themselves with mixing everything up, packing their beds and all their things together, in order to go "home," etc. The term "occupational delirium" is also used in this connection, but in the forms of senile dementia not complicated with alcoholism the picture is entirely different from that in delirium tremens. In the latter there is an uncertain complicated pseudo-activity in individual, not really connected parts. The patients believe that they are sitting in a bar-room, that they are writing, driving, while they may be lying on their backs in bed, or if they are walking about they do notice that something is wrong, whereas in the senile patients, it concerns mostly real acts, even if they appear decidedly purposeless.[22] Many, even those who are relatively clear, collect useless rubbish, they go to the street to look for things that the children have carried away, "they look for something, upset the bed, tear open the mattress, mix up the horse hair, tear up the linen, frequently cover themselves with it in a phantastically senseless manner" (*Fischer*). If they are not confined to the bed they busy themselves incessantly with something that, though producing little that is comprehensible, always pursues some idea. It is only with the complete decline, that the stereotyped movements come which correspond to the previous occupation (washing and sewing motions, etc.) The patients then often become unclean, not only because of carelessness and paralysis, if not carefully watched they readily begin to

[22] Comp. p. 237.

play with the excrements. Such conditions, which in their higher developments must be designated as severe deliria, occur at first most frequently at night or they last, as transient excitations, for days and weeks, or finally, near the end, they form a chronic condition that may continue for months and years.

Other accessory symptoms result from local disturbances in the brain which are not directly a part of the disease but naturally appear frequently as a result of the arteriosclerosis that exists at the same time; among these we have paralyses, aphasic and apractic disturbances. The spinal cord is usually also involved more or less, so that the sphincter muscles and the (lower) extremities also are no longer controlled properly.

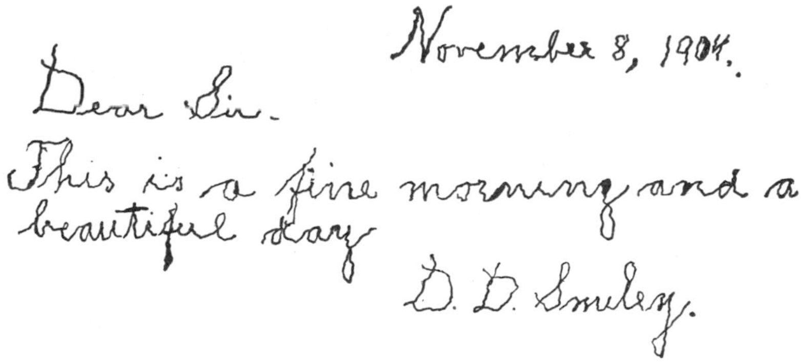

November 8, 1904.

Dear Sir—

This is a fine morning and a beautiful day

D. D. Smiley.

Fig. 9.—The handwriting of a simple senile dement of the lighter grade, showing regular tremors. The patient took great pains to write very carefully.

The physical symptoms are otherwise chiefly basic symptoms which correspond with the general cerebral atrophy among which we find: clumsiness, stiff weak motions, and finally marasmus. Metabolism is retarded very early, the appetite frequently disappears, the handwriting becomes shaky and in many cases is clumsy in other respects. Sometimes the tremor is entirely regular but rather coarse. Other manifestations, as the shrinking and the decrease in the elasticity of the skin, the *arco senilis* in the cornea, etc., are expressions of the general decrease in vitality, to which the brain atrophy also belongs; they are, therefore, parallel manifestations, which in relation to the brain disturbance may be developed to very different degrees.

On the basis of these accessory symptoms different forms have been distinguished.

If there are no accessory symptoms at all, we have *senile dementia in the narrower sense, or the simple form of dementia senilis*. The forms with affective displacements, such as the senile melancholias and manias, are probably the commonest among the institutional cases. That these names designate only the acute pictures with which the patient usually comes to the physician, need not be so important, because as indicated, the moods are usually still recognizable in the quiet period also.

The forms showing a clear sensorium with delusional formation and eventually hallucinations are designated as *senile paranoia* (or paranoid forms of dementia senilis); they are not frequent. Such people think they are spied on by neighbors, teased, robbed especially by those living in the same house, they find everywhere references to themselves, and confirmation of their ideas in voices, etc.

In dementia senilis, as in paresis, catatonic-like forms have been spoken of, inasmuch as one observes stereotype movements and attitudes, verbigeration, flexibilitas cerea, stupor, and echolalia. Many of these cases, as the anamnesis and other symptoms show, are undoubtedly (latent) schizophrenics that have become senile. In others the stereotype movements prove to be remnants of habituated movements (twisting the moustache, scratching). What gives the impression of verbigeration is often plainly nothing but the incessant expression of the identical feeling that always dominates the patient, as in such an expression as "Oh, God, help me!" or it represents an organic preservation in which the patients want to say something else but invariably slip back into the once trodden path. The echolalia may be an organic disturbance which is probably somewhat differently conditioned than in schizophrenia. But as yet we do not know enough, and can only insufficiently analyze these invariably severely demented patients, in order to make an exact differentiation in the individual case between schizophrenic and organic-catatonic symptoms.[23]

The *course* of simple dementia senilis is usually very slow; it may extend over a decade. The weakness sets in very gradually; not even the year in which senility merges into disease can be regularly determined. With minor fluctuations the dementia and the physical weakness gradually increase; extensive remissions are not to be expected here.

Also the paranoid forms with complete clearness usually run a decidedly chronic course, but the delusions are subjected to somewhat severer and more frequent fluctuations, so that really bearable conditions can sometimes alternate with those that are almost delirious.

Acute shifts with total confusion can appear very early and under certain conditions can disappear after a few weeks or months, so that

[23] Compare p. 236.

Wernicke e.g., may talk of cures. But even if the patients do not die soon, new and definitive exacerbations are to be expected.

Senile manias and melancholias can heal, the manias very often, the melancholias less frequently. But many of the latter are also disposed to gradual improvement. However, the senile dementia then remains, even though it is often noticeably of slight force. But as in paresis the affective forms tend to a lasting displacement of the affects, since after the storm has run its course a milder euphoric or depressive mood remains. Senile melancholia can even maintain itself for years, up to death, on the same plane of melancholic depression.

Anatomically senile dementia proves to be a *diffuse reduction* of the entire central nervous system. As in paresis the convolutions are narrowed, uneven at the surface, the ventricles are widened, at death the entire brain is reduced just as much as in arteriosclerosis.

The *pia* is clouded but hardly really opaque, just as little is it infiltrated.

The *ganglion cells* disappear in different ways. They dissolve, they undergo fatty or pigmentary degeneration, and vacuoles are formed in them. The glia hypertrophies, but more as to the number of the elements than in thickness of the fibres or in size of the

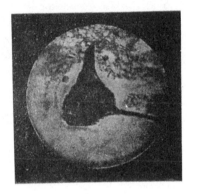

FIG. 10.—Pyramidal cell in a simple dementia senilis. The well preserved fibrils (clearer in the specimen) form a net about the fat droplets that fill up and bulge out a part of the cell.

cells; in contrast with paresis the cells usually remain relatively small and delicate, and the fibres remain thin; mitoses are rarely seen (except in acute lesions). In addition, debris and products of cells are naturally found.

The *causes* of senile dementia are still quite obscure; undoubtedly the hereditary disposition plays a part. The maximum of the disease lies in the *age* between sixty-five and eighty years. The disease afflicts both *sexes* about equally.

Early waning of the trophic energy of the brain occurs especially in *oligophrenics* (sometimes as early as in the forties), in *alcoholics* ("Dementia *alcoholica senilis*," *Forel*, with transition to *chronic Korsakoff* of earlier age), in manic depressives, and in *endocardiacs*.

Not rarely acute debilitating diseases, like pleuritis, or fracture of the neck of the femur, etc., occasion the outbreak.

Differential Diagnosis. The most difficult thing in the diagnosis is to differentiate it from "normal" senility. Where the line should be drawn is arbitrary. For forensic purposes one must depend on the practical considerations; all things being equal, a wholesale merchant should be declared insane and incompetent even if he shows less severe disturbances than a day laborer in the same state. Indeed, under rare circumstances a few harmless delusions will not yet induce us to declare the patient practically as mentally unsound, while naturally in the medical sense all such cases are pathological in the same way as those showing a noticeable affective displacement.

The disease is distinguished from *arteriosclerotic insanity* by the absence of arteriosclerotic and local manifestations, by the more general affection of all functions, and the greater steadiness of the course. But the frequency of the combination of both diseases may cause difficulties which are fortunately chiefly of a theoretic character only.

The melancholic and manic states are recognized as senile by the organic signs of the disease, the lability of the affects, and the senselessness of the delusions, etc. The weakness of the memory is sometimes revealed by the fact that the affects exert an abnormal influence over it. Thus a melancholic patient in the incipient stage of senility, whose memory otherwise appears to be still completely intact and who is also still capable of work to a considerable extent, may be noticed by the fact that he forgets (it is not a blocking) all pleasant experiences, while he retains very well all those that correspond with his mood.

Treatment: For the *prophylaxis* of senile dementia we know nothing that can be done except to avoid all the ordinary nervous injuries, above all alcohol. Besides the physician must be careful not to create situations that may act as causes. Old people suffering from a fracture of the neck of the femur, whenever possible, should not be long confined to the bed, etc.

When the disease has once broken out it naturally cannot be cured. The general principles of therapy in the senile psychoses should be symptomatic.[24]

PRESBYOPHRENIA

Presbyophrenia, the classification of which to be sure varies according to the author and even in the same author at different times, is, according to some, a special morbid picture, according to others a variation of dementia senilis. According to the present state of the question, a morbid picture is best called presbyophrenia which in its typical cases is very well characterized. It always presents the general

[24] See p. 279.

signs of dementia senilis, but shows besides a peculiar excitation and an alteration of thinking that extends beyond the ordinary senile disturbance. The patients are always engaged in an apparent activity; as long as they walk and can orient themselves at least in their immediate surroundings, they fuss about incessantly, things are misplaced, carried to another place, everywhere something is looked for, and all of this, without anything being really accomplished. If the patients are weaker, they cannot lie in bed decently; even there they are occupied, they sit in any old way, and stretch their legs out of bed. With uncertain but eager motions the bed clothes are pulled together, twisted together, tied into disorderly bundles or only moved and rubbed together (the patient "is washing"). Despite a good affective rapport with the surroundings, persons, places, situations, and times of day are mixed up, just as much as the bedding. As long as the patients can talk there is a certain talkativeness, behind which, however, there is no flight of ideas unless something manic exceptionally supervenes; at all events they readily lose the thread merely because of weakness of memory. For the most part they get a special kind of speech disturbance in which at times they no longer find the words, or misplace, repeat, and mutilate them, and cling to single syllables that either do or do not belong to the word, and produce alliterations and permutations, as well as logoclonus, etc., but at the same time, at least in the beginning and when stimulated, they give entirely correct answers.

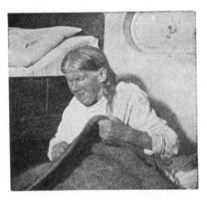

Fig. 11.—"Washing" presbyophrenic. In spite of the demented expression one can see the eagerness in the activity. Unfortunately the results of the occupation, the disorder of the bed, are not visible in the picture.

An example cited by *Fischer* [25] illustrates this best: "Mother of God, Virgin Mary, our lord, our dord thour dord, dord, dord dord, de—de—de—de—Oh now just listen, blessed fruit of the body, give us this day your our ours, holy Mary pray for usars, so that we much. . . . Our Lord our dord so that we shall do much. Come you lousy fellow come quly, dosoorly sanctify our lord, you lousy fellow, than art among women, the fruit of the body, Jesus well yes, that is the great

[25] Ein Beitrag zur Klinik und Pathologie der presbyophrenen Demenz. Zeitsch. f. d. ges. Neur. u. Psych. Bd. 12, 1912, p. 125.

one, but thou thinkesest holicst our Lord, our lord, then and here is certainly certainly sanctified himself himself, but thou felt for the sinners and have sanctifieth all sins and misdeeds our lord, our lord has made forbad and fruit of the body well he has give it ever. . . ."

Typical epileptiform attacks are not rare in presbyophrenia. Hallucinations and delusions, concerning which more exact information is naturally not easily obtainable frequently exist, but are not at all necessarily as a determinant for these peculiar confusions.

In the cases thus classified one finds in the brain regularly, and in especially large numbers, the senile plaques of *Fischer* (spherotrichia), the significance of which is not yet clear.[26] In the other forms they rarely occur, so that the morbid picture is kept together even anatomically to a certain degree.

Kahlbaum, who coined the name presbyophrenia, understood it to mean senile psychoses; *Wernicke* made a morbid picture of it which he identified symptomatologically with Korsakoff's disease so that the conception corresponds approximately to a "simple senile dementia," the torpid forms excepted. *Kraepelin* then required relative retention of the order of the mental process and even of judgment, without keeping strictly to these qualifications. *Fischer* found somewhat later in his anatomical *spherotrichia* a definite morbid picture, and he also put the disease parallel with Korsakoff, but in many of his cases it went beyond Korsakoff in the far greater alterations of thinking, and it corresponded in part with the one pictured above. But finally pretty nearly every dementia senilis which is colored to a considerable extent by accessory symptoms came to ·mean for him presbyophrenic dementia, thus the melancholic, manic, paranoid, and catatonic forms (everything with the exception of his "arteriosclerotic pseudopresbyophrenic dementia"), which correspond practically with the forms of our erethic arteriosclerotic insanity.

Not to be separated from presbyophrenia for the present is *Alzheimer's disease* in which one deals with a dementia, beginning early, in the sense of presbyophrenia, but which in a few years leads to a particularly high degree of dementia with aphasic, agnostic, and apractic symptoms and finally results in death. In exceptional cases it may break out in the forties. The anatomical findings correspond qualitatively about with presbyophrenia but it is very intensive; there is a general cerebral degeneration with destruction of the fibrils and numerous senile plaques; but cases are also included in which the one or the other of the last two distinguishing features is lacking.

Course. The presbyophrenic forms usually exhaust themselves

[26] See below anatomy.

within one or two years, often already in a few months after the disease has become manifest. The more acute the cases, the more are fluctuations to be expected; many of the slower ones run an entirely straight course until death.

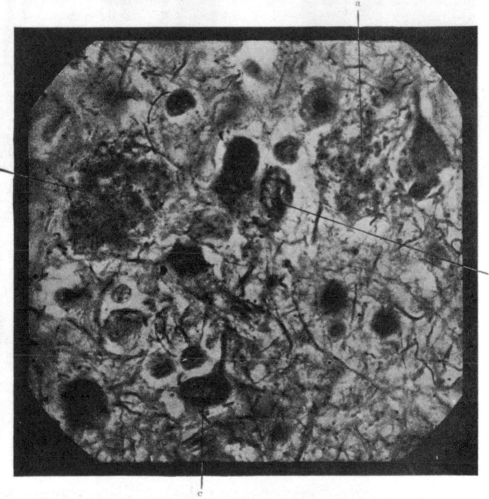

FIG. 12.—Cortex in presbyophrenia. a. Cross sections of large senile plaques. b. Degenerated fibrils stuck together. c. Fibrils stuck together into the form of a sling as the remnant of ganglion cell.

Anatomically besides the general brain atrophy with hypertrophy of the glia the senile plaques are characteristic (*Fischer's* "Spherotrichia," "senile plaques," *Simchowicz*). Their significance as yet is in no way clear. Formations are involved that appear threadlike or

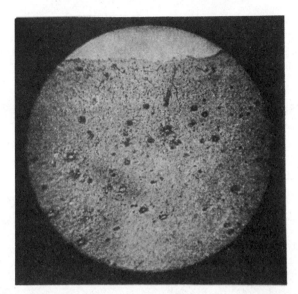

FIG. 13.—Presbyophrenia. Senile plaques in the brain cortex.

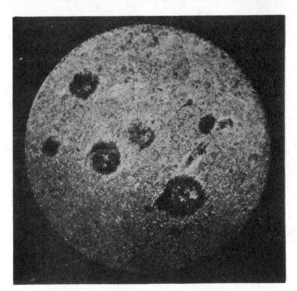

FIG. 14.—Presbyophrenia. Senile plaques. More strongly magnified.

roll themselves together in balls, and include nervous and gliose elements in a transformed condition; they usually form conglomerates that can far exceed a ganglion cell in size and are scattered everywhere in the brain.

In a large part of the cases with senile plaques one can see a severe disease condition of the fibrils which is not visible in ordinary senile dementia. The fibrils bubble up and drop together into irregular forms. Sometimes, e.g., in Alzheimer's disease, they form peculiar tangled bundles.

Differential Diagnosis. Pronounced presbyophrenia can hardly be mistaken. It is often compared with *alcoholic deliria.* In part the deliria are colored in that way by accompanying alcoholism. In most cases it is purely a question of imperfect differentiation. Deliria with hallucinations of sight are not necessarily alcoholic deliria. For this diagnosis all or, at any rate, most of the symptoms must be characteristic. But above all the state of consciousness and the reaction rate in both diseases is so different, that usually the diagnosis is made at the first glance. The alcoholic can be roused much more easily, and has a quick conception and rapid reactions; the senile demented rarely gets into proper touch with the environment and his perception is slow. Perhaps the good-natured rapport also, which is rarely entirely lacking even in the deeply confused senile but is rare in the confused alcoholic, can be utilized in the diagnosis. To recognize it immediately one must have seen the difference between the presbyophrenic eagerness for occupation and the alcoholic occupation delirium.

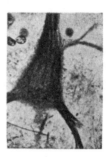

Fig. 15.—Normal cortical cell. Staining of the fibrils.

Especially the slower reaction capacity, the mood, and frequently also the age, distinguish the presbyophrenic as well as every other senile delirium from the alcoholic Korsakoff.

The *causes* of presbyophrenia are unknown.

The *treatment* of the unyielding disease is purely symptomatic.

VI. THE TOXIC PSYCHOSES

1. THE ACUTE TOXEMIAS

Among the acute toxemias *Kraepelin* includes *Uremia* which is important inasmuch as epileptiform attacks occur in it, and because it can stimulate any cerebral local symptoms. The uremic psychosis as such usually runs its course with a picture of various deliria, whose specific peculiarities, if they have any at all, are not yet known; it proceeds in the majority of cases to a rather sudden death.

Eclampsia of pregnancy and child bearing is recognizable by epileptiform attacks, besides which there are also occasional delirious conditions.

In carbon monoxide poisonings after the patients emerge from the narcosis, they may run their course with a picture of twilight states lasting for hours or days. Central and more peripheral paralytic manifestations often complicate the disease. If the patients do not recover entirely, then the organic symptom complex, accompanied usually by conspicuous severe memory defects and depression, remain as an expression of the diffuse destruction of the brain tissue. Between the first toxic sleep and the later developments of the symptoms several days or even weeks, free from disturbance, may intervene.

Of the remaining toxemias we unfortunately have more toxicological than psychiatric knowledge. Only alcoholic inebriation is more exactly known even though we should know still more about it. Its every day forms are ignored by psychiatry; but several unusual kinds of manifestations require special consideration:

Pathological Drunkenness [27]

The acute effects of alcohol are, as is well known, individual and very different according to chance circumstances. Sometimes such fluctuations lead to quite abnormal reactions which, as far as they are of practical importance, are gathered together under the name of pathological drunkenness.[28] Even "maudlin drunkenness" is an abnormal reaction but it is not included here. Pathological states of drunkenness are sudden excitations or twilight states set free by alcohol, usually with a mistaking of the situation, often also with illusions and hallucinations, and excessive affects, mostly of anxiety and rage. In individual cases the entire morbid process can transpire in hardly a minute but it usually lasts longer, up to several hours.

Among the *predisposing* factors that are regularly found, there are lasting and accidental causes. To the first belong all kinds of neuropathic dispositions, above all epileptic and schizophrenic, according to *Heilbronner*, frequently hysteria (e.g. among prostitutes), and cere-

---

[27] *Heilbronner.* Über pathologische Rauschzustände. Münch. Med. Wochenschrift 1901, S. 962.

[28] The name "complicated drunkenness" has been proposed because every drunkenness is supposed to be pathological. But the ordinary name, aside from its theoretical justification, is of practical value especially in the courts, because there it is a question of "morbid or not morbid?" Formerly one spoke of "mania ebriosa" and similar terms. "Senseless intoxication" differs from pathological drunkenness in the fact that in the former no qualitatively unusual symptoms have to be visible.

bral traumas. It is self-evident that the disposition is not to be mistaken for *alcoholic intolerance,* in which small quantities have a disproportionately strong effect but without the inebriation having to be qualitatively abnormal. Chronic alcoholism also can lay the foundation for pathological drunkenness since many drunkards first become disposed to it when they have reached a higher degree of alcoholic degeneration.

To the transient dispositions belong all influences that weaken the body, such as over-exertion, waking at night, excessive heat or cold, then, as is well known, affective excitations, sexual excitement, and "drinking oneself into a rage."

Under such circumstances very small quantities of alcohol, such as two glasses of beer, can often provoke an attack. At first one does not notice anything wrong with the patient, then he begins to be irritated or anxious in order to rave and storm against persons and things about him. The paroxysm is sometimes set free by any occasion, an exchange of words, an attempt to direct, the intervention of a policeman, or without visible cause the drunkard hurls himself at some one just entering. Thus a student suddenly hurled a full salad dish at a classmate's head; it was evidently due to a spasm of ocular accommodation; his comrade seemed to him so tremendously diminished in size that he wanted to make certain where he was and how big he was. It also happens that at first these persons go to sleep and then wake up in a rage, or when they are awakened feel themselves threatened and seize a knife. The confusion is sometimes begun by an epileptiform attack. Even though rarely, attacks of this character may occur also during the paroxysm; according to *Heilbronner* there are also pathological states of drunkenness whose motor manifestations consist chiefly of senseless rhythmic movements.

In these excitements alcoholic disturbances of coordination, such as paralysis of the tongue and staggering,[29] are lacking. Usually the head is extremely congested, and one may also observe the pulsation of the carotids. The expression of the eyes is often somewhat of a stare. Under the influence of illusions and hallucinations of sight, and more rarely of hearing, the conditions of the surroundings are mistaken. The patients are usually markedly disoriented, showing "anxious phantastic fears," and are dominated by terrifying delusions of reference. More rarely they act on the basis of some isolated, usually unclear conception, as in somnambulism, and set fire to a

---

[29] To be sure, this is partly due to the fact that one does not like to include drunkenness with coordination disturbances, among the pathological. But in this case, also, there are no sharp divisions.

house in a rather peculiar way, etc. (*alcoholic twilight state*). The picture may also resemble delirium tremens or acute alcoholic insanity.

Nearly always the scene is ended by a protracted narcotic sleep from which the patient awakes with a dizzy head, but as a rule, without any recollection of what has happened. In less frequent cases the *amnesia* is not complete, or it appears later, perhaps in the course of the following day, at times only after the patients have already admitted having committed a crime.

There are people who have such attacks only once in their lives; others, especially heavy drinkers, may be so afflicted very frequently. But, as far as I know, the above described alcoholic effects are always the exception in the same individual; he also has spells of normal drunkenness. To be sure there are drunkards who, finally, in nearly every drunken spell get *"drunken hallucinations,"* sometimes in the sense of delirium tremens, sometimes more in the sense of alcoholic insanity or of alcoholic jealousy, but here the reaction is usually a much milder one. Even where there is fighting, raging and stabbing, it does not occur so blindly but with a certain consciousness of purpose and with a consideration of real things and persons.

If pathological drunkenness recurs in the same person, they often have a great similarity.

The *differential diagnosis* is based on the demonstration, first, of the disposition, then of the disturbance of orientation (in which naturally the proper recognition of single persons, or of a single street, is not at all excluded), then of the externally unmotivated anxiety or anger (the latter can apparently originate in a quarrel preceding the drunkenness, which in reality caused the disposing affective agitation), then on the demonstration of false perceptions, the lack of disturbance of coordination, and perhaps the continued raging when the patient is put to bed (ordinary drunkards usually fall asleep very quickly). When the critical sleep is not followed by the amnesia, then it will be difficult to assume pathological drunkenness without other, very plain morbid symptoms, such as hallucinations and disorientation; on the other hand it must be especially emphasized that ordinary drunkenness not rarely completely wipes out the memory. If it can be demonstrated that the quantity of alcohol imbibed was so small that normally it does not cause any manifestations of intoxication, then the pathological element cannot be disputed, although this does not yet directly demonstrate the disturbances of reflection.

Treatment. In case the patient still raves when he comes to the physician, restraint can rarely be avoided. Efforts to convince the patient through talking does not help. In one case, however, a colleague was able to put a patient to sleep by hypnotism, while he was in the act of destroying his room, whom we had previously hypnotized into sleep. Of the narcotics only hyoscine (with morphine) is to be used; but even the largest permissible doses leave no certain effect. On the other hand, when necessary, one can resort to a real narcosis through ether or chloroform if the heart can be carefully watched.

2. THE CHRONIC INTOXICATIONS

A. Chronic Alcoholic Poisoning

The Simple Drinking Mania

Theoretically alcoholism and drinking mania should be distinguished. He who cannot abstain from spirituous drinks even when he realizes that it would be better not to drink, he who habitually oversteps the measure which he himself considers proper, is a drinking maniac; he who shows other psychic results of drinking or physical alcoholic signs, is an alcoholic. But the two diseases cannot, however, be sharply separated, if only because the drinking mania on the one hand, if it is primary, usually leads in time to alcoholism, and on the other hand it appears secondary as a symptom of alcoholism, so that both syndromes are mostly encountered in association.

In other drug manias [30] like morphinism, it is not so essential to distinguish the mania from the consequences, because only the chronic morpho-maniac takes too much morphine, and as a rule he also shows soon the other symptoms of morphinism. But as alcohol is generally taken for enjoyment and nourishment, there are plenty of people who become alcoholics who usually do not drink more than what they and the environment consider right, that is, they become alcoholics without being drinking maniacs. This becomes most striking, when such people get delirium tremens on the occasion of an injury or pneumonia, which, to be sure, one then prefers to designate as "fever delirium."

Under drinking mania we therefore include all those cases who on the basis of a disposition, or habituation cannot give up the enjoyment of alcohol, despite better insight, or cannot reduce it to a "harmless" amount, but who (still) do not show the symptoms described under the manifestations of chronic alcoholism. If added signs of chronic poisoning supervene, we designate the disease as chronic alcoholism. As in the case of any other mania the drinking mania afflicts particu-

[30] Psychological and national—economically it would be of interest to go deeper into the study of the "Tobacco mania." The latter, however, is of slight significance medicinally.

larly psychopaths of every description; but there is no question that the essential factor in many cases of simple habituation is based on our drinking customs and the false view of the harmlessness or even the usefulness of regular enjoyment of spirituous drinks. As a matter of fact one should not go too far in tracing things to "psychopathies." Is there any one in whom one cannot find some deviations from the normal or even verify them? We shall therefore speak of a *"simple drinking mania,"* where the mania is not yet complicated by other signs of poisoning, regardless .of some, though not considerate, psychopathically predisposing factors.

The *treatment* of the drinking mania is the same as that of chronic alcoholism.

The symptoms of chronic alcohol poisoning have since the time of *Magnus Huss* (1852) been described under the name of chronic alcoholism. There are physical and psychic symptoms, of which the former are of special importance for the psychiatrist, because proof of their existence can make the layman comprehend most readily that a "disease" is involved.

The *dilatation of the blood vessels*, especially in the face, which in milder cases also causes the skin to appear more red, is generally known. In some severe cases the dilatation of the veins on the nose and the adjacent parts of the cheek is especially conspicuous; finally the color may turn more into blue and in some cases acne rosacea develops. But in most alcoholics there is no such a marked disfigurement.

The excessive use of alcohol is mentioned as one of the causes of *arteriosclerosis*. I do not know whether this is right.

The heart shows an alcoholic fatty degeneration which may heal with abstinence and reappear with the resumption of drinking. It is the most important cause of the usual symptoms of inadequate circulation, irregular pulse and enlargement of the heart ("beer heart"); chronic myocarditis also is evidently found more frequently in inebriates than in others.

A disease that is usual in alcoholism but is otherwise not at all frequent is the real [31] *chronic catarrh of the stomach; cirrhosis of the liver* is practically always alcoholic, while *fatty degeneration* of the liver is frequently so. It is supposed that there is an *alcoholic atrophy of the kidneys*.

General *nutrition* varies greatly. In the severe cases there is either a bloated appearance or more or less pronounced marasmus, the former chiefly in the beginning, the latter in the later years of the disease.

[31] What is otherwise so called is usually a nervous affection.

The well nourished shapes are said to keep more to beer and wine the others are said to be whiskey drinkers.

In the advanced stages, *functional disturbances* are nearly always present. Well known is the *tremor* which under ordinary circumstances is regular and fine and only in severe cases develops into a coarse disturbance of motion; it is usually most marked when the patient is sober, and may force him to drink his first glass in the morning directly from the table because he might spill it with his hand. The patients often know instinctively how to render the trembling

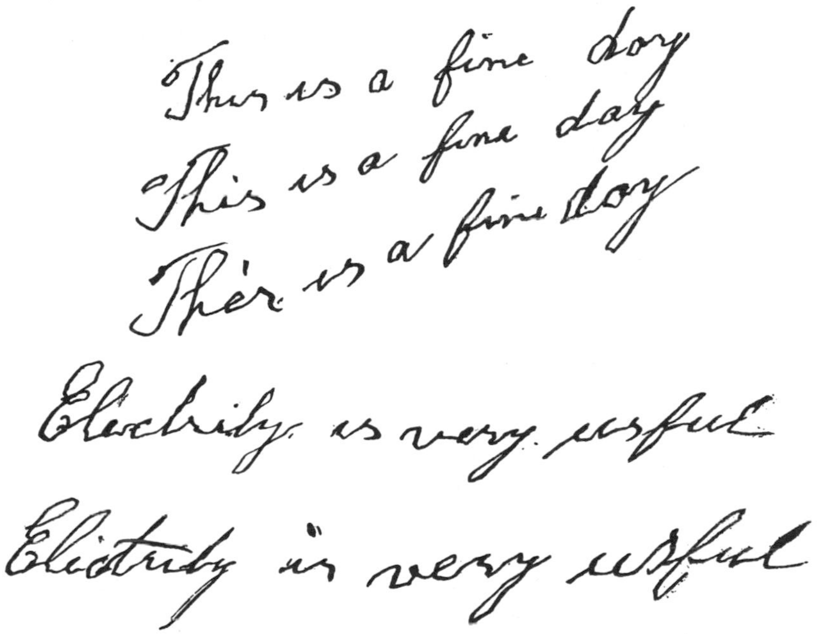

Fig. 16.—Handwriting of a chronic alcoholic of 63 years, who drank heavily, mostly whiskey for about 45 years. The characteristic tremors are plainly visible, and increase with fatigue, as shown in the last lines of the two examples.

harmless or to conceal it; thus if the physician extends his hands and spreads out his fingers and requests the patient to imitate him, he extends his hands but does not spread out his fingers because they would show a (greater) tremor; the patient has to be especially requested to do so. In some cases the affection can be completely neutralized for a short time by mere self-control.

The tremor rarely also affects the eye muscles in the form of nystagmus.

Besides, twitchings in various muscle groups are seen now and then, a tendency to cramps in the calves of the legs, and in the severer stages the drunkards become weak, their walk is unsteady, the face becomes as flabby as in the paretic.

In the stage where the patients come to an institution the *pupils* often react badly, they may also be unequal, but after some abstinence nearly everything is normal. Alcoholic *optic atrophy* with a paling of the temporal side of the papillae and color scotoma is known, though it is relatively rare. Still rarer are chronic *paralyses of the eye muscles.*

The *deep reflexes* are often increased according to the state of anatomical degeneration; more rarely they are diminished or absent.

In the *sensory* field one often finds on closer observation a local reduction of sensitiveness in individual skin areas, especially those of the lower leg, as a result of the degeneration of particular skin branches; more deeply vague pains appear which are likely to be treated as rheumatic. A heavy head, dizziness, *mouches volantes,* buzzing in the ears and similar affections are usually signs of the continued acute poisoning.

The *digestion* often becomes irregular. *Vomitus matutinus,* which is only produced by alkaline saliva, is a common and pretty sure sign of chronic alcohol poisoning (in women, pregnancy is to be excluded).

Sleep is irregular, at times poor, restless, at times heavy. Higher grades of alcoholism manifest themselves among other things also in the need of imbibing the necessary "night cap" before retiring.

Potency declines in the later stages and often sinks to nearly nothing; the libido, which in the beginning is usually strongly aroused, usually maintains itself longer. There is a diffuse atrophy of the testicles in the severer cases.

Single *epileptic attacks* may indicate the severity of the cerebral poisoning; they follow particularly after especially heavy drinking bouts, but in mere alcoholism they are not nearly so common as in delirium tremens.

In the descriptions of the *psychic disturbances* "ethical degeneration," the "blunting of the finer feelings," the "moral coarseness" are invariably emphasized. It is important to state that this characterization in the manner in which it is usually expressed is not true to facts. The alcoholic, who was originally decent, remains the pleasant, cordial companion in his singing society and in drinking circles; he can shed warm tears at his neighbor's misfortune, become wildly enthusiastic about political or any ethical purposes; not only can he state, but even feel what is good and bad; he can give wonderful advice to others; if he is an artist or poet, he can create works of art that indicate a fine sensibility even in the realm of ethics and good taste. On occasions where the affectivity is not involved, his judgment is quite good until a fairly advanced stage of the disease. But notwithstanding this, the description of the disgusting coarseness and the inconsiderate actions of the alcoholics is not mere fiction; *such people act thoughtlessly under the influence of the affect and are coarse under certain circumstances*, e.g. at home, where they have to feel the expressed or mute reproaches of the family, at work where they cannot hold themselves and which they subordinate to their drinking pleasures, and in a quarrel in certain stages of drunkenness. The great majority of inebriates is made up of those who were originally well disposed and who are still capable of finer feelings. Besides them there are others, who have "gone to the dogs" in all respects; some are weaklings who always permit themselves to be misled into following the customs of their environment and to whom vulgarity in this way becomes a habit; others are sick persons whom alcoholic atrophy of the brain has made into irritable and thoughtless children of the passing moment. The third class consists of those who are naturally coarse and generally morally deficient but who lose, through alcohol, the inhibitions that otherwise restrain them a little. To be sure most of our work as psychiatrists is with this class, but their vulgarity does not result from alcohol; it is only made apparent and increased by it. Only the last two categories correspond with the usual picture. The three mentioned constitute the main forms between which, and beside which, there are transitions and combinations that can be readily imagined.

It is because on suitable occasions alcoholics can command in all sincerity the finest sentiments, that these people become dangerous and attractive; they are not hypocritical in this respect. They can still occupy important public positions without attracting attention to themselves, even though at home they beat their wives, walk naked into the kitchen before their children, etc. They believe on appropriate occasions, that they want to do everything for their families, can show the loveliest remorse and can make still finer promises. Whoever does not know them well, must believe them because they themselves believe in their own uprightness. But with the first change in the external situation the fine feeling also gives way to another that is just as sincere and that takes hold of the entire man just as much.

A mother of thirteen children is stricken with cancer of the womb. The alcoholic husband visits her solemnly every Sunday in the hospital, bringing her flowers. Finally it is too much for him to spend the few pennies and he demands that his wife be sent back. At home he maltreats her as before and, as the carcinoma has a strong smell, he regardlessly indulges at the table in the gruesome joke that now they had potatoes and crab (cancer) for dinner.

The following was brought to light in a court case: After partaking of cider and four deciliters of whiskey an alcoholic had misused one of his children and had attempted to misuse the other in his wife's presence. He had boasted to his wife that on her communion day he had taken her innocence. He sent another child to the mother with the news that he was about to tear out all the hair from the pubes (this in the most disgusting expressions). He had beaten his wife's body black and blue, and wounded her head, scalded her with hot water and peed in her face (perhaps to treat the wound without a doctor). The beating lasted two days, in which time the children had to hold the mother once so that he could hit her with a rope. At last the woman could escape in her shirt to a neighboring house; the man remained at home. After two days a neighbor brought him some milk; one could not let him starve. Then the villain was so penitent and shed such bitter tears that the neighbor, a farmer, began to weep also, brought the wife and the children; then everybody deeply touched cried together. The affair with the children was brought before a court, where the man maligned his wife outrageously.—The above mentioned beating was not at all extraordinary, only the misuse of the children had been a novelty.

Because the customary descriptions consider completely only the naturally coarse group and present only the darker side of the far larger group of those originally decently disposed, the diagnosis is usually mistaken; one does not dare to designate as an alcoholic one whom one has just seen conduct himself so nicely and considerately. And, on the contrary, many coarse individuals, who among other things drink, are considered alcoholics which they are not, or in whom at least the unpleasant psychic characteristics are not the result of drinking.

The alcoholic ethical defect, therefore, does not consist in the loss of ethical feelings but in the abrupt change of the feelings generally and in the domination of the entire man, his mental stream and his will, by every momentary mood, by the affect of the present moment. We have the same condition as in the so-called ethical defects of the organics; only in alcoholics the duality is much more apparent because the intelligence in itself is still well preserved, while in the paretic the loss of ethical standards may appear as a partial symptom of the general dementia.

The most important change in the feelings of alcoholics is, therefore, their *lability* with which is always associated a heightened emotional coloring of all experiences and, with this, the complete domination of the affects. The patient can make himself endlessly sad over the condition of his business, over the misfortune that he has brought on his family, but shortly after he sits in the saloon, a carefree and cheerful companion, and a short time after that he can become enraged and with word and deed deeply injure his best friend. Practically, the ethical value of such a man is, to be sure, the same as that of a pronounced moral defective; because what good does it do his wife, if at one time he is tender, only to misuse her again immediately afterwards? To do good requires time; a clumsy act, maliciousness, a misfortune, can occur in the excitement of a moment.

One of *Benoit's* alcoholics at a dance gets into a jealous rage with a girl, so that she leaves him. In desperation he hangs himself, is cut down and immediately continues dancing.

The affective flightiness naturally also makes *steadiness of endeavor and action* impossible. Drunkards are easily inclined to take up new plans, to let the old ones fall and finally not to accomplish anything worth while. The lack of a consistent mood deprives them, in the realm of character, of the *endurance* and *perseverance* of their endeavors and, in the realm of intellect, of a consistent *purpose*. And because reflections also are under the influence of the affects, the reviewing of complicated situations, in which the affects play a part, e.g. the state of one's own affairs, must suffer as well; essentials and details are no longer differentiated because both are strongly colored by the feelings.

With this leveling of the feelings in the direction of enhanced vividness the *striving for something higher* must naturally suffer also or be completely suppressed. The gratification of immediate wants satisfies the patients. This also finds expression in the ethical reactions; the alcoholic who has celebrated blue Monday is ashamed to go to work on Tuesday and bums the entire week; he consider it a disgrace to enter an institution for alcoholics and overlooks the disgrace of his alcoholism.

Also the *weakness of will* of alcoholics is chiefly based on the affective lability. They can break the most serious promises five minutes later, have no endurance anywhere, and for the latter reason in the severer cases leave their positions so readily, partly to take another, partly without any definite aim, merely because work no longer suits them. The weakness of will naturally becomes apparent earliest and in the most pronounced fashion in relation to their appetites.

All of this and especially the alcoholic fickleness have still another cause, to wit, the *protracted euphoric attitude of the affectivity* which makes it possible for the patient to feel even misery as good, or at least as less evil than the normal person does. A circumstance as important as commitment into an insane asylum is treated by most drunkards for perhaps a week as a bad joke. The patient is "in the hotel where the big fools are treated"; "he has quarrelled a bit too much with his chamber maid (his wife)."

This euphoric mood is also indissolubly connected with the ideas of drinking. The great mass of filth and misery appeals to them affectively, even with clear insight after many months of abstinence, as something lovely which has to be "renounced." The contempt of society, and to be cast out among the lowest set which he formerly looked down on with disgust, all this no longer matters to the patient; his *sense of honor* is gone. To be sure a colossal *vanity* still remains but not in the right place. Such people boast with their mouths but not with deeds. They brag of the number of empty glasses, of their firmness toward their wives' admonitions, but also of things that do not exist, of their ability, knowledge and achievements, and of their honesty. As long as a drunkard still has this alcoholic fickleness of the euphoria in his system it is impossible to inculcate in him an honest pride in real and worth-while achievements. It usually disappears very gradually in the course of many months of total abstinence, although after a few weeks in the insane asylum one usually observes a somewhat heightened irritability which is due to a clearer realization of the enforced confinement.

By all these affective disturbances the *reflection* also is indirectly weakened: Whoever devotes his feelings to ever changing purposes, never succeeds in thoroughly thinking out anything to its conclusions; whoever lets himself be dominated by his affects, always thinks only in terms of these affects; whoever is led, especially by a morbid euphoria, to look at things only from the good side, cannot evaluate bad chances, and continually shows wrong judgments.

But there are besides *direct alcoholic disturbances of intelligence* that are not brought on in this roundabout manner, even though for many years they are not so evident. The associations become shallower and more of the external type; the typical bar-room jokes with their word associations illustrate that sufficiently. But in more extreme cases the associations become at the same time more limited; it is for this reason that the patients find it irksome to deliberate on complicated matters, even though there are no affective hindrances.

It is then difficult for the alcoholic to *reproduce* exactly. What he tells is easily distorted by changes and additions. Especially striking is the *need for a causal rounding out* of a situation. In the fable of the donkey loaded with salt,[32] e.g. many alcoholics inject a reason why the donkey went into the water (it was warm, he was thirsty, the burden was too heavy, etc.). This is connected with the greater necessity and the greater capacity for excuses. As is known, there is nothing that would not do as an excuse for drinking: Heat and cold, exercising and sitting still, every vocation without exception justifies indulgence in alcohol,—and it is peculiar that men with academic training as well as illiterates abate these reasons in the identical words and adhere to them with the same faith. But in other matters also the drunkard is distinguished by the great necessity for excuses and the great ability in inventing them.

Hand in hand with the heightened affectivity and dulness of thinking there is the tendency to morbid self-reference. Even people still quite well preserved take the donkey and the water in the above mentioned fable as a reference to themselves.

The exaggerated self-references form one of the roots of the *alcoholic suspicion,* which at first is directed toward relatives and then against all who would like to exert an elevating influence on the patients, or who have to suffer from their doings, while on the contrary in the society of even the most degenerate drinking companions a complete feeling of confidence holds sway which among other things leads to many business indiscretions. This characteristic becomes the more dangerous as alcoholics have an exaggerated positive and also negative *suggestibility,* corresponding to their affectivity. Whoever knows how to get in with them, can use them, as he pleases; in other matters, especially in regard to admonitions and related things, they are obstinate and stubborn.

The *memory* of alcoholics become inexact. In tests these people do not give fewer answers than ordinary people, often more, but among them more wrong ones. It is the same in life: often they are no longer capable of thinking of things exactly as they are. Only in the later stages of the severer cases there is added very gradually, as something radically new, the memory disturbance of the organic psychoses with its weakness for recent events. It is a sure sign of brain atrophy and, with this, of the impossibility of complete restoration.

This is sufficient to make *liars* of alcoholics. Numerous affective causes lead them to excuses, to misrepresentations; on the other hand, they cannot sufficiently imagine things exactly as they are. Justification of their own and other people's acts involuntarily enter into their thinking and the euphoric liveliness excites their ideational association

[32] See p. 189.

to such an extent that the necessary phantasy is never lacking, whereas moral and intellectual criticism is suppressed during this entire time. Female inebriates because of readily comprehensible reasons lie still more consistently than men. How many of the lies are conscious and how many they believe themselves for the time being cannot be readily determined.

A large part of the psychology of alcoholics is bound up with the *peculiar attitude of the patients toward their surroundings*. In spite of all their blustering it can easily be demonstrated that alcoholics always feel themselves to be on the defensive toward everybody who does not drink, an attitude which even many moderate drinkers evince in the presence of every abstainer, but which in immoderate inebriates in time actually dominates the entire psyche, and stimulates a real necessity for excuses and lies. They have reason to mistrust just these decent people and those who mean well by them, and to hate and annoy them; they are particularly sensitive and irritable in their presence, while with bums who cannot reproach them they feel at home. Thus they not only get into bad company and altogether away from decent people, but they are ruined more and more by being accustomed to intercourse with degenerate elements. Concerning the more intellectual field it should be added that the patients *cannot even dare* to see things as they are; otherwise they would appear too miserable in their own eyes.

The *attention* has a limited tenacity, partly because of the lability of interest, partly too especially because patients are *more easily fatigued* The latter shows itself everywhere, especially in their work.

In the uncomplicated cases *orientation* remains normal.

In severe cases *perception* also is disturbed in the same sense as in delirium tremens, only to a lesser degree; the patients easily misread, they mistake pictures on brief exposures, and they hear incorrectly.

Many alcoholics that have any sexual relationship show *delusions of jealousy*, which are quite peculiar in form. They fluctuate up and down in direct proportion to the amount of alcohol imbibed. In relatively sober times it may disappear entirely, in intoxication it becomes stronger and entirely senseless; not only chance spots on the bed but also those on the toilet can prove the wife's faithlessness. Illusions and memory deceptions often promote the delusion, rarely, and almost only during inebriation it is also helped by hallucinations, especially of sight; the husband sees that his wife winks at a man passing on the street; he has watched her through a hole. But at first these suppositions, produced with complete conviction, do not hold ground; they become uncertain or dissolve completely when one wants to ascertain what the patient has found out for himself. Jealousy delusions often lead to murderous attacks on the wife. But toward actual unfaithfulness many of these patients are hardly sensitive.

Many reasons are given for the genetic explanation of the jealousy delusions. The alcoholic loses his potency, while the libido still exists; the marital relations are bad; the wife's love is impaired, if it has not entirely vanished; through his absence in the saloon the husband gives her many opportunities to be with other men; he treats her badly and is not himself scrupulous in the matter of marital faithfulness. All these elements produce or increase jealousy under other circumstances also. But between jealousy and delusion there is still a difference that is not explained by all these reasons.

From another, though much rarer form of alcoholic delusion, originates the *self-surrender* to the police on the grounds of having committed some crime, usually one that was sensational at the time, rarely one that does not exist. The patients want to confess and demand punishment. In the cases that I could follow more closely, it was certainly or probably alcoholism on top of schizophrenia (this is to say, incipient alcoholic hallucinosis).

Morbid Picture. The drunkard is a man who cheers himself up, or forgets his sad thoughts with alcohol. Gradually he takes more and more time from other purposes, especially his work, and more money from his family and business. He is irritated by actual or merely probable reproaches, under certain circumstances he becomes senselessly enraged by them, especially when he has just been drinking. Later he regrets what he has done, but not deeply or for long, and ugly scenes recur more and more frequently. He "fluctuates between unmanly weeping and dishonorable indifference" (*Kraepelin*), the latter taking up the greater part of his time; a carefree humor of drunkards, which is easily transformed into irritability or pangs of conscience, dominates him most frequently. In his exalted self-conceit he believes himself to be something extraordinary, thinks he works harder than everybody. But this overestimation does not, however, lead to real delusions of grandeur.

More and more he forgets honor, good manners and decency; when he speaks and acts, he does not hinder his own dignity. He discusses the most intimate family affairs at the bar. The dignified man who was formerly faultlessly proper finally becomes outwardly untidy, and even loses his sense for the poor appearance of others.

In his more intimate dealings, that is, where it is not a question of established standards, the drunkard no longer considers the rights of others. From his wife, even when he admits a part of his faults, he demands as her self-evident duty all consideration and love, while he himself can do as he likes; if he conducts himself badly, it is only the result of her lack of understanding.

He has an entirely wrong conception of his cravings; it is right and necessary for him to drink; it is right because he earns money (even when the wife really supports the family) because he is the man, because one has to have some enjoyment;—it is necessary as otherwise one cannot work. As far as he indulges in it, drinking is harmless; other people drink too, and still more than he. In every case some one else is to blame, not he. If at times through some bad luck or perhaps through special enlightenment he is in a position to judge himself somewhat better, it only touches him in moments of moral dumps, an unpleasantness he seeks to remove as soon as possible with alcohol. Hundreds and thousands of times he promises either in all seriousness or in a hypocritical way to reform, "to be a better man," only to break his promises just as often.

With this all he ruins his family life. The children, whom he maltreats, are afraid of him. As a rule his financial condition suffers. In the lower classes the wife often has to support the entire family; the husband drinks up what he earns and extorts with threats and maltreatment the wife's hard earned pennies, for which she has deprived herself of sleep. No law, much less public opinion, hinders him in this. He is not dangerous to the public generally, he "only" maltreats his wife, one reads in the police reports. The wife is usually entirely at his mercy and leads a life that is worse than that of the average slave in very different times.

The worst acts, to be sure, occur during intoxication but many of these people do not come out of this state for days at a time.

Many of the patients get into jail intermittently. The hospital gives room to only a small part. Of those who live longer many spend their last years or decades in poorhouses and asylums.

The *female inebriate* differs not a little from her male companion in fate. She is also much more difficult to picture than the latter, not only because she is less frequent, but especially because as a rule she is much more seriously psychopathically predisposed. It then becomes difficult to isolate what is characteristic of alcoholism in the individual cases that are abnormal in the most different directions. To be sure, in the psychologic examination one finds the identical abnormalities as in men. But the attitude is different. Contrasted with the men the female patients are taciturn at least toward the people who are concerned with their alcoholism, they seek to conceal their inner thoughts, do not admit drinking at all or only to a very moderate degree, and when one does not believe them, they are accustomed to make the most definite and serious protestations, even when they have frequently been caught in the act.

This conduct, like the severer psychopathic condition, is readily explained by the absence of the drinking compulsion in woman; for her, custom does not transform a vice into a virtue. She must be much more abnormal before she drinks so much (if the modern bottle beer business is maintained at the present level, it will, to be sure, diminish the difference); furthermore she cannot boast of her "prowess" like the man; the entire situation shows her at all times that she is doing something that should not be done.[33]

In pronounced schizoids the drinking mania and alcoholism frequently show a special characteristic. Such people lead a secluded life, and create disturbances only in the form of outbursts of irritability, the affectivity as well as the contact with the environment remains inadequate, even in the higher grades of alcoholism, a real ability to discuss the mania does not exist. Nevertheless after a long sojourn in the hospital (at least a year) and proper treatment (consistent action without many words, for the rest to be left alone, no irritation) will produce an essential improvement in most cases.[34]

Course. The disease as a rule creeps in entirely unnoticed; in many cases one cannot tell within ten years when it really began. These people just gradually drink a little more or they gradually become less capable of resistance against the same quantities, and at all events the characteristic symptom complex is only formed in the course of years. With this all, many maintain themselves as good commonplace people as they only need continue living at the ordinary pace, they have nothing new to learn and need not exert themselves especially until the more or less premature death ends all. Only a small part get plain alcoholic dementia as a result of brain atrophy.

In this course there are often pretty strong fluctuations in part as the result of some insight and some effort toward moderation, in part, however, as the result of the intervention of third parties or other change of circumstances. But on the whole there is an unchecked decline, in many cases to the lowest human misery into which the patients usually drag their families with them; in more favorable cases the decline is only to a certain grade of feebleness which substitutes

[33] That description may not hold true for all American female inebriates.
[34] *Binswanger,* K. Ueber schizoide Alkoholiker, Zeitschrift. f. d. ges. Neurologie, U. Psychiatrie, 1922. Springer, Berlin.

bar-room gossip for recreation that elevates the mind and spirit, and finally also lets it take the place of work.

Prognosis. Theoretically most alcoholics are still curable at a time when their disease has long been obvious to the layman. Only when in spite of energetic attempts they are no longer capable of seeing and feeling the misery that they are bringing to themselves and their family, or when stealthy memory defects indicate brain atrophy or also when the innate disposition is ethically untrainable, then the inebriate must be given up because nothing can be done for him. To be sure, he usually has to be given up because the more intimate or distant connections do not want to intervene at all, or begin too late. Thus the majority of inebriates sink deeper and deeper and are ruined after they have for decades made the family which is tied to them unhappy in every respect; often the cause is alcoholism itself, more frequently it is other diseases to which they offer a diminished resistance. A small number spend their last years in a quiet or erethic form of alcoholic brain atrophy (dementia-alco-holico-senilis, see organic diseases). Not seldom the end is suicide, usually during an alcoholic depression, occasionally too during some other emotional state.

Anatomy. According to *Rose* the cranial bones are frequently thickened. In the cranial cavity one often finds in the more severe cases, that the pia is clouded and thickened; occasionally (but not nearly so frequent as in paresis) there is also pachymeningitis hæmor-rhagica. The brain itself in advanced cases is plainly reduced in size. The ganglion cells show at an early stage different forms of degenera-tion. The glia is increased as to the number of cells and fibres. The ependyma of the fourth ventricle often shows granulations. In some of the nerve and glia cells as well as in the walls of blood vessels, one finds, as a rule, much fat. The organs show in different ways alcoholic degeneration.[35]

Frequency. Depending on the methods of admission in the hos-pitals for the insane, male alcoholics constitute from 10 to 35% of the admissions (not of the population). But this is no measure of the distribution of alcoholism. Only a very small part of the patients get into institutions. A degree of alcoholism, recog-nizable on close inspection in Central Europe, is quite usual in the second stage of maturity. If one only wants to count the cases from where a noticeable injury of the individual is apparent, then there are naturally no figures at one's disposal; but whoever keeps his eyes open will probably consider alcoholism as the most frequent disease

[35] Comp. p. 303 ff.

of men, aside from cold and such trivial things. In Switzerland about
16% of the men dying between forty and sixty are designated by
physicians as alcoholics. Naturally the figure is in reality much
greater. In the remaining parts of Central Europe conditions are
probably the same! [36]

Causes. Hardly anywhere is as much known concerning the causes
of disease as in the case of alcoholism, and yet nowhere is there more
dispute than just here. In the first place there are two kinds of congenital disposition, upon which alcoholism thrives; the first represents
a disposition causing or impelling one to partake of spirituous drinks
in larger quantities, the second represents a lower degree of resistance
toward the quantity partaken of, in which case the resistance of the
brain is of especial significance for psychiatry.

The first group is not homogeneous. Under our conditions different dispositions cultivate the active impulse to drink and the weakness toward the ever-present temptation and seduction. Here one
finds in the first place those with a congenital weakness of will. Others
surrender to alcohol because they have no reason for not doing so;
they are coarse and morally dull and seek momentary pleasures. Less
offensive are the cheerful boon companions who fall victim to alcohol
in enormous numbers; most of these people not only are not psychopathic, but belong to those who react to life syntonically, who are also
free from inner resistances and inhibitions; *it is therefore absolutely
wrong to assert that only psychopaths become drinking maniacs or
alcoholics, and that they must drink because they otherwise cannot
adjust themselves to the world.* Others take to drinking for the opposite reason because they are not capable of getting out of themselves or
of ridding themselves of things disagreeable in some way. Alcohol enables them to forget or frees them from their inhibitions. As mere complex diseases in the psychoanalytic sense I have not to my surprise seen
any actual alcoholics in the hospitals for the insane and in the inebriate
sanatoria. Persons having pure complexes even if they frequently
narcotize themselves in a striking manner probably do not drink continually enough to become real alcoholics. Moreover, it is also possible
that the pronounced alcoholic, like the organic patient, loses the ability
to split off complexes. Many have some other difficulty of adjusting

[36] Only a person who has delved into the matter can form a proper conception of the social and economic significance of alcohol. For this purpose Germany spends yearly about two million marks pre-war currency; little Switzerland
spends daily nearly a million francs, much more than the costs of mobilization.
For these sums are purchased disease, misery, crime, reduced working hours and
weakened capacity for work. Comp. *Hoppe,* Die Tatsachen über den Alcohol,
3rd Ed.   Calvary, Berlin, 1904.

themselves to life; some have ambitions that are beyond their ability and never act because they are always planning, others do too much, but do it senselessly, the third has "nervous" troubles, etc. To this class also belong many that suffer from mild mental diseases, in whom alcoholism is not the cause but the result of the disturbance.[37] Contrasted with the class of weaklings we find the strong men who believe they can stand everything and thus indulge excessively in alcohol. Many, perhaps the greatest number of alcoholics, are the complete victims of our drinking customs; to be sure, the latter are rarely seen in institutions; but one sees them by chance all the more in the ordinary walks of life and as carriers of various other diseases.

The second group, those incapable of resistance, we can describe still less. We only know that there are peculiar dispositions (certainly not homogeneous ones) in which the brain reacts to the quantity of drink imbibed in the sense of pronounced chronic alcoholism. We cannot determine why in one, drink ruins the liver, in another the heart, in the third the regulation of metabolism, in the fourth the brain, in the fifth all these organs, and why many others can stand the same quantities of alcohol fairly well without becoming alcoholics in our sense.

Both dispositions are only exaggerations of weaknesses that human nature generally is liable to. A craving for poison like alcohol exists everywhere; but those races which in the course of their development through thousands of years have had at their disposal a certain quantity of this mode of gratification have adapted themselves to it; they are temperate. But modern industry and means of communication have nearly everywhere surpassed adaptation, hence the misery. Only a generation ago Italy was still a temperate country; now many of her insane asylums admit the same percentage of alcoholics as our own.

It is self-evident that it is possible that every brain could become alcoholic, not only because we can narcotize everybody with alcohol but because we see everywhere the identical toxic effects of alcohol. But I doubt whether the average capacity to resist alcohol has declined in the last centuries as many suppose.

The various dispositions manifest themselves also in *heredity*. In the families of drunkards we find very diverse abnormal dispositions, which in perhaps half of the cases become manifest as the father's alcoholism.

Among the predisposing causes the most important is our *drinking*

---

[37] *Ferenczi* is of the opinion that alcoholism is generally a substitute for repressed sexual desires (abstinence would then be a compensation for sexual weakness). In reality no one lives a better sexual life than the average alcoholic.

custom, which has developed from both these dispositions with the assistance of our specific social conditions. This custom represents the indulgence in alcohol as something lovely, useful, necessary, and self-evident, so that it requires some strength to withdraw from its influence. As a camp follower of the drinking custom, is the capital invested in the alcohol industry whose millions have organized very skilfully the inducements to drink. Of the well known opportunities and seductions that come into consideration for the individual I should like to emphasize only a few. By mothers of spoiled sons bad company is most often considered the criminal; but this is usually unjust because one is rarely compelled to associate with bad company. But in reference to drinking the accusation is too often true; drinking companions are, to begin with, so decent that the inexperienced neither notices the evil connected with them nor can he foresee the danger that is in store for him. One goes to these gatherings for a worthy reason, and does not consider how unworthy a few hours or perhaps a decade later, it may become; it is also said that trouble and misery can be drowned in alcohol; that is true only in exceptional cases; trouble and misery are the results of alcohol and then, to be sure, by means of a vicious circle they constitute an excuse to increase the evil with additional alcohol. I know of no case where increased wages have reduced the use of alcohol and statistics prove the opposite.

What quantities of alcohol are necessary to produce the disease depends on the personal disposition, perhaps also on the quality of nourishment and manner of living generally. One person may become physically and mentally a pronounced alcoholic while perhaps one of his companions drinks several times as much and nevertheless remains within the so-called norm. *The number and strength of the inebriations is immaterial.* Whoever gets drunk on small quantities will hardly ever become an alcoholic; whoever as a general thing lives moderately will never become so, even though every year he is found several times in the gutter. *But whoever regularly imbibes larger quantities, risks a chronic poisoning, even though he is never intoxicated.*

Differential Diagnosis. Alcoholism can be associated with every other disease and then one of the two is often overlooked. Other symptom complexes such as paresis, schizophrenia, fever deliria, etc., can be tinged by alcohol. Schizophrenics, who are at the same time inebriates, are most frequently mistaken for mere alcoholics. If they are sent to insane asylums, no great harm is done. The mistake is more serious in homes for inebriates, where they usually do not know how to handle schizophrenics, and in home cures, where the treatment of the patients should legally and medically be entirely different from that of mere alcoholics. Among the less noticed signs of the basic schizophrenia the unrealistic seclusion from social intercourse is important; the inebriate who does not know what to say and withdraws from the other patients in the institution is no mere alcoholic.

Many psychic symptoms of alcoholism resemble the paretic and organic symptoms generally; they may even *be* organic, because the intoxication also produces a kind of brain atrophy.[38] In older persons the question how much of the disease is senile and how much is alcoholic, can often not be decided on theoretic grounds.

Chronic manic patients are readily mistaken for alcoholics; more rarely the reverse is the case. The flight of ideas, the fluctuations of the disturbance independent of the use of alcohol, and its persistence even in abstinence or strict moderation makes the diagnosis of mania certain. The absence of these symptoms in spite of careful observation excludes it. Naturally the anamnesis often gives at once definite information.

The differentiation of alcoholism from normal health is most difficult. Regular quantities, which in Europe are considered moderate, plainly change the appearance of the aging person; whoever has a little practice can ascertain the same in reference to the psyche. With us a little alcoholism, therefore, belongs to the "normal" and since a Munich Court [39] has decided that to drink from six to eight liters daily is not yet immoderation, one must not imagine the "little" as being very small. I would, therefore, have alcoholism in the sense of medical practice begin there, where practical reasons demand it: *Whoever plainly harms himself or his family through the use of alcohol and who cannot be made to realize this, or who no longer has the will or the strength to better himself, must be considered an alcoholic.* Among the signs of harmfulness one naturally understands also the physical and mental symptoms of chronic alcoholism in the psychic sense. That this somewhat narrow, but for practical purposes valuable definition, includes also the drinking mania is not only true, because drinking mania and alcoholism condition each other, but also because practically and legally they are a unit.

There are people, also, who, without distinct signs of alcoholism, behave badly for other reasons, e.g., congenital disposition, and do not manage their affairs properly; alcohol only aggravates their condition still more. Such people must not be mistaken for alcoholics; the prognosis and treatment are entirely different here.

[38] Cf. alcoholic paresis.
[39] Internationale Monatschrift zur Bekämpfúng der Trinksitten, 1897, Jahrg. 7, p. 239.

It was said that he suffers from alcoholism who regularly imbibes alcohol before the effects of previous doses have disappeared. But this cannot at all be taken strictly, since in psychologic investigations such effects can be demonstrated twenty-four hours later and even much longer, and no one will want to designate as alcoholic one who drinks a few glasses of beer every twenty-four hours. Then again, he is to be considered an alcoholic who has a craving for alcohol and cannot resist it. But this cannot be a test, because the criterion is, in the first place, the evaluation of the reasons which should restrain from indulgence. The ordinary habitué of the saloon does not drink as much as he does because he cannot help it, but because he knows no reason, or cannot appreciate any, that should keep him from doing so.

That alcoholism should be measured scientifically with a different standard from that used in other diseases is naturally nonsense. In a medical sense every one is an alcoholic who exhibits sure signs of alcoholism; whoever shows mild signs is a mild alcoholic; whoever exhibits serious ones is a serious alcoholic. The consequences to be inferred from this vary according to the case: practice will be infinitely more lax than science, which cannot permit herself to be falsified by affective or opportunistic viewpoints.

Naturally the entire affective symptom complex is not in itself to be inferred with certainty from single symptoms, since organic diseases and congenital dispositions can have a similar appearance. One can most readily make a diagnosis from the liveliness of the reaction in many failures, from the characteristic evasions, and from the causal elaborations.

If one has a little time to observe the patient, then naturally his reaction to abstinence is important. Patients who improve after a few weeks in the institution, who plainly change their character for the better and quickly get worse after indulgence, are in the main alcoholics.

The diagnosis is very materially supported by physical symptoms and the anamnesis. But in taking the latter one has to be very careful, not only because nowhere except in sexual matters does one ever get such false reports as in the matter of alcoholism, but also because alcoholics who are brought to insane asylums have not always been psychopathics.

Erben [40] states that the alcoholic tremor has the rapidity and fineness of the oscillations in common with that in diabetes, nicotine

[40] Diagnose der Simulation Nervösen Symptome. Urban & Schwarzenberg, Berlin, Wien, 1912.

poisoning, lead, zinc, mercury, sulphuric oxide and in convalescence after serious diseases. These tremors are more severe when the fingers are spread, weaker when the fingers are moderately bent; as distinguished from paralysis agitans the fingers among themselves do not move synchronously; in alcoholism the tongue also trembles easily, but less so or not at all in metallic poisoning.

Care is also necessary in judging the dilation of the facial blood vessels. There are very temperate or abstinent people who have a red nose and only a very small fraction of inebriates can be diagnosed in this way.

Treatment. The experience of a thousand years proves that training to moderation is a utopia. In the first place the treatment has to solve three problems: Above all the quasi-physical dishabituation from the need of alcohol. This is easier than is generally supposed. It is only an exception when the alcoholic in the hospital for the insane feels a real need of indulgence, as does the smoker for tobacco or the morphinist for his alkaloid. Of the abstinence manifestations I only know the coarse trembling. Still others are mentioned, e.g. sleeplessness, and certainly among several dozen inebriates, one perhaps will not sleep as much as he would like, for the first few nights in the hospital for the insane. But in the first place there are other reasons for this; secondly, many inebriates slept irregularly previous to this, and usually under abstinence they not only sleep better but even normally. It is, therefore, necessary very decidedly to advise against giving soporifics merely because of this indication. *It is just these people who must be thoroughly rid of the habit of taking drugs for slight discomforts.*

It is still supposed that the sudden deprivation of alcohol kills these people. This is directly contrary to the facts. The omission of alcohol kills nobody, it is only the use of it that does. Protracted abstinence is not harmful; out of 279 patients discharged from the Ellikon Sanitarium who relapsed, 62 (22%) died in the first twelve years; of 295 cured and improved discharges 5 (1.7%) died.

Therefore the first indication is the *immediate removal of the injurious matter.*

More difficult is the *associative dishabituation,* i.e., the breaking of the association of ideas that incessantly impel toward drinking; in those better disposed, it is especially hard to break the associative identification of alcoholic indulgence with everything beautiful and ideal that has been experienced in the past (old college men!), and to form newer associations corresponding to realities. It is necessary on the one hand to associate the patient's misery and those of others with drink, and on the other hand to connect the conceptions of righteousness, ability, work, and happiness with the anti-alcoholic idea. Still more time is needed for the *training of character generally*, the habituation to regular work, the cultivation of resistance to the incessant temptations, the development of self-control, of joy in real achievement, and of pride of the right kind.

The best way to satisfy all three indications is a *sanatorium* which is not just a resort for inebriates but where the patient is skilfully treated by pedagogic and psychologic methods, and where the superintendent is imbued with the lofty purpose of his cause. The patient must persist on the average for about a year and should not be accepted if he does not bind himself in advance for this length of time. But with us he can leave in spite of his pledge, if he wants to; therefore, the superintendent must have personal influence enough to retain the large part of the patients. Brewers, saloonkeepers and others in the alcohol industry should only be accepted when some guarantee is given that the business is to be transferred to some one else before the patient leaves the institution; one cannot be an abstainer and saloonkeeper at the same time. The hopeless, or those with a morally defective disposition should be kept away from alcoholic sanatoria as much as possible, because they endanger the cure of others.

In milder cases associations for total abstainers under good leadership may suffice. But naturally they offer much fewer opportunities and, in addition, they have the *disadvantage which must not be underestimated, of dragging along until they are incurable, cases which in themselves are hopeful.* Where the danger of postponement is not too great and where admission to a sanatorium for alcoholics is difficult or impossible, one of these associations may be tried. If one has a choice of several associations, then, aside from the personality of the director, that one is to be recommended that is most consistent. In spite of the fact that the Blue Cross does a world of good, it has the fundamental error of demanding total abstinence only from inebriates and those who want to help them. This reduces it to a mere crutch and makes of the patient a second rate person who is in need of one. Whoever cannot adopt the platform, self-evident in the light of all the facts, "that drinking causes much misery and practically no benefit, and hence it is better for all mankind to dispense with it," such a man is always in danger of trying, by means of drink, to elevate himself to the rank of superior persons. The reformed drunkard must feel at ease in his decency and must not, like the turtle in the ball room, get homesick for the mire.[41]

[41] The Good Templars, the Opponents of Alcohol and, in most places, the Catholic Abstinence League are consistent abstinence associations.

These alcoholics who lack the insight to permit themselves to be cured willingly must be put in restraining institutions, that is, at present, in hospitals. It is a blessing for many a drunkard if he perpetrates something real serious or gets an attack of delirium tremens, because then for once, he can be subjected to treatment. Therefore, where the statutes do not make it impossible, and by way of exception, where there is an intent to cure the patient, one should make the most of such opportunities and recommend the hospital. But the patient hardly gets there before a drive is made against the "unjust" incarceration, either by himself or those like him, or by friends disposed to moderation. Then it is necessary to stand firm. Unfortunately the wife usually has the decision in her hands, i.e. the most unsuitable person; because she is the one who has most to fear from his revenge and who loves him or has loved him, and for that reason is most readily deceived by the solemn protestations that appear in quantity two or more weeks after the commitment. Then in addition, reasons are advanced that unfortunately seem to have weight with those not so close to the patient: "The man is not crazy at all and therefore does not belong in the insane asylum; among the insane he will have to become crazy; he has to be given a chance to show that he wants to do better and can do better," etc. Thus the wife usually weakens, even though at the time of commitment she gave solemn assurance of her firmness. But if she can remain firm, so that the husband never feels her doubts and if she avoids many visits as long as he is anxious to go home instead of to an alcoholic sanatorium, then it may still go well with those patients who are at all curable. To be sure, as a rule after the stage of facetious euphoria and solemn promises, there is a third stage of irritation and threats to be withstood, that gives the useful insight that the promises are in vain; one has to know this in order not to be frightened, because it is only a matter of firmness to make these manifestations disappear quickly. The ordinary threats of suicide are to be ignored.[42] After one to three months the patients are usually transferred to a sanatorium for alcoholics. To be sure, individual cases have to remain in the hospital for years and, if they have sufficient endurance, they may be cured anyway.

---

[42] There are only two sensible answers to threats of suicide: either to ignore them, that is to do the opposite of that which the threat seeks to accomplish, or commitment to the observation ward of an insane asylum. If one acts differently the threat becomes the worst sort of fetter that makes decent people the weak tools of brutal rascals. *It is well to think of this in the treatment of moral defectives also.* To be sure, one has to be able to take it upon oneself that in many thousand cases one useless and harmful life may find its end on such an occasion.

To be sure, the hospital must be equal to its task. In many places such patients still get alcohol, or it is made plain to them that only for them are the benefits of alcohol injurious, or they are given positions as bartenders, etc. It may be that such institutions are not bad in other respects, but at all events they are incapable of curing inebriates.

Guardianship also is a palliative when properly handled. According to the German and much more according to the Swiss code it should also be a factor in the cure. But as long as the majority of guardians feel themselves closer to the inebriate than to the abstainer, naturally not much is to be expected from this; but even now this device has a certain benefit if the right kind of guardian is found, and with the spread of better ideas this advantage will grow more and more if the court of guardians has the legal means to compel a cure. Naturally it is always a mistake if the wife becomes the guardian of the inebriate.

As a principal remedy or as an auxiliary to a cure *hypnotism* has been recommended. It has the danger of diverting physician and patient from the real problem. Therefore I do not use it here, although there may be cases where it is very useful.

The *chemical remedies* recommended are humbug.

Whether the patient is at home or in any kind of institution, the treatment of his environment is just as important as that of the patient himself. That so many curable inebriates are lost is the fault of the unfortunate patience of the wives who cannot, before it is too late, make up their minds to a measure that hurts their pride. The family physician should endeavor to direct to the right place the patience which here only does harm; furthermore he must take care that after recovery the patient's wife remains abstinent with him.

Incurable alcoholics are a terrible burden for their families and the community. *Kraepelin* recommends hospitals as a place of confinement. But to me the present arrangements of the hospitals do not seem suitable for the patients, nor do the present laws meet the scientific demands. *Forel* and others therefore demand that special institutions be arranged for them in which they are bound to earn by labor at least as much as they need. This would have the advantage of being a solemn warning to the attitude of the alcoholic that everyone is powerless over him. It would obviate many crimes and other dangers and disadvantages, and would offer the possibility of belated cures through protracted compulsory abstinence and training which might return to society after years and years many a man apparently lost.

Strange to say in the case of alcoholism the modern physician has to be told that the most important part of the therapy is the *prophylaxis*. But one must realize that here too only the right remedy helps: abstaining from alcohol. It is nonsense to recommend moderation: It is the very soil on which alcoholism flourishes. The limitation, even the complete eradication of alcoholism is possible, if the determination is there. There is no other avoidable disease that brings so much misery to civilized people. Therefore it is the physician's duty [43] to be informed at least as exactly in this matter as in the case of infectious diseases. The textbook of psychiatry can only point out this duty. There are people who are afraid of the result that a better insight would compel them to avoid spirituous beverages themselves. To put it mildly, this would be no loss to the individual physician; for many of his patients it would be a gain, because only the abstinent physician can cure inebriates; for the community it would be a blessing. Whoever avoids abstinence in spite of insight into its benefits, because it seems a sacrifice, lowers the medical profession which, as no other calling, is accustomed to sacrifice life and personal advantage for the benefit of others.

Unfortunately it is just the physicians, who in the matter of alcohol have to make good the much harm that previous generations have done. The theories that were advanced especially in the middle of the last century concerning the properties of alcohol as a strength and blood producer, as a preventative of infection and dispeller of fever, have, it is true, been given up by science, but all the more have they become part and parcel of common knowledge. And the charge must be made against physicians that, though at the time they eagerly disseminated the prejudice, they now do far too little to remove it and, instead, still do much to support it. Every (public) prescription of alcohol, even though in itself indicated,[44] is harmful, partly for the patient, partly for the community because it is irresistibly interpreted that alcohol is beneficial or necessary for the healthy. And unfortunately mistakes in practice are still being made where physicians instigate the cured inebriate to again indulge in alcohol and thereby lead him with his family into misfortune.

Delirium Tremens

There are several acute psychoses of a plainly specific character based on chronic alcoholism. The most important of these is *delirium*

---

[43] The study of drinking customs and everything connected with them is otherwise very useful also; it reveals a wonderful insight into human psychology, especially of the power of affectivity over thought.

[44] Proof is, as yet, wanting that there are indications for alcohol, i.e. that it cannot be substituted by something else.

tremens, drinker's insanity. It occurs almost only after many years of indulgence in alcohol; but occasionally we have seen it in young people in the early twenties who were addicted to drink from two to four years; so far they have all proved to be latent schizophrenics. Even in children and young people for whom the physician has prescribed large quantities of alcohol, the delirium may break out after a few years; but fortunately such cases are very rare.

The attack is usually precipitated by *special occasions:* any weakening factors such as any of the acute diseases, especially those with fever (pneumonia, exacerbations of alcoholic catarrh of the stomach, influenza, etc.), excessive and continued drinking, or a trauma may induce an attack. *Bonhoeffer* believes that the latter are less the cause than the result of the incipient alteration of consciousness and foresight; but the operating surgeon also does not fear the disease without reason.

Abstinence from alcohol is also said to produce delirium tremens. But this is very decidedly contradicted by the experience in sanatoria for alcoholics and in insane asylums, in which every alcoholic is kept abstinent from the time of entrance. According to my experience, and that of others, in hardly one case in a thousand does the delirium break out, which could not have been demonstrated previously with a fairly good anamnesis or examination on entrance, while, on the contrary, many cases, already clearly diagnosable, recover in spite of abstinence. As far as I know, the individual cases cited to prove the contrary are described and evaluated in an extremely uncritical manner. Only *Bonhoeffer's* statement is worthy of discussion that very frequently in the first days of confinement, especially in the case of tramps, the delirium breaks out; but since the same deprivation of alcohol in sanatoria does not have the same result, the difference must lie in the other circumstances, and these are really not far to seek; one can mention the psychical influence of confinement, the bad hygienic conditions, the forbidden nourishment, the sudden deprivation of liquids and perhaps still other factors. Have not many of these people permitted themselves to be caught because the delirium was already in the incipient stages? Sudden increase in the cost of whiskey brought with it a reduction of deliria, as did the whiskey boycott in Breslau in 1909-10. *Wigert* [45] ascertained that the suppression of the whiskey traffic during the general strike in Stockholm was followed by a small increase of cases of delirium tremens in Stockholm; instead of

[45] The frequency of delirium tremens in Stockholm during the prohibition of alcohol, August-September, 1909, Ztschr. f. d. ges. Neur. u. Psych. 1910, I. Bd. Orig. S. 556.

an average of 4, 6 and a maximum of 9, 16 cases came to notice in the first week, one in the following week, then no more until the re-opening of the saloons. But the author did not examine the individual cases, so that here too it is not even proven, first, that these delirants previously had days without alcohol and, second, that the addition of other factors (lack of work, hunger) is very probable. But if the improbable assumption that these were cases of abstinence deliria is to be taken as valid, it remains proven by this investigation that abstinence deliria, even when they occur, are so rare that it would be a mistake to consider them a factor: Among the many thousand inebriates who were suddenly forced into abstinence in a city which consumes 4.4 million liters of whiskey in a year, there were at the most a dozen cases.

Sometimes, but not always, delirium tremens is preceded for weeks or even months by *premonitions:* Sleep is cut short or disturbed by terror, moroseness, irritability and uneasiness appear; the last may be heightened to real anxiety which appears to be psychically unmotivated. Occasionally dizziness occurs. All actions are restless. The fine tremor quickly becomes coarser: single hallucinations usually of sight then occur, which are frequently in stable form; generally these prodromal sensory deceptions need not have the specific character of pronounced delirium tremens: A black dog follows the patient every time when he comes from his morning's drink, two policemen stand behind the closet whenever he comes home, etc. Sometimes the hallucinations plainly betray their origin in the irritated condition of the nerves. The patient sees shadows with high lights, he has sensations of itching or of being stabbed. These hallucinations scare the patient, although usually they are first recognized as such until they pass over into the hallucinations of the developed delirium.

The latter ordinarily breaks out rather suddenly at night, often awakening in terror or even in complete sleeplessness.

Hallucinations of a very characteristic coloring are most prominent and involve in the first place sight and touch. The visions are multiple, movable, mostly colorless and have a tendency toward diminutions. Furthermore, hallucinations of touch and vision both very frequently have the character of wires, threads, water sprays and other elongated things. Elementary visions, sparks and shadows, etc., are frequent. If auditory hallucinations are present, the patient most frequently hears music (especially often with a very decided beat), which is very rare in other psychoses. At the same time one also observes elementary hallucinations, especially in the form of reports and shots, but also buzzing, roaring, hissing, etc. Words and sentences are sometimes heard but never appear in the foreground; during the entire course of the disease delirious patients can visually enter into relations with hundreds of hallucinated persons that are all speechless. Whenever auditory hallucinations formed an important component of the morbid picture, then in our cases it has so far always been a question of a complication with schizophrenia. Now and then hallucinations of smell and, somewhat more frequently, of taste are observed. Not at all rare are hallucinations of the kinæsthetic sensations and of the sensations of position. When the patients sit, they suddenly feel the stool sway to one side, the floor moves under them; while they are lying in bed, they believe themselves at work in a sitting or upright position. The feeling that some real objects, that are at rest, seem to move is probably a part of these hallucinations. Individual somatic hallucinations can usually be accounted for on the basis of neuritic parasthesias interpreted through illusions.

At the height of the pronounced delirium the hallucinations of vision, in spite of a noticeably blurring of the coloring, are distinguished by great vividness and plasticity. This is particularly noticeable in neighborhoods where on the whole descriptions of visual experiences seem very colorless; but when alcoholics tell of their hallucinations, they usually describe them with a striking vividness and indicate the forms and movements with the hands as if they were still seeing everything before them. "A play is performed" for the milder patients; delirious patients always see the movies; scenes with ballet dancers, etc., are thrown on the screen for them.

But both the distinct and indistinct visions may suddenly disappear, especially if the patient, under a less lively concomitant hallucination of touch, grabs in the air when he wants to seize or strike at a vision. This gives an opportunity for all sorts of explanatory delusions. A delirious professor took great pleasure in proving to us what a shabby thing modern advertising is; one should just take notice, now he had in his hand the finest advertisement which he read to us; now he only made a motion, and everything had disappeared.

Small movable and multiple things are usually represented in reality by small animals, like mice and insects, hence these are among the most frequent hallucinations of alcoholics. Besides these one often sees here also animal visions of the most various kinds; pigs, horses, lions, camels may appear either reduced or in life size; sometimes, too, there may be animals "that do not exist" in extremely phantastic combinations. In entirely the same way I have noticeably often heard depicted on a board hallucinated on the wall, passing menageries of all kinds of animals, usually large ones, but in some cases reduced to about the size of a cat, which entertain the patients very well. People, too, are frequently reduced, but they may also appear life size.

The hallucinations of the different senses readily combine; mice and insects are not only seen but also touched when the patient grabs them or when they crawl over his skin. Money is gathered together and carefully placed into a hallucinated pocket. The patient sees passing soldiers and hears the band music; he sees and hears some one shooting at him; he fights with hallucinated assailants, whom he hears speak and more rarely also touches.

The optical sense deceptions of delirium tremens are livelier than in other deliria. In moments of hallucinating, reality does not exist; the patients take the window for the door, the stairs for the street, and consequently are in danger of falling; instead of the wall of the room they see the open field, bump their heads and get a mortal meningeal hemorrhage.

Besides the hallucinations visual *illusions* occur in vast quantities; those of the other senses are less frequent. The patient mistakes persons and things. He misreads, often producing complete nonsense, but frequently only inserting wrong words that have some logical connections with the real text, e.g. closet instead of box, eggs instead of butter, and similar things. It is peculiar that at times delirious patients that have read aloud disconnectedly or entirely senselessly, can, nevertheless, later repeat the real text correctly. Hallucinations and illusions can often be provoked and their content determined by suggestion; under certain conditions both at the beginning and the end of the delirium where spontaneous sense deceptions are not present. One presses on the eye ball (according to *Liepmann*) and asks the patient what he sees. If he sees nothing or merely elementary light manifestation, one asks him, for instance, if he sees the dog, which is often successful in making him believe that he perceives such an animal and he can then describe it exactly. One hands him an unused sheet of paper from which he usually reads disconnected nonsense but occasionally also whole stories or business letters. When requested to do so he carries on a lengthy conversation on a disconnected telephone with a distant place. It may also happen that three hallucinating patients who are in adjoining bath-tubs hallucinate about the same fish which they want to catch and which jumps from one tub into the other. *Perceptions* are disturbed in other respects also. The patients very readily mistake pictures after a brief exposure, and sometimes in this case as in reading they do it in a manner that hardly occurs elsewhere; instead of the correct object, they name another which has some relation to it but no external optical similarity. For instance, instead of spectacles, they think they see an opera glass; instead of a cat, a mouse; a bird's egg is designated as a nest; a shovel as "two picks." It is often very easily determined that paraphasic disturbances are not involved. This shows that the "actual perception" was correct but in its stead an overcharged associated idea comes into consciousness. Frequently the color of the picture is disregarded; the green head of cabbage in Meggendorfer's picture book "Nimm Mich Mit" is more often than not taken for a rose (moreover this is not rarely the case with non-alcoholics also). The cucumber in the same book has even been mistaken for a sausage.

Gregor and Roemer found in one case that perception was retarded. Contrasted with this it is striking that a brief exposure (uncovering and covering the picture with the hand without apparatus) in complicated cases does not at all, or not materially, aggravate the result as compared with the longer exposure.

It is self-evident that with the constant visual deceptions *orientation* as to place is disturbed severely. But this is not merely the result of the hallucination. In the last days of a somewhat drawn-out delirium one now and then sees orientation fail, without the presence of an hallucination and even without a memory deception which could explain this. Orientation as to time is also disturbed during the duration of the delirium, in severer cases even beyond this, so that the patients state the wrong year, etc. Often the length of the delirium appears much greater to the patients than it really was.

Autopsychically, all pure cases of delirium are oriented. They know who they are, what position in the world they occupy, what sort of family they have, where they live, etc.

Attention is profoundly disturbed. Left to themselves, the patients are occupied with their hallucinations and do not bother themselves much with what goes on about them. But if they are spoken to sharply, they can be distracted. Presented before students at a clinic they usually conduct themselves in such an orderly manner that it is difficult to show the coarse peculiarities of conduct. It is possible, if the attention which is constantly striving to wander is kept awake, to make even psychological experiments with alcoholic delirious patients. Left to themselves they are immediately occupied with their hallucinations. Even when they collect themselves, the field of thought is very narrowed, consequently the ability to concentrate, attention, tenacity, and vigility, as well as the limits of these are greatly reduced.

The mental stream in delirious patients has not as yet been sufficiently investigated. At all events far too few ideas are present. The patients talk according to the momentary need, without even feeling simple contradictions.[46] They are no longer capable of participating in complicated reflections, which accounts for the marked absence of the critical attitude as contrasted with the promptness of the answers. It is particularly striking in the case of the senseless hallucinations. A patient can very quietly state that somebody has chopped off his hands and head; another patient said that he has been decapitated four times, etc.

In contrast perhaps to all other cases of delirium and crepuscular states they show in conversation [47] an unusually quick reaction; excuses, especially, are evoked with an incomprehensible rapidity, and not alone in the matter of drinking, but in all other directions. Thus the patients want to get away; their attention is called to the fact that they have no trousers, whereupon they at once respond: "Yes, that damned office boy always steals my pants; I have often told him about it." Or his wife has taken away his shoes so that he cannot go to the saloon, etc. Another always trembles so severely "when the wind blows." To the question what the patient had done with his pants, I once received the answer: "They are at home. I never wear pants in summer."

If the delirium is complicated by epileptiform attacks or any severer organic disturbances, this readiness may then be lacking and, on the contrary one now observes a heaviness of perception and reaction.

Lasting delusions are rarely formed. These patients naturally believe in their hallucinations and endeavor to explain them; but usually the delusion vanishes with the change in the sense deception. Most frequently the patients retain for a longer period persecutory deliria accompanied by anxiety. They tell how different people have made holes in the wall and squirt water or poison through them, etc.

The *memory* is deeply disturbed. Even during the delirium the patients recall only a small part of all that they have experienced; above all the time sequence of the experience is invariably completely disrupted (except in cases that have originated on a foundation of schizophrenia. Here the most complicated experiences are reproduced for several days with great clearness, and the objective control, as far as this is possible, may be a sort of guarantee for the correctness of the recollection). Also *after* the delirium, the memory as a rule is very incomplete; but by mentioning experiences one can sometimes get

---

[46] See below among the excuses.

[47] As in perception laboratory experiment with associations shows a retardation of reaction. This is probably explained by the difficulties inherent in the experimental situation.

the patients to recall individual scenes. But even then larger or smaller distortions are rarely lacking.

Also positive memory disturbances are probably always combined with delirium tremens, having the characteristics of *spontaneous and despairing confabulations.* The patients tell a lot of things which they have experienced neither in reality nor in hallucination, and bring their real experiences into entirely new connections.

Recollections from the time preceding the delirium are usually good.

The *affectivity* has specific characteristics. In spite of the fact that the patients always find themselves in situations not suited to them, rarely attaining what they want (entirely similar to the dream state), and are bothered rather than entertained by their visions, they bear everything with an evident *humor*. Often they themselves feel the silly improbabilities (impossibilities for the spectator) of their hallucinations. They can take nothing seriously except for a moment, they behave in this manner in the case of some clumsy treatment that irritates them, or in the case of anxiety hallucinations that readily lead to dangerous attacks. The majority of these patients suffer from anxiety. *And this combination of anxiety with euphroic humor* (grim humor) *is present in most cases, and does not occur in this way anywhere else.*

Corresponding to the lively feelings and the lack of a critical attitude there exists a marked *suggestibility*. One can usually talk the patients into believing without any difficulty that yesterday they did this and that, and were in one place or another. The easy provocation of hallucinations has already been mentioned. The patients respond to requests with excessive acquiescence, they stretch their legs much too high when one wants to test the patella reflex, etc. But still other mechanisms must assist in the production of similar manifestations. For instance, in psychological tests one should be wary of presenting the same test units several times in the same sequence because otherwise the patients readily answer in the sense of this sequence. Consequently there exists in contrast to the memory disturbance an abnormal capacity for habituating associations, in a direction not more exactly known to us.

The *conduct* is so characteristic that the delirious alcoholic is recognized at a distance with practical certainty. He is incessantly restless; one can put him to bed a hundred time a day and yet he is always out of it: the patient "is on the run." In an uncertain trembling way something is always being done; pressing on real and hallucinated locks, knocking the bed around, bracing against the wardrobe because it wants to fall over, picking up money, mice and spiders are caught, hallucinated saliva threads or hair are pulled out of the mouth and rolled up, and other threads are spun off objects. With comical detail the patient treads over a stretched cord, avoids wires drawn through the air, clings to pieces of clothing, while he mistakes their different parts, takes a sleeve for a pocket, and wants to use the shirt as a pair of pants. He supposes people behind the door who keep it locked, bangs against it, calls "Open up," etc. He wants to go away, has to go at once to a certain street, where he has important business. But on the whole very little is said in contrast with the high degree of motor restlessness.

Occupation deliria are frequent which may be evenly divided as to content between business in the saloon and business in his line of work. The coachman drives a wagon or cleans the horses, the baker

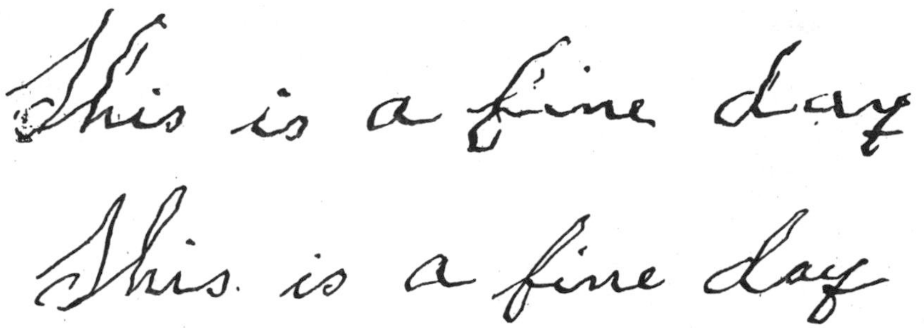

Fig. 17.—Handwriting of a delirious patient. Fairly coarse, irregular tremors and marked inequalities of pressure. The second line is more marked as the result of fatigue.

kneads the dough and takes bread out of the oven, the carpenter planes wood, handles boards, etc. Then again the ward is taken for a bar-room, the orderly for a waitress; the patient orders beer; sometimes he gets it by way of hallucination and can drink it with satisfaction. But frequently he gets angry that nothing is brought and scolds, only to forget his misconduct the next moment. A great many foolish things are done; the shirt is often torn. A saloon keeper at home took his big toe for a cork, screwed the cork-screw into it and began to pull at it for dear life.

Severer cases remain in bed longer but have the same ideas; the bed with its pieces of bed clothes then represents the largest part of the environment, falsified by illusions; it is a wagon with a horse, a carpenter's bench, etc. The patient has to catch little animals from the bed spread; occasionally he reads entire stories which are supposed to be on the linen.

If the weakness increases, the deliria become frothing, the patients only make coarse tremulous movements, which are difficult to interpret, pull at the spread or pick at the sheets. In fatal cases convulsive movements, gnashing of teeth, etc., may also be present.

The delirious patient *does not become unclean* except toward the end.

Among the *physical symptoms* which are never entirely lacking but whose severity is not always in proportion to the intensity of the psychical disturbances, *the most noticeable* is the coarse, irregular tremor which is evident in all movements, as well as in speech.

The *pulse* is usually rapid, fluttering, irregular and, at least in severe cases, weak. In spite of this the blood pressure is supposed to be increased as long as no collapse threatens. The heart weakness is not merely a case of the chronic disturbances of the alcoholic, but evidently of an unknown toxic substance that appears and disappears with the deliria. In contrast with the alcoholic facial congestion the face is usually pale and at the same time covered with sweat so that the patients often appear markedly troubled. The *urine* is always highly colored; at the height of the attack it usually contains a trace of albumen, in some cases larger quantities and for a longer time; not seldom some sugar is found.

The *pupils* often react poorly; they may also be unequal and even irregular. The deep *reflexes* are usually exaggerated; in case of neuritis they are naturally diminished; on admission to the hospital they are often still lively, on the following day diminished or absent.

The *temperature,* even when no complications are present, is usually somewhat high; in rare cases it rises to over 140° F. so that the patients die of hyperpyrexia (Delirium tremens febrile).

Typical *epileptiform attacks* may initiate or accompany the delirium; usually they are single attacks.

Sometimes there are evident signs of neuritis or at least neuritic irritations, thus one can elicit pain through pressure over the nerve trunks and muscles, there may also be weakness and even pareses. I have frequently observed inflammation of the optic nerve; also central organic signs such as disturbances of coordination or cerebellar ataxia; but they are often difficult to see on account of the marked tremor. In many cases there is a complete *analgesia* which is often very unpleasant especially in surgical cases: The patients want to walk about when their legs have been recently amputated or their bones broken, they tear off their bandages and dig into their wounds.

At the height of the attack *sleep* is entirely absent or is, at any rate, very brief. Moreover the excitements are invariably severer at night than during the day.

Course. The disease usually runs a course from two to four days and ends in recovery, often following a usually very long, critical sleep; in other cases recovery comes gradually. I have not seen a delirium tremens last longer than fourteen days. The slower the recovery proceeds, the more probably are organic disturbances in the sense of Korsakoff connected with it. Deliria, which are further protracted into the second week, are probably always complicated; this is especially true of those in which after improvement a sort of relapse occurs.

If the disease runs its typical course, the hallucinations gradually become more and more blurred and less numerous. Often, however, they at first lose the value of reality; the birds are no longer alive but stuffed, the scenes are especially performed and finally are thrown on the screen only optically as if by a magic lantern.

Perhaps in between one and two percent of the uncomplicated cases the patients die of *heart failure.* Moreover the initial diseases (pneumonia with pus, etc.) may naturally end fatally. The mortality statistics from different places are not comparable because, depending on conditions of admission, some institutions admit mainly complicated or mainly uncomplicated cases. But there are statistics in which the fatalities still reach 26 percent. I cannot account for this in any other way than by supposing that mistakes were made in the treatment.

After the delirium there naturally remains the chronic alcoholism. The anatomical findings justify the assumption that in every alcoholic delirium some components of the brain are destroyed. In severer cases the delirium is followed by alcoholic feeble-mindedness or Korsakoff's disease. Some delusions may persist for a longer time until they are forgotten rather than corrected. According to some, "alcoholic paranoia" and chronic hallucinoses may become superimposed.

The attack of delirium tremens may recur; in the course of several years the same patient may pass through a dozen or more deliria. But such people who relapse several times invariably become very demented.

Besides the typical cases there are *abortive* ones which show only few symptoms, such as very slight confusion and marked tremors or a few hallucinations. They pass away completely in one or two days. Then there are deliria which from the very beginning show a chronic character. The patients usually remain oriented, hallucinate almost only at night, even then not always, and sleep in between times; during the day they can, under certain conditions, even perform simpler tasks. Such deliria can last four weeks and are to be differentiated from the fully developed attacks in which a complication with Korsakoff's disease is responsible for a protracted convalescence.

In *schizophrenics,* delirium tremens is somewhat modified. The deliria often expose complexes. Auditory hallucinations are prominent (somatic hallucinations are, as far as my experience goes, not exactly frequent). But above all the deliria are more connected; for days the patients experience complicated scenes.

Such a patient very dramatically described his experiences in prison and in the insane asylum in thirty-six pages: "What I suddenly had to see there, made my hair stand on end. Forests, rivers, oceans with every kind of dreadful animal and human figure, which no human eye ever saw before, whirled by incessantly, changing off with the work shops of all callings, in which horrible spirit figures were working. —At both sides the walls were nothing but a single ocean with thousands of little ships on it; the passengers were all naked men and women who indulged themselves to the tempo of music, whereat every time a pair had satisfied themselves a figure stabbed them from behind with a long spear so that the ocean was colored blood red; but fresh droves always came. . . . A train from which many people alighted. Among these I heard the voices of my father and my sister K. who came to deliver me. I plainly heard them converse with each other. Then I heard my sister whisper again with an old woman; I called to her for dear life to deliver me. . . . She called that she would do it but the old woman did not let her go, warning my sister that thereby she would bring misfortune on the entire household, but that nothing was happening to me. . . . Amid prayerful tears I awaited my death. The silence of the grave prevailed and spirit figures surrounded me in droves; at last one of the spirits came and held his watch in front of my eyes at a certain distance merely indicating to me that it was not yet three o'clock as none of the figures were permitted to speak." Then there were long negotiations among the relatives of the patient who wanted to ransom him, at first with smaller sums, then with larger ones. Other voices debated how they would do away with the patient. Then the relatives were induced to go on ladders and thrown into the castle mote where they were heard crying and choking. The wife of the jailer came, cut off his flesh piece by piece, beginning at his feet and going up to his breast, fried and ate it. She poured salt on his wounds. On a wildly swaying scaffold the patient was drawn into the various heavens up to the eighth, past choruses of trumpets, who proclaimed his fame. At last because of some terror he was again consigned to earth. . . . People sat at a table and ate and drank things with the most marvelous aroma; but a glass was handed to him, it disappeared into nothing and he suffered great thirst. Thereupon he had to count and figure out loud for hours (objectively: verbigeration). In a little flask a divine drink was handed to him; but when he wanted to take it, it broke *and the content flowed between his fingers like threads of glue.* Later a great battle was fought between his tormentors and his relatives of which he saw nothing but heard blows and groans, etc. Then *scorpions* came, *drawn on long threads.* During the entire journey to the institution, which was also not recognized by the patient, his sister sat on the roof of the wagon and always cried out the same words. In the institution was a man who always *squirted him* with *urine* so that the patient had to freeze severely.

Anatomy. As a sign of the poisoning one finds throughout the entire brain diseased and degenerating ganglia cells and fibres, which are not, however, evenly distributed. The fibres are said to degenerate in large numbers especially in the motor centres and in the cerebellum. Punctiform hemorrhages are frequently seen and belong to the degeneration of the blood vessels. As a result of death from heart failure there is also a venous congestion of the entire cranial content. Naturally the clinical signs of chronic alcoholism are found in the brain and the other organs. The sclerosis and discoloration of the heart muscles is probably connected with the acute disease.

The *causes* were mentioned at the beginning. Protracted drinking must have prepared the ground, and the disease afflicts chiefly, even though perhaps not entirely, drunkards who indulge in whiskey,—either exclusively, or in addition to other alcoholic liquors.

The most frequent *age for the disease* is accordingly between thirty and fifty, and the maximum is closer to the latter figure than the former, many cases even occurring after fifty.

The *pathology* of delirium tremens is still entirely obscure. To be sure, it is not a question of direct alcoholic poisoning, but of a toxin (apparently clinical), which in consequence of a protracted indulgence in alcohol in the case of a definite personal disposition, is set free as a result of fortuitous impairments. At all events not only is the nervous system poisoned but also the heart and perhaps also the kidneys, and other organs.

The *character of the hallucinations* is fully explained by the irritating states of the optical and tactile apparatus. The slight participation also of the psyche indicates a more peripheral origin of the sense deceptions. Complex hallucinations are very rarely involved. If most of the sensory disturbances are auxilliary to the complexes, complications with schizophrenia may with great probability be inferred. In most cases the patients are hardly or not at all participating spectators of their hallucinations, or they conceive of the annoyances that the animals cause them as comical misfortunes.

Only the anxious hallucinations have a different significance. They are evidently the expression of the somatic fear, caused by weakness of the heart and perhaps also directly by the poisoning, the anxiety expressing itself as in a dream or in fever by hallucinations. The accompanying euphoria and the ready humor are a part of chronic alcoholism.

The *diagnosis* is usually very easy. The following points are to be considered: In the first place, the entire appearance, which one must have had an opportunity to see; then the anamnesis, in which, moreover, the drinking is sometimes denied in every way; the physical signs of alcoholism, the coarse tremor; the type of hallucinations, a combination of visual and tactile; in both fields one frequently finds threadlike structures; in the visual field the hallucinations are multiple, moveable, and colorless, manifesting themselves especially in the form of animals with a tendency to dimunitiveness; the retention of auto-psychic orientation; the promptness of the psychical reactions; the (relative) capacity of being aroused from the delirium; the scarcity of complex contents, and the intermingling of humor and anxiety.

As far as I have seen, the *fever deliria*, that are so often mistaken for delirium tremens, are invariably complex deliria in which the rapid reaction is lacking. But there are many kinds of fever deliria, and psychiatry does not as yet know them all.

It is important to note that because of accompanying alcoholism any other conditions may obtain "alcoholic coloring." The connected hallucinations of schizophrenics which are also visually especially plastic have been mentioned above. Living visions, etc., mingle with other morbid pictures, e.g. in epileptic twilight states.

Treatment. Unfortunately delirium tremens usually must be treated at home or in the general hospital. But the physician must not forget that to cure the alcoholism at the same time would only be possible if the patient is brought to a suitable hospital for the insane.

The prime condition of a proper treatment is *supervision*. The patients can very readily do harm. In the first place, because they hallucinate differently than any one else; [48] or they consider themselves attacked or insulted; they are jealous of their wife and resort to weapons; or they handle weapons in such a manner that they accidentally injure themselves or others. One of our patients jumped into the manure hole to hide from the animals. In surgical cases the

[48] Comp. p. 328.

analgesias constitute the most serious danger. The orderlies should try to keep the patients in bed. To be sure they always get out again but if they are permitted to wander at will in a room not specially adapted, too much damage may readily be done. If the patient becomes weaker, he is kept in bed more easily—fortunately so, because just at that time the stay in bed conserves the strength. The incessantly repeated request that they remain in bed and go to bed is an excellent means of diverting them *that does not irritate much*. Instead of the bed the tepid bath is often recommended. This is naturally also a good place for the patient to stay; but it is questionable whether by itself it shortens the delirium or has a quieting influence. With proper treatment the patient is violent only in exceptional cases; to be sure he may tear his shirt, damage the door, etc. It only comes to a real fight in case of clumsiness or impatience on the part of the attendants, or in case of severe anxiety hallucinations; but these too are amenable to quieting influences.

The second important point is the *nourishment*. The patients are near a collapse, the heart is poisoned, the urine is too scanty, the functioning of the stomach is disturbed by the catarrhal condition; the patients do not take the time to eat, or refuse nourishment because they fear they will be poisoned. All these indications call for a milk diet, which needs not be exclusively so, except in case of complicated cirrhosis of the liver or nephritis. One should offer the patient milk in addition to the ordinary foods, from one to several quarts a day. Since they are used to swallowing fluids, a drink is the easiest thing to get them to take; the milk is at the same time nourishing and relatively easy to digest. It promotes somewhat diuresis and thus probably has the effect of tending to rid the organism of poison.

Everything else is secondary. In a private home one will usually be compelled to give hypnotics. They do little good, probably not at all, until the crisis is passed, which practically means when they are no longer necessary; to be sure, one can perhaps at this time induce the critical sleep a few hours earlier. Chloral, sulfonal, trional, methylal, amylene hydrate, and paraldehyde are used, of which especially the last is to be recommended.

For the threatened collapse cardiac *stimulants* are also given. If I found this necessary, I would, e.g., prescribe digalin.

The question has been much discussed whether *alcohol* should be given. It is certain that since the larger quantities of alcohol have been dispensed with, the mortality has decreased greatly; if one really did help individual patients with alcohol, a greater number would be killed by it. Consequently in more recent times delirium tremens is treated without alcohol. But it is not to be denied that at times one of the severer cases, which with us are to be seen only in people that come from East Europe, might be carried through the crisis by alcohol. In a single case that I observed myself, I can interpret the result in that way. In other cases where I permitted myself to be influenced by relatives or other circumstances, no benefit but probably harm could be noted. But I assume that only the larger doses, which nowadays are hardly ever used, are directly dangerous.—*If one feels compelled to give alcohol, the taste should be disguised as the patient will otherwise carry over into the chronic alcoholism the professional sanction of his conviction that the stimulus is necessary for him.*[49]

Alcoholic Hallucinosis

(Kraepelin's hallucinatory insanity of drunkards)

(Wernicke's acute hallucinosis of drunkards)

Alcoholic insanity is in many respects the opposite of delirium tremens. It manifests itself chiefly in auditory hallucinations, which have a peculiar character: In most patients it is a case of the voices of several or many people not present who discuss the patient in a dramatically elaborate dialogue; that is, they discuss him in the third person; much more rarely do they speak to him.[50] These voices threaten him, remind him of his sins, scold him, make plans as to how they will catch him and perhaps torment and torture his family also. Some egg the other on, or some of them side with the patient, try to defend him and save him. In very acute cases the connection is usually less organized; in place of more quiet scenes there is a confusion of voices. Sometimes the voices are rhythmic, partly synchronous with the pulse, and partly with an external sound, e.g. the ticking of a watch, as "You are a fool, you are a fool" (*Bonhoeffer*), or they take the form of rhymes and satiric verses about the patient. Frequently the patients hear their own thoughts or answers to them, or one ascertains what they are doing or criticizes their actions.

Besides, especially in the beginning, one seldom fails to note sounds, such as buzzing, snapping of gun triggers, striking of rifle bullets, cracking, and sounds of horses' hoofs, all of which is related to the patient.

[49] For prescriptions see p. 223.

[50] However, even in the most pronounced cases, it is also quite usual for the patients to try to communicate with those hallucinated persons who take their part, and to obtain answers from them.

Of the hallucinations of the other senses *visual deceptions* occur most readily, one of the acting persons is seen behind a door or somewhere in the dark. Visions similar to those in delirium tremens may also appear intermingled with the others. Skin sensations, being squirted at, or blown at, are also said to occur; hallucinations of smell, taste, and especially somatic hallucinations, probably belong to a fundamental schizophrenia.

Delusions of persecution correspond to the hallucinations. There are people present who mock the patient, punish him, want to do away with him, and under certain conditions there are also some who take his part. Usually the patient does not feel entirely innocent; besides enormous and unjust accusations, real mistakes are held against him, among others, e.g., his drinking; but everything is exaggerated. Invariably there are delusions of reference, this or that real person, but especially this or that event, being brought into connection with the machinations against the patient. *Isolated ideas of grandeur* are very rare. The delusions do not constitute a compact, carefully thought out picture, the patients are just being persecuted by a gang; but the improbabilities are not noticed, much less explained. To be sure, at times there is an explanation. Their enemies have machines, with which they listen in on the patients and through which they speak to them; they want to poison them in some way. Supernatural accomplices, such as God, angels, devil, hardly ever occur.

At the same time the patients remain *oriented* and in spite of the delusions they generally remain *clear*. They do not mistake the real environment into which they put the hallucinatory experiences.

Attention appears to be nearly normal; one can carry on a systematic conversation with the patients; to be sure they are easily diverted by the voices. Normal thinking, as far as it can be tested, appears not to be changed outside of the delusions.

The *dominant affect* is anxiety, which is not lacking in any case and usually dominates the whole behavior, which at most only temporarily corresponds to the situation which subjectively is often altogether desperate. The patients are *relatively* indifferent, often resigned to their fate; or, instead of defending themselves, they go to the police and demand the punishment of their persecutors. I cannot decide whether this incomplete reaction is an expression of the superficiality characteristic of drunkards, or whether there does exist anywhere a consciousness of the unreality of the experiences. At all events in a large number of cases as in delirium tremens the *alcoholic humor* remains at the same time with the anxiety. In spite of this suicide is not rare, especially in the first stage. In cases taking a chronic course *irritability* also appears; but I have not seen real outbursts of violence.

The *suggestibility* so pronounced in delirium tremens is wanting here, at least in regard to the hallucinations. The patients do not let themselves be diverted from anything; on the contrary, they feel the necessity of proving their ideas to others.

Memory is in all cases good, even better than could be expected in the confusing variety of experiences. During the disease and after it the patients can recount a number of details in an orderly manner. Confabulation is rare.

The *behavior* of the patients is to all appearances proper; whatever strange thing they do is a defense against supposed attacks. In all other respects they retain their composure. Many even travel about, to evade their enemies, when to be sure they may barricade their room in the hotel. In the asylum they submit to the regulations as far as they are not prevented by the hallucinations. The physician is recognized as such, and does not belong to the enemies, and the hallucinated scenes are, in contrast with delirium tremens, outside of the room in which the patient is situated. Bonhoeffer actually speaks of a "clear-minded delirium."

The *physical symptoms* are insignificant. It is a striking fact that the symptoms of the basic chronic alcoholism are sometimes not visible at all; at all events, they are on the average far less pronounced than in all other alcoholic diseases. In very acute cases, which in other respects also have a tendency to mingle with delirious symptoms, coarse tremors and similar signs of alcohol may also be present.—*Sleep* is invariably disturbed but hardly ever entirely lacking as in delirium tremens.

Course. Alcoholic insanity usually breaks out very acutely; premonitory signs need not have preceded but may be present in forms similar to those in delirium tremens, the hallucinations always appear rather as noises than as visual deceptions, in addition there may be anxiety, and irritation; furtive transition of the prodromal symptoms into the real delirium in the course of a few days or even weeks occurs only rarely. The outcome is probably always by lysis, it may be after a few days or after months.

Repeated attacks in the same patient are not rare.

As a rule the disease passes over into recovery. Korsakoff's syndrome never follows typical alcoholic hallucinosis. It is a question whether the delusions and hallucinations can continue to exist in a chronic form. At all events it rarely occurs, except when there existed previously a paranoid or otherwise a latent schizophrenia.

According to the course one can distinguish with *Kraepelin* an *acute* and a *subacute* form, the former of which lasts from several days to several months, the latter about two or three months. But transitional forms are not rare. The two types are also plainly differentiated symptomologically; in the subacute form every indication of confusion is usually lacking; the hallucinated scenes are in this case elaborated to the greatest extent and may be carried on for months in a very consistent and unified manner. The remaining alcoholic signs are very apt to be lacking here. On the contrary, in the acute cases the alcoholism is more pronounced; even coarse tremors and gastric symptoms also are not so rare. The voices are more confused, more peculiar, fragmentary, and speak to the patient oftener, e.g. in case of denunciations; here the rhythmic expressions and repetitions occur, and finally only mixtures with delirium tremens symptoms are present which may predominate to such an extent that one cannot tell to which disease the case should be ascribed.

Thus the *symptom picture* of alcoholic hallucinosis is much more changeable than that of delirium tremens. The cases taking a slow course behave themselves outwardly in an orderly manner so far as they do not react to the delusions; they can run about without being at once conspicuous. But anxious restlessness, defensive measures, or stories of persecutions easily betray the patient. The most acute are so dominated by their delusions and hallucinations that they take too little consideration of their surroundings and on superficial inspection appear confused without being so.

The disease is *not frequent* and, disregarding the different classifications of psychosis in different places, occurs rather irregularly. According to *Kraepelin* the proportion to delirium tremens is 1 to 3, according to *Schroeder,* (Breslau), 1 to 20, with us in Switzerland about 1 to 44.

According to *Kraepelin* alcoholic hallucinosis afflicts *women* relatively frequently.

The *age* of the patients is on the average less than in delirium tremens, according to *Schroeder* between 30 and 35 years.

The *cause* and *pathology* are still entirely unclear.

In cases with the ordinary sub-acute course which I have seen so far, I could always demonstrate with certainty or great probability that besides the alcoholism a long standing schizophrenia was present. The (rare) acute attacks in my experience were all at least a little abnormal in the direction of schizophrenia, although the connection here was less plainly pronounced.[51]

The *differential* diagnosis of alcoholic hallucinosis as such is usually very easy. As a rule the anamnesis alone points to the disease, but the diagnosis is further confirmed by the vivid and connected hallucinations. I know of no psychosis with dramatically connected and elaborated auditory hallucinations, which speak of the patient in the third person, in which there is no alcoholism. Also the particular vividness of the hallucinations with persistent clearness and orientation indicates the alcoholic coloring with certainty. The only difficult question is whether a pronounced schizophrenia is in back of it. Where neither in the anamnesis nor in the picture itself pronounced schizophrenic indications are found (lively somatic hallucinations, affective disturbances), the prognosis should not be considered bad, even when the schizophrenia is certain; the latter is very rarely subject to an exacerbation during the insanity.

Treatment. Because the patients, at least in the beginning, are very strongly inclined to suicide, and during the entire course are very burdensome, treatment in an institution is nearly always indicated. Under favorable circumstances the alcoholism can then be treated at the same time.

Alcoholic Psychoses with Organic Symptoms

Even delirium tremens is a distinct poisoning of the nervous system with indications of peripheral neuritis, frequent organically conditioned eye symptoms, and acute alteration of nervous elements in the brain. However, here the psychic manifestations predominate and they are apparently more the expression of a functional poisoning of the central nervous system than of the slight destruction in it. In contrast to this are the purely alcoholic neuritis and the (rare) alcoholic myelitis, where only an anatomic disturbance seems to be present and where, at the same time, the psyche remains entirely or almost entirely intact. Now the acute injury to the tissue may chiefly afflict the brain or it may be localized only in the brain, and we then deal with a *Korsakoff psychosis*, the main characteristic of which is the organic symptom complex, usually combined with neuritic manifestations. In other cases the process, besides being localized in the cortex, is also localized in the centers that control the inner eye muscles and speech coordina-

---

[51] Alcoholic hallucinosis could therefore be a mere syndrome of schizophrenia induced by alcohol. This would be borne out by the circumstance, that under other conditions the generally disjointed auditory hallucinations of schizophrenics readily become connected through indulgence in alcohol.

tion, which produces a picture similar to paresis, or *alcoholic pseudo-paresis*. Between these borderline cases, distinguished as types, there are all kinds of transitions and mixtures, and the number of the combinations is further increased by the fact that such processes may also be chronic or sub-acute; this is especially true of the degeneration of the cutaneous nerves and the rheumatoid pains which regularly take an entirely chronic course. Neuritis in individual nerves, especially in the peronei, may begin in sub-acute form; also psychoses of the Korsakoff variety, and still more frequently of the pseudoparesis variety may take months for their development. To be sure there are also mild, "abortive" cases.

In reality we therefore meet all kinds of combinations of chronic and acute neuritis, and cerebral organic and toxic manifestations (the organic syndrome corresponds to the organic-cerebral processes; the delirium tremens syndrome corresponds to the toxic-functional process); the entirely pure cases are not even the more frequent, but as a rule one of the syndromes stands in the foreground. Delirium tremens is especially often connected with the diseases having an acute onset; they may be neuritic or pseudoparalytic or of the Korsakoff variety.

The division of the acute forms into *delirium tremens, Korsakoff,* pseudoparesis, polioencephalitis superior does not therefore presuppose a distinct and fundamental separation. It is not yet known whether differences in the localization, intensity, and the time of development are due to the influence of the identical poison, or whether they are due to combinations of different poisons.

On the more neurological side two forms are conspicuous that must be mentioned: The internal and even the external *eye-muscles* may be especially severely affected. The cases that I have seen ran their course with a somewhat protracted and not very pronounced delirium tremens. They healed in several weeks or months.—Then *Charcot* distinguished the (two sided) *alcoholic neuritis of the peronei* with paralysis of the anterior foot muscles and consequent sinking of the points of the feet (steppage gait). It seems to occur chiefly in those that drink the higher grades of liquors.

The Alcoholic Korsakoff Psychosis (*Chronic alcoholic delirium according to* **Kiefer** *and* **Bonhoeffer**).

The Korsakoff psychosis [52] in the majority of cases begins with a delirium tremens that recedes somewhat slowly and leaves behind the organic syndrome. It does not correspond with the facts to designate only the "amnestic symptom complex" as the characteristic feature; all other organic symptoms belong to it.

[52] See p. 230.

Nevertheless the *memory defect* is in the foreground. In pronounced cases the patients forget from one moment to another what they have experienced; at every visit they tell and ask for the same things. But sometimes single elements, especially confabulated ones, are retained for a long time. In most cases at the beginning there is a plain boundary line at the period of the onset of the disease in which what happened previously is still remembered. But the line is usually blurred in time; as in other organic diseases the memory defect can finally extend back very far. For example, some live again in the time of their military service and, with the exception of smaller islands, have forgotten what happened after. Only when the disease has improved a little do the patients sometimes notice the memory defect and endeavor to help themselves with memoranda. Previously they conceal it from themselves with the most flourishing confabulations; they never appear at a loss for words, narrate spontaneously, and on occasion, all sorts of invented experiences, usually such as are still conceivable.

The general opinions which the patients have formed in the course of their lives are not lost, neither are the simpler acquired aptitudes, etc. In the ordinary cases, also, the patients have no difficulty in finding words.

In the beginning the mood is usually alcoholic-euphoric; after months or years it may change in various directions and become morose or indifferent. In other respects the affectivity is very labile and easily stimulated in all directions.

Orientation is disturbed to a high degree. The patients no longer have any conception of time relations and as to location, also, they only get along somewhat after a longer time. In spite of this the patients move about entirely free from care, because they do not notice their deficiency.

The *apperception* of sense impressions is retarded and is readily falsified.

Active attention seems very good in conversation; the passive is reduced.

The patients tire very easily of all mental exertions.

In the beginning the patients are fairly active; but they retire more and more, and their initiative, as well as their interest in their surroundings and sometimes even in their own welfare, declines.

There are also somnolent and stuporous cases, usually as a result of more severe organic affection, especially in the region of the corpora quadrigemini.

On the whole only the symptoms of deficiency become chronic

(such as the organic dementia, and not the delirium, the stupor, etc.), but now and then one also finds later on states of confusion, and especially individual passing, or more protracted, but not elaborated, delusions, preferably those of being robbed or persecuted, and at times also a grandiose idea. In patients that are quite demented these delusions as well as the confabulations may appear senseless; the patient is "Emperor of Rothschild" (*Schroeder*). In a few cases I have seen pictures of a schizophrenic variety following later, but these patients were previously already abnormal, so that it was probably a case of a combination of alcoholic Korsakoff and schizophrenia.

The *physical symptoms*, aside from the signs of chronic alcoholism, are those of a general neuritis, thus we have: pains, paralyses, atrophies, contractures of the muscles of the eyes, of the vagus region, of the nerves of deglutition, and more rarely of the bladder and colon. During the delirious stage *sleep* is naturally disturbed; afterwards it is usually normal.

In the beginning the *metabolism* is usually disturbed. In the chronic stage it is normal, or the patients actually weigh more than before.

Frequently, especially in the beginning of the course, *epileptiform attacks* are found.

Course and *prognosis*. Ordinarily there are premonitions of the disease, which are the same as in delirium tremens. The delirium then breaks out, usually with a pronounced tremens character; in single cases it takes other forms also. With slow fluctuations it subsides, leaving behind the simple Korsakoff. Rarely, there is a chronic development that takes several months or even more than a year. Such cases, too, may improve decidedly or even recover.

The stuporous form is probably always acute.

In the course of about a year, sometimes a little longer, sometimes sooner, a part of the manifestations invariably disappear but least of all the affective disturbance. In some cases the recovery reaches as far as complete ability to work and practical rehabilitation. But most of the patients remain more or less organically demented even though they can be used in the institution for many tasks

The neuritic manifestations disappear much more frequently, sometimes with remarkable rapidity. But at times atrophies of individual muscle groups persist.

Some patients die in the acute stage, in part from weakness of the heart, in part from paralysis of the vagus or from choking and similar accidents.

Anatomy. Anatomically one finds as the sign of the Korsakoff psychosis a diffuse disintegration of nervous elements in the brain; in severer cases this is connected with an inflammatory reaction of smaller vessels that form offshoots and whose cells proliferate. Other vascular changes occur also, e.g. hyaline degenerations. As a result of the vascular disease one notes numerous small hemorrhages. Besides these one naturally finds also the disturbances of chronic alcoholism.

Pathology, and cause. Compared with the more functional delirium tremens the anatomically conditioned Korsakoff is the severer disease. It also appears a little later, chiefly in the forties or fifties. It is striking that relatively it afflicts the female sex severely; according to *Chotzen* there is one case of Korsakoff to about twenty cases of male delirium tremens, but only two female cases. With our conditions the difference is still greater in that Korsakoff among men is decidedly rarer. It has also been noticed that infectious diseases, marasmus, higher grades of alcoholism, seem to favor the disease, and that it frequently appears after repeated delirium tremens, which indicates that a poor resistance of the nervous system is a concomitant factor in the disease. But one can also think of the kind of poison; of the women that I saw, most or all consumed cordials, and it is known that the essences of the liquor can cause neuritis.

The *differential diagnosis* is usually easy. Even during the initial delirium tremens one usually notices a reduced ability to be aroused, the absence of quick reaction, and a difficulty in grasping simpler questions which does not readily occur in the simple delirium. Compared with the other organic diseases the course is important, in so far as it shows on the one side improvement with abstinence, on the other side progressive dementia, even though there be fluctuations; then, too, the delusions and confabulations only rarely become senseless. Against paresis is the negative spinal-Wassermann. It becomes impossible to keep apart the influence of the different causes, when arteriosclerosis or old age contribute to cerebral changes. As against the Korsakoff-like complex in head trauma, it is to be noted that usually the latter begins in an acute form and improves quickly or heals, whereas the trauma may also be the result of the incipient Korsakoff. An exact anamnesis is therefore of special importance.

Treatment. A lasting deprivation of the responsible poison is naturally necessary and this can almost only be achieved in a hospital. Moreover, the excitement at the beginning, and then especially the disturbance of orientation and memory, which make the patient incapable of taking care of himself properly, usually necessitate treatment in a custodial institution. After partial improvement some cases can be cared for in public almshouses, but the tendency to alcoholic indulgence remains which readily causes new shifts.

Alcoholic Pseudoparesis.

As alcoholic pseudoparesis we designate a Korsakoff which as a result of special localization imitates the physical signs of paresis, especially the pupilary and speech disturbances. The differential diagnosis from paresis enters into consideration especially when the patients are brought to the hospital because of delirium tremens and the organic symptom complex remains after the delirium has passed away. In most cases, probably always, the flourishing ideas of grandeur are lacking in pseudoparesis. Real manic states probably do not belong to it; the continued progress of the disease in the institution speaks for paresis; however, in the beginning of the disturbance only the spinal Wassermann can definitely decide the differential diagnosis. Alcoholic paresis may improve and in some cases the recovery may be complete.

Kraepelin designates as *"alcoholic paresis"* the simple combination of paresis with alcoholic symptoms, especially the hallucinations of delirium tremens. Others use the expression in the sense of alcoholic pseudoparesis.

Probably because the concept of paresis has become clearer we have not seen for ten years any disease that we could designate as alcoholic pseudoparesis.

Polioencephalitis Superior.

The encephalitic changes, even in the ordinary Korsakoff, show a certain preference for localizing themselves around the third and fourth ventricles, from the caudate body to the anterior part of the red nucleus, especially in the nuclei of the eye muscle nerves. In some cases a hemorrhagic encephalitis of this region constitutes the sole or, at least, the chief disturbance. The corresponding morbid picture belongs rather to the pathology of the brain than to psychiatry. Nevertheless these cases not seldom get into insane asylums because in the beginning they are confused and at times somnolent and comatose. Paralysis of the external, and occasionally of the internal eye muscles is especially noticeable, and at the end of the first week or in the second the patients usually succumb to general paralysis. Some cases remain alive and may then recover or go over into a symptom picture similar to Korsakoff. It is difficult to designate it from *encephalitis lethargica.*

Alcoholic Leukencephalitis of the Corpus Callosum

Marchiafava and his pupils have described an alcoholic disease in which the fibres of the inner two thirds of the corpus callosum in their entire extent disintegrate after a while. Other brain localities also, especially the anterior commissure, may also be slightly affected. In Korsakoff, similar processes are said to have been found occasionally, so that here too, perhaps, there may be nothing new.

But the affliction is rather chronic and results in death in from two to six years; first a gradual organic dementia appears, often combined with epileptiform attacks; later there is also confusion; death results in coma and marasmus.

Chronic Delusions of Jealousy in Alcoholics and Alcoholic Paranoia

Alcoholic delusions of jealousy usually fluctuate with the quantity of the imbibed liquor and ordinarily disappear quickly with enforced abstinence in the institution. In very rare cases it appears to survive the misuse of alcohol and even to become incurable.

Additional delusions and hallucinations, especially of hearing, may also attach themselves to it so that a complete "alcoholic paranoia" is present. This, nevertheless, cannot be differentiated from the paranoid forms in which the specific schizoid symptoms are not very pronounced. At all events, this outcome requires a special predisposition, and what is more, it must be one that even previously expressed itself in distrust, stubbornness, or characteristics evidently of a schizophrenic variety. By far most of the cases diagnosed elsewhere as alcoholic paranoiacs I had to consider with certainty as schizophrenics, who also were alcoholics, and whose hallucinations and delusions had in part an alcoholic coloring. As a matter of fact they were really sick before drinking made itself felt. Nor is it conceivable that the alcoholically conditioned insanity could take root and that especially the alcoholic delusions of reference could persist independent of excessive indulgence; but the material at present available makes the assumption of an actual alcoholic paranoia unnecessary. At all events it would be relatively independent of the quantity of drink consumed.

Dipsomania

There are psychopaths with decidedly differing tendencies who from time to time become moody. If they endeavor to help themselves out with alcohol, the symptoms in time become more intense and frequent, and at the same time so closely associated with the alcohol idea that at those times the patients succumb to an absolutely irresistible impulse to drink. These moods are difficult to describe and are not at all the same in different patients. A certain world sorrow, a sort of anxiety, and irritability toward everything that comes along are rarely lacking, but do not constitute the essential element; an indescribable feeling of dreadful discomfort, a condition "that cannot be endured," overpowers the patient. Thinking becomes circumscribed, perhaps also a little unclear; whether merely because of the affect or independent of it as a concomitant manifestation, I do not know. To counteract this condition large quantities of alcohol in the most different forms, preferably concentrated, are consumed, occasionally also other things, such as ether and even petroleum. But as a matter of fact the condition is improved little or not at all by indulgence in alcohol. Some have the drink brought home to their rooms most of them go to the saloon; those whose sense of shame is still retained go to one that is distant or secluded, where they do not meet friends; others go from one saloon to another. Most of them, while drinking, are shy; a few bluster or quarrel. Real inebriation does not occur. After about from two to eight days the attacks pass over; the patients find themselves, usually after a sleep, anywhere at all, either in a saloon, or in the gutter, or in the police station. Whatever they carried with them has usually been converted into alcohol; sometimes they have only the most necessary clothing left. Recollection is usually imperfect; the head is confused as after an ordinary severe drink. They are now ashamed of the past, make the best resolutions but without success.

In the intervals, that may last several weeks but also many months, most of these patients are temperate, and some are abstinent. But there are also chronic alcoholics who at the same time are dipsomaniacs or who, as it seems, have become dipsomaniacs through alcohol. The better class among them can retain their positions or obtain new ones when necessary.

The *disposition* for dipsomania we do not understand as yet; it is probably not uniform. The majority of the patients are psychopaths who cannot as yet be classified. Others are epileptics or at least in their entire psychical make-up epileptoid; there are also schizophrenics among them. Furthermore depressions of brief duration may provoke similar symptoms in cases that we must number with maniac depressive insanity. Brain trauma, also, may obviously constitute the foundation of the moods; in one of these cases we observed that the symptoms were connected with poriomanic tendencies.

As *exciting causes* of the individual case, anger, and at times over-work are mentioned; whether rightly so, I cannot decide. At all events the disturbance usually comes entirely from within.

Age. The first moods are often noticed soon after puberty; most of the patients come for treatment in early or late manhood.

The *differential diagnosis* is as a rule easy. The patients ordinarily describe the compulsion very clearly, and the difference in conduct in the good and bad periods is uncommonly striking. Nevertheless very many alcoholics are sent to us as dipsomaniacs, which they are not; they are people who commit excesses only on certain occasions, perhaps on pay day, and who can otherwise control themselves, or they are unrestrained and wavering natures who simply at times go wild and at times take hold of themselves.

Without treatment the affliction grows worse as time goes along. But our intervention also is not any too successful. In cases that seem epileptic bromide is only exceptionally effective, at times, perhaps in depressions of another kind the results are better. The best results are obtained when the entire manner of living is regulated as far as possible and the patient is permitted to undergo a large number of attacks *without* alcohol, under the protection of a closed institution. The depressions then gradually become weaker and less frequent. But since it takes years to accomplish this, one usually loses patience before a cure is attained and after the first new excess one has to start again at the beginning. One, therefore, often tries to keep the patients outside the institution during the intervals, with the intention of watching or interning them as soon as the attack is impending. But even this does not get one very far, because at the given time the patient has insufficient insight and, above all, no will power. And the relatives also no longer summons sufficient energy for immediate action when the last bad attack has been somewhat forgotten.

Alcoholic Epilepsy

In particularly predisposed persons acute alcoholism excites epileptiform attacks; in cases of chronic alcoholism we frequently see some typical attacks, especially when any accessory brain disturbance, such as delirium tremens, Korsakoff, Leukencephalitis supervene. Here the attacks are probably nothing but symptoms of the alcoholism. But occasionally one finds alcoholic epilepsy appearing in their mature years, which in other respects runs a course about the same as the ordinary genuine epilepsy and usually develops very slowly into dementia of an epileptic character.[53]

It is probable that the ordinary attacks in alcoholics, which are especially brought along by delirium tremens, do not come from true epilepsy, but from other poisons which are of the same nature, as, e.g., that of delirium tremens. For the other cases one must presuppose a particular disposition to epilepsy and often the presence of the two diseases may be accidental, or the epileptic character may have produced the disposition to alcoholism. Among those stricken with epilepsy in later years, say after thirty-five, men are in a large majority and as a rule they are alcoholics; furthermore cases which otherwise closely resemble the former still seem to be cured in the beginning by abstinence. One is therefore probably compelled to recognize in alcoholism the essential casual force of such diseases, that is, to presuppose an alcoholic epilepsy in the actual sense.

The *treatment* is the same as that for ordinary epilepsy,—abstinence, eventually also bromides; in those cases which I could observe for some time, which to be sure were not numerous, the latter remedy accomplished nothing.

Alcoholic Melancholia

Not very rarely alcoholics suffer from depressive conditions which cannot be distinguished symptomatologically from a melancholia of manic depressive insanity, even though the delusions usually remain merely rudimentary. But they do not last so long, only about two weeks. Perhaps still briefer attacks are not so rare but they naturally hardly come to the notice of the physician.[54] Some of the suicides of alcoholics may be attributed to this depression. The attacks may recur several times in the same patient. The alcoholic character is established by the fact that with abstinence, even with temperance, they do not develop.

B. Morphinism

The chronic use of morphine usually leads to a number of disagreeable manifestations. Productive ability in all lines is reduced, it

---

[53] If others assert, that the "alcoholic epilepsy" does not present the psychic signs of genuine epilepsy in its course, they probably have a broader concept of the disease than is indicated here.

[54] Prolonged "drunkard's misery," and severer "moral remorse of the morning after," cannot be distinctly separated from alcoholic melancholia.

becomes especially unequal; with increasing fatigue endurance can be artificially forced only by incessant doses of the alkaloid. Memory becomes inexact. Even in organically well disposed characters there appears an astounding tendency to prevaricate which is not at all limited to obtaining morphine and to whatever else is connected with the craving. The morphinist who comes to an institution swears by everything dear to him that he has no morphine with him. But one usually finds very considerable quantities of it divided in the clothing, in the soles of the shoes, in any of the accessible body cavities, or in any utensil. With every powder or flask that one finds, the protestations are repeated: that is positively the last one. And they lie to themselves just as well, because they submit to the treatment to be cured, but they at once make every arrangement in advance so that they can be cured only against their own exertions. The character also changes for the worse in other respects. The sense of duty is dulled or at least yields to even slight difficulties; the patients become careless and weak willed in other respects also. The *affectivity* is fluctuating but rather from within than from without as a reaction to certain concepts. The mood is very varying on the whole, corresponding to the distance in time from the last injection. Anxiety feelings may occur also. In severe cases delirious conditions are said to occur, somewhat similar to delirium tremens. But it is probably a case of mixed effects from other poisons, especially alcohol or cocaine.

The *physical symptoms* consist of tremors, in severe cases also of slight disturbances of coordination which are general, affecting the organs of speech, and even the eye muscles. Parasthenias of all sorts appear, pains or indescribable sensations, buzzing in the ears, and sensations of heat and cold. The pulse becomes irregular in the various conditions; beating of the heart is frequent; digestion is irregular; diarrhœa may alternate with constipation. In severe cases a definite marasmus develops in the course of years; the skin becomes grayish and sallow. *Sleep* is poor in spite of frequent tiredness during the day. *Libido* and *potency* decline, under certain conditions to zero; *menstruation* ceases.

All subjective complaints except in very severe cases are banished at once by a new dose of morphine. Slowly or quickly, according to the constitution, the body always finds weapons to destroy the poison, increased doses of which are consequently necessary. With this the complaints increase and the possibility of obtaining a sufficient amount of the alkaloid and injecting it in sufficient quantities becomes less. The increase of the dose, therefore, has practical limits which most frequently, perhaps, fluctuate around one gramme a day, and very rarely exceeds a few grammes, even though daily doses up to twenty grammes are said to have been observed.

But with the larger doses the patients are severely injured physically, socially, and especially in their productive ability. They make attempts to reduce the doses, but few succeed to any considerable extent. The *manifestations of abstinence* are too unbearable. They consist of pains in any place at all, often in the entire body, trembling, yawning, perspiring, nausea to the extent of vomiting, diarrhœa, palpitation and poor pulse to a degree endangering life, and then a feeling of anxiety and unrest which is perhaps the worst feeling of all. Deliria also are said to result from abstinence. Such a craving for morphine must be one of the most painful conditions possible. If no more morphine can be obtained, taking nourishment remains almost impossible, and there is loss of weight; only after several days does the recuperation follow.

We do not know positively on what the abstinence symptoms are based.

Causes. Most morphinists are psychopaths from the beginning. Even highly gifted and famous men have succumbed to the craving, and some of them retained their elevated station for a long time in spite of it. It is strange that one has to call attention to the fact that they, no more than the alcoholic geniuses, are famous *because* they have taken to the poison, but that men of genius are simply *different* from ordinary men; on the one hand they are geniuses, on the other they are inclined to various abnormalities which we may designate as weaknesses. The *accidental causes* that lead to the habit are usually pains which are treated with morphine; but then, too, there is a certain euphoric reaction brought about immediately by the first dose, that tempts to repetitions. Naturally the majority of the patients are medical people; the lower classes contribute only a small number because morphine is very expensive. In a large number of cases the doctors are at fault, who give useless injections of morphine and even place the syringe in the patient's hands. Physicians addicted to morphine are especially dangerous, because in the alkaloid craving as in alcoholism there is a desire for similarly disposed associates and for proselytizing. For example, we used to have women's clubs in which indulgence in morphine was the binding tie; whether they still exist I do not know.

As the morphinist usually either specifies another disease or does not go to a physician at all, one is rarely in a position to make the *diagnosis* from the symptoms. But one must always have morphinism in mind when one meets people who are very differently disposed, at times, appearing anxious, run down, weak and trembling, at other times,—especially after they have absented themselves for a few minutes,—being cheerful again. The sallow gray skin often indicates the disease. One finds the injection scars the more readily because many patients do not take the time for aseptic measures, even injecting through the clothing and thus inducing abscesses in large numbers. The morphine cannot always be detected in the urine. If one wants to examine former morphinists to ascertain whether they are cured or relapsed, nothing can be done except to institute a close surveillance.

The *prognosis* is discouraging; definite cures occur but constitute a small minority. To be sure, a number of these people maintain themselves externally in their positions; but few are still completely efficient, they oscillate between suffering and euphoria, and even when they can work it depends only on the morphine syringe. Many are ruined physically and socially. Their entire energy is consumed in obtaining morphine. When there are obstacles in the way of this, they are overcome with astonishing skill in which lying, theft, and fraud are not feared.

The *treatment* demands in the first place the deprivation of the morphine. The most rational way should be the sudden deprivation; but I cannot bring myself to cause any one such suffering; besides it involves some danger to life. If one takes a few weeks, in milder cases only one week, one prolongs the suffering but reduces it very considerably; this can be done if one takes the pains to control personally every request for morphine either during the day or during the night and when necessary, but then only, to administer himself the effective dose immediately.

If cocaine has been taken at the same time, it can nearly always be omitted at once with benefit. In the beginning of the treatment one seeks to ascertain whenever possible the patient's previous daily dose of morphine in order to reduce it at once to one third or a half. The patient will usually greatly exaggerate the size of the dose. It is to be recommended that the patient be informed from the very beginning that the size of the injected dose will never be told to him. Then one does not have to lie to him, one puts a stop to all grumbling and above all one avoids the anxious excitations and worriment as to whether the patient can get along with a certain quantity, questions which arise as soon as the patient sees that one does not let him suffer unnecessarily.—It is most earnestly necessary to warn against sanatoria with which one is not thoroughly acquainted.

If one wants to do anything for the abstinence manifestations, one should prescribe prolonged warm baths for the restlessness and sleep-lessness. Local cold applications may under certain circumstances reduce the heart action; vomiting and hyperacidity of the gastric juices are combatted with pieces of ice and alkaline water; milk with ice, later with concentrated nourishment, can sometimes still be fairly well digested; the diarrhœa should also be treated, e.g., with tannalbin injections. Hypnotics should be given only in extreme cases. But cocaine and similar drugs should never be substituted for the morphine which would only be adding the devil to Beelzebub.

One cannot expect much assistance from the patient. Even the bravest are dominated by the fear that one will let them suffer too much and therefore readily demand in every way possible more morphine than they themselves find necessary at the time. Attempts to obtain the alkaloid for themselves, especially by bribing the attend-ants, are very common. A hermetic and absolutely reliable super-vision is therefore necessary. Outside of a closed institution the deprivation cure can only be carried on in exceptional cases.

None of the chemical remedies that are supposed to mitigate the deprivation have proven of value; most of them are simply frauds.

After the dishabituation from morphine there remains the more important and difficult task, the training of character to overcome the disagreeable without the aid of a chemical crutch. To be sure it is rarely possible to remove altogether the firm disagreeable association, namely, morphine; it seems as if not only psychic but actually chemico-organic changes in the nervous system had built up mechanisms that compel the indulgence in morphine. Relapses are consequently very common. A certain hold is obtained by the promise, recom-mended by *Kraepelin,* to place oneself in confinement for a few days each year for careful observation. If possible, one should naturally try to regulate external conditions so that depressive influences are avoided. When physical diseases threaten, the patient should, if possible, be put to bed, in order to reduce the temptation to obtain morphine. It is self-evident that all other poisons, especially alcohol, are to be avoided.

In incurable cases it has been recommended that the indulgence be kept at a moderate amount which might be accomplished with patients who cooperate a little by having them take treatment each year in a sanatorium, in which the dose which has grown slowly in the interval is again reduced. But one must carefully consider whether one wants to enter on such a compact with evil, which really is calculated to make the physician, the patient, and those about him indifferent to a serious and infectious mania.

The *prophylactic measures* should be self-evident; one should never use morphine without a very exact indication and especially never for any length of time, and under no circumstances put the hypodermic needle in the patient's hands. It is also inadvisable to tell him that he is getting morphine when there is no necessity for doing so. Where there is danger one should write on the prescription, *"Ne Repetatur."* Furthermore no one should prescribe morphine for himself or give himself morphine even though he has it in his possession. At all events every physician addicted to morphine, as long as he is not cured, should be excluded from practicing.

Related to morphinism are *opium eating* and *opium smoking.* Neither is of any importance with us. The manifestations and treatment of opium eating do not differ essentially from those of morphinism. Concerning opium smoking we know little that is certain.

C. Cocainism

Several different types of cocainism can be distinguished which, however, cannot be sharply distinguished, and also do not exhaust entirely the manifoldness of the pictures. There is a *memory disturbance, similar to Korsakoff,* coming after a relatively brief misuse of from a few weeks to a few years, with excessive irritation, lack of will power, facile flight of ideas and a preoccupation with various tasks that leads to nothing. Under certain circumstances disturbances of coordination similar to those resulting from a state of alcoholic intoxication are also observed, there is a decline in strength, the skin becomes sallow and flabby, potency vanishes, and sleep becomes very disturbed. The picture can show a great similarity to paresis but one regularly misses the rigidity to light of the pupils. All symptoms, even the memory disturbance, disappear pretty quickly with abstinence.

In many cases there develops a *cocaine insanity,* characterized by extremely small hallucinations of sight and touch, in the form of mites and other parasites, which the patients sometimes want to demonstrate to us through a microscope under the impression that they have made a great discovery. One of our patients saw the cells of his retina functioning and drew scientific and therapeutic conclusions therefrom. Voices are rarer in these conditions and some delusions of persecution are sometimes present. But in other cases the latter are in the foreground, especially also in the form of uncontrollable delusions of jealousy (*Kraepelin*), in which the voices play a more important part. But in both conditions the patients are mentally clear and orientated; the persecuted patients may become dangerous.

The psychosis usually develops within a few weeks, the hallucinations disappear in from about one to two weeks after the deprivation of the poison; the delusions may last considerably longer.

As sudden as an explosion *cocaine snuffing* has spread as an epidemic of unsuspected danger; this is especially seen among the demimonde and artistic circles but also among university and college men. It is brought about usually by being led into it by others, more rarely by the snuff powders for coryza which contain cocaine and can be obtained without a prescription. This should be forbidden. Since the dose is usually raised up to several grammes a day, on the one hand large fortunes may be endangered and on the other hand, those that gather the large profits are induced to become eager tempters.

According to *Hans W. Maier* the manifestations after the first doses are usually slight dizziness and headache which, however, is quickly supplanted by a feeling of extraordinary well being. With this the patients feel mentally stimulated and more productive than usual, which they really are, but as there is a lack of endurance the practical results usually amount to very little. A slight flightiness of ideas may also be noticed. Many then lie for hours in vivid dreams without, however, losing altogether their critical attitude toward them. In others illusions and hallucinations, above all those of sight but also of hearing, quickly appear. Rapidly changing small objects predominate. A splitting of consciousness, similar to that in schizophrenia, permits the addict of the poison a certain insight into the morbidness of the perceptions but in the next moment they again believe in the reality of these morbid manifestations. A strong suggestibility brings it about that entire groups may enjoy themselves with hallucinations that the members have in common. At the height of the poisoning the phantasies are usually wish fulfilments. During abstinence the phantasies assume a threatening and fearful character which, with stomach troubles and creeping skin sensations, lead to new doses. Only after protracted use does the critical attitude disappear altogether, the associations become disconnected and develop into the above described cocaine insanity.

The libido sexualis disappears quickly in the man, while in women, on the contrary, it is heightened to a desire for all sorts of perversities. Physically the large, slowly reacting pupils are noticeable; nervous palpitation annoys the patients; dryness in the throat often compels them to drink excessively; the appetite disappears and finally there results marasmus with fatty degeneration of the liver: Heart collapse, paralysis of respiration, and suicide at times end this sad condition.

The *prospects of a cure* for cocaine taking are still darker than those for morphinism because relapses are even more common.

There are no serious *abstinence manifestations. Withdrawal of the cocaine* is therefore regularly to be brought about at once. But usually still other poisons, especially morphine, have been used in addition, which then necessitates an even longer protracted withdrawal treatment. But even in plain cases, the after treatment, the education, requires a long duration with close supervision (for over half a year).

VII. INFECTIOUS PSYCHOSES

In cases of infection the activity of the brain may be disturbed by an unlimited number of different influences, such as many kinds of toxins and antitoxins and a normal metabolic products induced by these, perhaps also weakness, fever, etc. Our observations cannot at all follow the manifoldness of the pictures that must result from these influences. We know only coarse differentiations which, however, corresponded so little to the differences of the causative factors, that the monograph on these conditions (*Bonhoeffer*) had for weighty reasons distinguished only syndromes. The author proceeds on the theory that we can distinguish different symptomatological steps while the individual infections can in no way be brought into connection with the clinical pictures. Thus he distinguishes deliria, epileptiform excitements (appearing and ceasing suddenly), twilight states, hallucinoses (hallucinatory states without noticeable disturbances of thinking and orientation), amentia pictures; the latter are at times more hallucinatory, at times catatonic, and at times of an incoherent character, then the Korsakoff type, and delirium acutum. For details I must refer to the original.[55] *The only thing to be emphasized as of practical importance is that in fever psychoses symptoms may occur which according to our present methods of investigation cannot be distinguished from the catatonic. A catatonic morbid picture may, therefore, under certain circumstances be a fever psychosis (Amentia in the sense of the term employed by Bonhoeffer).*

As of theoretic interest it may also be mentioned, that *Bonhoeffer* observed a recovery from infectious Korsakoff which came suddenly after a few weeks.

Kraepelin does not like to surrender entirely the conception of the connection of cause and effect. The following division follows his classifications.

[55] *Aschaffenburg.* Handbuch der Psychiatrie, Deuticke, Leipzig u. Wien, 1911, Spezieller Teil III. Abt. 1. Hälfte.

A. Fever Deliria

At the height of febrile diseases we see deliria break out, which unfortunately have been examined very little from a psychiatric point of view. Four grades are distinguished: 1. The *prodromal* state with discomfort, dullness of the head, sensitiveness, anxiety dreams, etc. 2. Illusions and hallucinations, especially of sight and also of hearing, in which the patients, either spontaneously or by being spoken to, become capable for a time of orientating themselves and in a general way of becoming relatively clear. The hallucinations are often transferred into the real environment, thus the mother may see her little children at her bed. The patients become restless and are usually cheerful or moodily depressed. 3. In the third grade the entire environment is mistaken. There is complete confusion with lively emotional outbursts and marked pressure activity. 4. Manifestations of paralysis gradually appear. The strength to move and express feeling declines; the patients remain lying on their backs, mumble to themselves, pull at the bed clothes, and pick things until they die, often in a complete coma.

Individual epileptic attacks are rarely seen.

The content of the deliria is as a rule dreamlike. Usually it is a case of complex deliria which intimately concern the patient's ego. In pneumonia and perhaps also in other diseases the transition to anxious conceptions indicates the incipient cardiac insufficiency. In alcoholics the delirium is alcoholically tinged, animal visions are especially frequent, etc.

The fever deliria, like most infectious deliria, are usually more pronounced at night than in the day.

Prospects. Children become delirious relatively easily, so that the psychic disturbances are not of particularly great significance in them. Women, also, are said to become delirious sooner than temperate men. But in adults the completely developed deliria indicates as a rule the special severity of the infection and with it the danger to life. However, the first stage is of little significance and many patients recover even from the third, since, parallel usually with the decline of the fever, they become clearer and lose the hallucinations. But sometimes the delusions outlast the disease a long time; I know a colleague who long after an attack of typhus requested a friend on the street to return the money which, since the fever delirium, he believed he had lent him. The duration of the delirium depends on the disease; as it is usually a case of acute infections and the psychosis, as a rule, only appears at the crisis of the disease, it usually ends as early as the second week either by recovery or death.

The *treatment* is naturally that of the fundamental disease. Sometimes ice on the head seems to have a quieting effect, as do small doses of opiates. Due to the fundamental disease hypnotics should be given with care. In many cases cool baths which should naturally be of short duration are effective. To be sure, supervision is necessary; the patients may come to grief or do harm.

B. INFECTIOUS DELIRIA

Besides the deliria that come and go with the severity of the fever there are others that seem to be independent of the fever itself since they appear before or after it, or do not run parallel with the fever in their fluctuations.

Mostly in typhus but also in other diseases we observe the *initial deliria* which *Aschaffenburg* has divided into two groups: a paranoid with delusions of reference and persecution, hallucinations, and depression that is usually anxious or sad; and a second form that quickly rises to a complete delirious confusion with flight of ideas, sense deceptions and vague delusions, more frequently anxiety, and above all senseless pressure movements. The two forms are not sharply differentiated; the first may go over into the second. They usually last only a few days and may disappear or become ordinary fever deliria. I have seen a paranoid form in typhus persist far into the period of convalescence.

The *differential diagnosis* is not easy; but such initial deliria do not quite fit into any other symptom picture. In the excited form one might think of catatonia or epilepsy; the existence of flight of ideas guards against the second diagnosis; the absence of schizophrenic symptoms makes the former improbable.

Like *Kraepelin* I saw several *influenza deliria* of a typical neuritic character, in which parasthenias were interpreted illusionally. At all events, in grippe psychoses it is mostly a question of a schizophrenic sort of dissociation of the mental stream, which appears all the more similar to the schizophrenic because irritations of the nervous system readily give occasion to a kind of physical hallucination; the affectivity invariably, however, continues to fluctuate. Optical illusions sometimes make one think of delirium tremens. States of febrile deliria readily become mixed, as many patients lose orientation when they are left to themselves, especially at night. The content of the deliria and delusions is regularly taken from emotionally toned complexes.—Fever deliria without a schizoid character, often with motor restlessness and a tendency to violence, also occur.

In my experience all *grippe psychoses* which do not look from the very beginning like schizophrenia are curable (that is to say if the schizophrenia does not just happen to appear at the same time as the infection).

The typical picture of the *Chorea Minor Psychosis* [56] seems to present a fairly uniform picture. In the beginning one notes sensitiveness, irritability, lability of the affects, and fatigue; vigility and tenacity of attention decline. The memory becomes poor or at least the patients appear very distracted. Thinking then becomes very laborious, and suddenly interrupted; sense deceptions and delusions supervene, and in severe cases it may go as far as complete confusion and disorientation. In spite of the severity of the disease, which permits the choreatic movement to become especially pronounced, most of these cases, as far as I know, are cured, the delirious state disappears first, and the chorea a long time after. Cases of *chorea gravis* show their character from the very beginning in the sudden rise of the disease and in the initial prostration of strength. Paralyses soon appear and death follows after two or more weeks. In cases not quite so severe it may sometimes result in a state of psychic deficiency.

The *treatment* for all cases of infectious deliria is that of the fundamental disease, with careful supervision, avoidance of excitement and occasions for doing harm to oneself. In *chorea gravidarum,* which is not to be taken lightly, abortion is indicated, at least when there is a physical breakdown, this is often followed by a cure in a few days. Some, however, recover without any interference.

The *delirium acutum* belongs to the infectious deliria of a different origin.[57]

A condition appearing with the febrile attack and developing a violent state and high grade confusion with dreamlike sense illusions, flight of ideas, change of mood, lively motor excitation, and disconnected delusions, is called *collapse delirium* by *Kraepelin.*

C. Acute Confusion, Amentia

In infectious diseases, puerperal fever, and especially in chronic nephritis which may not always show itself through examination of the urine, one finds states of confusion, which ordinarily last for weeks or months and as yet have no certain positive diagnostic sign. They are designated with the name of *Amentia* which formerly included all

---

[56] Naturally only the real chorea is referred to here which originates on the basis of a bacterial infection (Rheumatism). Unfortunately hysterical epidemics in schools manifesting themselves in abnormal movements and similar things are also still called chorea. The medieval Chorea St. Viti, or chorea magna, was also psychogenetic.

[57] See p. 163.

possible kinds of confusion, especially also many belonging to schizophrenia. They may disappear, but as a result of the basic disease, they may also lead to death. The diagnosis can only be made by exclusion. The conception of confusion or of incoherence are altogether too equivocal to be used in differentiation, especially from schizophrenia. Where *Kraepelin's* conception is combined with the name of dementia praecox, the disease is very rare. Besides infection and autointoxication, *exhaustion* was formerly considered as one of the factors.

Biswanger classifies the "exhaustive psychosis" as follows: 1. *Exhaustion stupor* in mild grades, and *acute curable dementia* in severe grades.   2. *Exhaustive amentia*.   3. *Delirium acutum exhaustivum*. These forms, too, cannot be characterized sufficiently. The names give an idea of the external picture.

D. INFECTIOUS STATES OF WEAKNESS

After infectious diseases some patients recover very slowly. For weeks or months they remain morose, easily exhausted, have difficulties in thinking, and do not like to exert themselves either mentally or physically. They are, however, mentally clear and externally adjusted ("acute dementia"). In most cases recovery still takes place, but now and then the condition is serious. Hallucinations, delusions, and rather severe anxious or depressive moods supervene and the patients remain permanently demented.

The anatomy of these psychoses is insufficiently known. But there are cases, e.g. after typhus, smallpox and scarlet fever, with circumscribed brain lesions, which have also often manifested focal symptoms. Sometimes diffuse disturbances are present, especially after influenza and sepsis, and at times, also, after typhus. It is then a case of infectious Korsakoff, usually with polyneuritis, which is distinguished from the alcoholic form by less vividness of the psyche—stuporous confusion is not rare—and if life is preserved, is said to disappear more frequently than in those of alcoholic origin.

VIII. THYREOGENIC PSYCHOSES

PSYCHOSES IN BASEDOW'S DISEASE

Basedow's disease is not rarely accompanied by psychoses which, however, have no uniform picture. Hysterias often accompany the basic disease and the frequently present syndromes, similar to neurasthenia, may become so severe that the paralysis of energy takes on the character of a psychosis. Besides, one also observes depressions with anxiety states and milder forms of mania. Most frequent, however, one finds pronounced chronic states similar to catatonia with marked excitements, dissociation of thoughts, confused and sometimes symbolized delusions, hallucinations of hearing and sight, eventually of smell and taste, and perhaps even of physical sensations. Neither in the descriptions nor in the few cases that I have seen myself can I distinguish them absolutely from catatonic states, as the difference consists only in the absence of a pronounced schizophrenic coloring. The affectivity remains livelier, the stream of thought is not so disconnected, catatonic symptoms are rare or not so pronounced, etc. All of this may also occur in patients who have no Basedow and who after a year or more become demented in the typical schizophrenic manner.

The hysterical and neurasthenic syndromes improve usually with the Basedow. The depressive and manic forms may also disappear regardless of the Basedow, and rarely accompany the entire disease, although moods of some sort naturally are hardly ever lacking. The catatonic variety does seem capable of improvement, but it may not fluctuate at all and readily becomes incurable.

The causal treatment depends on the Basedow condition, whereas the symptomatic treatment is that of the special psychic syndrome.

Myxœdema

(Cachexia Strumipriva)

When the thyroid is completely removed, or severely damaged anatomically or functionally by a disease, a very definite physical and psychic symptom complex results. The subcutaneous cell structures proliferate and degenerate in a specific form. Thus the skin then becomes generally thick and puffed, but especially in the face and on the back of the hands and feet; even the nose and tongue become bigger. This gives the face a plump expression. Pressure of the finger leaves no fingerprint as is the case in simple œdema. The skin takes on a muddy pallor, it becomes dry, and scales easily; the hair on the head, but especially on the body, falls out; the teeth also become brittle or fall out; the extremities become cold; the body temperature sinks below normal, and the pulse becomes slow and weak.

Also movements become slow; the same is also true of the facial mimetic expression which makes the patient look still more stupid. The finer movements under certain circumstances are also disturbed in their coordinations, as, for example, writing. The voice becomes grating. Muscular strength is diminished, sensibility is dulled; sometimes actual hardness of hearing occurs. Paresthesias very often supervene, especially headache, and later a feeling as if the limbs have gone to sleep.

The essential psychic symptom is the retardation of all processes of thinking, of decision, and then especially the translation of the latter into movement; even very simple functions may require many times the normal time, thus putting the hands on the neck may require 45 seconds. Memory for recent events becomes bad. The patients notice their deficiency and are consequently depressed in their moods; occasionally real depressions occur but the other affects are clearly retained. Sometimes one also notices dissatisfaction and distrust which may rise to the extent of delusions. In severe cases illusions and hallucinations of hearing, sight, smell and taste also occur, under certain circumstances even compulsive states. The severest cases finally develop into hallucinatory confusions; at the same time the physical strength declines and the patients die, often in convulsion.

Treatment. Continued administration of thyroid extract, best in the form of ready made tablets, may cause a total disappearance of the symptoms. It is given first in doses of 0.1 to 0.3 g. of the gland per day, but the physical strength and the heart have to be watched very carefully. If necessary, the dose may be increased. If the disease disappears, the effective minimum dose should be ascertained.

ENDEMIC AND SPORADIC CRETINISM

If the thyroid gland is already absent in childhood or if it functionates insufficiently, a specific kind of idiocy develops. Such children remain torpid, psychically as well as physically; they are slow and awkward in thought and movement. Initiative is reduced, and in high grade cases it is almost entirely lacking. Nevertheless the patients have feelings, and remain good natured, even though at times they are stubborn. A certain timidity can be demonstrated in most of them and this accounts for one of the reasons why such children are slow in learning to walk; but talking also is hindered. As far as our present knowledge goes the intelligence is not as characteristic as in the other forms of oligophrenia of which this disease forms a causal subdivision. Further details will therefore be found in Chapter XIV. The patients have too few associations, not ·sufficient over-sight; during their whole life they give the impression of a non-intelligent child. Because of their awkwardness and their lack of initiative they can only perform easier kinds of work. The memory remains good as far as the patients have a conception of the happenings about them.

They love and fear and hate on the basis of their experience, they take a lively interest in their environment, and are grateful if one occupies oneself with them. Thus one can get a very good affective relationship with them. The sex impulse in the higher grades is weak or zero. Some cases may show suspicion, delusions and hallucinations, but such accessory psychoses which usually have a chronic character are not at all frequent.

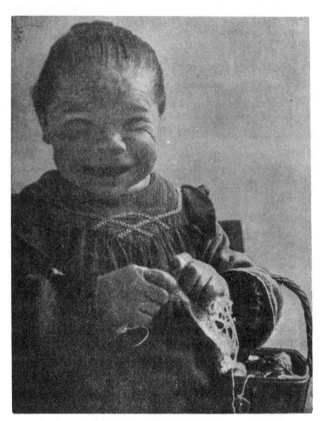

Fig. 18.—A Cretin. Age 30 years. Height 112 cm.

On the *physical side* their small stature is most noticeable. Some remain less than a yard high. The rump and the extremities contribute about equally to this anomaly although the extremities sometimes appear especially short. The skull and facial formation is characteristic. The base of the skull remains short, the root of the nose is deep and broad; the nose is very short; sometimes the length is less than the breadth. The ethmoid bone is strikingly broad on account of which the distance between the two eyes becomes large. The upper jaw often remains relatively short. During youth the skin has all the signs of myxœdema [58] that sometimes disappear in the third or fourth decade; the skin then becomes wrinkled. But even

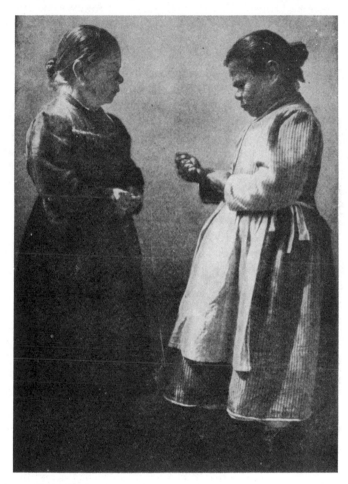

Fig. 19.—Two Cretins in profile. Height 118 (left) and 120 cm. (right). 50 and 49 years.

earlier marked horizontal wrinkles in the forehead are rarely lacking. The genitals as well as the secondary sexual signs develop late anatomically and functionally, or remain at a childish stage. Menstruation may not appear. In men the beard remains thin or is usually entirely

[58] Cf. previous chapter.

absent; the voice is rough and rasping. In many cases there is hardness of hearing or deafness, in part as a result of middle ear trouble, in part also as a result of some trouble in the labyrinth. In endemic cretinism the athyroid signs are on the average less pronounced; dwarfishness is especially less extreme. The hypophysis is in many cases enlarged, but not always. Usually there is a more or less enlarged goitre; in rarer cases the thyroid is reduced; it may even be entirely absent. The latter is the usual thing in "sporadic cretinism."

According to the degree and relative conditions of individual cases different forms may be distinguished. Extreme cases are those cretins

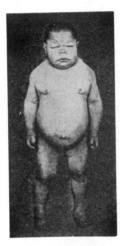

FIG. 20.—Extremely myxœdematous cretin woman, 44 years old. Height 99 cm.

which are purely physical, purely psychical, purely deaf and dumb, and those in which all three symptom groups are developed to the same marked extent. The merely deaf and dumb are usually not classed with the cretins although according to all we know they belong to it; however, it is impossible in individual cases to separate them from other congenital forms of deafness. According to the grade one speaks of a *full cretin, half cretin,* and *cretinoid* or *cretinous types.*

Course. Some of these patients are born cretins; but in most cases the disease is recognizable only in the course of the first or second year, reaching its climax in a few years and then becoming stationary. The patients remain children mentally, and the physical indications for estimating age are lost to a great extent. The greatest change is the disappearance of the Myxœdema in the milder cases. They offer very little resistance to other diseases and rarely attain old age. Sometimes brain atrophy with the symptoms of senile dementia appear very early; I could diagnose them in patients in the forties.

Pathology. There is no doubt that a part of the symptoms of cretinism, especially the physical symptoms, are the result of the hypofunctioning or a-functioning of the thyroid. Myxœdema is identical with the same manifestations in athyroidism. Endemic cretinism occurs only in goitre regions. Thyroid medication may cause an improvement in all manifestations. On the other hand, it is striking that the psychic symptoms do not at all run parallel with the physical symptoms. There are physical cretins, even of real high grade, who are psychically still well developed. In *goitre regions* we meet imbeciles who exhibit the psychical character of cretinism but who are physically regularly developed. Hardness of hearing and deafness, which in endemic cretinism afflict at least half of the patients, are absent in other forms of athyroidism, but are common in goitre regions, among the non-cretinous inhabitants. Hence, between goitre, psychical cretinism, and hardness of hearing, there is an etiological connecting link, or besides the goitre an additional cause may be assumed, or both manifestations have a parallel origin in a common cause. *Wagner von Jauregg* assumes that not only a quantitive, but a qualitative disturbance of thyroid function also plays a part.

The retardation of bony growth is connected with the very late ossification of the diaphysis cartilage (until within the fourth decade) and the long period of open fontanelles.

The *causes* of endemic cretinism like those of goitre are not yet known to us. It probably has some connection with the drinking water, of what kind we do not know. Other factors also are probably involved. A general improvement of the social and hygienic conditions without other changes invariably produces a decrease of cretinism. In most recent times many believe that there is an infection from one person to another or a transmission through infected material that clings to the house or to a dirty bed.

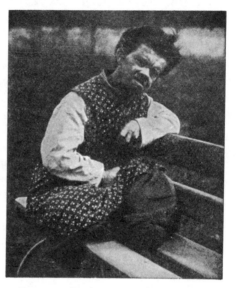

Fig. 21.—Cretin woman in a state of excitation, mostly irritation. Hence the contemptuous challenging facial expression (very rare for a cretin woman). She could only grunt but for several decades she fooled nearly all new doctors in the institution with simulated diseases (scratch wounds among others), need of care and by attracting attention to her own personality.

Sporadic cretinism probably has various but not exactly known causes. In most cases the athyroidism is congenital; but the thyroid gland may also be injured subsequently, e.g. by infectious diseases. It may occur everywhere, but it is evidently particularly frequent in certain places, e.g., in England. In cretinous neighborhoods it can hardly be diagnosed.

The *differential diagnosis* is very easy in pronounced cases; whoever has seen a cretin can always recognize the type. Formerly the term had a broader and less distinct application, and other forms of idiocy with physical malformations were also included. The *Mongolian types* that also have a broad nasal base can be mistaken in youth for light cases of cretinism; but their adipose layer has a different character from that of myxœdema. Later, as contrasted with the cretins, they become very active. In *Nanosomia,* or *Nanism* the entire body remains small without any great change in the proportions and as such is not accompanied by idiocy; in *Micromelia* ·the retardation in growth almost only affects the extremities; *fœtal rachitis* causes entirely different deformities and, like all the above mentioned forms, lacks the myxœdematous degeneration of the subcutaneous cellular structure.

In infantile cretins the *treatment* may still achieve very much. Thyroid in doses of about 0.5 g. daily or every other day is given, in larger children naturally a correspondingly larger dose. With this medication the patients may develop entirely normally; the mental condition, to be sure, often remains impaired even though it improves; in older cretins an increase of activity but not of intelligence may be attained. Growth may set in even at the end of the twenties. It is interesting that in endemic cretinism a thyroid cure often has a lasting effect while in the sporadic where the gland is entirely missing the remedy must always be repeated.

Good *hygienic* treatment is also important in all cases.

IX. SCHIZOPHRENIAS (DEMENTIA PRAECOX)

After paresis was excluded from among the "functional psychoses" and the other organic forms followed of themselves, for seventy years theoretical psychiatry stood entirely helpless before the chaos of the most frequent mental diseases. *Kraepelin,* following *Kahlbaum's* ideas, was the first to find symptomological differences between the acute forms that passed over into "secondary dementia" or "secondary paranoia" (dementia præcox), and the mild forms (manic-depressive insanity), and these differences were to the effect that in the severe forms symptom groups occurred that were lacking in the others but not the reverse. But a number of diseases taking a chronic course from the beginning, which were formerly regarded as something entirely different, proved to be identical with the acute psychoses which terminated unfavorably. Moreover, a large part of the acute syndromes which did not run into dementia, which in the beginning were exactly like the malignant forms and in the after stages showed, on exact inspection, more or less pronounced anomalies which only differed quantitatively from the severe secondary forms, were also identical with the same psychoses. All these pictures showed more or less numerous examples of these symptoms, very differently grouped in the individual cases. But whereas, a manic depressive attack turns out favorably, one might say always, the prognosis of an attack of dementia præcox is really not always bad, since in very many cases after the exhaustion of a shift only slight changes of the psyche call attention to the disease. But these peculiarities have the identical character in severe and mild cases, i.e. the course of the prognosis of the entire group is the same, while the degree of dementia to be expected or the extent of the prognosis is not determined by the mere recognition of the disease. As the disease needs not progress as far as dementia and does not always appear *praecociter*, i.e. during puberty or soon after, I prefer the name *schizophrenia*.

This disease may come to a standstill at every stage and many of its symptoms may clear up very much or altogether; but if it progresses, it leads to a dementia of a definite character.

Even though we cannot as yet formulate a natural division within the disease, nevertheless schizophrenia does not appear to us as a disease in the narrower sense but as a disease group, about analogous with the group of the organic dementias, which are divided into paresis, senile forms, etc. One should, therefore, really speak of schizophrenias in the plural. The disease at times runs a chronic course, at times in shifts; it may become stationary at any stage or may regress a certain distance, but probably does not permit of a complete *restitutio ad integrum*. It is characterized by a specific kind of alteration of thinking and feeling, and of the relations with the outer world that occur nowhere else. Moreover, accessory symptoms, with a specific coloring in part, are something very common.

A. THE SIMPLE FUNCTIONS

Among the *basic symptoms* the disturbances of association [59] are especially important. The normal associative connections suffer in strength; any other kinds take their place. Thus links of association following one another in sequence may lack all relation to one another so that thinking becomes disconnected. The following associations are typical:

"I found the money.// "Doctor, doctor, doctor.// Please give me some ice water.// "No, I was never here, no, no. The bastard

[59] See pp. 77-78.

swiped my handkerchief.// Oh, oh, oh, Jack (attendant) you think you're smart.// "I've eleven of National Baking Powder. Hell, no! Take that thing away. Lucille, stop crying. Who the devil cares if he eats. What did you do with Jennie? My word, my word, the devil you did," etc.[60]

At the places designated with // in this example the chain of thought is entirely broken, perhaps at other places also. This makes the whole thing illogical and incomprehensible. The formal coherence is also torn asunder. Nothing was said to the patient to stimulate this production; it seemed as if he reacted to hallucination. This patient who had a good education used good English when his attention could be held; this entire production corresponds to the dislocation of the whole stream of thought.

Another example is the following: "Sea water, deep lake, foundation, Interlaken, Davos, Switzerland, I will get there too, I have a high inland lake, please, please, do we have high tide. Inland water very cold and quiet. High lake, deep lake, negligéant." [61]

The lack of connection frequently finds expression in the answers to questions: "Why don't you work? (at house-work)." "I do not know French." Here only the form of an answer to the question is preserved; the content lacks every connection with the latter.

Sometimes only some of the numerous threads that bind our thoughts are lacking. This may find expression in the changeableness and unclearness of the conceptions, even of the commonest; the father may speak of himself as the mother of his children. This idea forces itself, for example, into the place of the proper father idea because he is just speaking of the loving care of the children, which is more frequently associated with the mother than with the father; at the same time the difference between himself and the mother (his wife) no longer exists.

The ideas "land" and "globe"—or their connections—are treated in a peculiar way in the following illustration: A patient is given four small pieces of card board which can very easily be put together to make the figure of a church. He makes a senseless figure out of it and calls it a new land—a new "globe." [62]

In regard to the progressive stream of thought compare "Brutus was an Italian" (p. 77), where the relations with ancient times are supplanted by relations with recent times, or: "Have you any sorrow?"

[60] Given by Editor.
[61] *Pfersdorff*, die Gruppierung der sprachlichen Assoziationen. Mon. Schr. f. Psych. u. Neur. Bd. XXXI. 1912. S. 356.
[62] *K. Schneider*, Ueber einige Klinisch-psychologische Untersuchungsmethoden usw. Zeitschr. f. d. ges. Neur. u. Psych. O. 8. 1912. S. 586.

"No." "Are your thoughts heavy?" "Yes, Iron is heavy." "Heavy" is here suddenly used in a physical sense with a disregard for the actual connection. Thus the chain of thought and the entire mode of expression become somewhat *bizarre*. There is also a separation from the situation when a seamstress thinks she throws a kiss every time she wets the thread with her mouth.

The incompleteness of ideas facilitates the formation of *condensations* which are consequently unusually frequent in schizophrenia. Various lovers, various places of residence are no longer kept apart; sometimes one lover and one place are the representatives of the entire total conception, at other times others. But in this connection the expression "total conception" (Sammelbegriff) is used in another sense than the ordinary one. No collective ideas originate for the patient through such condensation; he thinks he has an individual idea and only the observer is conscious of the fact that in the idea are concealed different separate entities. Further examples of condensations are "Steam sail" from steam ship and sail boat, and "grucsor" from gruesome and sorrowful or the sentence: "God is the ship of the desert" where ideas from the Bible about God, the desert, and camel, with the figurative expression elsewhere obtained for the useful animal, are slung together into a senseless sentence.

Often one idea appears for another: *displacement of ideas.*[63]

A patient had left in disgust her position as "support" of the housewife; now she gets an uncontrollable antipathy toward everything that resembles a support or a cane. In these cases the displacement takes place in the affects; but it can also originate in any associative manner: two men are mistaken for each other because they have some resemblance: the superintendent of the insane asylum is substituted for the superintendent of the training school. A paranoid female "is a Billy-goat," i.e., she is united with her beloved minister: Minister = Christ = lamb = Billy goat.

A special form of displacement is the *symbol* which plays an important part in dementia præcox, not in its ordinary application but in such a way that it takes the place of the original idea without the patients noticing it: thus the patient sees fire or is burnt, that is, he hallucinates as realities these things that to the normal person are symbols of feelings and thoughts of love. He has "heard" that the superintendent "has stuck his tongue out at him." This is taken literally (to mean that the tongue was stuck out), although he only hallucinated that he was laughed at.

A catatonic woman hears the stork clapping in her body; that

[63] Comp. p. 118, the hornformed things.

means she is pregnant. A patient is the moon, the wife is the sun. The wife and the sun represent the thora and justice; the moon is the sword. The relation of the woman to Dr. B. *is* Psyche and Amor. The woman is the goddess of love; she can heal the sick.

Not only may there be an absence of secondary threads of the mental stream but also of the *central idea.* There is no visible purpose for writing "Blossom time of Horticulture." [64] Thus one frequently receives letters from patients that describe everything imaginable that is about them or happens to them; they even mention the trade-mark on their pen; but neither the reader nor the patient himself knows why such commonplace things are written down. Besides letter writing comprehensible and incomprehensible things are expressed orally and in writing without any purpose, and in the same way all sorts of unmotivated acts are performed. Through this change of objective and of the inner association, the train of thought sometimes resembles the *flight of ideas;* but the *absence* of an objective becomes noticeable through the lack of an emotional value while in flight of ideas the objective is merely *changed.*

As a result of the lack of an objective, the train of thought readily merges into *by-associations* so that at times mere alliterations become the deciding factors as in "boots—beauty." Naturally in this case some other idea besides the alliteration has influenced the train of thought but since the same patient, like others also, was accustomed to make similar associations the alliteration cannot be an accident.

Sometimes apparently senseless associations are explained by connecting links that do not come into the patient's consciousness but nevertheless may be guessed by the observer. Thus when a young woman answers "sweat shop paradise" to the stimulus word "tree," she refers to her unhappy love affair in a sweat shop, where she "sinned" for the first time—tree of knowledge—paradise, the complexes of her disease. Such *mediate associations* become evident much more in the association experiment than in ordinary thinking.

Through all these disturbances thinking becomes illogical, unclear, and, when many such mistakes follow one another in a series, thought becomes *dilapidated and incoherent.* This dilapidation is still more increased by a peculiar kind of *distractability.* In conversation the patients sometimes appear difficult or impossible to divert because they enter very little into what one tells them; in spite of all injected questions they continue their train of thought, but, on the other hand, they are brought to a topic, totally irrelevant to the subject in hand,

[64] See p. 78.

by any accidental things that happen to affect their senses, such as the ink-well, or a noise. The normal directives through questions from without and purposive conceptions from within are incapable of holding the train of thought in the proper channels. If the patients are governed by an affect, if they begin to scold, distractability is often entirely lacking.

Conspicuous also is a morbid tendency to *generalizations*, the transference of a thought, or of a function generally to other spheres. Delusions that could only originate concerning a particular individual are transferred to others with whom they have no inner connection at all. The patient has been irritated and strikes the guilty person but he does the same to others who happen to be near. A stereotype action is not only provoked by definite circumstances in which it has a comprehensible significance, but later it is also performed without a recognizable occasion and finally it is repeated continually for years. An obstruction that originated as the result of the influence of a definite complex also spreads to other subjects, frequently to the entire psyche and also outlasts the occasion any length of time.

Thus reasoning is naturally impaired to a great extent. *Logical operations* with incomplete or improperly limited concepts and ideas readily give the wrong results. Deviations from the ordinary train of thought given by experience also usually lead into wrong directions. When unrelated ideas are brought together in any connection, wrong results always follow; this is especially true in the every day senseless motivations in which any chance idea is supposed to offer the reason for a morbid act. The patient breaks windows, "because the physician is just coming"; he laughs "because the physician is just clearing out the dresser"; when confronted with the fact that he had already previously laughed, he says he did it because the things were still in it. All sorts of bad actions are motivated by the fact that the patients are held in an institution and it never does any good to tell them that the causal connection, if there is any at all, is just the reverse.

It is especially important, that in this weakness of associations as in every other, the *affects* obtain a greater domination over the train of thought. Wishes and fears control the trend instead of logical connection; thus the most senseless *delusions* are formed and the road is cleared for exaggerated *dereistic* thinking with its turning away from reality, its tendency to symbolism, displacements, and condensations.

Among the formal disturbances of the mental stream the *obstruc-*

tions (deprivation of thought) are the most striking [65] and when they occur too readily or too often or become too general and too persistent, they are positively pathognomonic of schizophrenia.

The feeling of *"thought pressure"* should then be mentioned, in which the patient has the feeling that he has to think, where against his will "it" thinks within him, and where thoughts are incessantly "made" for him; all of this is usually accompanied by an unpleasant feeling of strain.

In many cases there is a tendency to *perseveration*, the patients do not get away from one topic or from one or more words and thus, aside from a sensible adherence to the same idea, series like the following may occur: "Love, dove, name, dame, sane, love, dove, names, dame, same, love, dove, going back, going back, going back, going back, same. . . ." In such cases thinking is usually temporarily or permanently very impoverished. It is not yet known to what extent this disturbance of association is connected with the tendency to stereotyped expressions that show themselves in thinking as in acting.

In moody states one naturally finds *flight of ideas* or *inhibition*. But besides this in acute cases a non-depressive inhibition is not so rare, which obviously arises from a general aggravation of the central processes through some chemical or physical anomalies such as cerebral pressure or inflammation.

In such inhibitions, but even otherwise, we find rather frequently abnormal *brevity of the associations*. Such schizophrenics are always quickly finished with every train of thought without its being thought out in a normal way. This also accounts for *impoverished thinking*, but this is less in the sense of a limitation of the themes than in the sense of incompleteness of the individual ideas.

Affectivity. In the severer forms of schizophrenia the *"affective dementia"* is the most striking symptom. In the sanatoria there are patients sitting around who for decades show no affect no matter what happens to them or to those about them. They are indifferent to maltreatment; left to themselves they lie in wet and frozen beds, do not bother about hunger and thirst. They have to be taken care of in all respects. Toward their own delusions they are often strikingly indifferent.

In less severe cases we still see affective expressions, sometimes quite a number of them; but they are circumscribed. Especially often we find only *irritability* which is pathologically exaggerated. The negativistic patients are therefore impossible to maintain outside of the institutions because they quickly become enraged about everything

[65] See p. 79.

and yell and fight.   The mild and latent schizophrenics on the outside are simply considered sensitive and moody people who are hard
to get along with.

Sometimes—but not always—in otherwise totally indifferent women,
mother love is completely retained, and in more intimate association
with the average patient one still sees many affects, e.g., pleasure in
festivals and games at the institution, laughing at jokes, even joy in
artistic performances.   But the finer feelings, based on complicated
processes, are naturally more impaired than the elementary.   The
ethical sense does not seem to be especially affected although it
suffers from the general indifference and obtuseness.

In those cases also where we see livelier affects, the entire conduct
generally has the character of *indifference,* especially in important
matters; their most vital interests, their own future, as well as the
fate of the family leaves the patients entirely cold while cakes brought
at visits are often eaten with relish.   In the beginning of the disease
in very mild cases and in late forms the weakening of the affects is
not always visible; on the contrary in individual cases an *oversensitive-
ness* in various directions may be observed.   Then there are active
schizophrenics who with great zeal improve the universe or at least the
health of mankind, etc.   But on closer inspection one finds in all these
cases at least partial defects of affectivity, indifference in certain
important matters, temporary reduction of emotivity or contradictions in the interplay of the finer feelings.

Therefore one cannot sometimes speak of simple indifference,
because there exists a plain *fundamental mood* of euphoria or depression or fear.   Nevertheless the schizophrenic clogging usually makes
itself felt under these circumstances also since the mood shows no
modulation; entirely independent of the train of thought the patients
remain in the emotional state determined from within; nothing is
important to them, nothing is sacred to them.   The general attitude is
"I don't care," sometimes purely so, at times with a depressive or
especially with a euphoric coloring.

Moreover one of the surest signs of the disease is the *incapacity
to modulate the affects, or an affective rigidity.*   One can speak with
the patients about the most various subjects without noticing a change
of affect, which is especially noticeable in manic moods where one
usually finds very marked emotional fluctuations, while in the less
mobile depressive moods, the schizophrenic peculiarity is not so
conspicuous.

If affects are present, they often do not last.   In acute stages
it happens, that without any external reason, patients cry and whine

and rejoice and scold in immediate succession. It is a case of a chance association of ideas which are followed for a short time and are connected with affective expressions that correspond qualitatively but are exaggerated quantitatively, just as if an actor were to present all his emotional rôles one after another. Real inability in the sense that the affects might change very quickly with the mental trend, directed from within or without, does not belong to the picture of schizophrenia. A sudden outburst, e.g. of anger, may be frequently observed but then it is not very easy to divert the affect, even though one has the feeling that it is "skin deep."

If a change of affect occurs it often takes place more slowly than in normal people; the affects follow slowly after the ideas or they appear very capriciously. One does not quite know why they appeared just now and why they took this form.

Under no conditions has the affectivity disappeared altogether. By touching on the complexes one can very often provoke, even in apparently very indifferent cases, lively and adequate reactions, and in the dereistic ideas of apparently merely vegetating patients one finds fulfilments of active wishes and endeavors or even of fears; the analysis of schizophrenic delusions and logical mistakes shows that thinking is dominated more by the affects than it is in healthy people. The entire affectivity may also reappear when an organic brain disease (senile atrophy, apoplexy) complicates the schizophrenia. Hence it may be assumed that the morbid process as such does not attack the affects, but they are functionally only prevented from appearing, somewhat in the same manner as a child that is suddenly placed in a strange environment may merge into a stupor without an affect.[66]

The affects may also appear changed qualitatively in such a way that what should produce joy provokes sadness or anger, and the reverse—*parathymia*. But sometimes only the manifestations are inadequate; the patients experience joy from a present but complain at the same time—*paramimia*.[67]

Moreover the affective expressions are usually somewhat unnatural, exaggerated, or theatrical. Consequently the joy of a schizophrenic does not transport us, and his expressions of pain leave us cold. This becomes especially plain if one has occasion to observe the reaction of little children to such expressions. Just as little do the patients sometimes react to our affects. Thus one speaks of a *defect in the*

[66] Comp. Livingstone, Baelz, p. 127.
[67] Concerning the schizophrenic unmotivated laughter—see among the automatisms.

emotional rapport, which is an important sign of schizophrenia.   One feels emotionally more in touch with an idiot who does not utter a word than with a schizophrenic who can still converse well intellectually but who is inwardly unapproachable.

The affects themselves, like their expressions, have frequently lost their *unity.*   A patient who had murdered her child, which she lo̱ved as her own but hated as the child of her unloved husband, afterwards for several weeks was in a condition in which she wept in desperation

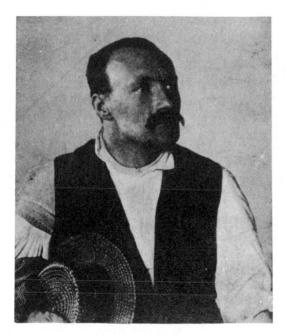

Fig. 22.—Hebephrenic who dictated "Epaminondas" (p. 78), the affected imagination of the facial expression which usually has nothing to express is significant.

with her eyes and laughed with her mouth.   Once I even saw such a splitting of the emotional expression shown on the two sides of the face.   Milder disturbances of the unity of the feelings are more frequent.

Affective disturbances in the form of acute manic, depressive, or anxiety moods, are not rare in dementia præcox.   But they belong to the accessory symptoms.

Parathymias are often indissolubly connected with the *alteration of the impulses.*   Coprophagia and the most various other aberrations from the normal nutritive instinct, previously unnoticable sexual perversions, lack of the impulse of self-preservation are very frequent manifestations.

Ambivalence. The synchronous laughing and crying are a partial manifestation of *schizophrenic ambivalence.* The schizophrenic defect of the associational paths makes it possible that contrasts that otherwise are mutually exclusive exist side by side in the psyche. Love and hatred toward the same person may be equally ardent without influencing one another (affective ambivalence).[68] The patients want at the same time to eat and not to eat; they do what they do not want to do as well as what they want to do (ambivalence of the will; ambi-

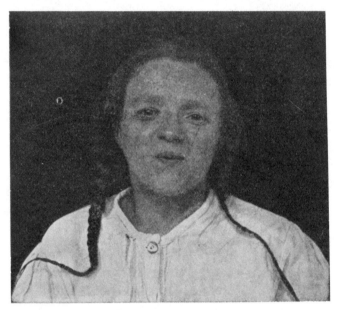

Fig. 23.—Rigid, benign mimicry in an erotic catatonic patient.

tendency); in the same moment they think, "I am a human being like you," and "I am not a human being like you." God and Devil, parting and meeting are the same to them and fuse into one idea (intellectual ambivalence). In the delusions too, expansive and depressive ideas very frequently mingle in multicolored confusion.

The "unimpaired" functions. Sensation, memory, orientation as to place and time, and motility are not directly disturbed according to our present methods of investigation. To be sure one frequently obtains wrong answers to simple questions, e.g., about orientation, but this is due to special causes: The patients answer incorrectly because

[68] See p. 125.

of negativism, or because of sheer mental laziness they talk nonsense, or they falsify orientation and memory as a result of delusions or the requirements of complexes.

Perception, as well as *orientation,* may be indirectly falsified by hallucinations and illusions. But it is strange that schizophrenics even in the deeper deliria and twilight states usually show the proper orientation together with the morbid. Although they imagine themselves in a prison or in hell or in a church, they nevertheless know in some other connection that they are in the ward of the insane asylum; although they look on and treat the visiting parents as devils, nevertheless they can later tell that their parents have been there; the patients know that the wife and child whom he murders are his household relatives; but he knows "also" that both are devils ("double orientation").

Thus while orientation as to time and place are not disturbed at all or only indirectly and temporarily, *orientation as to the patient's own situation* is very frequently disturbed, in asylum patients it is as a rule practically disturbed, deficient, and falsified. Only in exceptional cases can the patients understand why they have been interned. They consider themselves improperly treated, take an entirely wrong view of their relations to their family and to their social standing. That delusions, especially those of persecution, befog the conception of their own situation, is self-evident. The autopsychic orientation also suffers sometimes in which case the personality [69] is changed.

Memory. The patients usually reproduce their experiences just as well as normal persons do, frequently even better inasmuch as they take note indiscriminately of all details, while the normal person does not take the irrelevant into consciousness at all. Paranoid patients can often tell the dates of all sorts of trifling happenings. School learning is retained as well as in the normal who no longer apply it. Accomplishments like piano playing, etc., may after an interval of a decade be practiced as if nothing had intervened.

The registration of experiences is therefore very good. But reproduction may be disturbed; much that is related to the complexes may be blocked or the momentary general condition (lack of clearness and similar feelings) does not generally permit of a free disposition of the material. Besides, the patients very frequently appear "forgetful," as they do not remind themselves at the right time of what they should do; the housewife forgets to cook, the man forgets to go to business. But these are not disturbances of memory but the results of the schizophrenic "distraction."

[69] See below.

Motility also does not show any disturbances either in respect to strength or in respect to coordination. We notice in the most delicate movements, e.g. violin playing, no motor disturbances (the frequent tremors and catalepsy are here disregarded, some of the latter having been classed with the disturbances of motility).

B. THE COMPLEX FUNCTIONS

(α) *Dereism.* Schizophrenics lose contact with reality, the mild cases inconspicuously in one respect or another, the severer cases lose it completely. A patient believes the physician wants to marry her. He tells her the contrary every day, but this is entirely ineffective. Another sings at a concert in the hospital but much too long. The audience jeers; but this does not bother her and when at last she has finished, she takes her seat completely satisfied. The patients make countless requests of us, orally and in writing, to which they do not expect any answer at all, although very often immediate necessities, like their release, are involved. They want to get out; daily they press the door-knob hundreds of times and when the door is opened it does not occur to them to go away. They insistently demand a certain visitor; when he comes, they do not bother with him.

In place of this they live in an imaginary world of all kinds of wish fulfilments and persecutory ideas. But both worlds are a reality to them; sometimes they can consciously keep the two kinds separate. In other cases the dereistic world is the more real to them; the other is an imaginary world. Real people are "masks," "hastily constructed people," etc. According to the constellation, in cases of medium severity, at times the one world, at times the other is in the foreground. Indeed there are patients, though they are rare, who can translate themselves at will from one to the other. The milder cases move more in reality; the severest can no longer be torn out of the dream world, even though for the simplest purposes like eating and drinking a certain contact with reality is still retained.

(β) *Attention.* Naturally active attention is as a result of lack of interest often permanently very weak. It is all the more striking that passive attention is usually not only not disturbed but appears more active than normally. At any interval or external occupation the patients usually register excellently what goes on about them, and can make use of the material perceived.

Sometimes, especially in the beginning of the disease, the patients make every effort to collect their thoughts, but they do not succeed. This probably involves in part functional disturbances, about like those in cases of distraction, but besides there are certainly also general impediments to thinking. In the latter case intensity as well as extensity of attention are disturbed, but here, too, the passive invariably less than the active. The tendency of individual cases to exhaustion also permits the function to weaken readily.

In other respects, corresponding to the character of the disease, attention is very variable. Tenacity as well as vigility may fluctuate upwards and downwards. Patients, who for a long time cannot give attention in any way, are suddenly capable of planning a complicated plan of escape, etc.

(γ) *The Will.* A good many of the patients suffer from weakness of will, in the sense of apathy as well as in the sense of lack of persistence of the will. This is frequently accompanied by a fitful stubbornness. But under certain conditions definite aims can be held to with great energy, so that the term hyperbulia is really applicable. In overcoming pain, e.g. in cases of self-mutilation, the will sometimes appears abnormally strong.

In addition to thinking, the obstructions naturally also inhibit willing and execution. But the inner splitting of the will is most significant. The patients want something and at the same time want the opposite or when they want to execute an act, a counter impulse or cross purpose intervenes; subjectively the will often appears shackled. The patients believe they think and act under the influence of strange people or powers (being hypnotized; compulsive acts, automatic acts, command automatisms, etc.).

(δ) *The Personality.* Aside from very severe hallucinatory states, the patients know who they are. Sometimes, to be sure, the belief that they are some one else predominates, and does not permit the recognition of reality to appear.[70]

(ε) *Schizophrenic Dementia.* Schizophrenic dementia gets its stamp in the first place from the disturbance of affectivity: indifference on the one hand, uncontrolled affects on the other; then from the associative disturbances, which on account of obscurity and aimlessness and the interference of by-paths, lead to inadequate, incorrect, senseless, bizarre, and silly results. But even in severe schizophrenics many associations still take a proper course and though naturally, other things being equal, more complicated and finer functions are more readily disturbed than the simpler and coarser ones, nevertheless the ordinary failure of a particular function does not depend on its difficulty. A schizophrenic may be unable to add correctly two numbers of two digits and immediately afterwards extract a cube root. The severer

[70] For the severer disturbances of personality see among the accessory symptoms.

schizophrenic dementia is distinguished from the milder dementia not so much by the fact that it also afflicts the simpler functions as by the fact that numerically there is a decline of functions, be they difficult or easy. The so-called intelligence test may turn out excellently, but the patient may nevertheless be utterly incapable of managing himself properly in the simplest relations. Under certain conditions he may understand a philosophical treatise, but he may fail to understand that he must conduct himself decently if he wants to be discharged from the asylum. Where his complexes are involved he is impervious to argument, insensible of the most obvious contradictions of logic, as well as of the conceptions of ordinary reality. The schizophrenic is not downright demented, but he is demented as to certain times, certain constellations, certain complexes.

The products of pronounced schizophrenia in literature and art usually have the character of the demented or bizarre, which is not rarely concealed by a hollow pathos. In individual cases a slight degree of deviation from the normal gives the work of art a peculiar attractiveness, or the patients can utter truths which the normal person does not dare exhibit in their nakedness. Not rarely schizophrenic excitement produces at first a certain impulse to poetic activity, and even a certain ability otherwise lacking.

(ζ) *Activity.* Schizophrenic activity may be readily deduced from the disturbance of the affects and the associations. Where the affects are prostrate, little or nothing is done, where—in the very severe cases—dereism dominates the patient, he no longer bothers with the outer world. Lack of initiative, the absence of a definite aim, the ignoring of many factors of reality, dilapidation, sudden notions and peculiarities, characterize the middling severe cases. The milder cases live like other people, only now and then the abnormality is noticed. In all cases we find an insufficient motivation of individual acts and of the entire attitude toward life. The patients change their position and calling, or without reason fail to appear at their work, are irritable, moody, and inclined to pout and scold. In the organization of the asylums many can be very good working machines, but even on the outside, many whose view has been narrowed by the disease are still considered ideal workers, until a stupid act reveals their condition. A teacher suddenly lies down in a well, a young woman sews stockings to the carpet, etc.

Where accessory symptoms as, for example, hallucinations, delusions, manic or catatonic syndromes are present, these primarily determine action and conduct.

The excited cases in asylums are very unpleasant: Yelling, scolding, fighting, destroying, all sorts of uncleanliness, are every day occurrences with many; special peculiarities, coprophagia, scraping the walls and beds, refusal of food, impulse to suicide, self-infliction of injuries, make the treatment of individual cases especially difficult; but with the improvement of the technic of treatment, and with increased understanding of the patients these matters are becoming more rare and of shorter duration.

C. The Accessory Symptoms

The accessory symptoms complicate the fundamental picture, at times permanently, at times only in transient appearances.

(α) *Sense Deceptions.* Characteristic of schizophrenia are the *hallucinations of bodily sensations in clear mental states;* besides there exist a *pronounced preference for auditory deceptions in the form of words* (voices). *Visual hallucinations* are very frequent and lively in the acute stages, otherwise rare. *Tactile hallucinations* occur almost only in combination with bodily hallucinations and as partial mani-festations of a complicated perception (snakes, being struck). *Deceptions of smell and taste* and of the *kinæsthetic* senses occasionally obtrude themselves.

The patients *hear* blowing, roaring, humming, rattling, shooting, thundering, music, crying and laughing, but above all whispering, speaking, calling; they *see* individual things, landscapes, animals, people and all sorts of impossible figures; they *smell* and *taste* all sorts of pleasant and unpleasant things; they touch things, animals, and people and are struck by rain drops, fire, and bullets; they *feel* all the tortures and perhaps all the pleasant things also that our bodily sensations can transmit.

Elementary hallucinations of hearing are rare and influence the patient little. The voices usually speak in abrupt words and short sentences; long, connected scenes are signs of accompanying alcoholism or, in rare cases, of twilight states, and hysteroid additions. They scold, threaten, console, they criticize as "voices of conscience," or also say the opposite of what the patient wills or thinks. In the case of *the thoughts becoming loud,* on the contrary, what is thought at the moment by the patient is spoken out. The voices come from all sorts of places, from heaven and hell, or from ordinary places, where people are; but they are also situated in the walls, in the air, in the clothes, or in the body of the patient himself. Perhaps they use only one ear, or the good voices are heard in the right ear and the bad ones in the left.

The *hallucinations of bodily sensations* offer an endless variety.

The patients are clubbed, burnt, stuck with hot needles, their legs are made smaller, their eyes are pulled out, the lungs are sucked out, the liver is taken out and put into another place, the body is pulled apart and pressed together like a harmonica, a bullet runs along the top of the skull from the base to the top, the brain is sawed apart, the heart beat is decreased or increased, the urine is drawn out or held back. But above all the joys of normal and abnormal sexual satisfaction and, still more frequently, all sexual indecencies that can be imagined are felt; the semen is drawn off, the outer and inner genitals are burnt, cut, torn out, women are violated in the most refined manner, are forced to intercourse with animals. The sexual element in the sensations is often disguised; a female patient feels, instead of the sexual act, that a hobby horse is in the bed. Sexual experiences are transferred to the heart, to the mouth, to the nose, etc.

Hallucinations of sight are rare in chronic conditions and when present are usually fragmentary and disconnected; a head, angels as large as wasps, and hands appear before the patient, sometimes also a sexually symbolic animal, a snake, an elephant, a horse. In acute delirious conditions an entire background is hallucinated; paradise, hell, a castle, a dungeon, all with acting inmates. At the same time, reality may be hallucinated out of the way, or illusioned to correspond with the hallucinated milieu; in more clear cases some of the pictures are injected into reality, and in an altogether clear consciousness all are so injected.

Where it is possible to hallucinate, *illusions* also appear; but they are less important than the hallucinations. Sometimes the two forms of *sense* deception cannot be distinctly separated.

The deceptions of the different senses, especially in acute syndromes, *combine* very readily with one another. The patients experience scenes, see persons act, hear them speak, feel their influence, smell or taste their poisonous or pleasant presents. In mentally clear chronic stages, usually only voices and somatic hallucinations combine. The sense deceptions appear most frequently when the patients are left to themselves. But there are exceptions; now and then they appear especially disturbed during 'work. They are often provoked by another sense impression: the patient sees the physician come into the ward and at once hears him utter a command that concerns himself; the key turned in the lock is felt painfully in the breast (*reflex hallucinations*). Not so rarely the hallucinations are dependent to a certain extent on the will; the patients ask questions out loud or in thought; they are answered for them; they put themselves into certain situations where the sense deceptions appear, or into others, where they are free from them.

The *intensity of the hallucinations* may assume all degrees, from the least whisper to the terrifying thunder tone, from the slightest abnormal feeling to the most unbearable pain.

In the same way the *clearness* fluctuates within maximum limits. Frequently the false perceptions are really very obscure. But the patients do not notice it because the meaning of these perceptions is plain to them in advance; they hallucinate the meaning much more than the word. When they are pressed to reproduce a voice word by word, they often do so using different words in immediately successive times; but the sense, e.g. of the denunciation, remains the same; a distinct smell comes from snake-poison *or* from morphine, etc.

The same is true of the *projection to the outer world,* which is quite indefinite for the patient, much oftener than he at first notices. On closer inquiry it often turns out that the patients do not differentiate between vivid thoughts and real voices, between ideas and prepared pictures and (hallucinated) objects, and do not feel the necessity of doing so. Extracampine hallucinations occur most frequently, especially in schizophrenia.

In spite of this, the value of reality of the hallucinations for the patients usually holds as self-evident. They usually believe in the voices with unshakable conviction, and when these come in conflict with actuality, it is the latter whose reality they reject, or at least doubt. Hallucinations, the morbidness of which is recognized in spite of the vividness of the deceptive perception (pseudo-hallucinations), occur most readily in the visual sense.

Thus the patients cannot readily evade their hallucinations, while in ordinary life one can ignore a large part of the normal sense impressions. Only after a long while some of the more intelligent learn to pay no attention to the sense deceptions. Most of the patients, who in spite of all hallucinatory annoyances gradually become quieter, in time adjust themselves to them in such a way, that they transfer themselves into another world, into a separated part of the ego, which is decidedly cut off from reality. Thus they can work quietly or otherwise adapt themselves to the asylum routine although they hear voices incessantly and are tortured physically.

Contrasted somewhat with this persistence of the schizophrenic hallucinations there is the peculiarity that, as soon as another train of thought is present, they are readily *shut off or split off.* Even patients who are almost incessantly occupied with their hallucinations and are influenced by them, consequently cannot even with the best intentions give any account of them when they are questioned about them.

The patients have the most various conceptions of the *manner in which the hallucinations originate.* Often they are tortured with complicated machines or telepathic influences. Formerly it was witchcraft. Special talents also, "second hearing," enable the patients to hear voices. Not rarely the need of an explanation is entirely lacking.

The attitude of schizophrenics toward their hallucinations is most varied. Many adjust themselves to them, others even quietly amuse themselves with them; but very many react with excitements, threats, and violence. In acute twilight states, schizophrenics sometimes occupy themselves in accordance with their imaginings or they submit passively to everything; they lie around catatonically, partly with a consciousness of the absence of reaction, partly as a result of kinæsthetic hallucinations with the belief that they are doing something, like the normal person in a dream.

(β) *Delusions.* The schizophrenic delusions show in most cases the impress of the illogical. In the delusions themselves contradictory and absolutely unrelated ideas can exist together; the most decided contradiction of reality is not felt. The physician is at the same time their friend Jones, but besides "he may come as Thomas or Smith." The patient himself is long since dead but he lives in the asylum. A catatonic woman swallowed the whole world with every gulp; a patient has had his head cut off many times. Often the ideas are extremely indefinite. He has one hundred thousand dollars, which occasionally, without noticing the contradiction, he estimates as ten dollars. Many ideas are intended entirely symbolically; a female patient "is" the cranes of Ibycus because she is "free from blame and error," and "free," that is, she should not be confined.

The individual delusions have little or no logical connection among themselves; they often constitute a real "chaos of delusion." But usually they readily become organized in accordance with affective needs. The patients want to be more than they are and this then results in the delusion of grandeur. They do not get what they wish for, and as they themselves do not want to admit that they are incompetent, the result is the delusion of persecution.

In respect to *content* the most prominent part is played by persecutions. Particular individuals, relatives, superiors, the physicians in the asylum, but especially complete plots, the free masons, the Jesuits, the "Black Jews," mind readers, "Spiritualists," persecute the patient with voices, slander and annihilate him, subject him to all the tortures which objectively we ascribe to the bodily hallucinations (physical delusions of persecution).

The delusion of grandeur permits the patient to be a genius or some other great person, such as an inventor, count, Kaiser, pope, Christ, or prophet. This delusion is rarely altogether pure but is usually mixed with that of persecution. Erotic aspirations are nearly always present in women, and very frequently in men. If they are in the foreground there is usually at the same time involved, at least in women, an exaltation of rank; they have a lover who is socially above them; envious people are at fault that he has not as yet married them. ‹ The delusion of jealousy also may be schizophrenic. ‹ The delusions of poverty and sin usually exist only in depression. However, delusions of self-accusation may also be the expression of suppressed wishes or merely the result of chance associative connections. Thus a patient falsely accused himself of having violated a girl. In a village, where there had been several fires, a schizophrenic got the idea that he had caused them. People who in case of a sensational crime falsely surrender to the police as the criminals are usually alcoholic schizophrenics.

Autopsychic delusions are very frequent; the patient is not at all the person for whom he has been taken, but an entirely different person; his name is not the one shown in the documents, he was frozen in a bathtub and is here anyway; a young woman "is interchangeable, at times a virgin, at times a woman." Other patients are changed into animals, a delusion which to be sure rarely persists in clear states. Sometimes the ego also is changed. Then again it is not the patients at all who think and act, but strange powers in them (Demonism).

All schizophrenic forms of delusions, above all the delusion of persecution, draw their sustenance in large part from an uncontrollable *delusion of reference*. Everything that happens can have some reference to the patient, not only what people do, but external events also: a thunder storm, a war, etc.

Usually the delusions are self-evident truths to the patient. Some patients, to be sure, themselves feel in a certain connection the absurdity or the peculiarity without, however, being led to make a correction. The reaction to the delusion is sometimes adequate, in the sense that the persecuted ones complain and defend themselves, or the megalomaniacs want to carry out their presumptions; one wears a high hat to show his dignity as "inspector of the asylum"; another strikes any person at all whom he considers a persecutor; or to ward off the secretive "influences," counter measures of a magical character are resorted to. But much more frequently the conduct of the patients is inadequate. They really do nothing to attain their goal; the emperor and the pope help to manure the fields; the queen of heaven irons the patients' shirts or besmears herself and the table with saliva.

Delusions formed in acute states may be carried over into the quieter states as *"residual delusions" (Neisser)*. But usually they disappear with the other acute manifestations even though a schizophrenic hardly ever attains an entirely objective attitude toward a delusion. A delusion formed in chronic states is usually retained a long time, often for life, even though it is rare that it does not in time experience additions and transformations which, however, only in exceptional cases change it materially. At all events in the stages of higher dementia, where the withdrawal from reality clouds the judgment most seriously, we find the wishes most frequently gratified by the delusion of grandeur, while previously the impediments to wish fulfilment came more into consciousness and occasioned ideas of persecution. One of the commonest and often very rapid transformations is the one where the beloved becomes the persecutor.—With a change in the surroundings delusions that are attached to them are sometimes forced into the background for a short time; but soon the new environment seems the same as the old and attracts the previous delusions to itself.

The delusions, in large part, turn up in the form of hallucinations, others as visual deceptions; many suddenly spring from the unconscious as primordial ideas; many originate in a dream in which case it is significant that the patients often know the genesis without on this account entertaining any doubts as to the correctness. To be sure, manic and melancholic shifts of mood form corresponding ideas.

(γ) *The Accessory Memory Disturbances.* Occasionally *hypermnesias* appear, in which individual recollections turn up with special vividness, sometimes with the character of compulsion. Memory gaps or amnesias occur, more frequently, e.g. after deliria, but also after merely psychically conditioned excitements. But *paramnesias* are most common, in the form of illusions as well as in the form of hallucinations of memory. A patient who inwardly is not entirely satisfied with her husband accuses herself of having slandered him dreadfully. Many find in print what they have thought some time ago. What others have written, they have written about long ago. It is very common that patients who do not get along with those about them believe afterwards that they have endured many hardships on their account, while in reality they were the aggressors, or nothing special has happened at all. Memory hallucinations are very common. Suddenly, while playing cards, a patient becomes excited and complains that yesterday at a particular time, which he really spent very quietly, his clothes were taken off him and he was beaten.[71]

Memory deceptions through identification are much rarer.[72] But when they are once present, they may be consistently retained many years, so that e.g. a patient imagines every time something happens that it occurred exactly in the same way on the same date of the previous year.[73]

(δ) *The Personality.* Loss of a feeling of activity and the inability to control the thoughts often rob the schizophrenic ego of essential components (*depersonalization*). Disturbance of associations and morbid bodily sensations make it appear entirely different from what it formerly was, so that their changed condition is made conscious to the patients; they have become a different person, or they must at least "find their own self for short periods." The restriction of the ego when contrasted with other persons, even things, and abstract conceptions, may be obliterated; the patient can identify himself not only with many other persons, but with a chair, or a staff. His recollections are split into two or more parts; the one set of his experiences he ascribes to the real John Smith, the other to his new personality which was born in Charenton and is named Midhat Pasha. Others become a new personality at a definite moment.[74]

Objectively the personality suffers from the marked independence of the individual complexes. On ordinary occasions a patient may appear normal. If he is brought around to his delusions, he is altogether different, with a different character, with a different logic, with a different expression. On the other hand many severe catatonics may be completely opened up, by a discussion of their complexes and change their conduct, so that temporarily the disease can hardly be demonstrated. Towards some persons many schizophrenics are outwardly normal, toward others they are brutal, or shut-in, or negativistic. But in this case it is not as if the change were willed or even conscious. There simply exists an entirely different shift; feelings and impulses, and even associations, which dominate in one picture are inhibited in the other, and in their place others substituted. Both dissociation products of the personality can exist side by side. I observed this most clearly in a patient who, as a rule, while she listened to a reading and comprehended it faultlessly, or even while con-

---

[71] Compare further p. 105.
[72] See p. 108.
[73] For *negative memory hallucinations* see p. 101.
[74] Comp. p. 391, the autopsychic delusions.

versing with us, entertained herself with her pathological creations by whispering quietly or making gestures.[75]

Transitivistic manifestations are nowhere so frequent as in schizophrenia. Very commonly, the patients are convinced that those about them also hear their voices, sometimes even that they undergo the physical persecutions with them. A patient has holes in her hands and maintains that the nurse also has holes in her hands. A patient strikes himself twenty times in the belief that he is striking his enemies. A hebephrenic patient believes when he does anything, e.g. scratches his face, that he does not do it at all, but some other person whom he sees in front of him.

Appersonifications are rarer. A woman who nursed her husband, who was suffering from intestinal cancer, believed that she had the same disease, whereby her disease first became manifest. The bed neighbor of a woman patient died; she, thereupon, considered herself as having died.

In twilight states, or in attacks of rage the patients are often entirely different people as to character and ideas. Change of personality of the most different kinds are often indicated, not only by attitude and conduct, but occasionally also by different speech; one personality speaks in a low tone, the other in a loud tone; one articulates childishly, the other normally.

(ε) *Speech and Hand-writing.* Most schizophrenics do not show anything striking in their speech, but among our asylum patients disturbances of this function are not rare. Frequently the speech impulse is changed: the patients speak a great deal, often without saying anything and without a comprehensible reason; others no longer speak at all (Mutism). and for different reasons. At times they offer the information that ideas of sin forbid them to speak. But that the delusions should have just this content requires a cause lying further back, e.g. negativistic tendencies; speech may also be temporarily hindered by obstructions. The most important reason for protracted mutism is undoubtedly, that the patients have lost contact with the outer world and have nothing to say to it.

If the patients speak, the tone may be abnormal, too loud, too low, too fast, too slow, falsetto, humming, grunting, staccato, rushing, etc. It also happens that patients do not open the mouth to speak, as a result of which understanding is naturally reduced to zero. Then again speech may be without any affect, monotonous, or embellished in some way.[76] Speech mannerisms often express a definite complex,

---

[75] Compare also the double orientation, p. 111.
[76] For verbigeration see under stereotypism.

the child complex in diminutives and high voice, social aspirations in the use of foreign words and intonations, that are supposed to be superior. A catatonic woman, even in her clear states, usually spoke

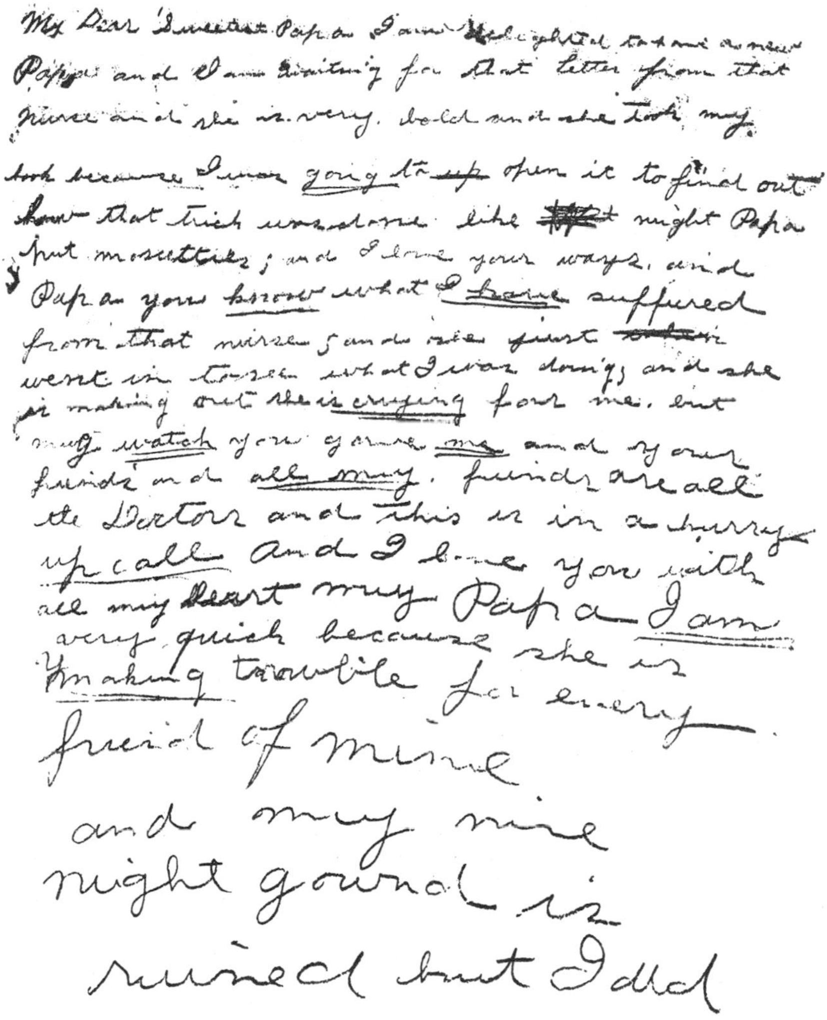
My Dear Sweetest Papa I am delighted to have a new Pappa and I am waiting for that letter from that nurse and she is very bold and she took my book because I was going to open it to find out how that trick was done like night Papa put mosquitoes; and I love your ways. and Papa you know what I have suffered from that nurse and she first went in to see what I was doing, and she is making out she is crying for me. but my watch you gave me and your friends and all my friends are all the Doctors and this is in a hurry up call and I love you with all my heart my Papa I am very quick because she is making trouble for every friend of mine and my nice night gownd is ruined but I did

FIG. 24.—Writing of a hebephrenic. The script changes from small to big hand, words are frequently underlined and some changed and scratched out.

an ordinary Zurich German, but concerning her disease always in the St. Gall dialect; when her husband was discussed, she used vulgar expressions and curses; on the subject of "America," which

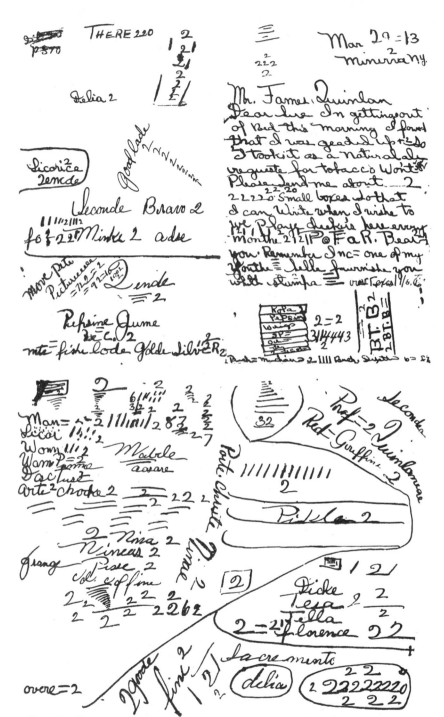

Fig. 25.—Letter written by a schizophrenic patient. Incomprehensible, containing stereotype expressions, neologisms, of words and numbers, and peculiar figures.

was connected with her aspirations, she used educated, decent expressions.

Frequently ideas are designated by other words, "courageous" by "rowdy," a wall clock by "buffet," or neologisms are formed, in part

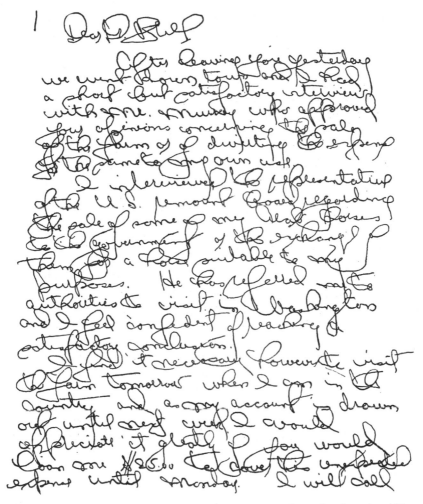

FIG. 26.—Flourishing writing of a paranoid præcox patient who shows grandiose feelings of the aristocratic type.

for existing ideas, in part for the designation of new conceptions. "Double polytechnic" means the inclusive idea of all the patients' aptitudes and the rewards belonging to them; one gives the patient pain "on the cosmos path." At times grammar fails them (*paragram-*

matism). Many words are used incorrectly, thus e.g. frequently the word "murder" that designates all the tortures that the patients suffer. "I am England" means: "England belongs to me."

At times only words are used or written, which have no meaning for us (Word Salad) or the patient speaks a particular "artificial language," sometimes with the pretense that it should be understood.

The *written* expressions correspond to the oral. Abnormalities of style of all sorts are frequent. The handwriting is sometimes over decorated or entirely affected; it not rarely changes very much suddenly, as if it came from another person; it contains repetitions of letters, of words, of all sorts of signs (written verbigeration), omissions, or excessive use of punctuation, and peculiar orthography. The arrangement of the writing, and the folding of the paper are often striking. In catatonic "unclearness" accidental mistakes occur, especially the omission of letters, the contraction of two words into one (In't instead of I not), contamination by later words that the writer already has in mind.

(ζ) *Physical symptoms* are usually not pronounced; but sometimes one comes across signs of cerebral pressure which is to be ascribed in part to an œdema in the skull, and in part to a special "brain inflammation."

The *weight of the body* shows large and unaccountable fluctuations; a marked addition of fat is especially frequent during reconvalescence from acute attacks. During catatonic states we frequently have a severe disturbance of metabolism; the picture looks like an infection: thickly coated tongue, tremors, rapid decrease of weight and strength even when sufficient nourishment is given, and sometimes also slightly increased temperatures. The metabolic disturbances, as well as the cerebral inflammation, may become fatal.

The *functioning of the intestines and the different glands* in most chronic cases is, as far as we know, normal, but under certain conditions very irregular; constipation may alternate with frequent movements, polyuria with penuria. High grade ptyalism and parched mouth occur in the same way.

The functions of the *vaso-motor system* are perhaps most strikingly *changed*. Without comprehensible reason the pulse may fluctuate; *livor* and *cyanosis* often occur, which in rare high grade cases may go as far as blue-black coloration of the hands and feet. Then again the head or any other circumscribed part of the body is overheated, another part is cold. Œdemas of a striking consistency appear on the feet, in the face, on the wrists, occasionally also on very unusual places. Menstruation is often disturbed, but more in the sense of

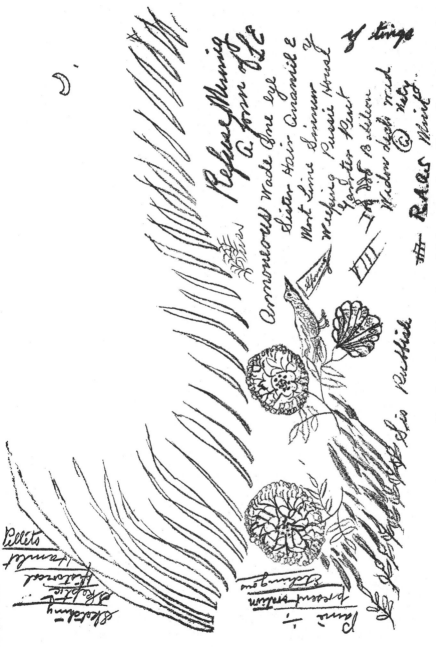

Fig. 27.—A drawing made by a paranoid patient who at times shows definite catatonic reactions. One notes stereotype expressions and neologisms.

reduction than in hyperfunctioning. Especially in acute stages it usually ceases for a time. But the subjective menstrual troubles common in mentally healthy women hardly occur here, an important sign that they are psychically conditioned. Men are sometimes impotent or there is at least a reduced libido.

Naturally during acute shifts *sleep* is usually disturbed; in contrast with this one sees at times a protracted desire for sleep. Chronic patients sleep normally at times, at other times they are kept excited through the night by hallucinations.

The *manifestations of exhaustion* vary greatly; especially in the beginning they form at times a prominent symptom. At every task, especially thinking, the patients immediately become tired and consequently fall back on as complete an inactivity as possible, sometimes after a hard struggle against the evil. On the other hand others hardly feel any tiredness, either at work or at the exertions caused by the excitations or the hyperkineses.

Of the *motor symptoms* there are still to be mentioned the frequent aggravation of the idio-muscular contractions and fibrillar or muscular twitching in the face, then fine tremors. Coarse tremors occur only in acute disturbances with weakness.

The *gait* in severe cases is often striking as aimless, and irregular in respect to length and duration of the step. Organic paralyses do not belong to the picture of schizophrenia, but hysterical forms of all kinds do, even though they are not particularly frequent.

The deep *reflexes* are usually exaggerated. In acute conditions the *pupils* are often pathologically dilated, rarely and probably only in chronic patients excessively contracted; more frequently, but transiently and variably, the pupils are unequal. Usually the psychic pupillary reflexes are absent.[77]

Besides the hallucinations of bodily sensations *parasthesias* of all kinds are very frequent and often constitute for a long time the only symptoms of the disease. Worthy of note is an *analgesia* which occurs not too rarely and which is sometimes quite complete. It is responsible for the fact that the patients readily injure themselves purposely or accidentally.

Sometimes *catatonic attacks* occur which show two extreme types with every possible intermediate forms. On the one side one observes attacks that appear purely psychical, evincing a hysterical form; on the other side there are organic attacks with disturbances of consciousness, interference with the thought processes, involuntary evacuations, and occasional residual mild paralyses of speech, facial

[77] For catalepsy see below among the catatonic symptoms, p. 403.

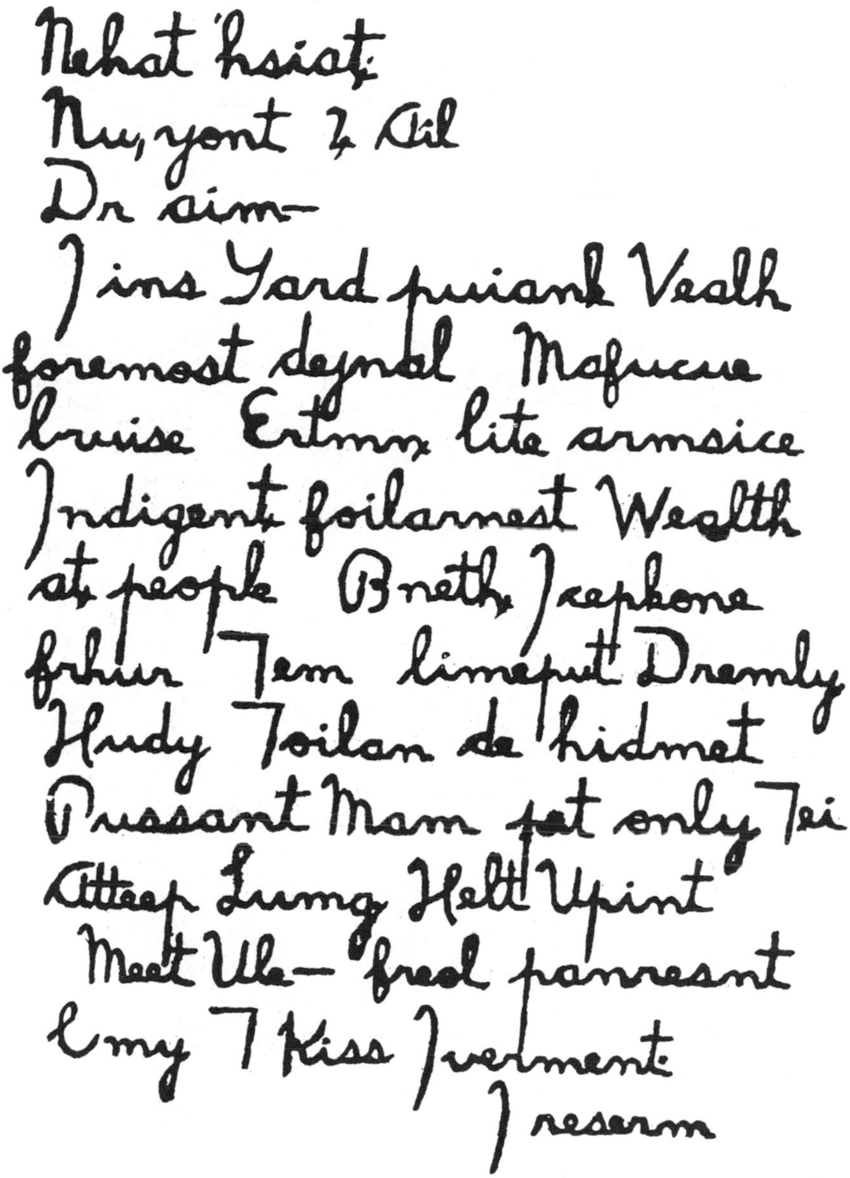

Nehat 'hsiat:
Nu, yont 2 Ail
Dr aim—
Jins Yard puiank Vealh
foremost deynal Mafucue
bruise Ertmn lite armsice
Indigent foilarnest Wealth
at people Breth Jcephone
frhur Jem limeput Dremly
Hudy Toilan de hidmet
Pussant Mam fat only Tei
Atteap Lumg Helt Upint
Meet Ule— freal panreant
Emy T Kiss Jvelment
Jresarm

FIG. 28.—Letter written by schizophrenic patient who is controlled by senseless ideas of grandeur. The patient has invented a new language which one can, however, occasionally decipher. Thus for Manhattan State Hospital he writes, "Nehat ' hsiat." One can also recognize in the 2nd line, the words "New York," the 2nd of April; and in the 3rd line "Dr. Heyman" (the superintendent of the hospital). Occasionally one can also find correct words. The patient is a native American.

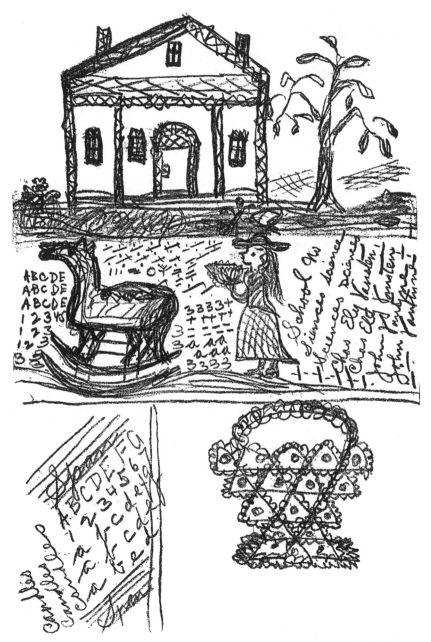

Fig. 29.—From the note book of a chronic catatonic. Verbigerations in letters, childish drawings in spite of the fact that the patient can really draw quite well.

nerve, or hemiplegia. If the patients are not entirely unconscious with this, they are delirious in the sense of a more or less perceptible hysterical twilight state. Besides there are *fainting spells*, and especially typical *epileptiform convulsions* also.

Physical deformities (stigmata) are obviously somewhat more frequent than in the normal persons but much less frequent than in *idiots, epileptics* and *criminals*.

(η) *The Catatonic Symptoms.* With this name a number of symptoms were designated which at the time helped to formulate a definite conception of catatonia. They may readily occur singly, but it is not improbable that they nevertheless have an inner connection in the sense that they occur most frequently with a certain condition of the brain that is at the foundation of catatonia.

1. *Catalepsy* (waxlike flexibility, pseudoflexibility, and rigid catalepsy).[78]

Most of the severer cataleptic schizophrenics assume definite attitudes for months and years; one stands at the window on the tips of the toes of one foot, holding up the other leg and both hands. Others assume a particular attitude in bed, etc. Usually these forms are associated with rigid catalepsy.

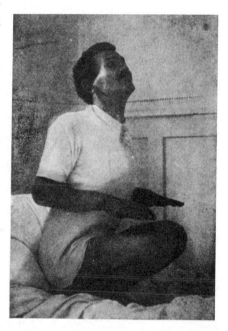

FIG. 30.—Spontaneous attitude of a catatonic, at first lasting, then only assumed when the physician appeared.

2. *Stupor.* Stupor of varying origin is very frequent in acute conditions but may also characterize a chronic stage for decades. The patients move little, speak little or not at all, and generally limit intercourse with the outer world as much as possible. Cataleptics are naturally all stuporous. Many appear depressed ("Melancholica attonita"). In severe cases there are usually very numerous hallucinations of all senses with a falsification of the outer world and the environment; the patients are in a dream land.

3. *Hyperkinesis.* Many catatonics are in incessant motion: they

[78] See p. 153.

nod the head, hop, hammer on the bed, throw themselves about, dash themselves on the head, let themselves fall backwards over the foot end of the bed, climb up wherever they can, all in a peculiar manner that seems purposeless.

4. *Stereotype Expressions.* The inclination to stereotype expressions is prevalent in all fields. It may just as likely be transient as it may for decades provoke the identical movements and the identical attitude.

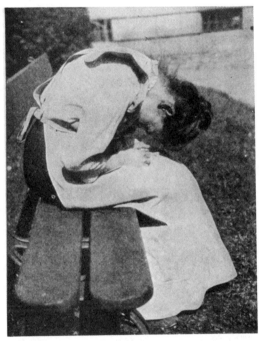

FIG. 31.—Permanent attitude of a catatonic, who in spite of all measures finally suffered from a pretty severe kyphosis.

Stereotype Movements: Rubbing the right hand over the left thumb for decades; continuous rubbing with the right hand over the middle of the breast; running the finger along all edges; tapping with the foot on certain places; knocking on a particular part of the bed; turning about the vertical axis with a particular position of the arms, etc. Some stereotypes have the character of senseless acts: pulling out the hairs at certain places, sticking the finger into the anus, smearing in a particular way, twisting the clothes, ripping off the buttons.

Stereotyped Attitudes: many catatonics who lie in bed hold the head away from the pillow in a position which the normal person could not endure very long, or they draw the knee up to the chin, or stand rigid like an Egyptian statue; they hold the legs spread apart, stare for weeks at the same spot, under certain conditions with an extreme awry position of the eyes.

Stereotypes of Place. The patients want to remain only in one particular place, always walk exactly the same paths in the garden, so that these become trodden down, or they touch the wall at certain places, thus leaving marks of this constant wear and tear.

A particular stereotype is the "snout cramp" in which the lips are held protruded forward.

The stereotype of speech, or *verbigeration*, always repeats the same words or sentences, often entirely senseless ones. This is not to be confused with such incessantly repeated ejaculations as "Oh God! Kill me!" etc., which are the expression of a persistent depressive affect. In those playing music one finds repetitions lasting for years of the same figure (*musical verbigeration*).

Thoughts, wishes and *hallucinations* may also become stereotyped.

Some of the stereotype expressions have a comprehensible content: one will represent the movements of a shoemaker because the lover was a shoemaker; another the balancing in the quadrille because the lover was first met in a quadrille. In two cases snout cramp was the expression of contempt for the surroundings. Usually the patients are not conscious of the meaning, and at least during

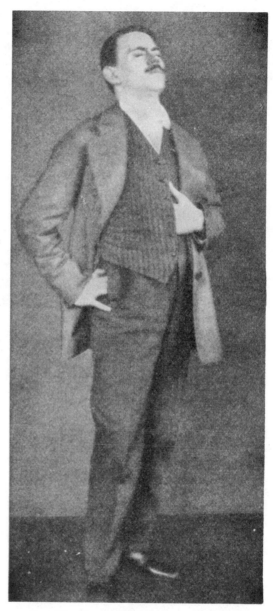

FIG. 32.—Stereotype, catatonic attitude with closed eyes. It imitates some complex of greatness. The expression of the face is vapid.

the phase when stereotypes were present, I

have never obtained direct information about them. Only the association experiment, subsequent or indirect remarks of the patient, an exact objective anamnesis, and similar things, can enlighten us.

5. *Mannerisms.*[79] Many patients assume certain poses; e.g. one will for years try to imitate Bismarck; others want to represent something else that is extraordinary, nearly always in a pompous, artificial, caricatured manner. But sometimes only particular acts are changed or over-embellished in some way: Before partaking of food the plate is struck three times, food is taken on the fork seven times and thrown off again before it is taken into the mouth; in dressing, before making any slight movement, the cloth is rubbed

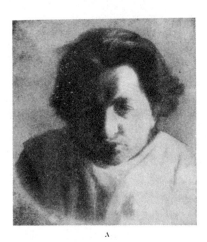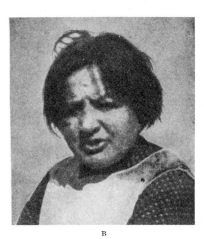

A　　　　　　　　　　　　B

Figs. 33a and 33b.—"Snout cramp" in a catatonic with alternating manic and melancholic days. Change of phase very decided, often from one minute to the other. (a) on a melancholy day, (b) on a manic day.

several times; the patient walks about the chamber three times before she sits down on it. In talking diminutives or foreign words are used with affected intonation. To all words an "is" or an "ism" is attached. The hand is improperly extended in greeting or only the little finger is offered.

6. *Negativism*[80] is a very frequent and very disagreeable symptom of schizophrenia. When the patients should get up, they want to remain in bed; if they should remain in bed, they want to get up. Neither on command, nor in accordance with the rules of the hospital do they want to get dressed or undressed or come to meals or

[79] According to Ziehen "Variational stereotypes." (But all mannerisms need not become stereotyped.)

[80] See p. 154.

leave their meals; but if they can perform the same acts outside of the required time or somehow contrary to the will of the environment, they often do them. Of their own accord they do not go to the toilet; if they are brought there, they hold back the excrements, in order to soil the bed or the clothes immediately afterwards. They eat the soup with a fork or with the dessert spoon, the dessert with the soup spoon. Many resist all influences with all their might, often with excited scoldings and fighting; thus negativism becomes a source of attacks of rage. It can develop into a real impulse to tease, into an active impulse to anger incessantly those about them in the most ingenious manner; the patients hide their things and then maintain that the orderlies have stolen them or have not given them to them, etc. In some cases one can with certainty bring the patient to do the desired act if one forbids him to do it, or orders him to do the opposite (*command negativism*).

Many patients are negativistic toward their own impulses (*inner negativism*); as soon as they want to perform an act, an inhibition or counter impulse appears so that they do not perform the simplest acts like eating. The spoon is arrested half way up to the mouth and must finally be put down again.

In purely intellectual matters also, negativistic tendencies are very disturbing, since with every thought the patients must also think the opposite: "I am in the hospital, no, I am not in the hospital" (*intellectual negativism*). Even the voices can continually say the opposite of what the patients want or think, or they can recite the two contradictions.[81]

However, even the most pronounced negativism is not absolute; toward certain persons it is usually greater than toward others. Often it only becomes apparent in the intercourse with the personnel of the hospital, but not with the other patients. Sometimes it is provoked when the complexes are touched.

Negativism is a complicated symptom. To a certain degree "negative suggestibility" is a normal characteristic, which is often disagreeably conspicuous especially in little children, in that they reject all sorts of things. That negativism in schizophrenics is especially pronounced, may be due to a fundamental cause of which we are ignorant. But it is undoubtedly connected with dereism which makes every external disturbance felt as unpleasant. But the deficient understanding of the environment, the enduring of counter measures such as the confinement, naturally produce a

[81] See also ambivalency, p. 286.

hostile attitude. Sometimes, especially in women, sexuality with its marked ambivalence contributes its influence, and leads the patients to reject what they really want.

The patients themselves can usually give no explanation of the negativistic attitude. The explanation by means of voices or delusions is naturally not sufficient because usually the reverse is the case, in that the content of these symptoms is conditioned by the existing negativism.

7. *Command Automatism and Echopraxia.* As an outward contrast to negativism there is sometimes found in our patients an automatic obedience to given commands, even when the patients really resist, e.g. if one orders them to stick out their tongue and threatens to pierce it. Besides, in confused as in twilight states, echopraxia and echolalia occur at times.

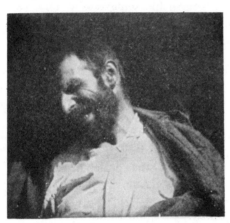

8. *Automatism* (including *compulsive phenomena*). Nowhere do we find automatic action so frequently as in schizophrenia and in the most various degrees of connection with the conscious ego.[82] Apparently insignificant movements such as lifting the arms, assuming the position of the crucified, screaming, then real "actions" as breaking windows, tearing clothes, smearing, often take place without the conscious will of the patient. To be sure, occasionally it goes as far as arson, murder, or suicide; some of these serious anti-social actions are performed so clumsily that one gets the impression that an inner resistance prevents the actual attainment of the purpose.

FIG. 34.—Grimmacing catatonic.

Automatic impulses may also change a normal willed action, e.g. a complicated piece of knitting is made incorrectly against the will of the patient who knows the pattern well.

Automatisms of speech lead only rarely in schizophrenia to combined utterances; instead they sometimes produce incomprehensible hodge podge. Verbigeration may also be classed with these as *generally the greater part of the stereotypes run off automatically. Coprolalia* often has the distinct character of compulsion.

[82] Comp. p. 150.

There is also a schizophrenic compulsive thinking, a compulsive remembering, even a compulsive cessation of thought. Among the affective disturbances compulsive laughter is especially frequent; it rarely has the character of the hysterical laughing fit, but that of a soulless mimic utterance behind which no feeling is noticeable. It may often be provoked by allusion to a complex. Sometimes the patients feel only the movements of the facile muscles ("the drawn laughter").

Contrasted with hysterics and compulsive neurotic patients, schizophrenics usually give little thought to their automatisms. It simply happens, they cannot help it, and with that they are satisfied. To be sure, some struggle against it and feel the obsession, and still more believe themselves possessed and influenced by their persecutors. In the latter case they not rarely adopt defensive measures to prevent themselves from carrying them out, e.g. sticking a piece of wood into the mouth to prevent the utterance of unseemly words.

The automatisms are to be conceived as actions of the unconscious; the complexes on which they are based can be often demonstrated in the analysis of accessible patients.

9. *Impulsiveness.* Schizophrenic

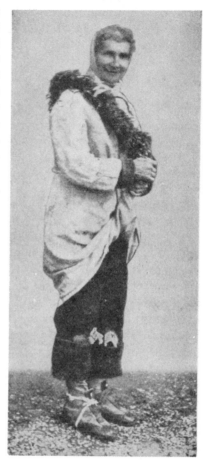

Fig. 35. — Manic schizophrenic woman who has made herself a wreath out of grass and twigs and besides holds with both hands the lower part of her dress which has been twisted into the shape of a sausage. In bed she holds in front of herself the linen twisted in the same way. Interest in the process of photography conceals the otherwise rigid facial expression.

impulsiveness is not a uniform symptom but a frequent method of manifestation of the morbid actions which originates in different sources.

Some of the impulsive actions are automatic, others are affective actions, "unloading" in the case of an emotional tension in which the patients feel more and more uncomfortable. Something must then give way; they scold or fight or tear up only to quiet down after minutes or days. With this may also be included the "explosion in prisons" observed in latent schizophrenics. In the same way the sudden outburst of rage, which is frequent in schizophrenia, leads to impulsive acts. Many sudden acts are based on the disturbance of association; it is a case of unmotivated notions which are carried out without resistance.

(ϑ) *Acute Syndromes.* The course of schizophrenia is frequently interrupted by acute appearances of entirely different manifestation and origin. To these belong: *Shifts of the pathologic process,* frequently with catatonic-hallucinatory or stuporous manifestations; *simpler exacerbations of the chronic condition,* mostly with paranoid or catatonic syndromes, *abnormal reactions* to emotionally toned experiences, especially in the form of hysterical twilight states or attacks of scolding. A part of the manic or melancholic *displacements of mood* are probably by-products of the morbid process. Then also there are naturally conditions that do not depend at all directly on the disease but complicate it or at the most are released by it, as perhaps periodic moodiness which may belong to an accompanying manic-depressive insanity. The acute appearances may last hours or years. Severer forms also, that give the impression of independent psychoses, may break out suddenly, one might say from one minute to the next. An exacerbation of the schizophrenic process favors the appearance of psychogenic symptoms; thus the manifestations combine indiscriminately.

Melancholic and manic states often constitute the first manifest syndrome of the disease, but they may also supervene later. They usually last months or years and appear as a combination of the melancholy, or it may be a manic triad with schizophrenic symptoms.

The depressive affect in this case is frequently combined with anxiety, but it appears rigid, and superficial, the utterances being exaggerated and often pathetic; the delusions strike one as altogether too senseless. Occasionally one finds a combination of senseless delusions of grandeur with the depressive delusion. The disturbance of thinking is very extreme and may lead to an absolute monideaism, which probably does not occur in simple melancholias.

The *manic states* are similarly characterized. The fresh joyousness of the manic is lacking; outbursts of rage often appear completely unmotivated. The rigidity of the affects is particularly noticeable in this case. With the flight of ideas one observes dilapidation, and bizarre schizophrenic associations. The manic pressure activity readily becomes an incomprehensible pressure motion; silly tricks may be added to the peculiar actions. Hallucinations and delusions are generally present. But the delusions are usually more flighty than in the depressive states.

Of special importance are the *acute catatonic pictures* in which catatonic symptoms mingle indiscriminately. In akinetic forms of attonity, of stupor, of flexibilitas cerea, the patients move little or not at all; they do not take care of themselves, let the saliva dribble out, never swallow spontaneously, and soil themselves. Peculiar poses are sometimes retained for a long time. Usually complete mutism exists. But such conditions are now and then amenable to temporary psychical influence so that an act may be performed or an answer given. Mutistic patients at times make themselves understood in writing. Often this is accompanied by a coated tongue and fuligo. Vasomotor symptoms most frequently and severely, complicate just this picture.

In the pronounced hyperkinetic forms the patients are in motion day and night:

They climb around, turn somersaults, hop over the beds, knock twenty times on the table, then on the wall, balance themselves, bend their knees, throw themselves into the air, strike, destroy, force the arms in the most twisted position possible between the radiators of the heating apparatus, and they are unmindful of burns; they scream, sing, verbigerate, scold, laugh, cry, spit, make faces, sad, terrible, or cheerful; they take any object into their hands, move it in any way at all, lay it down in another position and make a thousand other movements, of which, to be sure, the individual patient usually limits himself to a certain number. The movements are always somewhat abnormal. If the patients lift an object, they do it in a particular way as it is not ordinarily done; they climb into bed from the head end and with most unusual acrobatic flourishes or they let themselves fall into it, etc. The movements are often made with great strength, nearly always with the exertion of unnecessary muscle groups; indifference to themselves sometimes appears as great as that toward the animate and inanimate enviroment.—Many patients are also always in motion but it is slower, more clam-like, and more dream-like. The akinesis may be interrupted by sudden catatonic raptus, in which the patients do some kind of harm, from the breaking of a pane of glass to a brutal attempt at murder or suicide.—*Analgesia* often increases the danger and indifference of these patients, to themselves and others.

In severe catatonias the psychic state is usually altogether unclear. Many give no account of themselves or even lie in a complete dream-world. The affectivity is usually difficult to make out. Often there are indications of various contradictory feelings but none seem to penetrate. Subjectively also no describable mood exists except a frequent indifference.

The *buffoonery syndrome* is not always easily separated from catatonic states. In this syndrome the entire picture is taken up with playing demonstrative striking tricks, and with giving wrong answers; like the Ganser twilight state it probably only occurs as a reaction to a situation from which unconsciously one wants to escape through insanity.

If in an acute appearance hallucinations and delusions prevail to the extent of fully disturbing clearness, and if the catatonic symptoms are absent or insignificant, we call the condition *schizophrenic insanity.* Here the affectivity is usually less injured than in the preceding group. The mood frequently has definite coloring and is often slightly modifiable.

In the face of unbearable situations, most frequently in disappointed love, schizophrenics retreat into a *twilight state;* the unpleasant reality is split off and exists for them only secondarily; in its place another world, frequently with frank wish gratification, is imagined. The patient marries her lover, he visits her every night, she becomes pregnant and bears a child. But not nearly all of these patients are happy. They cannot flee entirely from reality and, consequently, come into conflict with it outwardly. Shutting off succeeds most intensively, and the imagined happiness is therefore least disturbed in the religious *ecstasies.*[83]

The behavior of those in the twilight state varies. Some live their dream quietly in bed or even under the covers. Others stalk about like ghosts in an unintelligent manner, as they have a false conception of the environment and hence get into conflicts. Invariably double orientation plainly exists. The outcome is usually by lysis. While the twilight states in hysteria or epilepsy usually last only hours or days, the schizophrenic sometimes extend over months, under certain conditions into the second year. Nevertheless, corresponding to their origin, they much more rarely leave behind a serious aggravation of the permanent condition than do other acute syndromes of the schizophrenia.—In prisoners held for examination, but occasionally in other cases, the condition manifests some signs of Ganser's syndrome.

While the twilight states are formed on psychic foundation, there is a form of "unclearness" which has an organic character and has to be noticed because of its particularly bad prognosis. The patients are in an unclear twilight state, they do not let themselves be aroused

[83] See p. 113.

by psychical influences, in spite of the fact that one is in intellectual contact with them, and they often make every effort to answer our questions. The train of thought is slow, unclear and fragmentary. These patients fail even in simple calculations; in writing they unwillingly make orthographic and grammatical errors, contractions, contaminations, etc.: at the same time hallucinations and disturbances of orientation may be lacking. Affectivity also may be relatively well preserved. Nevertheless the condition is very difficult to distinguish from the more psychogenetic forms.

We still have to mention *states of confusion* in which the incoherence of the train of ideas dominates the whole picture, and where one observes exogenous and endogenous *attacks of rage, delirious syndromes,* and *states of wandering* (fugues), at times as a result of a special brain disturbance, at times more of an hysterical nature or as a reaction against unpleasant experiences or merely as a pathological fancy. A considerable part of army deserters are schizophrenic wanderers. Dipsomanic moodiness may also appear occasionally on a foundation of schizophrenia.

D. The Subdivisions

Although schizophrenia is probably not a homogeneous disease, we are not yet able to divide it into natural subdivisions. Nevertheless in order to orient oneself in the external forms of the constantly changing morbid picture, four forms have been distinguished, according to the presence or absence of definite symptom groups. They are not nosological units and from patient to patient and in the same patient pass over into one another, so that a schizophrenic may be admitted into the asylum, e.g. as a hebephrenic, may remain there for years as a catatonic and may finally be released as paranoid. But most patients remain permanently within their group.

1. Where delusions and hallucinations—the two symptoms usually go together in schizophrenia—are in the foreground, one speaks of the *paranoid* type or *dementia paranoides.*[84] The paranoid type can develop after any melancholic, manic, catatonic acute initial onset ("secondary insanity" of the older authors), or can begin immediately as such. In the latter case the entire course is as a rule chronic throughout. During a stage of discomfort in which ideas of reference gradually become more definite, there develops in the course of years a

---

[84] The latter term, up to the eighth edition of *Kraepelin's* manual, does not mean all paranoid forms of dementia præcox but a particular sub-group which quickly forms confused delusions but no catatonic changes of the external attitude.

complicated pile of delusions, which are only connected by the general tendency of persecution or (much more rarely) of grandeur or of hypochondria. However, the beginning may also manifest itself by finished primordial delusions that seem to come from a clear sky, which then increase and are only later followed by distinct ideas of reference and hallucinations. Many of the patients keep out of asylums for a relatively long time, others alternate between freedom and commitment, and others again lose the external control so early and so severely that they have to remain in asylums the greater part of their lives. Especially in the last, single or even many catatonic symptoms very easily complicate the picture.

To this class belong some of the *litigious* schizophrenics who demand police protection against imagined injuries, and in spite of all refusals cannot cease with their complaints. Others may be classed as cases of simple schizophrenia because their attitude seems to rest more on the determination to be always right than on a real delusion.

Some of the cases mentioned by Kraepelin among the *pre-senile delusions of injury* are according to our conceptions belated paranoid forms.

Paranoid. Railroad employee. Medium intelligence. At first spinner, then railroad worker where he rose to train conductor. Always particular, silent. Toward the end of the thirties he began to be mistrustful toward his wife. At the same time a better position with the owner of a factory who was a free-mason was offered him by intimation from a workingman who was very "sympathetic" toward him; finally other positions right in the lodge were also offered him. Years ago he was supposed to have seen a free-mason in a compromising situation (in reality a woman had merely entered a railroad compartment after him); some allusions were supposed to be made to it in the newspapers. But he had kept quiet about it and now the free-masons want to reward him for it. Because he did not accept the reward, they persecute him. Furthermore years ago he once made unfavorable remarks about the free-masons. All sorts of things are said to him on the street in passing; remarks are also made elsewhere which he only understands later. At night he hears voices. In a mysterious way his thoughts are read. The free-masons are after women; they use his wife also. He demanded from her with threats the money that she had obtained in that way; once he wanted to cut open her stomach with a razor. His sister-in-law is sometimes pale and sometimes red; that is on his account. Theatricals and thoughts are made for him while awake and especially while dreaming. During the night he is questioned; only in the course of the day does this come into his consciousness. Because he maltreated his wife and did not work any more, he was brought into the hospital. There he showed the same picture for years, at time quiet and capable of work, at times in milder excitations with scolding and incessant complaining about persecutions. All sorts of poisons are put into his food; he feels them working in his body; they want to murder him; especially at night, sperma, human blood, urine, "pollen," and horse manure are put into his body in various ways; one spits into his mouth; one hypnotizes and magnetizes him, and brings him into a "latent" state where one cannot breathe. The people here have a staff like a magnet staff; with this they make him powerless, rob him of his potency. They want to castrate him, extract his semen, cut up his lungs, smash his urethra, distend the sexual canal, cut up his buttons, burn up the inner sexual organs, and pinch him all over his body. Voices threaten to cut out his eyes;—against his will, his daughter has been admitted to the masons; he is accused of having used her in various positions; the government, the church, the whole international society, his wife and his own mother and the physician are combined with the free-masons; the physicians have obtained millions to hold him in the asylum; he himself demands 30,000 fr. damages per day for the con-finement and he figures up everything exactly. He keeps a record of all the hallucinatory maltreatments; they demand that he become a free-mason; he does not want to and therefore they persecute him. At other times he wants to become a free-mason but then they will not admit him at all. For a long time he said in a stereotype manner to everybody a hundred times a day, "If you please," by which he meant to say on the one hand nothing, and on the other, he put various interpretations into it. He should be admitted to the free-masons or he should be permitted to have intercourse, etc. When he sees a woman, he is compelled to prove his potency; then he can join the masons. Then he can only be prevented by force from undressing himself. He wants to enter an aviation race from Petersburg to Mos-cow, he invents flying machines, improves trolley cars, makes count-less contributions to the physicians and officers of the hospital. Once he tore away a toe nail because the scissors were not good enough to cut it off. For a large part of the time the patient is in the quiet ward. He shakes hands with visitors in a friendly way, even though often with a slight, superior smile.

Schizophrenic Litigious Woman. Excellent worker in a hat busi-ness. Was a good pupil but wanted to get somewhat higher up in the world; as a farm girl she attended a vocational school for women to learn finer work. Then she had various places as cook and housemaid; at thirty-two she was housekeeper for a doctor who was just establishing a practice. Now she affirms that on the very first day he became intimate with her and promised to marry her. The further details are still more improbable or entirely impossible. His relatives wanted to prevent him from marrying her. He should make an arrangement with her. On the first day he told her she had the right to object if he married. (These can be only memory deceptions.) She would have to make good her claim or be silent. After about nine months the physician discharged her, according to her version, because the people were talking too much about their relations. She then worked in different places, at last mostly with a hatter and from time to time reminded the physician of his promise. When thirty-four years old she once had a headache, pains in the eyes, an "attack like a stroke," trembling all over the body. She was treated by the physician who was supposed to have renewed his promise. When thirty-six she read the announcement of the physician's marriage. Then she demanded "her rights or a good payment" and took a position in his neighborhood. He was supposed to have had a simple wedding to indicate that he really loved the patient. Then she wrote to him frequently, called him names and then also preferably his wife, at last on post-cards. "Jail-bird," "shabby hotel frequenter," "whore," "Mrs. Louse," are among the better expressions. She became unreliable in her work and even when she made big mistakes she claimed to be right. Then she began suits in all the courts which naturally could not entertain a complaint without evidence of probability, when it concerned entirely abstruse demands. The courts were then vilified: "His Honor the Judge is idiotic." Finally the physician was compelled to sue for slander whereupon the patient was examined. During the examination she was absolutely incapable of discussing her complaints. She was not fully certain of the time sequence of all her experiences but otherwise she had a good memory and good orientation. She recounted impossible assertions of the physicians and the judges, who had said she was right (memory deceptions). She really did not want anything from the physician "she only wanted the physician's wife to have a chance to get away with an honorable reputation." Since the physician did not answer, he admitted her claims. Either he had to do that publicly and send his wife away, or he had to dispute it and keep his wife." She stoutly maintained that as long as he made none of these declarations, his marriage was void and his wife was a concubine. The doctor had made her (the patient) a promise of marriage that held for life; with the other he was only engaged. She was incapable of seeing that the doctor's wife was entirely innocent toward her.   Presented at a clinic she began at once to talk about her affair, taking for granted that the auditor knew everything.   Of course she had to be pronounced irresponsible; she was placed under a guardianship and released.   But she did not want to accept the verdict or pay the trial costs which led to a number of scenes with much noise and spitting at the marshal, etc.   She scolded us too in various missives.   Nevertheless she was not brought in for four years until she forced her way into the police station, made a big scene and, after being thrown out, continued it with increased energy.   It was reported that she had worked regularly and had spoken sensibly about indifferent matters.   But as soon as she touched on her affair, she became confused, excited and hard to understand.   She did not want to work until she was put to bed and ordered to cease her written litigations. There she pulled herself together and after a stay of six months could again be discharged.   But in the following year she came back because she had made a scene before the justice of the peace and promised she would do it every day until the doctor was summoned to court. This time with us she did not cease her protesting, made a lot of noise, ran after the physician in her shirt in order to scold him.   She was taken out by the poor relief society, which should long ago have taken charge of the impoverished invalid, and as yet she has not returned. Her last greeting was: "Sow dogs, sons of bitches, alienists send me my clothes to X. St. . . . , promise of marriage belongs in the courts. I will reproach the poor relief society until the matter is brought to court."   Hallucinations were not observed, on the other hand many illusions, perhaps also memory hallucinations.   She also told many things about us that we had never done; e.g. that the physician in charge of the division had said that she did not belong in an insane asylum.   The schizophrenia shows itself, among other things, by the confused nonsense of her representations in court, the absolute incapacity for discussion and also, by the decline of the strength to work, and by the occasional incapacity for discussion even in her work.—All this counts all the more because she was formerly intelligent.

2. If catatonic symptoms are permanently in the foreground the picture is called *catatonia*.   A large part of these forms begins with an acute attack; under certain conditions the psychosis is revealed from one moment to another,—other cases begin with a chronic attack, with some catatonic peculiarities, e.g., mutism or mannerisms, and remain chronic, while in others chronic and acute conditions alternate.   Following acute catatonic attacks a tolerable condition may again recur; the cases that begin furtively all have a bad prognosis without any remissions that are worth mentioning.

Catatonic State. Nineteen years old. At first a bar-keeper; then he worked in many different places; at last in a dye factory. In spite of the fact that he was a Catholic, he had recently joined the Salvation Army. He came into a meeting in shabby, dirty clothes. He began to pray but very incoherently. He had learned something wonderful; Noah's ark was coming; he was compelled to speak. It was difficult to silence him. Then he told that he had previously run after the sun. In the factory he had refused to touch any other colored silk but white. Some days later he came to a musical rehearsal and began suddenly to read a psalm. He was requested to be silent. Suddenly he stood up, stood in front of the others and said with a staring expression: "Do you believe that the devil is tied? Do you believe that the devil is tied? He is tied; he is tied." He repeated the last words several times, becoming louder each time. When he saw that the others did not join in, he exclaimed: "You are enslaved; tomorrow I will go into the heart of the city and begin to pray." Then he became quiet again. The following day he did not come to dinner and began to pray in his room with a roaring voice. At night he went to a friend's room, stood there rigid in a peculiarly twisted pose, the one arm stretched out straight, the other held over the head, and made a stiff, peculiar face. Then he suddenly wanted to write in the friend's memorandum book. When the latter refused, he called him Judas. Had he come to betray Christ with a kiss? He tried with all his might to kiss him. He then got down on his knees and began to pray in a dreadfully loud voice. Getting up suddenly he said: "Now all is over," and had a normal expression but immediately continued that he was crucified, he had been called for something special, he was Christ. He told that when he was in bed a spirit had come from above and another from below, and a great power had come over him. He demanded that all present eat of his bread. Then they would understand him. When brought to the clinic, he quieted down quickly, became half aware of the impropriety of his conduct and thinking, but remained indifferent, did not want to leave the asylum, and had to be transferred to another.

Depressive Catatonia. Continuous hearing of voices. Teacher, who had previously seemed quite normal. At thirty-four for the first time he was irritated and sleepless, and occasionally had dizzy spells for a year; then there was a delirious stage. After a stay of twenty-eight weeks in a sanitorium he was "cured." After a year and a half he had a similar attack. Then he was once more a good teacher, felt well and cheerful. During a trip to Tyrol with friends when forty years old he felt that his ideas were getting hazy, he could not speak any longer, and again entered the sanatorium. Here he was in a stupor most of the time and believed they wanted to bury him alive. He had many hallucinations of hearing. He believed his dreams were real experiences, ate poorly, vomited. After a temporary improvement in the fifth month he wanted to go through the window, and reproached himself; at the command of the voices he threw his wedding ring out of the window, whereupon he was taken to the clinic. Here he lay in bed in a deep stupor, maintaining a peculiar position. He saw pictures on the wall, children and women, who were kissing; but most of all he heard voices and felt that something was being done to his body. He had threads about his hand, especially on the ring finger, that drew together. His penis was being operated on "so that the indecent sensations would disappear." The voices tell him that he had denied his God and had perpetrated a lust murder. "Lust murder is sexual desire." He is not a human being; he is decapitated. Depressed but rigid expression. Catatonic raptures; jumps up suddenly, breaks a window, etc. After eight months' duration of the attack there was a sudden reversal to a euphoric mood and orderly conduct: he spoke and wrote of his gratitude to his creator and the physicians, of how he was drawn to his home, how unutterably glad he was to stand again in the school room, a disciple of Pestalozzi, of the bursting energy of youth, and the plans of a returned spring tide, etc. But he did nothing to get out. Eleven months after the beginning of the attack he was discharged, took up his school work and for six years always remained euphoric and apparently a good teacher. Since then a similar attack, lasting only three months; then he returned to his former state. The voices warn him in school when he want to say something silly. Thus, objectively and subjectively, he gets along well.

Manic Catatonic. Unmarried woman, a chambermaid from a psychopathic family. Intelligent, has read much. Twenty-nine years old. After her mother's death she suffered from over-exertion and money losses. She believed falsely that a cousin wanted to marry her and always waited for him. After several months, manic excitations occurred which increased during eight days. She sang in an unseemly way, wrote a note to the effect that her brother-in-law should not bother her all night. Violent. She said she had to die all the time and was not being buried. She believed all men wanted to do her violence. Following moods of marked excitement, she cried. In the reception ward of the clinic she lay down on the floor and described a beautiful vision (ecstasy). Nevertheless she permitted herself to be diverted, and then she became completely oriented, felt very happy, declaimed that she had faith, which would help her withstand all trials, etc. She spoke in the same tone of the fact that she wanted to die; in the bath she tried to dive under the water. Then again for some time she remained rigid, the arms stretched upward, with a tense facial expression. When touched she jumped up enraged, stuck out her tongue, etc.; pronounced flight of ideas. At times the schizophrenic element could not be recognized in the manic; then again pathetic expressions that were repeated endlessly. The nurse was sometimes her brother, at others her sister and at the same time a third person. She was most quiet when isolated. Tore up a great deal. Indications of negativism; did not shake hands with the physician but handed him her cup that he should hold it. For a time she climbed about on the edge of the bed with a tense face and tightly pressed lips (she later maintained she had to play the part of a monkey). In the room she ran around in a circle, waved her hands to keep time. She has been made insane by powders; she was being electrocuted. After a while she quieted down; after six months she could be discharged, and by outsiders was considered cured. After another six months she returned in a similar condition. Now she became rapidly demented. Though she remained euphoric but irresponsible, she breaks windows, tears things, fights, turns somersaults, hears many voices, and becomes less and less capable of doing the simplest task. If one has voices, one calls it "Stirking." The voices say that one should "stirk," that is, one should "rattle" the windows.

Catatonia with Religious Delusions. A farm hand, twenty-one years old; came to the asylum because he had assaulted the minister of his village, as he declared because the minister had designated his own son as "Messiah," while the patient had in the last few years "undergone the Messiah's suffering" and now wanted to be the real Messiah. The patient had been a quiet, not unintelligent boy. A few years previously he had become pious, went often to the minister and recently had told, in writing and orally, of visions (angels, Messiah, and God). Once he demanded urgently that the minister change his (patient's) name, that is, take him as his son. In the asylum he at first spoke much of the minister and his family, but chiefly in another sense; even since his school days he had been in love with the minister's daughter. The angel materializations have the features of his daughter. The God materializations resembled in part the minister, in part the patient's grandfather. As Messiah he had the right of sexual intercourse with several women and with all the minister's daughters and also with his wife. Once he saw himself married to the daughter. Once the voice of one of the daughters called: "Oh, that he would kiss me with a kiss from his mouth." Later he hallucinated the daughters as being successively in his bed and having intercourse with them, wherein he experienced heavenly raptures. Occasionally he was also "Priest King" which signified possessor of the minister's daughters.—But he felt the minister's resistance more and more. He thought the latter wanted to leave him only his wife, and himself beget a Messiah with the daughters, so that the Messiahnic dignity would remain in his family. In materialization he saw the

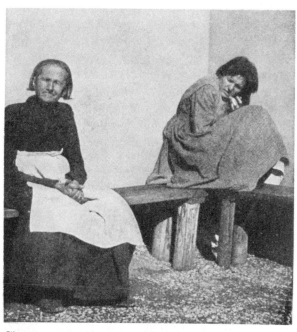

Fig. 36.—Chronic catatonic women. Both react to the taking of the picture with a sidelong glance. The patient at the left has a pronouncedly compressed mouth. The one crouching at the right half closes her eyes. The entire picture (aside from the attention to the picture taking) is one of continuous repose.

minister's daughters pregnant. A voice told him he should assault the minister. Finally he was impelled by the spirit to take a club and strike the minister, "because he would not let him have his daughters." In this connection his arms raised automatically.—As usual (or always?) the morbid religious aspirations are a symbol of sexual strivings. In addition another complex was satisfied: Tuberculosis raged in the family and the patient himself suffered from lung trouble; the penetration of the spirit within his breast at times made him well.

—The patient very quickly wove himself into his sexual religious phantasies, stood mute for several years in peculiar positions and died five years later of tuberculosis.

Catatonic after Castration. Wife of a physician. From a family of high standing but somewhat peculiar. At nineteen a fall from a stair. "Traumatic hysteria" of short duration. Engaged at twenty-two, while taking a walk she wanted to jump into the water because of a little discussion with her fiancé. During her first pregnancy often depressed. Bladder and bowel trouble without apparent cause. Always particular, but cheerful, was a little afraid of housework, excited when contradicted.—At twenty-eight "hysterical ovary trouble," later ovariotomy because of bilateral cystic degeneration with a normal recovery. At home after eight days she acted as usual. Then went to a resort to recuperate from which she returned depressed: She could no longer be a real woman and mother, she was a perjurer, justice was pursuing her, she saw and heard the district attorney, etc. Attempts at suicide. Then stupor, mutism, refusal of nourishment; *at intervals there are times when she speaks normally.* After several months she came to the asylum: mutistic but going about excited; at times she took the physician to be her husband, at times for the asylum physician. She heard her mother and children in the corridor. Rigid position for days, staring into the distance, mutistic. Between times excited, strove to get out of bed to the window or the washstand. Refusal of nourishment. Sees a horse's hoof. After a few days suddenly pleasant, clear concerning the environment, sensible conversation but often sudden obstructions. From now on continuous change of condition: sometimes quietly inhibited, at others excited; also clearer moments with conversation and music. She wants to write but sometimes does not get beyond the beginning. Expresses sometimes love, sometimes hate for the physician, both with a strong sexual element. Often retention of urine to the extent of catheterization. Frequent refusal of nourishment. Always many voices; her husband's head has been knocked off; she is at the North Pole; especially frequent is the idea, "I have been robbed; everything has been taken away from me, my money, my name." She feels a key in the genitals, wants to take the keys from the nurses. Her husband is married to the nurse. Then for several months incessant change between timid agitation with frequent violence, hits and bites, mild stupors. Scratches her face and feet. Special agitation on the anniversary of her marriage and on the anniversary of her last attempt at suicide. Later negativism, marked shrewishness, rigid face, uncertain walking, back and forth, usually without any purpose, then again times with verbigeration:

"he, he, he, now" or "no, no" or "de, de, de." After sixteen months she was discharged at first to a physician, then home. There she was very changeable, at times cheerful and apparently normal, then for hours verbigerating while walking up and down stairs; ran to the street, spoke to strange children as her own, then for days excited, violent. In the meantime at the table she can be the hostess to perfection. Sometimes unclean. After nine months she returned to the asylum where for years she has been very dissociated. Her mood is usually elevated but rigid. She is married to the doctors and all the other men of station. Goes through countless confinements. The nurses are at times her daughters, at times the wives of her husband, and should, therefore, be beaten. She prepares for her engagements to be married, in that she paints her eyelids and brows with shoe-blacking. She dresses her hair peculiarly. She has an engagement to sing Mignon. At other times she is continually under the bed-clothes.— Memory deceptions: The nurse once had an affair with her husband. Patient has once been proclaimed queen of Switzerland at Basle. Frequent mistaking of persons. After a while she became incapable of any work; nevertheless at intervals she still has good days when she occupies herself somewhat. Psychologically it is interesting that she always was peculiar. Her husband was ambivalent to her. (Attempt at suicide while taking her first walk with him. Depressions when her first child was born. Later her husband has been beheaded, has other wives. She has other husbands. When visiting she is hostile toward him, when staying at home she is usually very kind.) Hysteroid troubles of the ovaries after the fall, and after the births. After the castration there was an aggravation clearly connected with the mutilation; she is no longer a woman, no longer a mother. She has been robbed of everything, of the keys also, which are the symbol of the power of the house-wife but at the same time evidently of the genital of the man and of the man himself. The nurses have robbed her of the key and they have robbed her of her husband; these are identical for her. Then we observe the compensations: She marries the most distinguished men; she bears countless children, becomes young again as Mignon, becomes queen of Switzerland. Excitements during commemoration days.

Catatonia with a Cycle of Two Days. Intelligent girl, but always reserved, after puberty to a striking degree, in spite of a cheerful disposition. At twenty-four an apparently happy marriage with a very patient man; but she herself was stubborn and irritated. At the birth of the third child, being thirty-eight years old, a melancholic condition with ideas of sin; she had not taken care of the child. At forty-seven she lost her husband; for the first few days there was no reaction. Then a stuporous condition for two weeks in which she remained practically motionless, then changed into melancholia with unclear, fragmentary ideas of sin, she was being punished; heard many voices; very rigid expression; at intervals cataleptic; then attacks of fear with noise and a striving to get away. About a year later the patient begins to alternate regularly with days on which she is negativistically rigid and stubborn and others on which she is relatively approachable and pleasant, sits at the table and pulls silk. For a long time there was a three day cycle instead of a two day, there was one depressive-stuporous day, one irritable day, and one euphoric. Otherwise the two day cycle has lasted twelve years. Besides there is a negativism, varying in degree with different persons. She tries to shake hands but withdraws again; she is erotically jealous when others are greeted pleasantly; she is married to the physicians in the asylum. Very brief associations. An attempt to take her home had to be given up on the second (irritable) day.

Catatonia with Rapid Dementia. Teacher. The mother was temporarily and is now again in an asylum; in the interval latent schizophrenia for about twenty years. The patient was always somewhat peculiar; at school uneven; many pranks; kept to himself very much. Busied himself with different problems, such as socialism, and Schiller's Robbers. Was apprenticed to store-keeper but did not stay long. Then worked in various places. Once for nine months in a business school, then he went to a high school. Once went suddenly to Berlin where he stayed a month without doing anything. Then he entered a normal school in another canton, where he managed to stay for the final examination (age twenty-two). At first he was a teacher in a private institute, then in a primary school which he had to leave because the pupils did not learn anything and "had nose-bleed if he merely touched them." Then he wandered about Zürich and was arrested and brought to the clinic because he broke into a tramway station to sleep there, although all his brothers lived in the neighborhood. At first he was entirely indifferent, then much excited. Presented at the clinic he came in laughing loudly with his hand to his nose. During the recital of a story he saw on the table the story of the "Miser's Piece," and then wove a disconnected word mixture with the word "Miser." When coaxed he becomes quiet, lets himself drop heavily into a chair, sits there disinterested. Then he rocks on the chair, smiles to himself, suddenly remains rigid and stares in front of himself. Then he gets up, makes a lot of noise, sits down. When I described his conduct he remarked: "That is so." At the mention of word mixtures he added, "It is an Italian ox-mouth dish. The only thing in the room is worms. I am the director of the seminar. ("Where are we?") In an evolving hemisphere. C'est monsieur Jardin. I am a patient. That is a palandes versus plassus." Stands up and stamps hard on the platform, screams in an oratorical tone: "Oh, my dear Blapsen, you are my dearest Klapsen." He must go away; he walks away singing quietly, "One has left." Hops down from the platform, makes a lot of faces, lies on the floor, permits himself to be shoved and smiles blandly. After this he remains mostly quiet, and mute; he stays in all sorts of positions, partly in bed, partly up. Makes all sorts of faces. Once he urinated in front of the toilet-door; then he made a noise and prattled absolutely disconnected nonsense. To a visiting schoolmate he never said a word. Once he fell down suddenly and lay there quite rigid for some time; flexibilitas cerea. Then again he made extremely affected speeches of incomprehensible word salad. After a while he became quieter, sat around, sometimes verbigerating. For a long time he asked the visiting physician the stereotype question: "Isn't Aunt Grite coming yet?" To the aunt he wrote:

> Today, in the seventh
> of July, 1914.

To our dear Aunt Grite
          from
Hans Jacob and Max.
Dear Kind Aunt Schüfeli:

I hope you no longer have to work so hard for the capitalists in St. Gall; because here in Burghölzli (hospital) I still hope to find in the socialistic centre of the world in Zürich—wiedikon, a position as upper grade teacher for Italian children; although I was brought here against my will per (police automobile) "by the watch dog of clericalism for the Zürich ministers (K)" and here I have to perform work of not the least use; although it is known that I am a licensed practicing teacher of the Swiss Confederation.

Brother Hans has helped me in forming the sentences of this letter as he is as you are aware a very faithful abstinent resembling you personally and individually more than I.

Signaturely I can only then excuse it as I got here in a milieu, in which my own love of nature was violently stolen only with technical devilish means and in contradiction to the laws of the milieu. So long as I don't get the power over these "accursed" laws and conditions (As Hans calls them) I can accept them only hypothetically as technical-devilism."

Chronic Catatonia. A good house-wife of retiring disposition, marked by few peculiarities, begins to speak less and less and in the course of a few months ceases to speak altogether. Notwithstanding this she takes care of her housework very properly for another year. Then other difficulties appear: she becomes irritated, untidy; negativism prevents her from doing just what she should do, or she does it wrong. In the hospital she at first works very decently, keeping silent, but loses more and more weight, becomes more negativistic, unclean, tears things up, begins to fight and after about three years sinks into a state of stolid negativism so that she remains only an object of care, and rather difficult care at that. Among other things she had taken on some mannerisms, had some hallucinatory excitements in which she scolded loudly.

3. *Schizophrenics with accessory symptoms* of different kinds and varying strength have retained the old name Hebephrenia, although it no longer fits the present conception.

The *Kahlbaum-Hecker* Hebephrenia was a dementia which began relatively quickly at the time of puberty; it usually ran its course with various affective disturbances, e.g. it began with a manic attack, and besides, as was supposed, was further characterized by the symptoms of callow youth, that is affectation, pathetic expressions and mimicry, delight in boyish pranks on the one side, affectation of mature wisdom and the desire to be occupied with the highest problems on the other. But we can also find these symptoms in schizophrenias of other varieties that break out late, if their complexes signify an attempt at self-elevation and being great.

In the present conception of hebephrenia the age of the onset is unimportant, even though most of the cases become sick during and soon after puberty. It now constitutes the big trough into which are thrown the forms that cannot be classed with the other three forms.

Hebephrenia with Manic and Depressive Attacks. She had lost her mother early and was brought up in an institution where she remained as an attendant. Always retiring and rather particular but with pleasant manners. At thirty-six, when the father had to be taken care of, she reproached herself for not doing enough for him and that she had sinned by him. There was no improvement after a stay at a sanitarium; thoughts of suicide; once she stole around a fish pond, remained all night in the woods and then returned unobserved to her asylum. When brought to the clinic, she at first seemed rather stiff and apathetic, then depressed, but complained that she was the poorest of all the inmates, lost and abandoned by God and man. She did not sleep and was confused in the head. The upper part of her face looked depressed, the lower was rather smiling. She showed frequent obstructions. There were many voices. Stereotype striking about with the arms. She identified various things, e.g. the different physicians with one another. She was only three days old. The first day was "when the first immoral act occurred" as a small child, "the second corresponded with the second immoral act, the third is the present when she has to die." She is also "here three days or three weeks." The director of Burgholzli is also the head of her former institution. Whomever she sees now, she has seen previously but as another person. All mankind must become different (probably first as a very small child). The body is poisoned. She will be murdered and the murderers will go unpunished; at first she will be put in hot water and then cut into pieces. Her sins have earned immortality for her. Incessant voices concerning which she can give no account. Obstructions. To indifferent questions she gives prompt replies. Many paresthesias of the intestines. In the course of a year gradual improvement up to complete capacity for work. Two years later, twenty-nine years old, there was a manic attack, in which she gossiped about her relation with the director of the institution so that he lost his position. As a manic depressive she was brought from another institution to us but after one month she could already be discharged. A year later she returned in a manic condition after having been at different places. She states she had worked too hard, had had stomach bleedings, had been contradicted too much; she wants everybody to obey her. Rigid mania with dancing and singing, tearing of clothes and scolding. But her face does not change whether she jokes or scolds. After half a year she could again be discharged and remained away fourteen months. Then she merged in a new euphoric mood with great indifference toward the commitment and everything that happened or was said to her. At times she was extremely manic, noisy, smearing and tearing. She began consciously to annoy physicians and nurses. At intervals she was again very decent. Between laughter she can suddenly cry. "She would not marry Doctor M. (former asylum physician)." After seven months in a rest resort she was discharged, returned a year later for the fifth time with rigid euphoria from which she soon calmed down. She has now sat about for years inactive but quiet.

Depressive Hebephrenia. Nurse. Pleasant, intelligent girl. Refused several offers of marriage; she was afraid of marriage, of births. Nevertheless she blames her sister because of the latter's warnings for the cause of the failure of a certain relationship with a man. From her twenty-ninth to her thirty-second year she was with us as a conscientious nurse. Because of physical diseases she resigned and then held various other positions. After a while she became tired, sensitive, considered herself annoyed, in part rightly so, because she angered others because of her irritability. She felt herself getting weaker and weaker; work became too hard for her. When she was to take over another ward in the hospital where she worked, she became afraid and left. She was dissatisfied with the reference. She planned suicide and consequently at thirty-seven was brought to us. Here she was more or less depressed, had entertained mild ideas of reference. Now and then she heard some voices, was at times bothered by memories of her youth that crowded up in her. Then she was better; she was afraid to leave the hospital; but after thirteen months she could be discharged to take a position. She did her work well but soon found it too hard, took several other positions, but could make up her mind with difficulty and after eight months had to be brought back to the clinic. She had lost much of her energy, had a certain insight into her disease but only at times, spent much time in bed, worked little. Work was too much of a strain for her; at times she spoke listlessly of going away, but was always afraid when it came to the point, was very sensitive even toward her relatives. After about a year she was again discharged. Since then she has been in different positions but has been in difficulties (four years).

Hebephrenia with Transition to the Paranoid Form. As a child somewhat apathetic. Lost her parents early. While in a foreign boarding school a "nervous disease" appeared for which she was treated unsuccessfully for a year, with persuasion. But she was seized with a morbid feeling for the physician and had to be taken away from him almost with force. She came to another physician's house, then to a relative where she busied herself with house-work. At twenty-four she went to England to board where she had several sentimental and pious friendships. "For convalescence and also for work" she returned to Switzerland at thirty-three, then went to a relative in America, let a friend of his cheat her of her money, but returned in time to Switzerland, because she had lung trouble. Later she was operated for an intestinal growth. In the hospital she was depressed and cut her throat with a pen-knife, whereupon at thirty-five she was admitted to the clinic. Here she was fearful, liked to stand at the door in her shirt, called to everybody that passed that she had to go on the street in her shirt. Finally she did not want to put anything on, tore her shirts because they were too beautiful. She had to be tube fed, and slept very little. When the door opened, she always thought now some one was coming to torture her to death. She did not want to urinate because she was being watched through the windows. Active auditory and somatic hallucinations concerning which, however, she spoke little. After four months she was somewhat quieter. But the voices forbade her to speak loudly. She always was glad to return from visiting relatives. The voices tell her they are not the right relatives. She has to be assured that she has not a cat and a dog in her bowels. During sleep she is transported to many places, once with the room and all to a river, then again to a place where there is snow. "The furniture has wilted because of the rays from her green eyes." After a while the sad mood changes to a mildly manic which in the course of a year makes way for a very apathetic one, but always with brief fluctuations upward and downward. She is to be destroyed purposely, she hears many voices, mistakes people, is afraid to go into the open where there are people who shoot her; the physicians do dreadful things to her body. Nevertheless with mild protesting she is very pleasant, as far as her indifference permits. The friend from America, in the form of a nurse, has sneaked up to her. She is given poison and disagreeable things to eat. Her uncle was in a tree opposite her window and wanted to shoot her; but an angel protected her. She is being hypnotized, cats' eyes have been put into her. The nurses talk about her. Her passport has been forged. An illegitimate child has been put over on her. Men, dressed as nurses, come in, bind her, hit her on the head, hypnotize her, pour poison into her eyes, throw stones at her. Aside from this she is very quiet, busies herself with womanly tasks and copying.

Hebephrenia with Fatal Results. Intelligent business woman. At nineteen a melancholic depression. Afterwards a good worker but never very energetic. At thirty-eight work became too much for her. Attacks of insomnia, anxiety, and reticence; when making purchases she often could not find words at all, or could not speak on other occasions. Then showed ideas of fearful observation and reference. A stay in a private institution did not help, nor did her leaving it help any. After two years the patient was brought to the clinic, where within a few days she became euphoric. At the same time she was indifferent, untidy, concealed books, played a few bars from sheets of music and then threw them on the floor, etc. Nevertheless she maintained herself in the best ward where she worked a little without doing much. Once she wrote home a verbigerating letter. An attempt to take her to her family failed since she did not work at all and was very untidy, did not even dress herself and did not comb her hair. Brought back to the asylum she remained mildly euphoric but always worked less, became more and more untidy, kneeled or lay down on the floor when she thought herself alone. She endeavored to give her laziness an aristocratic tone. Later she was occasionally unclean, deposited her feces in unsuitable places. After a stay of six years in all, being forty-five, she rather suddenly became anxiously depressed with a desire to go away, to hold on to things, to make a noise in long and endlessly repeated sentences; with this there was sexual excitation. In the course of two months there was a return to the status quo ante. But soon she became sick again with fever without any physical signs. She had a temperature of 104° F., which subsided after five days and gave way to subnormal temperatures (down to 96.8° F.) Her strength failed rapidly. To be sure her pulse even shortly before her death was noticeably strong, not rapid but often irregular. Rigidness of the neck (or negativism); patella reflex very changeable, at times diminished, at times exaggerated. No Babinski. Several times analgesia. Rapidly spreading decubitus in spite of all preventive measures. Coma. Death after a duration of twelve days of the entire acute stage. In the brain, nothing was found maroscopically; microscopically marked increase of the glia in the cerebrum in all parts without any changes in the ganglion cells.

Schizophrenic Hypochondria. Very able farmer's girl, intellectually and physically above the average; for obvious reasons she did not have much schooling. Father and grandfather had suffered for years with "stomach cramps." Patient was a very good silk weaver; she had the more difficult work as well as the accounting; she lived with her brother. She positively refused offers of marriage; "she could not make up her mind,"—"was afraid of marriage." A few intimate friendships with girls; even in the asylum she composed a poem of "friendship" that betrayed strong homosexual components. When she was forty-seven, her brother died. Now she was "overworked," and had stomach trouble, soon had to give up altogether. She went from one doctor to another, obtained the most different diagnoses, stomach and bowel weakness, decay in the stomach, membranous colitis, multiple gall stones, cirrhosis of the liver, floating kidney, later also hysteria. The medicines that she took "were poison to her" and with electrical treatment, massage, persuasion and other nice things, within a few years wasted her fortune of 10,000 francs so that she became a public charge. At last she came to us from another asylum where they could not get along with her. She was fifty-four years old, physically perfect and strong. She complained about sluggishness of the bowels, blocking of all secretions, enlarged womb, which presses on the bowels, the contents of which were rotting; terrible pains, valvular trouble of the heart, etc., etc. Treatment by ignoring or diverting her brought it about in the six years that she was with us that she again worked daily and usually resigned herself not to ask for treatment. Nevertheless with the reservation that we did not understand her serious malady. If one speaks to her about her disease, she scolds about her suffering and the treatment. But within a few seconds she can be made erotically friendly. For instance, she lies there half dead in pain; one asks her to dance and she joins in until she is dizzy. While talking about the disease she sometimes has a pronounced paranoid look and always a strong *Veraguth* sign; both disappear immediately when she is diverted. Once I let myself be persuaded to give her a laxative because she maintained she never had a movement. She persisted in maintaining this in spite of several stools daily; she got a little thin —and never complained as much as at this time. She did not return from a walk, and has since remained with relatives (two years). She masturbated very much. Distinguished from hysteria: Complete indifference to everything that does not belong to her disease, *and to the disease* also if she is not given the opportunity to talk about it. The only rapport with her is concerning the disease and then it is of a simple erotic nature which is in marked contrast with her intelligence in other respects and her good manners. In the ward she lived on entirely dereistically without making herself noticeable, associating altogether with the other schizophrenics. If she complained of the nurses, she did not make a scene. Sometimes she plainly showed rigid affects. The hypochondrical delusions were too senseless for a hysteria. Absolute inability to discuss or be influenced in regard to her disease (the slight improvement was only gained by indirect means).—Psychically, her libido remained attached to her brother, to whom she usually associates, as soon as she talks of marriage. In contrast with her usual indifference toward everything that does not concern her disease, she can cry when she remembers him. When he died, she lost all emotional connection; work also became too much for her; "over-exertion" with subjective troubles of the stomach and bowels. Some chance remarks of the patient indicate almost certainly that the imagined uterus enlargement sprang from the desire for children and that the bowels, as is frequently the case, represent the uterus.

Hebephrenia with Alcoholism. Baker and formerly a saloon keeper. Medium intelligence. Always given to rage, is coarse. At twenty-six he had his own business, which gradually declined. At thirty-eight he heard voices, became anxious, barricaded the doors; at night looked for man that pursued his wife; found her bed in disorder, suddenly saw heads. Attempted suicide for the reason that his license would be withdrawn, because many unclean things walked in his saloon. For this reason he was brought to the hospital; came home improved, drank nothing for a while, worked well but reproached his wife for having been interned. Then he began to drink again, again had the jealousy ideas, but only when he was drunk. Worked irregularly. Because of violence, he was again brought to the clinic. He could not understand a fable clearly, had all sorts of drunkard's excuses, but was less capable of discussion than ordinary drunkards, and sometimes made very peculiar movements. Affectivity was at first still labile: tears in his eyes over the interning, then again rigid and indifferent. Now and then peculiar movements. After seven days he went to another hospital with the diagnosis of hebephrenia and alcoholism. From there he was discharged after twelve weeks. This time, too, at first everything went well for a short time while he abstained from alcohol, then he continually became worse. Jealousy delusions and acts directed against the wife. He had to give up his business because, while drunk, he threw bread and other things out of the window and insulted his customers. He worked as a baker's assistant and then for weeks not at all. Now and then it was noticed that he did not speak. The jealousy ideas became steadily worse. In the vilest words he asked the children about his wife's infidelity. Furthermore, he laid match sticks together in a particular way and said mysteriously that meant something. Because of maltreatment of the wife he was brought back (aged forty-seven). On admission he showed complete blocking. Later acted as formerly. After a few days he went to another hospital. The next year he was brought in again with mutism, and compressed lips. On the outside he had called attention to himself by all sorts of senseless acts; e.g. he had stood in front of the street car and had waved his handkerchief. Discharged again, he was conspicuous, worked very little, made all sorts of faces so that people were afraid of him, beat his wife and children. Nevertheless only after nearly five years he was returned in a state of alcoholic and schizophrenic dementia. He was transferred to another hospital.

4. Where only the basic symptoms are visible, we speak of *schizophrenia simplex* (the primary dementia of earlier authors). It is usually a case of a dementia in the sense of schizophrenia that increases gradually in the course of decades. The anamnesis invariably indicates that the disease has been mistaken for many years; it was a latent schizophrenia. But since this form also, like every other, need not progress to the point of recognizable dementia, there are undoubtedly latent schizophrenias, too, that never become manifest. One not

rarely meets with it in relatives of the manifestly diseased, or in visits with patients who come because of some "nervous" trouble.

Schizophrenia Simplex. Teacher. Intelligent but always somewhat peculiar, retiring, had various hobbies. At school in the course of time matters became worse. His discipline relaxed. But not until he was fifty was it pointed out to him that matters could not go on in that way. Instead of seeing it in this way, he demanded several increases in salary from the authorities. At last he had to resign and then entered into incessant litigations "about his rights"; the authorities had to get him a good position. He was completely incapable of seeing the material and formal impossibility of this fulfillment. At last he threatened to thrash the authorities, and was sent to the clinic as dangerous. Here he permitted himself to be somewhat calmed externally, and after eight months could again be discharged. On the outside he has been getting along for nearly twenty years, by occupying himself with subordinate farm work.

Kraepelin recently formulated a somewhat more exhaustive grouping:

1. *Dementia simplex,* corresponding to the hitherto established group. 2. *Foolish dementia,* corresponding generally to the Hebephrenia of *Hecker* and well designated by the name. 3. *Simple depressive* or *stuporous dementia* often has a preliminary stage lasting for years in which the patients retire, become peculiar, and brood. Only in about twenty percent does a milder schizophrenic depression with ideas of sin and persecution and often too with catatonic symptoms break out without such an introduction. A fairly large number of the patients afterwards merge into a tolerable condition without severe dementia; but the attacks may recur. The stuporous dementia includes many of our catatonics with a depressive stage, but perhaps also the Hebephrenics. 4. *Depressive dementia* with delusional formation have similar symptoms but on the average run a more chronic course, have a somewhat worse prognosis and show the delusions more conspicuously. 5. In the *circular form* excitations and depressions alternate; they usually lead to severer dementia. (There is another formation to which, perhaps, this name might better apply, since it runs its course in evident manic and depressive attacks which are sharply differentiated from better intervening states, or from those which, in the beginning, are very good). 6. In the *agitated form* one observes continuous excitements with compulsive acts, senseless movements and a general exalted mood. (This form seemed to Kraepelin the most frequent with the natives of Java.) 7. Forms with periodic attacks of confused excitation that usually begin and end very acutely, which

usually do not last long, only a few weeks, and are combined with a marked loss of weight. Not rarely they are associated with menstruation. 8. *Catatonia,* including the severer cases of the disease hitherto designated by this name by *Kraepelin.* 9. The *paranoid forms,* corresponding to our paranoids and divided into *dementia paranoides gravis* with a severe decay of the psychic life, disturbances of the feelings and will, as well as loss of external bearing, and into *paranoid or hallucinatory feeble-mindedness,* in which the hallucinations are in the foreground, but in which the fundamental personality has suffered less (dementia paranoides mitis). 10. As the tenth form, speech confusion (*schizophasia*) should be distinguished, running its course with very severe speech disturbance up to a complete word salad, but with relatively slight impairment of the other faculties, so that the patients are still fairly capable of work, at least within the asylums.

E. The Course

It is impossible to describe all the various courses of schizophrenia. Pretty nearly all imaginable combinations of courses may occur except the recession of a severe dementia. Nevertheless two types recur with special frequency; the course which is chronic from beginning to end, that requires many years for development, and the manifest type, beginning with an acute onset, and leaving behind secondary demented or paranoid states. But the acute syndrome need not leave behind an increase of the dementia, and on the other hand, the dementia as well as the formation of delusions may progress after, as well as between, the acute attacks. Forms taking an entirely chronic course belong especially to the simple schizophrenia and to certain catatonic ways of manifestation, also to the typical paranoid forms.

In every course exacerbations may appear at any time, but after the disease has lasted from two to three decades they are pretty rare. Complete arrests of the diseases are not frequent in asylum patients. In the course of decades an increase of the dementia can usually be noted. Among the more mildly afflicted, who maintain themselves outside of asylums, some seem not to go beyond a certain stage of the disease.

Improvements also may occur at every stage; but they relate primarily, to the accessory symptoms. Schizophrenic dementia itself no longer actually regresses. But to be sure all acute syndromes show a tendency to disappear, and chronic hallucinations and delusions may also regress, though much more rarely. *Psychoses which, from the beginning, run a course with a picture of a chronic catatonia, are quite hopeless.* Excited patients calm down as a rule in the course of years, in part because inwardly and outwardly they become used to the hallucinations and to the dissociation, or also because the sense deceptions decline in numbers and intensity.

The sudden and transient akalmias in the severe acute as well as in the chronic conditions are noteworthy. A highly excited, especially a confused, patient may, with or without external cause, appear entirely normal from one minute to the next, only to fall back after hours or days into the previous condition.

The qualitative course is somewhat more regular; the majority of cases from the beginning to the end remain within their category, even though a change from catatonic to paranoid forms and in every other direction is more frequent than in the various forms of paresis.

The *beginning of schizophrenia* is in reality usually furtive. Even though the disease often becomes obvious to the relatives first through an acute attack, a good anamnesis usually reveals certain previous changes of character, or other schizophrenic signs. Whether the inclination to retirement, often noticeable even in childhood, combined with a certain degree of irritability, is an expression of a disposition, or the actual beginning of the disease, cannot be decided. In many cases the disease itself makes itself felt by a gradual decline of acquired skill and of capacity to work; *in others, neurasthenic, hysteric, or compulsive neurotic symptoms are for years mistaken for the disease and treated unsuccessfully.* Anomalies of character and single immediate acts are much more conspicuous.

In a small number (under one percent) the *outcome* is death from cerebral inflammation or from the cessation of metabolism. Other patients die from the indirect consequences of schizophrenia, from injuries that are intended, or result from carelessness, and suicide. Usually phthisis is also mentioned but with satisfactory hygienic measures it is no more to be feared in asylums than in those mentally sound.

A small part is "cured" to such extent that only a very careful inspection shows any signs of the disease; one may observe a certain irritability, some remnants of the delusions, some peculiarities, etc. Nevertheless there are a great many "social cures." Under the conditions in our hospital one can figure that only about one third of the more severely demented and more than half of the others remain fairly capable of work for a considerable time, or permanently. Catatonia, especially in men, has a somewhat poorer prognosis than the other forms; pupillary symptoms also seem to occur chiefly in the more serious brain affections; and whenever it is ascertained that the patient showed previously an "abnormal" character the prognosis is less favorable. The twilight states regress the more completely, the purer they are. But aside from what was said we unfortunately have no basis at the beginning of the disease for the prognosis of its duration.

Terminations according to Kraepelin

Among the terminations *Kraepelin* mentions the following forms, which naturally are not clearly defined from one another.

1. In *simple feeble-mindedness* the defects above all influence the affectivity, whereby a certain ability to work is retained. 2. *Hallucinatory feeble-mindedness* is similar, but is permanently accompanied by individual sense deceptions the nature of which the patients recognize more or less, so that their external conduct may, in the main, still be orderly. 3. The *dementia paranoides mitis* is characterized by delusions and hallucinations, which, as distinguished from the previous group, are very numerous. 4. The *drivelling dementia* shows a severer unsteadiness of the train of thought with senseless delusions and senseless speech. 5. The *dull dementia* approaches the quiet of the grave, even though individual patients perform simple tasks, and occasionally excitations and more positive symptoms like stereotypisms, etc., are hardly ever entirely absent. 6. The *silly dementia* expresses itself in greater activity with a usually cheerful mood and silly actions. 7. The *dementia with mannerisms* is similar; here, however, peculiar deflections of volitional acts (like hopping about on one leg, stereotype positions, etc.) stand in the foreground of the morbid picture. 8. *Negativistic dementia* is characterized by the strength of the impulsive resistances.

F. What Is Included under the Term

Under schizophrenia are included many atypical melancholias and manias of other schools (especially nearly all "hysterical" melancholias and manias), most hallucinatory confusions, much that is elsewhere called amentia (our idea of amentia is much narrower), a part of the forms consigned to delirium acutum, motility psychoses of *Wernicke*, primary and secondary dementias without special names, most of the paranoias of the other schools, especially all hysterically crazy, nearly all incurable "hypochondriacs," some "nervous people" and compulsive and impulsive patients. The diseases especially distinguished as juvenile and masturbatory forms all belong here, also a large part of the puberty psychoses, and the degeneration psychoses of *Magnans*. Many prison psychoses and the Ganser twilight states are acute syndromes based on a chronic schizophrenia. If we still come across reactive psychoses included under this head, then it is due to defective diagnoses, not to the classification of a system.

Latent schizophrenias are very common under all conditions so that the "disease" schizophrenia has to be a much more extensive term than the pronounced psychosis of the same name. This is important for studies of heredity. At what stage of the anomaly any one should be designated as only a "schizoid" psychopathic, or as a schizophrenic mentally diseased, cannot at all be decided as yet. At all events, the name latent schizophrenia will always make one think of a morbid psychopathic state, in which the schizoid peculiarities are within normal limits. Social uselessness, catatonic symptoms, hallucinations, delusions make certain the practical diagnosis of the acute mental disease.

Paraphrenias. Kraepelin attempted to separate from the paranoid forms of schizophrenia, as a special morbid group, those in whom the personality was better retained, and whose feelings, will, and the external behavior are directly slightly changed; the incorrect actions are determined by delusions. In the *paraphrenia systematica* more or less connected delusions are conspicuous; they show, in the first place, the character of persecution, but later, beginning with a definite period, they become associated with grandiose ideas. *Paraphrenia expansiva* presents a light manic lasting mood, and, corresponding with it, luxurious ideas of grandeur from the very beginning. In *paraphrenia confabulatoria* the delusions appear as memory deceptions. The *paraphrenia phantastica* (paranoid dementia in the old narrow sense) [85] frequently develops even in a few months into quite a stable picture with a number of alternating senseless ideas of grandeur and persecution, with an enormous number of somatic hallucinations, often quite senseless speech, but a less conspicuous outward behavior, and under care a more or less continued productive capacity. A diagnostic differentiation of the paraphrenias from the other acute or chronic mild paranoid forms was never possible. Moreover our investigations, as well as the course and heredity, show the definite relationship of most, if not all these cases, to the schizophrenias.[86]

G. Combination of Schizophrenia with Other Diseases

Schizophrenia may be combined with other psychoses; it may undoubtedly originate on top of oligophrenias (Propfschizophrenia),[87]

---

[85] See p. 413.

[86] Comp. Schizophrenia, p. 177.

[87] Moreover, many Propfschizophrenias represent probably a distinct disease. At all events intercourse with most of these patients is maintained by way of the affects.

and may be followed by senile psychoses. Occasionally also a paresis, more frequently alcoholism, eventually with delirium tremens or hallucinosis, complicate the picture. There is probably also a mixture of manic-depressive insanity, and of epilepsy with schizophrenia. The associations of these two diseases with dementia præcox are undoubtedly multiform and not at all clear, no more than the delimitation of the combined from the simple forms with only apparent mixture symptoms.

H. Diagnosis

The diagnosis of schizophrenia in the ordinary cases is very easy. The peculiar, moody, abrupt, and scanty affective rapport often points to the disease at the first glance; furthermore, the inability to discuss matters that deal with subjects that the patient is otherwise conversant with. Also many accessory symptoms like the above described delusions, the hallucinations characteristic in their way, especially the physical sensations, pronounced catatonic symptoms, all make possible a quick recognition. If the examination does not yield definite indications one should carefully ask whether there are people who annoy the patient, whether there is anybody in his neighborhood who is hostile to him. Often a secretive persecutory mania will then come to light. *But nowhere as much as in schizophrenia are all individual symptoms to be evaluated in terms of their entire psychic environment.* In case of cloudiness of consciousness the identical manifestations are not nearly so valuable as evidence as in the case of apparent clearness. Catalepsy also occurs in epilepsy, in hysteria, then again in cerebral diseases, and as a concomitant manifestation of bodily diseases, e.g. uremia in children. In negativism the impulsive variety has to be differentiated from those forms of rejection based on other reasons. In any schizoid character any other psychoses can easily bring to light a few schizophrenic symptoms.[88] Beginners are then easily inclined to see only the schizophrenia. Of the physical symptoms only the lack of psychical pupillary reaction has a more definite significance. *One may never directly exclude a schizophrenia.*

Only prolonged observation will often guard against confusing schizophrenia with *manic-depressive insanity.* All manic-depressive symptoms may appear in schizophrenia but not the specific schizophrenia symptoms in the former disease. The simultaneous existence of grandiose ideas and depressive delusions indicates schizophrenia. From *paresis* and *dementia senilis* it is definitely differentiated by the absence of the signs of the organic psychoses (eventually by the exam-

[88] Comp. p. 177.

ination of the cerebro-spinal fluid). Coarse cerebral lesions may sometimes simulate a schizophrenic picture for a considerable time. A stupor may occur in an *imbecile* as a result of an unusual situation, e.g. in case of a judicial examination. From *epilepsy* it is differentiated especially by the striking schizophrenic anomalies of the affects, then on the other hand by the absence of the epileptic hesitating mental trend, the epileptic speech, and by the adhesiveness of the feelings. In the anamnesis of epilepsy the picture is usually dominated by the attacks, in the dementia præcox, even when attacks are present, it is dominated by the psychic disturbances. Epileptic catalepsy usually persists only a short time, e.g. a fractional part of an hour, never a month, as the schizophrenic. In epileptic cloudings of consciousness, especially when brain lesions are the basis of the disease, paresthesias sometimes occur which are elaborated in a dream-like manner and may simulate schizophrenic hallucinations of the organs. The various *alcoholic* psychoses not rarely originate on a schizophrenia which they then complicate. The differentiation from *hysteria and neurasthenia*, which at the beginning of the disease involves many pitfalls, is negative, as in manic-depressive insanity. As psychogenic symptoms occur in all three diseases, we presuppose schizophrenia when specific symptoms of this disease are demonstrated; we presuppose hysteria and neurasthenia when a minute examination has brought to light hysterical or neurasthenic but no schizophrenic symptoms. Dementia, disturbance of ideas, auditory hallucinations and permanent delusions with unclouded consciousness exclude the neurosis.[89]

Especially difficult is the delimitation of reactive syndromes, or logical peculiarities in *psychopaths*. As yet we have no standard to tell us how pronounced the symptoms must be to enable us to assume, or exclude, a schizophrenic process. In these cases one will assume schizophrenia only when more definite signs of it are present, but will be careful not to want "to exclude" it. Young people are nearly always schizophrenic who want to become something out of the ordinary just at the time that they are really failing, and who then believe that by particular tricks (thinking out something to the end, etc.) they can free themselves from the situation and then neglect the essential thing in favor of the means.

Oligophrenics who get symptoms that are of a paranoid nature or similar to those of catatonia are sometimes impossible to differentiate, because just here the diagnostic standard for such manifestations and even the limitation in principle of oligophrenia[90] are still uncertain.

---

[89] Compare the differential diagnosis in chapter on hysteria.
[90] Comp. paranoia, limitation.

I. Prognosis

The course of the disease runs in the direction of the described dementias. The special *directional prognosis* is decided with some probability by the assignment of a case to one of the sub-groups. The *extent prognosis* is much more uncertain. Many cases after the first shift, under certain conditions even later, show such a slight defect that they may be considered practically cured; others become demented quickly and to a high degree. To the latter belong with certainty all chronically beginning catatonias, probably also the rarer cases of mental confusion in the sense previously explained. All acute syndromes may regress to the former state. Very severe acute conditions with profound disturbances of consciousness are, therefore, not in themselves hopeless. But the cardinal symptoms regress very little, and of these, the disturbances of association least of all. In acute conditions the most important consideration is to determine how far the actual schizophrenic process has progressed. The more the schizophrenic picture of associative and affective disturbance protrudes from behind the transient acute symptoms, moods, stupor, and hallucinations, the worse the prognosis; the more a picture resembles a pure mania or melancholia, the better the prognosis. Naturally this does not make it very good because this observation only determines that as yet no dementia has set in, but not that it cannot set in. The anamnesis also often gives important basic points. Good remissions after earlier shifts warrant, with considerable probability, the expectation of another extensive improvement. On the other hand, the confirmation of an extensive dementia already existing before the actual shift excludes any considerable improvement, because improvements over the earlier conditions are only rarely found after an acute onset; exacerbations of the various grades are very common.

A favorable sign, especially plain in women, is the retention of decency in acute conditions, while a visible loss of the feeling of decency in a clear sensorium and otherwise orderly conduct is a sign of poor prospects. But the reverse inference would not be at all justified, namely, that absence of a feeling of decency in acute conditions indicates a bad outcome, and that the presence of decency in a state of mental clearness indicates a good one.

Actual chronic conditions are capable of little improvement; only we do not always know what is chronic. There are patients who for many years are at the same stage of excitement but still give the impression, more or less, of being acute and are then again surprisingly capable of improvements; after ten or twenty years in rarer cases, apparently entirely unsocial patients may be discharged as again capable of work. Moreover the increase of dementia is often to be taken externally as an improvement; the patients gradually become more indifferent toward their delusions and voices and consequently quieter; under certain conditions they even become more capable of work. In many cases the hallucinations decline after a while to the point of disappearance.

The tendency to relapses is hardly to be estimated. The longer an interval lasts, the less a new shift is to be feared. After a standstill of two decades there may still be a quietly progressing decrease of ability to work but only rarely new attacks. The climacterium, pregnancies, and especially the puerperium, present a certain danger to women.

K. Causes

Great importance is undoubtedly to be attached to *hereditary burdening*. Among the direct ancestors of the patients, psychoses, especially schizophrenia, are much more numerous than with the healthy. Most frequently one find in families schizoid characters, people who are shut-in, suspicious, incapable of discussion, people who are comfortably dull and at the same time sensitive, people who in a narrow manner pursue vague purposes, improvers of the universe, etc. Naturally nervous diseases also occur in the families of schizophrenics, *often because many milder schizophrenics are so called.* Some family relationships with a certain kind of epilepsy, that as yet cannot be characterized more definitely, seem to be present. Besides there are schizophrenias where an hereditary disposition is not to be found in spite of exact information concerning the family.

In probably three fourths of the cases the *personal disposition* already expresses itself during youth in an dereistic character inclined to seclusion, then in other peculiarities and deviations from normal thinking. A small percent of the pronounced diseases themselves go back into childhood. Most of them become manifest from puberty up to the twenty-fifth year; from thirty on, the morbidity sinks rapidly to rise again, in women, to a low second peak at the time of the climacterium. Only the chronic paranoid forms show a preference for breaking out rather late, especially around the fourth decade.

Among the external conditions pregnancy and, more readily, confinement at times precipitate attacks of schizophrenia, also perhaps acute infections, but not frequently, then any psychic factor, especially an unfortunate love-life. But we must assume that the disease is not engendered by such conditions but only made manifest. Onanism and over-work are both blamed as causes, absolutely without any justifiable reasons. Neither the grippe nor the war have added to the existence of schizophrenia.

L. Frequency and Prevalence

Aside from the oligophrenias and alcoholism, schizophrenia is the most common mental disease. In our asylums it is found in 23 percent of the men and 39 percent of the women and the difference in the relative numbers is due almost entirely to the excess of paretics and alcoholics among the men. As the schizophrenics are at the same time the incurable and the long-lived patients, they may constitute three fourths of all the inmates in any asylum that does not admit many cases of idiocy.

The disease occurs in all races and in every stage of culture. But it seems that among primitive people it assumes less frequently the character of catatonia.

M. Anatomy and Pathology

We do not know as yet on what the pathologic process is based. In acute stages various kinds of changes in the ganglion cells are found. In old cases the brain mass is reduced a little; many ganglion cells, especially in the second and third layer, are changed in various ways; sometimes the fibrils of the cells and the axis-cylinder look diseased. The glia is regularly involved: various changes of its cell varieties, increase of the small cells; there is a deposit of pigment and other catabolic materials, increase of the finer glia fibres and other things besides. The findings cannot as yet be lined up together nor interpreted as to their causes and effects.

Naturally one thinks first of toxic disturbances, especially of the influences of the sex organs and the thyroid also. With the *Abderhalden* reaction it was supposed that signs of the reduction of these two organs were pretty regularly found, naturally with the reduction of other organs, especially of the brain and then the suprarenals.

The supposition of an (hereditary) schizophrenic predisposition, which at present is being considered most, meets with many difficulties. Our total knowledge would be completely comprehensible if it were a case of a chronic infection or intoxication by means of a generally distributed agency or of something teratological.

In certain acute conditions the morbid picture is evidently conditioned chiefly by the anatomic or toxic processes, in the manner of the deliria in meningitis, fever, or intoxications. Also the rarer, general or localized, paralytic symptoms and the manifestations of brain pressure, originate in an organic process which is indicated in the more chronic course by only a few symptoms like tremors, pupillary disturbances, and irregularities of metabolism. In other respects the process seems to set free some associational weakness,[91] which, however, in its results may fluctuate from one moment to another from zero to maximum; and hence already shows the influence of some psychic factor; furthermore the schizophrenic associations have not as yet been differentiated from the functional changes of the mental trend in the dream and in distracted attention. The remaining symptoms of schizophrenia are secondary.[92] The content of the hallucinations and delusions is conditioned katathymically by the complexes; unpleasant complexes are repressed, as in normal people, into the unconscious and from there cause delusions and sense deceptions. Affective rigidity is also seen under such conditions in normal people, and all other affective disturbances occurring in schizophrenics are also noticed especially in the dreams of normal people.

N. Treatment

Most schizophrenics are not to be treated at all, or at any rate outside of asylums. They belong in asylums only when there are special indications, which to be sure appear frequently, e.g. in acute attacks, because of disturbing conduct, violence, danger of suicide, and then especially temporarily for purposes of training. They should be discharged as soon as possible, because later they are gotten rid of much less easily; because not only the patients but the relatives perhaps still more adapt themselves too quickly to the sequestration. The loss of affective rapport makes itself felt in this respect also. Expensive treatments, that are of no use anyway, should be cautioned against, above everything. Moreover the economic and moral interests of the healthy members of the family should not be sacrificed for a hopeless treatment. On the other hand, the supreme remedy which in the majority of cases still accomplishes very much and sometimes everything that can be desired is training for work under conditions that are as normal as possible. In seriously affected patients one must not be afraid to prescribe such unremunerative work as cutting wood, carding wool, making boxes, copying any sort of simple work. It is self-evident that psychical obstacles to improvement, as irritation by impatient treatment, arousing jealousy by having them live with a happily married member of the family, etc., are to be avoided. In addition the following details should be considered. For young

[91] Bleuler, Störung der Associationsspannung. Zeitschr. f. Psychiatrie, 74, S. 1.
[92] See p. 55.

schizophrenics capable of work simple vocations should be selected that lead to life and practical activity, and not to theory and dereism. Schizophrenic whims for some calling or activity should not be mistaken for special qualifications. Sometimes a quiet discussion of the frequent conflicts concerning onanism may contribute to produce calm and probably also in the future, to the avoidance of severe pathogenic complexes.

When the sensitive spots of the disease have been discovered, not only can the physician more easily exert a calming influence, but those about the patient can avoid many exciting influences (conversations about the sister's marriage, visit of a particular man whom the patient loved, etc.).

After the outbreak of the disease those about the patient are to be informed that the delusions and sense deceptions, as far as they do not lead to unpleasant actions, are to be taken quietly and without discussion as merely morbid manifestations. Some of the patient's physical complaints are of a purely psychogenetic nature and are to be treated by suggestion; others, like some headaches, sleeplessness, accumulated pollutions, probably depend more directly on the morbid process and may be treated with medicines, as long as the patient is not habituated to drugs. Bromide will often help to remove the state of general nervous excitability, even if not the real excitement. If after the decline of an acute shift the patients continue to act senselessly, and especially if their nutrition becomes reduced so as to excite apprehension, an 8 to 12 days *Somnifen half sleep* sometimes produces excellent results. To avoid any unpleasant initial manifestations it is best to begin with an injection of Hyoscine 0.001, with Morphine 0.01. When the patient is narcotized, that is, about half an hour later, the patient is given one ampule of Somnifen in both left and right arms, injecting it deeply under the skin or into the muscle. After 6 to 8 hours another ampule, and later according to need. Sleep is maintained so deeply that the patient, left to himself, is drowsy or asleep, but is either spontaneously or through instigation sufficiently aroused to take nourishment, to attend to his wants, and especially for psychic treatment. The latter is most important; one can get the impression that in his helplessness the patient has the need to appeal to some one; negativism and refusal of nourishment can thus be made to disappear or can be markedly weakened. In some cases the remedy seems to bring about directly acute hallucinatory shifts, which have not yet been thoroughly described; here sleep will have to be maintained to a deeper degree. Poor physical condition seems to be no contraindication; the patients usually gain in weight during this treatment. When a shift of the disease has run its course and the patient is nevertheless not freed from delusions or impulsive acts or from his fear of life and work, a change of residence often has a good effect, but not to a sanitarium where one gets accustomed to laziness. Even mild cases should not be left entirely to themselves. They need some one who busies himself with them in a tactful way without irritating them, who watches them unobtrusively, gives them support, and trains them as much as is necessary, and as much more as is possible. In more serious cases the tendency to become automatic can often be used and the patients held at least externally to an orderly existence if not at useful work. With increasing dementia, more and more simple kinds of work have to be found.

There are cases where abortion may be resorted to, followed under certain conditions even by sterilization, for which, however, there must be such very definite indications, as visible aggravation through pregnancy, uncontrollable sexual inclinations, etc. I never saw any good results but sometimes bad ones from the persistently proposed castration.

X. EPILEPSY

In a number of diseases that run their course with psychical symptoms the *epileptiform attack* is the most striking manifestation; we call them the epilepsies. Among them a fairly well characterized group includes about three fourths of the cases; the others are insufficiently known and were really more plainly differentiated first by an anatomical study by *Alzheimer*.[93] The main group, which is the only one that we can give attention to here, is called *genuine epilepsy*, a name that should really include the other forms too and distinguish all of them together from "symptomatic epilepsy," or the epileptiform attacks in other diseases. Such attacks may occur in all grain diseases (e.g. tumors, scleroses, paresis, arteriosclerotic insanity, presbyophrenia, and schizophrenia), as well as in toxic conditions, e.g. through alcohol, lead, ergotin, and in eclampsia and uremia. Genuine epilepsy is characterized not only by the chronically repeated epileptiform attacks, but it also develops a considerable number of psychic symptoms peculiar to it. Furthermore it frequently shows "abortive" or other variously formed attacks, from which the disease may be diagnosed just as clearly as from those attacks designated as epileptiform. The

[93] Die Gruppierung der Epilepsie. Bericht der Jahresversammlung des Deutschen Vereins für Psychiatrie 26/28 April 1907. Allg. Ztschr. f. Psychiatrie, Bd. 64, S. 418.

latter, considered as "typical" attacks, may altogether be in the background or may be totally absent without making the diagnosis impossible for that reason. Nearly all cases of genuine epilepsy also show a common anatomical finding. Nevertheless the differentiation from other forms of epilepsy is not yet sharply defined, and it is easily possible that the group thus delimited will also, on closer examination, be separated into subdivisions.

In cases in which the symptoms of epilepsy and schizophrenia are mingled clinically, *Tramer* also found anatomical signs of both diseases.

What is typical in the attacks designated as epileptiform is the *sudden, often actually "lightning-like" onset of a convulsion of the entire muscular system, which has at first a tonic, and then a clonic character; it lasts not more than a few minutes,*[94] *and is associated with a profound disturbance of consciousness, which leaves the impression of a complete loss of consciousness.*

The attack is often preceded by prodromata which last a few hours, more rarely days; most frequently they are represented by "moods," but also by any ill feeling, more rarely hallucinations and twilight states. In most cases these prodromata disappear in a trice with the attack.

The attack itself is often initiated by an *aura*. This most frequently consists of any kind of paresthesias, a pain, a feeling of cold, or being blown at (hence the name), which, however, is not so frequent; "a wheel is turning in the stomach"; then it may be initiated by real hallucinations, especially of sight and also, noticeably often, by those of taste. The visions often show the tendency to approach the patient and get larger and larger; the moment they touch his breast, consciousness disappears. In the rare "reflex epilepsy," whose attacks are set free by the irritation of a scar or some other pathological focus, the aura may begin as a sensation in the particular part of the body. In some cases complicated scenes are hallucinated. The psychic aura may also consist of sudden moods or subjectively felt disturbances of thought. There is beside a motor aura, consisting of all sorts of clonic and tonic, usually circumscribed, convulsions, lightning-like twitches, or complicated automatic movements, as, especially, aimless running (aura cursoria); it rarely goes as far as complicated acts like undressing, etc.

As the muscles of expiration and those closing the glottis are

---

[94] Relatives often speak of attacks of longer duration. This is due primarily to the fact that the terrible scene leaves the impression of a longer duration. Moreover the intermingling of the two phases with the stuporous after-effect, or the confusing of the attack with the status epilepticus, also contributes to this idea.

stronger than their antagonists, at the beginning of the general convulsion the air is usually pressed out through the closed vocal slit, thus causing the characteristic *scream*. Much more rarely it is a terrible scream of fear, belonging to the psychic, that is to say, cursative aura. With the scream the patient usually drops like a log without any regard for danger. An absolute immovable rigidity probably never occurs; a more strongly contracted group of muscles overcomes the opposing muscles and thus produces a slow movement; often one side especially predominates, then the other. In the tonic state livor naturally occurs, in severe cases, up to a terrifying dark blue; after about a half a minute one sees jerks in individual muscles that spread rapidly and go over into wild clonic convulsions. After a while one usually notices, in the chaos of movement, a certain purposeful coordination becoming visible, especially in the sense of defense. At all events, the movements become weaker until complete quiet takes place; usually some jerks of declining severity follow. Coordination, and to a certain extent the ability to move, usually return only gradually, in the course of minutes or also after a much longer time. Only in exceptional cases does consciousness appear suddenly or as early as the cessation of the motor attacks; usually the thoughts are gradually collected and with numerous fluctuations in the degree of clearness. Orientation, at first falsified, becomes clear first in respect to individual things, later on being spoken to, and then in other respects. The patient does not awaken as if from nothing, but as if he were coming out of a dream state. Sometimes circumscribed paresthesia, and more rarely paralyses, remain for some time.

In severer attacks the saliva is whipped into *foam* by the movements of the tongue and also by the strong mouth-breathing that appears after the tonic convulsions; this foam is frequently colored with blood because the tongue gets between the teeth. If one can examine the *pupils* during the attack, at the very beginning one usually finds miosis, but later pronounced mydriasis and rigidity, which after the attack make way with varying speed for the normal reaction. During the attack some patients sometimes involuntarily pass urine, very rarely feces. During the attack and usually even at the beginning of the stage in which movements and facial expression indicate a dream state, the patients do not react to external stimuli; the reflexes too disappear for a considerable time; the Babinski sign is often present. When the post-epileptic clouded consciousness lasts for hours and days instead of a few moments or minutes, or when noticeable actions are committed in this state, it is considered an independent *post-epileptic twilight* state. After the clouding of consciousness but often also immediately after the attack a stupor or actually a coma usually appears, sometimes also flexibilitas cerea. After the awakening a feeling of perfect well being is decidedly rare; on the one hand the patient usually feels nervous irritation, and on the other, he feels "knocked out," even when he has not really hurt himself. The pulse often keeps fluttering for hours. The Babinski sign may continue into the next day.

In the same patient the various attacks may have a photographic resemblance. In falling the patients land on the same part of the body; the aura is as a rule of the same form; in the post-epileptic twilight state the identical sense deceptions are perceived, and the identical acts are performed in the same succession.

The attacks may become *abortive* in the most diverse ways; this is especially true with the development of dementia when everything as a rule becomes less vigorous. Furthermore the tonic or clonic states may be reduced to a mere indication; the movements may from the beginning have the character of an action, even though it be irregular. Mere fainting spells also may be abortive epileptic attacks. If consciousness disappears for only a few seconds without the patient falling down, and is usually accompanied by pallor, more rarely blushing, and if it is often combined with a staring gaze, sometimes also with some movements of the lips or tongue, one speaks of *absences* or *petit mal*, in contrast to grand mal, or the pronounced attack. Sometimes the disease shows itself in rapidly disappearing *attacks of dizziness*. Besides these most frequent "attacks," there are many other minor symptoms of the same significance that cannot all be enumerated. In all these minor attacks there is hardly ever an absence of a disturbance of consciousness, which appears suddenly without a prodromal stage, partly in the form of an (apparent?) diminution of consciousness, and partly in the form of twilight thinking, or in the obtrusion of a certain thought, etc. Thus a patient suddenly gets up from a meal and masturbates; another urinates in the ticket box. Concerning pure hallucinatory states we get information only when the amnesia is lacking: thus the entire surroundings suddenly disappear for the patient, and instead he sees some rapidly moving cats.

The typical attacks at times follow one another so quickly that the patients do not recuperate in the interval: *status epilepticus*. In severer attacks of this sort the temperature then rises to unusual height (109° F.) and the patients die in coma or from aspiration pneumonia.

The *psychical disturbances*. Epileptics are as a rule psychopathic, even before the disease has left its characteristic mark on them. A large part of them, especially of the forms afflicted while young, actually have brain disease or are imbeciles. But specific psychic peculiarities are connected with epilepsy, which as a rule increase with the duration of the disease. According to the degree one speaks of an epileptic character, epileptic psychopathic constitution,[95] and in severer cases, of epileptic dementia.

The most conspicuous anomaly concerns the *affectivity*, which reacts to a morbid degree, and at the same time shows the peculiarity, that an existing affect lasts a long time and it is difficult to divert it by new impressions; *it is not merely irritability that shows itself in this manner but the other affects, as attachments, or joy, all take the same course.* The patients as a rule have a very decided mood,[96] and the unimportant very readily takes on as strong an emotional tone as the important. It is not true that some feelings, as, e.g. the moral feelings, atrophy. On the other hand, there is found a disproportionately strong affective coloring of conceptions that concern "righteousness." An increased interest is devoted to the patient's ego. But the egocentric trend of thought also has an associative root besides the affective.

All psychic functions, and most noticeable of all the *mental stream*, are markedly retarded and run heavily, and if the flow of speech may be taken as a measure, they preferably take place in a hesitating and jerky manner. The contextual peculiarities of the mental stream are most plainly revealed in the experimental associations where one observes: retardation, poverty of ideas, a tendency to repetition in form and content, to form definitions, difficulty in reacting with a single word, frequency of egocentric references, emotional accentuation of the preferred ideas, and the selection of reaction words that are indicative of emotion; in this respect, there is a particular preference for affective evaluation, as seen in the frequent use of good, beautiful, bad, dreadful; one also notes a difficulty in finding the expression with a tendency to awkwardly formed expressions of their own invention.[97]

Not only the manner of speaking, but epileptic thinking also has something *unclear* and *indefinite* about it; the limitations of conceptions and ideas become blurred; general notions supplant the special. Two different apprehensions cannot be kept apart. The definite

[95] Many mere psychopaths have the same affective habitus as pronounced *epileptoid* or as the less correctly designated *epileptic* character, especially when the patients come from families with evident epileptic members.

[96] Concerning moods that come like attacks see below.

[97] For illustrations see p. 83.

virtue of frugality is designated by the phrase, "Where one does the right thing." A squirrel "is now a rabbit or a cat or a fox." Even in mathematics 16 + 16 is "about from 32 to 34."

In *speaking* and *writing* we have the same peculiarities: The patient does not get anywhere with his talking, not only because of its slowness, but especially because of its circumstantiality, which must depict all trivialities in repetition and in manifold expression of the same idea in different forms. Besides this the manner of speaking is verbose and clumsy, and always vague. As to content the patient clings to the simple and the present. The ideas are limited to what immediately concerns the patient; his personality including the disease; then the members of his family ("family gossip," "family boasting"), his clothes ("whining about clothing") and a number of trifles which the patients, if permitted, like to carry about, usually packed carefully in many papers or clothes, each carefully tied with a string, as photographs, letters, a worthless ornament, etc. Affectively and hence associatively, the patients are to a high degree egocentric. The consciousness of their inferiority, the need of support and of putting the salvation of their personality in the foreground, of clothing vague ideas with pathetic, beautifully coined phrases, and also with intense feeling—all these give them the opportunity of assuming a vapid piety in religious circles, and of dressing their weal and woe in corresponding formulæ ("God nomenclature"). With the unintelligent this succeeds the more readily, because in their indistinct concepts and ideas they are satisfied with generaliites to which they attach an affective rather than an intellectual content. The *egocentricity* shows itself, among other ways, in the fact that they are incapable of evaluating the interests of others; whatever causes them joy and anger, they consider similarly important and emotionally colored for others. It is quite characteristic that frequently they take the physician aside with a solemn mien to tell him secretly something commonplace or something that was known long ago.

Perseveration and the difficulty of diverting them to another subject are illustrated in the following conversation reported by Wernicke: "What is your name?" "Martha Glockner." "How old are you?" "Martha Glockner." "Where are we now?" "Martha Flockner."— "How old are you?" "Twenty-two years old." "Where are we now?" "Twenty-two years old." "What is your calling?" "Twenty-two years old." "Who am I?" "Cousin George."

Circumstantiality and the tendency to tautology are shown in the following letter (whose dialect and orthography have been extensively corrected):

"My dear Director: I send you my best regards from the bottom of my heart and wish you from the bottom of my heart good health and God's blessing and I respect you and I thank you from the bottom of my heart and I wished all of this for the director and the minister, and I wished this all for your relatives all of this and I beg you from the bottom of my heart that you send the letter to Rüti which I handed in last week and the parents in Rüti I send. I sent my heartfelt wishes also and I respect them too and thank them too and wish them from the bottom of my heart good health and God's blessing and the sick and the healthy also and I have the greatest home sickness for his services and sermon and bible lessons and all prayer books were in me. . . ."

Ulrich gives a brief illustration of the unctuous emotionalism:

"I am the dear young lady Miss X. X. from X., Parish of X., Canton X., Switzerland." She wanted the physicians to explain to her daily that she was the dearest and best Miss X. X.; she pressed people's hands as much and as emotionally as possible, the left as well as the right. She always wished one a dear good Sunday, a dear good day of the week, whatever it might be, a' dear good night's rest; if one responded to her good wishes, she answered with satisfaction: "That is the right way."

The egocentricity shows itself in the following answer to the question, "What is the significance of Christmas?" "Last Christmas I received an apron, I wanted a skirt from my mother; she did not give it to me."

Thus the *conduct* of epileptics is to all appearances well regulated; but to those about them it readily becomes somewhat trying, as much because of their fussiness, as their adhesiveness and their clinging to trivialities. However one can very readily establish a satisfactory and not unpleasant rapport with them; where one does not get on with the average epileptic, there is some mistake in the treatment. They are as clinging in their demonstration of affection as they are persistent in their affect of offense. They do not release for a long time the proffered hand; if one forgets to greet them, it can dampen their spirit for days. They busy themselves as long as they possibly can even though not very much is produced; in the wards the more demented patients actually become a nuisance on account of their clumsy readiness to help; during the war the same zealousness showed itself in their "war spirit"; it made them forget any consideration of their disease and led them to try again and again to reach the front. When left to themselves, their unsteadiness is very great. Because they take everything to be too important and especially because of their moods, they cannot remain anywhere permanently; many become tramps.—The momentary mood also dominates primarily their attitude toward the disease, which is at times regarded as something very bad and then as improved or cured. However, their main afflictions as well as their various secondary ailments are always a matter of extraordinary importance to them, which they like to discuss incessantly, be it to obtain sympathy or help, or to boast of how well they are getting on. But in the main the "epileptic optimism" (*Rieger*) prevails, that is, even the more intelligent, in spite of all accidents and warnings, never take permanent consideration of their disease; they get into situations that are dangerous to themselves or undertake work and responsibilities that they cannot possibly carry out.

The *attention* of epileptics, corresponding to their affectivity, shows a reduced vigility (distractibility), but a good tenacity; at the same time it is very uneven at different times.

Even though many details, especially affective experiences, are remembered for a strikingly long time, nevertheless the *memory* after a while becomes bad but not in a recognizable systematic way; recent and old impressions are equally forgotten. Besides, it becomes blurred; experiences are associated with other connections; frequently it goes as far as actual *memory illusions* (the amnesias belong to the paroxysmal state).

Orientation, except in conditions of most advanced dementia which only a few attain, and in twilight states, is good.

Perceptions readily become unclear; like organic cases the patients require more time than normal persons and easily make mistakes. Furthermore, the after-effects of previous influences interfere (*Perseveration*). For example, they mistake a picture in terms of a previous visual impression. But the unclearness of the perception is not a result of inadequate peripheral sensory functioning; the patients are at least capable, despite their fussiness about minutiæ, e.g. of distinguishing the differences between two similar lines, much better than are healthy people. Often the patient cannot follow complicated relations and rapid changes of ideas. Sometimes there is a big difference between the conception of single words and an entire sentence.

The *speech* of epileptics is often so characteristic that the diagnosis can be made from it; it is slow, hesitating, in which case syllables are often repeated several times and the patients cannot make any progress.[98] Because of the slowness, and because the individual vowels

[98] To differentiate it from stuttering it does not show any spasmodic manifestations of the speech muscles.

often show a rising and falling and the unaccented syllables are stressed as much as the accented, their speech becomes somewhat sing-song. With this the tonal modulations are clumsy and rare, hardly ever finely shaded, so that the speech at the same time seems somewhat monotonous. The degree of these speech disturbances may vary decidedly in the same patient: at the approach of an attack or in a twilight state it is usually particularly pronounced.

Chronic hallucinating hardly ever occurs in epileptics. On the other hand, under the affective influence *delusions* are very frequently formed, especially of being treated unjustly. As a rule they are forgotten or corrected in the next opposite mood, but, like the delusions produced in the twilight states, they may, in exceptional cases, have a longer duration.

Besides symptoms of permanent epileptic degeneration, we regularly find in the psychical field also *transient manifestations* which, at least in part, are certainly equivalent to the attack. In the course of these, the permanent symptoms are especially pronounced.

In the first place we find the *twilight states* which most frequently occur post-epileptically, but may also take place pre-epileptically and instead of the attack ("Equivalents"). They usually begin quickly, often very suddenly, and disappear again within a few minutes or hours, after having lasted for hours or days. Epileptic deliria, lasting for weeks or even months, are rare. The most frequent form is the hallucinatory delirium. The patients hallucinate and have illusions, especially of sight, but also of the other senses, concerning another environment, or at any rate, other influences from without, and react to these. Among the hallucinations red ones (partly as fire or blood) occur with noticeable frequency. The content, in other respects, is very similar to our dreams. A part of the deliria is affectively indifferent. More frequent are those with an anxious or angry affect which readily lead to brutal acts of violence against the individual himself and others; sexual excitements are the basis of Ripper murders, or frequent exhibitionism. Besides fearful visions of hell and the devil, there occur much more rarely ecstasies which are completely beyond the reach of reality and blissful erotic-religious hallucinations of all the senses. Pronounced twilight states can be influenced very little; but under certain conditions one can get in touch with the patient; however, one gets few answers, and few sensible ones. Thinking is usually profoundly disturbed; [99] very simple answers are more easily obtained than complicated ones; under certain conditions the patient can figure 7 plus 18, but no longer 7 times 18, because he can

[99] See also p. 83.

no longer add 56 and 70. The associations run toward side-tracking as in dreams, while in other respects the heavy, everywhere halting, epileptic train of thought is strongly differentiated from dream thinking and schizophrenic thinking in spite of its inexactness in disarrangements of ideas and words. Sound associates also occur in many patients but not actual flight of ideas. The twilight states leaves, in most cases, a partial or complete amnesia.

Between the attacks, *milder states of obnubilation* are most frequent, in which sensory deceptions are entirely absent, orientation as to place and time is disturbed little or not at all; on the other hand, the relation with surrounding persons is usually falsified. Hostile attitudes are very common. In the most common types there is a feeling of pressure to talk, together with strongly retarded thinking and impeded word selection, and vague, unclear, poorly defined ideas. At the same time sound associations and the reception of chance material from without into the trend of ideas which never leave the same circle may simulate flight of ideas for the beginner. Perseveration and the absence of real distractibility readily reveal the true condition. Vagueness of apperception leads the patients to mistake persons, so that they even identify themselves with others in transitivism.

Outwardly very different are the *clear twilight states* in which the patients seem clear to the observer but are, in reality, extremely restricted associatively and carry out any dreamlike action.[100] But with *Heilbronner* I would like to attribute most of these conditions to hysteria, even when they occur in epileptics as they not seldom do. Sometimes a patient suddenly finds himself on a street where he did not want to go. Mere anxiety attacks are often epileptic equivalents.

With a slightly clouded consciousness *pseudo hallucinations* (especially of sight) may also appear in the form of attacks, e.g. figures who with long arms reach for the patient, an animal, the devil, or when in a pleasant mood, angels, or beautiful women.

A twilight state may also take on the form of a stupor of varying degree, or continuous identifying *memory deceptions* may dominate the picture.

Furthermore *somnambulism* may be a (rare) epileptic symptom.

Of especial importance are the *moods* which are probably not lacking in any epileptic (but which also occur in other psychopaths, oligophrenia, and in schizophrenia). There may be *euphoric* moods of especial good feeling, often with the idea of being finally cured of the epilepsy, but without flight of ideas (usually as a precursor of

[100] See p. 112.

attacks). Or *depressive* moods with or without fear which resemble completely a melancholic mood, relatively seldom with a suicidal impulse but very frequently with the emphasis on the incurability, or it manifests itself in the best known mood, namely *irritation*, in which, on the one hand, the patients are irritated by everything that takes place and, on the other, conduct themselves in a very presumptuous and impudent fashion so that conflicts are unavoidable. The moods may appear suddenly and be suddenly brought to an end (especially by an attack, the precursor of which they then were), or they may appear furtively and last hours or several days and rarely even longer.

Mere *paresthesias* are also common, especially headache, pains here and there, and any kind of nervous manifestations which distinctly show the paroxysmal character; furthermore, one observes stomach troubles, that appear and disappear suddenly, attacks of passion with or without impulsive onanism or attacks on others, also twitchings and other manifestations of spasms. The irregular fluctuations of a more severe tremor which are frequently found in the graphic registration of epileptics are also included here.

All these syndromes may occur in isolated form or irregularly intermingled; furthermore, like the attacks, they often repeat themselves in a similar or actually identical form.

In the *physical field* also we find anomalies that belong to epilepsy. In the first place a number of congenital malformations show the "degeneration" or the brain disease.

In the *blood* are found cytological and especially chemical peculiarities which, however, fluctuate greatly in the same patient, and still more in different cases so that as yet no clear picture can be obtained. The entire *metabolism* and with it the chemistry *of the urine* is abnormal, but cannot as yet be described in a uniform manner. It seems fairly certain that after the attack poisonous substances are excreted. It is not known on what the sensitiveness to *alcohol* in the most various ways is based; however, it can be connected with the intolerance of alcohol after injuries to the brain.

Like the other nervous processes, *movements* are often performed slowly, clumsily, and perhaps also with uncertainty. But bodily strength remains for a noticeably long time either good or very good.

The *course* of the disease is, on the whole, progressive, at least in respect to the permanent psychical condition. The attacks need not increase; often they even become milder or rudimentary in time. A direct connection between the number and severity of the attacks and dementia does not exist. Marked dementias may also appear with a simple petit mal. Some cases remain stationary, others become cured, especially with suitable treatment. Pauses extending over years or decades are not so rare; it is well known that there are patients who have attacks in earliest childhood, then seem cured, only to be afflicted again during puberty. Among the milder cases many recover definitively, others only from the attacks while the epileptic character remains, or under certain conditions even develops more strongly together with intellectual dementia. There are also epileptics who have quite a number of attacks every year and nevertheless—with or without therapy—do not become demented and whose character remains relatively good.

The *number of attacks* differs greatly. In milder cases only a few convulsions and twilight states may occur during their whole life; others produce several in a single day; in especially bad times they even have many, rarely a hundred and even more. Many patients, especially in the beginning of the disease, are stricken, only or chiefly, during the night and do not at all know that they are epileptic. In some the attacks are scattered, in others they appear more in series.

The prospects in case of a pronounced, interparoxystical dementia are naturally bad, even though at times a regulated therapy produces improvement to the extent that the subsidiary manifestations disappear. A certain percentage, especially of those afflicted after puberty, lose the attacks spontaneously and become little or not at all demented.[101] Undoubtedly a *timely* interference may extensively improve many a case or even cure it and prevent further decline. *Here the prospects depend especially on the psychic condition.* Extensive improvement or cure can be expected only in case of a slightly affected psyche.

The *duration of life* is considerably shortened by the disease. Many meet with an accident during the attack, others die from an early marasmus which is regularly connected with more severe dementia and cerebral atrophy. Epileptics who from birth were afflicted with some brain disease naturally have a weak physical endurance.

Anatomical Findings. Epileptics are comparatively rich in stigmata of degeneration [102] and other dysplasias; strikingly frequent one observes in the brain among other things ganglion cells in the white substance, Cajal's (foetal-) cells in the upper cortical layer, as well as *other disturbances of development.* As a foundation of the later dementia one finds a distinct, even though not a high grade atrophy of

[101] I have a decided distrust of the diagnosis of epilepsy in Mohammed, Socrates, or even Napoleon.
[102] Cf. pp. 159-160.

the brain with different forms of degeneration of the neurons, and as characteristic, an increase of the glia fibres, which, as distinguished from paresis, remain on the whole fine, usually arrange themselves in bunches in the interior of the brain and cover especially the surface with a thick felt of chiefly tangential fibres, which have little connection with the deeper layers. The glia cells are changed in different ways, readily increased and carry many catabolic products. What relation these findings have to the disease is still entirely unknown as is the significance of the frequently found sclerosis of one or both of the ammon horns with degeneration of the nerve cells and hypertrophy of the glia.

In death following status epilepticus one finds, as a rule, a higher pressure in the cranial cavity partly because of cerebral œdema and especially of the meninges, partly, too, probably because of cerebral inflammation.

Causes. Epilepsy has its roots in the congenital constitution. Hereditary burdens with mental diseases, psychopathic conditions with familiar nervous degeneration and especially with epilepsy itself, show the connection with a diseased kin. That the "epileptic characters" in such families often represent milder forms of the same disease is to be assumed. The various kinds of epilepsy, also, have unfortunately not been kept separate in the investigations of heredity. An important rôle is played by the alcoholism of the parents, probably that of a cause and not merely as a sign of a morbid family disposition.[103] According to more recent investigations epilepsy is supposed to have a connection with the familiar left-handedness, and not merely because left-sided brain lesions at the same time dispose to left-handedness and to epilepsy. As the Wassermann reaction shows in early epilepsy, many cases are based on hereditary lues. In the individual life epilepsy may be acquired from every possible brain disease, from the uterine porencephalus, the infectious encephalitides, and the traumata up to arteriosclerosis (the latter, however, is relatively rare), and from all sorts of poisons, especially alcohol and lead. Whether an epileptic disposition must have existed in such patients is not yet known. If a brain lesion is once present, *cocain* can precipitate an epileptic attack which may then repeat itself. (Caution! According to *Ulrich*, Novocain may on the contrary be used as a local anesthetic.)

The causes of the individual attack are, as a rule, internal; never-

[103] *Stuchlik*, Über die hereditären Beziehungen zwischen Alkoholismus und Epilepsie, Diss. Zurich 1914, und Korrespondenzblatt f. Schweizer Aerzte. Basel 1914.

theless psychic influences can hold back and precipitate attacks (a festival, remedies with a suggestive effect).[104] However, ordinarily the anger which is supposed to have released the attack is not the cause but the precursor of it. In his moodiness because of impossible demands, presumptuous conduct and irritability, the patient has brought about the anger.—Individual attacks are often precipitated by excesses of all kinds and even by relatively slight alcoholic indulgence. The famous moon phases have no influence; on the other hand atmospheric conditions seem to be able to effect slight fluctuations in the frequency of the attacks.

Forms, Range. As yet we have too little anatomical experience to differentiate the described groups sharply from other diseases with epileptic attacks. Especially must the question be raised whether all the "curable" cases, or those running their course with unnoticeably little dementia, or the very mild cases, generally are identical with the inevitably progressive ones. As an uninterrupted shading from the most favorable to the worse cases is perceptible, it is possible but not certain that all or many of the curable and (apparently) stationary cases represent only milder forms of the same disease. Cases with entirely different symptoms (more acute degeneration of the nervous substance) are naturally to be excluded *eo ipso*.

Traumatic epilepsy as a result of injuries to the brain frequently resembles the forms described, but it is quite evident that the organic dementia frequently contains an admixture of the psychic and physical signs of cerebral trauma. There are also milder cases which improve or remain in a quiescent state.

The *reflex epilepsies* cannot as yet be assigned to any classification.

Jacksonian epilepsy is not an epilepsy in our sense; but it very often is transformed into such as the attacks assume the epileptic type and the psychic manifestations change their nuance in the sense of epilepsy.

In *arteriosclerosis* and *presbyophrenia* the epileptic attacks are probably only partial manifestations of the main disease although in one case of arteriosclerosis I also found the epileptic gliosis.

In the same way the epileptiform attacks of *schizophrenia* naturally belong to this disease. But there are noticeably many patients from whom one gets the impression that schizophrenic and epileptic symptoms have intermingled.[105]

---

[104] According to *Hauptmann* one observed (that is, in the milder forms) no epileptic attacks in the war during an alarm or charge attacks (differs from hysterical attacks).

[105] Comp. p. 446.

Kraepelin also distinguishes a *"Residual epilepsy,"* recurring epileptiform attacks without a progressive course in brain scars and similar disturbances.

The *eclampsia* of children often resembles the epileptic attacks; but the tonic stage is often more strongly, the clonic much more weakly, pronounced. But as most of those children do not become epileptics, it is not known whether the two diseases are connected and in what way they are related. Spasmophilia is no primary stage of epilepsy.

Dipsomania and alcoholic epilepsy.[106] Most dipsomaniacs do not seem to become severely demented, even when they have the epileptic habitus.

On the basis of two clear cases *Kraepelin* would like to class with epilepsy the *running amok* of the Malays, in which the patients suddenly run through the streets with drawn daggers, cut people down at random until they collapse or, which is more frequent, are shot down or made harmless in some other way. The monotonous repetition of the same psychic syndrome in the various patients seems to me to point to the material influence of a psychogenic factor.[107]

Friedmann's Disease, which the author wants to designate with the already assigned name of Narkolepsy, consists of very frequently recurring attacks of prolonged psychic rigidity or confusion without loss of consciousness with a turning upward of the eyes. It occurs in children and disappears with age without dementia. *Kraepelin* would like to class this disease with hysteria. At all events it does not belong to our genuine epilepsy as some authors suppose.

Many also want to include *Migrain* with epilepsy. But it is a syndrome which may occur in the most varying functional and organic diseases of the nervous system.

On the other hand, the *affective epilepsies (Bratz)* or *reactive epilepsies (Bonhoeffer)* are important psychopathic states with strong affectivity, in which psychic influences may more or less frequently lead to epileptiform attacks. *Kraepelin* observed them especially in unsteady people who were inclined to wander and swindle, and he calls these *epileptic swindlers.* Bromide does not seem to influence affective epilepsy in the same specific way as it does the genuine form.

Occurrence. Epilepsy—in the older, wider sense of the term, to be sure,—is a frequent disease in all ages and in all races. With us undoubtedly several per thousand of the population suffer from the

---

[106] See Alcoholism, pp. 351-352.

[107] Cf. Brill, Piblokto or Hysteria Among Peary's Eskimos. Journal of Nervous and Mental Diseases, Vol. 40, No. 8.

disease. According to whether or not one includes the infantile convulsions, most cases begin in the first or second decade. The male
sex predominates considerably, particularly when the disease appears
in mature manhood; here it is evidently a result of alcoholic effects.

Recognition. In many cases the patients report nothing, or nothing
characteristic, concerning the attacks. They come to the physician
because of nervous symptoms, changes of character, unrecognized or
abortive twilight states; then the recognition is not easy. But frequently they bring with them a complete diagnosis or a clear anamnesis.
Even though the individual attack does not permit of recognition,
nevertheless a disease in which for years such attacks have occurred
in somewhat definite intervals is invariably an epilepsy, and if there
is nothing important in addition, it will be a genuine epilepsy. The
positive findings of the psychic symptoms will in most cases quickly
confirm the diagnosis. Typical absences, except at times in brain
tumors, occur almost only in epilepsy and are, to that extent, more
characteristic than the big attacks. During epileptic excitations, but
also in more advanced chronic conditions, the slow, hesitating reaction
is usually especially evident as against other disturbances (except
the organic) : [108] "A patient who responds quickly to all my objections,
is not an epileptic" (*Vogt*)! Often the anamnesis can contribute much
to the clarification. It offers evidence that the attacks already existed
earlier, or narrates experiences that point in that direction, such as
isolated bed-wettings in later years, falling out of bed during sleep
(usually without waking up), feeling knocked out in the morning,
tongue bites of unknown origin. But one must not expect to find
frequently tongue scars; even severe wounds of the tongue sometimes
heal without a mark; scars from injuries to the body are more frequent. Heredity of a similar kind may also be considered.

Under certain conditions the differential diagnosis from an
organic mental or brain disease may for a time be difficult, because,
aside from the convulsive attacks and absences, the psychic symptoms
(associations and attacks of confusion) of the two morbid groups
may also be similar. In this case, after a minute physical and
psychic examination, the discovery of the specific signs of one or the
other disease must finally decide.

From *dementia prœcox*, aside from the mentioned mixed or transition forms, the diagnosis is usually easy. In the twilight state one
should notice especially the hesitating speech; furthermore the uniform,
clear and real affective state in the epileptic, as against the artificial
state of the schizophrenic which is difficult to interpret. The difficult

[108] Cf. also brain injuries.

distractability must not be mistaken for affective rigidity: if I can violently deprive a person in a euphoric twilight state of his beloved trifles without his changing his affective attitude even a little bit, this behavior differs from the schizophrenic attitude by the fact that the epileptic defends himself but in reality is not distracted at all, even intellectually. He has therefore no reason for changing the affect. Minor traits by themselves may also often facilitate the diagnosis or make it certain; thus an apparently totally confused person in motion, who in this state continually handles in both hands a carefully folded handkerchief without disarranging the folds, is probably always an epileptic.

Among the more striking symptoms the following are common to both diseases: the tendency to symbolism, unclear ideas, and neologisms. But as a rule the symptoms are plainly distinguished by different nuances. The symbolism of epilepsy does not lead to the fixed delusions or even to hallucinations, as in schizophrenia. It remains rather a peculiarity of thinking. In schizophrenia the indefiniteness of the ideas and conceptions is altogether unbalanced. Besides the most senseless conceptions many entirely normal ones occur, while the demented epileptic finds it difficult at all times to create clear limitations. The epileptic neologisms consist rather of poor word formations than in genuine new creations; "unquitted love" is probably an epileptic formation: "Dossier path" for the secretive manner of persecution and "Anona" for morphine are schizophrenic.

Mistaking an epileptic crepuscular attack of rage for the *manic destructive impulse* is avoided, among other things, by the absence of distractibility and flight of ideas (but one must not associate the circumstantiality in which the patient is not distractible and does not forget his goal as well as the liability to interruption, with the goal-shifting flight of ideas).

The attacks are well distinguished from the *hysterical;* it is especially important to think of the tonic-clonic type, the brief duration of these phases, the tongue biting and other injuries, and the rigidity of the pupils. Involuntary passing of urine and feces hardly occurs in an hysterical attack. Ankle clonus or the Babinski sign after the attack excludes mere hysteria. According to *Bosshard* [109] in a pronounced epileptic attack there is regularly found a leucocytosis which differs from the "work-leucocytoses," by the early appearance of lymphocytosis and mononucleosis. Under certain circumstances the pulse, remaining good in spite of an apparently serious condition, gives evidence of hysteria; also the facts that the patients are accessible

[109] Über Leukocytenvermehrung bei epilept. Anfällen. Diss. Zürich 1917.

to influences, the consideration for themselves and, others when struggling and falling, as well as the reacting pupils,—all these elements are foreign to the epileptic attack. The marked dependence of the hysterical attack on external influences, and the slight dependence of the epileptic syndromes, can with a careful evaluation of circumstances often alone suffice for the diagnosis. In all other respects it should not be forgotten that in epilepsy all hysterical symptoms may occur.

The same signs help to distinguish the attack from *simulation*. Attacks of dizziness may also occur in the *nervous, arteriosclerotics*, and generally in all *brain diseases*, even though rarely in the same development as in epilepsy, with the brief duration, and the sharp, sudden limitation.[110]

Under certain conditions it is impossible for the moment to distinguish the epileptic twilight state from the *pathological drunkenness*, especially because epileptiform attacks occur in both, and alcohol may precipitate epileptic syndromes.

From the epileptic twilight state to the *moods* and *excitations of oligophrenics* there are so many transitions, that under certain circumstances the question has to be left open for some time, whether mere oligophrenia or combination with epilepsy is present.

In judicial cases one can resort, with the patient's consent, to the remedy of having the patient take bromide in medium doses for about three weeks, then suddenly stop the drug and give him well salted foods, or besides the foods, at least one ounce of cooking salt in one day. In latent epilepsy this may sometimes provoke an attack.

The *pathology* of genuine epilepsy is, in spite of all the works devoted to it, still entirely unknown. It may be a constitutional degeneration of the brain, something teratological; the frequent physical stigmata of degeneration, the Cajal cells and the other brain findings, which may, however, be secondary, would point to this. In accordance with the present humoral pathological views, it—or at least the convulsive attack with its equivalent—is to be considered a result of an autointoxication. The chemical examinations of the blood and urine favor this in spite of their lack of uniformity, but above all the observation, that when in patients that have preparoxysmal moods the attacks are suppressed with bromide, these moods are easily prolonged until an attack is permitted. The convulsive attack, therefore, seems to have the significance of a crisis, and as the urine is said to be more poisonous immediately after the attacks than otherwise, this crisis might be chemical.

[110] For absences, compare above, pp. 447-448.

One can also think that the brain pressure which can be verified in the status epilepticus may have something to do with the epilepsy; but it is well, however, to differentiate the known clinical manifestations of brain pressure from epilepsy.

Physiologically one must conclude that the brain cortex and deeper locations together participate in the production of the attack.

Treatment. Nothing can be done by way of prevention except to hinder the marriage of degenerates, and work against alcoholic indulgence.

In the treatment of the disease itself *bromide* is the most important and the only chemical remedy of significance. It is given as potassium bromide (the cheapest) or as sodium bromide, which avoids the effects of the potassium which, however, are not very noticeable, or it may be given in the form of a mixture of ammonium, sodium and potassium bromides in equal parts in doses of from 3 to 8 grammes a day (in children, of course, correspondingly less). One tries the dose after which the attacks disappear or are reduced to a minimum; in the beginning, perhaps in the course of the first year, it may be reduced a little, but later this dose is retained continually for years; best of all forever. Omissions and variations are soon paid for in the cases that can be influenced. *A fatal status epilepticus often follows a sudden omission.* It is important that the salt be given largely diluted, about two decileters per gramme, because otherwise the stomach is affected, and the patient too easily becomes tired of the remedy.

The effect can be increased by the reduction (not deprivation) of table salt (from 5 to 10 grammes per day). As a large quantity of it is taken up in soup, about 20 grammes, the latter may be salted with bromide or most palatably, by substituting a bouillon of *sedobrol*, a combination of sodium bromide and soup spices. In this form the remedy is gladly taken, does the least harm, and otherwise, too, seems to have the best results. In severe cases *Ulrich* gives successfully Sedobrol combined with Chloral-hydrate 0.5 to 1.5 grammes daily, given in the evening, especially in night attacks.

Bromism is usually better combatted by doses of table salt than by larger reductions of the bromide or its withdrawal (furthermore by arsenic; in case of open wounds mercury plaster or mercury ointments).

Not only the regular taking of the remedy but the *regulation of the whole manner of living* is important, in which excesses in all directions, in work, food, drink, recreation, and affective stimuli, must be avoided. Alcohol, even in small doses, must be forbidden. Other stimuli like caffein and strong condiments, as well as meat diet, should be restricted; in many cases a diet with large quantities of milk seems useful. To recommend marriage, as is often done, and not only by the laity, should be branded as a crime.

Some cases which do not respond to bromides may improve by *Luminal* taken evenings in *one* dose of 0.05-0.01. It can eventually be combined with bromides. But one must not continue to give this narcotic for years, and like bromide it should not be suddenly stopped.

As without confinement epileptics readily make the rigid enforcement of the treatment difficult because of their moods and fits and strong reactions to light discomforts, it is often wise to have them put into an asylum where the stay should last many months, a year, or even more.[111] If one sees that a substantial gain can no longer be obtained with bromide, which is usual in the advanced cases, who e.g. hang on in the insane asylums, it should be given up. Where medications do no good there is always occasion for friction with these moody patients, and when a status makes the use of bromide necessary it is obviously more effective in patients not habituated to it.

Of the numerous *surgical interferences* already undertaken against epilepsy, there have survived only the operations for irritating peripheral scars (a very rare cause of epilepsy), of brain scars and exostoses of the inner cranium, and "pressure relief" by trepanation with the greatest possible prevention of new bone formation. But these cases too must be treated with bromide before and after the operation.

In epilepsy after brain injury severe physical and mental exertion favors the appearance of attacks. Therefore, when possible, the patients are kept busy much under the maximum of their capacity.

In exceptional cases the single attacks may be checked by binding of the member in which the aura appears with an Esmarch bandage, or by extending an aura convulsion. Other interferences, from without or from the patients themselves, are at times successful only in exceptional cases. Usually the attack must be permitted to run its course. Against the status epilepticus amylenehydrate (in form of an enema in some vehicle) in doses from 5 to 6 grammes is effective; perhaps still better is bromide plus chloral hydrate (e.g. Potassium Bromide 2.0, chloral hydrate 1.0 to 2.0, to be repeated every half hour up to the maximum dose of chloral), perhaps combined with baths of almost body temperature.[112]

---

[111] For details, see *Ulrich*, Beitr. zur Techn. der wirks. Brombehdlg. Korresp. Bl. für Schweizerärzte. Basel 1914, Nr. 21.

[112] In the local asylum for epileptics as a result of the bromide treatment with a reduced salt diet no status has occurred for years.

Against injuries during the attack nothing much can be done prophylactically except to warn the patients—usually in vain to be sure—not to get into situations in which an attack may become dangerous. When a certain part of the head is repeatedly injured, it can be protected by a protective covering. Careful supervision can naturally prevent many accidents, but not all. Patients whom the aura warns of the proximity of the attack often still have the time to get themselves into a secure position or to call the protecting orderly. Besides obvious measures he has to be especially careful that the patient does not choke in the state of sopor when the tongue falls backwards.

XI. MANIC-DEPRESSIVE INSANITY

GROUP OF THE AFFECTIVE PSYCHOSES [113]

In not a small number of psychoses, displacements of moods are in the foreground and the remaining fundamental symptoms can frequently be so exactly deduced from the affective anomalies that mild cases cannot be distinguished symptomatically from normal affective fluctuations. On closer inspection, to be sure, other cases show that this explanation is nevertheless not sufficient, and that the disturbance of the affect represents merely the most conspicuous symptom of a general transformation of the psyche that cannot as yet be comprehended. The diseases are not progressive and never lead to a dementia that could be compared with that of the organic, epileptic, and schizophrenic forms. As to the affection of the intellectual activity it is a question of equalizable disturbances, which for the most part look like the accompanying intellectual manifestations of exaggerated affective fluctuations.

According to our present knowledge the basic symptoms are:

1. *Exalted or depressive moods.*

2. *Flight of ideas or retardation of the mental stream.*

3. *Abnormal facilitation or retardation of the centrifugal functions of resolution, of acting, inclusive of the psychic elements of motility.* Euphoria, flight of ideas, and pressure activity on the one hand (mania); depression, associative and centrifugal retardation on the other hand (melancholia), are the most frequent combinations. In the cases that reach the psychiatrist these syndromes nearly always occur in the forms of attacks and the intervals seem to be about normal; but it may also be a case of a persistent peculiarity which is then invariably of a lesser degree. *As accessory symptoms there*

[113] Not to be mistaken for the reaction psychoses.

occur also delusions and hallucinations (almost only of hearing and sight), and "nervous" manifestations.

The Manic Attack. The mood of the manic attack consists of an exalted feeling of self, euphoria, and cheerfulness. The patients feel happy, "overjoyed"; and experiences are colored with pleasant feelings; they are insensitive to depressive experiences; minor "unpleasantnesses" are more readily felt, and especially everything that hurts the patient's enhanced feeling of self; and because in his over-estimation of himself he is constantly making demands that cannot be fulfilled, he is always in a state of discord, *anger* and *rage*, with his environment. Moreover, the mood of the manic is very *fluctuating;* with great outbursts it follows every slight variation of the imagination, but in pronounced mania it does not easily descend by way of reaction to the depressive or anxious. On the other hand, endogenous reversals to depression, that last a quarter of an hour, an hour, or sometimes two days, are not at all rare.—*Sensitiveness to physical pain is not directly reduced.* To be sure, the patients frequently do not notice pains; when, however, they have e.g. to be subjected to a slight operation when the attention is directed to the injury, they can even be very tender.

The *thinking* of the manic is flighty.[114] He jumps by by-paths from one subject to another, and cannot adhere to anything. With this the ideas run along very easily and involuntarily, even so freely that it may be felt as unpleasant by the patient. In severer cases the patient is also bothered with a consciousness of unclearness, and an inability to arrange his thoughts and think them out. Aside from the severest forms only, where it looks as if the patient's speech and finally the listener's intelligence could not follow the wild racing of the ideas (flighty confusion), one finds as a rule the thread that connects the individual ideas. It is not a case of incoherence, at least not in principle. The thinking is incomplete and flighty but not "unclear" in the sense of psychopathology. Up to advanced stages of the disease one can converse with the manic, and more than in his normal times, he displays a rapid grasp and evaluation of the opponent's weakness, giving quick, witty, or sarcastic answers, or pettifogging logic.

Transiently in the course of an attack one may observe a *disturbance of thought having a certain similarity to a dream.*[115] It may persist for hours or days, in exceptional cases also during the entire phase, and shows subjective or objective unclearness of all ideas and logical connections, the nature of which has not yet been studied.

[114] See p. 71.
[115] To be distinguished from complicating hysterical trance-conditions.

Disturbances of apperception do not become noticeable in ordinary intercourse. Reactions to remarks and changes of situation generally are rapid and from the patient's point of view correct. To be sure, in an experimental test, the patients make many errors, which, however, are to be accounted for by "flightiness," and not by an actual disturbance of perceptions. The *orientation* as to time and place, except in the severest cases of flighty confusion, also remains undisturbed. Naturally, the situation is invariably incorrectly estimated, inasmuch as the patients usually consider themselves "particularly well," and in any case cannot understand the restrictions of their freedom of action.

The attention is characterized by an extreme distractibility from without and within.

Just as the ideas readily appear and crowd up, *they also translate themselves readily and of necessity (but without a subjective feeling of compulsion) into resolutions and actions.* Interest in everything is at the same time leveled upwards A thought is aroused; without any consideration for the object of thought at hand, it is pursued until it is supplanted by another. The patient sees something and grasps it; he notices that the physician wears a glass eye and at once calls out in the first moment of meeting: "But you only have one eye," which the one-eyed Dr. Jolly Sr. makes use of in diagnosing his cases; the idea crops up that something should be done, and without the noticeable intervention of consideration and resolution, he acts. Obstacles are not felt. The patients cannot be without occupation; they suffer from *pressure activity.*

The *external picture* varies according to the severity of the disease from mild manic excitability to "frenzy." In the *submanias* the patient is more active than usual; in small and big affairs he gets many plans that he at once seeks to carry out; he gets up especially early to take long walks or take part in some athletic sport; he makes inventions, poems, wants to improve something in the universe, mixes in everything imaginable that does not concern him, travels about, or enlarges his business; his mother's burial becomes an extraordinary festive arrangement. A bank employee, when war threatened, made proposals to his government for securing the supply of silver, and succeeded in being sent to Rothschild in London. A young girl for the first time comes to a federation of women's clubs and as a president of the federation is being sought, she at once indicates that she is prepared to accept. In associating with strangers or persons of note, the sub-manic may conduct himself as if with intimate friends. Because of lack of restraint and his presumptions he gets into trouble.

Often during the entire duration of the attack he indulges in *litigations*. But his good nature also manifests itself in a particularly lively fashion; a bug alone on the street arouses the patient's sympathy, and he carries it to a bakery where he buys a trifle in order to let it loose there. Against excesses of all kinds, especially sexual, alcoholic, wastefulness, inhibitions are lacking. When called to account, the patient not only has excuses but "good reasons" for his conduct ("folie raisonnante"). Because of the more rapid flow of ideas, and especially because of the falling off of inhibitions, artistic activities are facilitated even though something worth while is produced only in very mild cases and when the patient is otherwise talented in this direction. The heightened sensibilities naturally have the effect of furthering this.

If in the rather higher grades, institutional treatment becomes necessary, the patient keeps the ward, the physicians, and the attendants constantly on the go. He makes jokes, wants to help, finds many arrangements very fine, but wants to make improvements; he protests against the "restraint" even to the extent of severe outbursts of rage with the destruction of everything within reach; but violent acts toward persons are noticeably rare, except perhaps occasional slaps in the face, etc. At night the patient keeps on singing, or makes a doll of life size out of the bed, etc. Female patients, in greater numbers and more regularly than the male, are conspicuous for their marked eroticism, going as far as the most shameless acts. In spite of all, one can easily get a good rapport with the patients, as if with spoiled children, whom one likes. ("How goes it with you?" "Very well. Everything pleases me and I can run well,"—"Run" being a flighty association to the verb "goes" in the question.)

In the highest grade of mania *frenzy* (Tobsucht) appears permanently; the patients are in "incessant activity," tear up, destroy, in order to construct with the remains anything at all, a costume, a statue, a relief of Switzerland; they smear, scold, howl, sing, hop; nothing is completed, one "fragment of an action" supplants the other. The expressions do not become really senseless.

In all forms, it is only by way of exception that one does not find a great *talkativeness* up to incessant *logorrhœa* as a partial manifestation of the pressure activity. In severer cases the sentences are no longer completed, because before that can be done there is always a new idea to be expressed. Citations from all available languages are intermingled; occasionally, too, a new language is invented. The *hand-writing* shows the same disturbances, there is flightiness, unevenness, mixture of various languages; the writing is helter skelter, all sorts of things are sketched with it; in spite of many attempts at æsthetic decoration, something very dirty and disorderly is finally produced. But above all the hand-writing shows the patient's *excitability,* a very important attribute in respect to the treatment: a large part of the writing is in the beginning, entirely or relatively, well arranged and then becomes more and more morbid. Excitability is a very general attribute in mania. The patients are quieter, the fewer the stimuli affecting them, and the fewer their opportunities to express the impulse to activity. The curve of hand-writing pressure shows energetic and rapid movements. More exact examination of *motility* shows that the movements progress easily and quickly; the maximum of strength, at least in ergographic tests, is less than in the healthy. It is the lack of consideration for everything and the psychical energy of the movements that make the patients appear stronger; this is especially accentuated by the *endurance and the absence of a feeling of exhaustion.*

As accessory symptoms in these ordinary forms of mania, there are also illusions and hallucinations of sight and hearing, more rarely of smell and taste (touch or bodily sensations are hardly ever present) ; but they have little influence on the picture. *Ideas of over-estimation* are rarely absent, and frequently it goes as far as delusions of grandeur, the content of which does not really become senseless, but remains at least imaginable. The most absurd grandiose idea that I saw was that of a Swiss who thought he would become emperor. But one must take great care not to mistake ordinary playfulness for delusions, for which the patients very readily give occasion, especially so in their every day *"mistaking of persons."* The patients designate the people about them with other names, which is often based on any slight internal or external resemblance, and retain the fiction for a long time; but if one remains suspicious one can probably offer proof in all cases that it is a case of some kind of joke. On the other hand, the feelings of being injured and unjustly treated may often resemble a delusion of persecution, which, however, at the first glance is usually distinguished from the paranoiac and paranoid delusion of persecution by a lack of fixations and by the whole manner of expression.

Nervous symptoms are very rarely lacking in the manics, but obtain little significance in the euphoria.

If hallucinations dominate the picture, or if the thought disturbance advances to unclearness and to the formation of confused delusions, we speak of *manic insanity,* even though the euphoria is mixed with transient states of anxiety and depression.

There are also cases (very rare), where delusions and hallucinations merge into the background, but the *disturbance of thought* deviates

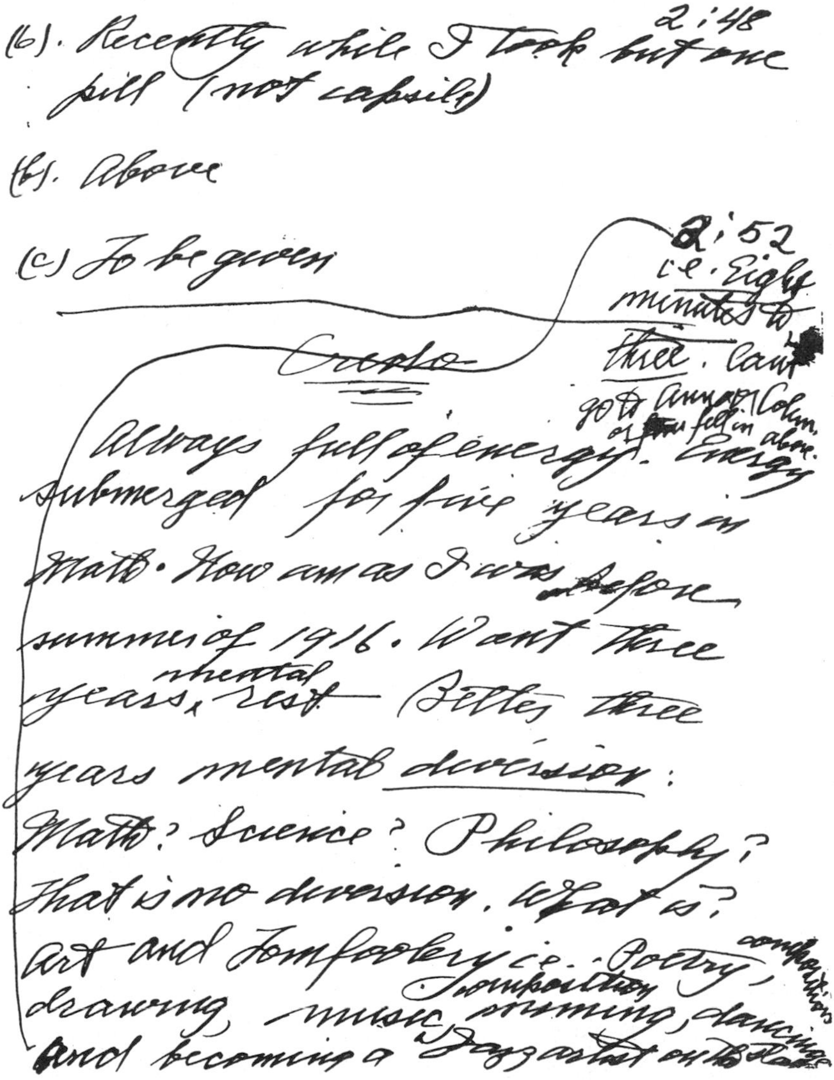

(b). Recently while I took but one 2:48
pill (not capsule)

(b). Above

(c) To be given 2:52
i.e. Eight
minutes to
three. Can
go to Anna of Colum.
of you felt in above. Energy

Always full of energy. Energy
Submerged for five years in
Math. Now am as I was before
summer of 1916. Want three
years, mental rest. Better three
years mental diversion:
Math? Science? Philosophy?
That is no diversion. What is?
Art and Tomfoolery i.e. Poetry, compositions
drawing, music swimming, dancing
And becoming a Jazz artist

Figs. 37 (a) and (b).—Marked excitability and

I(a). Time 2:45; Place Broadway
110th St; Cash: one nickel.
Bank closes 3:00. Going out
that night. Bank books home.
Taxi to home. Get book. To
Bank. Get there 2:55. Draw
out money. Calm and
collected (so did the drivers joke)
all the time.

(b). Time 8:55; place home; condition
as my mother had me; duty
class at 9:00. Called up
assistant's office that could
arrive 9:10 or 9:15; have students
work any problems they chose or
assistant to leave room. Arrived by
taxi 9:25. Began lecture while removing hat.

pressure activity in a very flighty manic patient.

at the height of the disease from the flight of ideas. One cannot really get in touch with the patients; in incomprehensible ways they become violent, externally they have a certain resemblance to excited catatonics but all schizophrenic signs are absent, while the thought disturbance cannot yet be characterized.

Melancholia. The depressive phase colors all experiences painfully; often anxiety is added (sometimes in the form of *præcordial anxiety*); however, the patients like to complain that they have no emotion; everything seems colorless, and strange. "Colorless" also

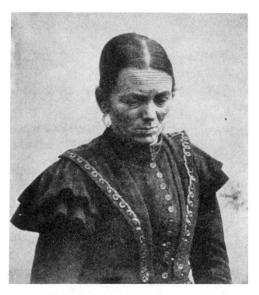

Fɪɢ. 38.—Facial expression of a melancholic. Position of the head and the glance are lowered. The furrowed skin of the forehead is drawn more strongly than ordinary.

often refers to perceptions, but the ability to distinguish colors remains normal. The *mimic expression* is painful, desperate, anxious usually with very little mobility; but as the conceptual content changes just a little, one cannot speak of the "rigidity" of the affects as in schizophrenia. In more severe cases the mimic secretion of tears invariably fails to function; the patients distort the face, sob, all just as in crying, but the eyes remain dry.

A particularly noticeable mimic sign of depression generally originates when the main fold of the upper lid at the edges of its inner third is contracted upward and a little backwards, so that the arch is there changed to an angle (*Veraguth*).

The *association of ideas* is retarded.[116] Thinking becomes slow
and laborious to the patients; it revolves monotonously about their
misfortune. "I think but do not get anywhere. I busy myself all the
time with something and torture myself because I cannot progress"
(*Wernicke*). But to the extent that the affect does not cut off certain
ideas, the melancholic patients can more readily get a proper view of
the more complicated relations than can the manics, when—in milder
cases—a certain objective interest induces them to do so. All psychical
activities are retarded. In more severe cases even retardation of
sensory perception can be demonstrated. As to content, all thoughts
are made difficult that do not harmonize with the psychic pain, so
that it comes to a pretty complete monideism.

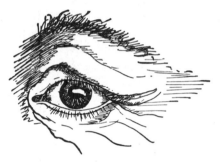 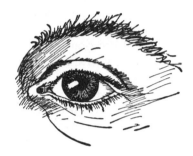

FIG. 39.—Veraguth's fold of the upper lid in depression.   FIG. 40.—Normal fold of the upper lid.

Apperception also is less defective than in the manic. Melancholics
do not make mistakes in reading. To be sure, the threshold values
in apperception tests seem, according to *Kraepelin*, to be heightened.

Orientation is good except in the dreamlike cases into which
melancholias seem to merge more frequently than the manias.

Attention remains concentrated on the imagined misfortune; distractibility is difficult or impossible; even within the melancholic
idea, attention moves with difficulty; it does not pass readily from
one topic to another.

The *centrifugal functions* are very seriously impaired. Irresolution
may grow to an unbelievable extent; a patient may want to change
her place at the table, lift up the chair, and then require half an hour
to decide whether and where she should place it.

Movements become trying, slow, and weak. The limbs are as
heavy as "lead." Movements require just as much exertion as does
thinking.

[116] See p. 74.

More frequently than in mania *one observes* as *accessory symptoms* delusions and hallucinations (of sight and hearing). The devil appears at the window, makes faces at the patients. They hear themselves condemned, they hear the scaffold erected on which they are to be executed, and their relatives crying who must suffer on their account, or starve or otherwise perish miserably.

But the *delusions* especially are never absent in a pronounced case and always as delusions of economic, bodily, and spiritual ruin. The patients think that they became poor, and it does no good to show them their valuables or their balance in the bank; that has no significance for them. Debts are there anyway, or demands are to be expected that will wipe out everything. The patients have a severe, incurable disease acquired through sin, naturally not a melancholia. This delusion is supported by feelings of uneasiness in the digestive tract. The convulsive contraction of the throat connected with the depression and difficulties in swallowing prove to them that there is a closing of the œsophagus, inactivity of the digestive tract, and a number of other severe disturbances. The patients have sinned in a dreadful manner; even the Grace of Christ cannot save them; they have perpetrated especially the sin against the Holy Ghost which can never be forgiven. "Even when I drink a little cold water, it is stolen and I have eaten and drunk so much." They involuntarily examine their whole life to find such crimes; they transform slight mistakes or even entirely innocent acts into the greatest sins. In the form of *delusions of reference* they sometimes attach new ideas to what goes on about them. It is their fault that the other patients are sick, that one has died; because of them the war broke out, because of their sins people must despise them; every one talks about them; in this world and the next they must be punished, usually in the most terrible way. The melancholics have deserved their tortures in contrast with the "persecuted." In a milder melancholia the feeling may appear now and then that things are not so bad as all that; an expected punishment may appear unjust. In other cases also there may sometimes appear, in the endlessly complicated workings of the human psyche, a real idea of persecution, e.g. even in healthy people—*but to melancholia belongs only the depressive delusions,*[117] *whose variations in genesis, in diagnostic, and prognostic significance are entirely different from the katathymic delusion of persecution.*

Not at all rare are *compulsive* fears, transitory or lasting throughout the entire phase, e.g. doing some harm to the loved one, or com-

[117] See p. 92.

pulsive thoughts, often of a coprolalic or sacrilegious nature. Unjustifiable self-reproaches may assume a compulsive form before belief in their correctness comes in and transforms them into delusions.

Among the other *accessory symptoms* the nervous ones should be mentioned again which, however, in connection with anxiety, the tendency to ideas concerning diseases, and the painful coloring of all experiences take on a far greater significance than in mania; the patients often complain chiefly about all sorts of weaknesses, black spots before the eyes, roaring in the ears, headache and other parasthesias. The beginning of the disease often gives the impression of *"Neurasthenia"* (as do the mild forms during the entire course.) Passing hysteriform syndromes also occur, e.g. fainting spells, attacks of dizziness, and crying spells.

Their *behavior* corresponds to the disease. In certain relatively milder cases, the patients try by mechanical, incessant work to keep away the anguish and probably at the same time make up for their supposed derelictions. But usually the ability to work declines rapidly, which, in turn, naturally increases the patients' pain. Even in moderately severe cases hardly any work is done. It may become too complicated for the patient to get from one bed to another (*Kraepelin*); they sit or lie about, and move only very little; it may even go as far as stuporous immobility. Sometimes they still reply to questions, but hardly spontaneously. Under certain conditions they can still copy but can no longer write a letter. In severe cases orthographic and grammatical errors also occur. But a letter often shows the preservation of intelligence, by its correct form, and by the clear inquiries concerning all situations even in patients with whom intellectual contact is prevented by retardation.

Even when a decision has been put in operation, the patients are not satisfied with it; whatever has been done, has always been just the wrong thing.

Where anxiety predominates it often expresses itself in restless movements such as striving to get away, or clinging to people; more rarely in loud wailing, etc. (*Melancholia agitata, activa*). But in regard to other actions and thinking these patients are retarded nevertheless. There may also be impulsive masturbation and, under certain conditions, attacks of excessive hunger as observed in the nervous, are not rare accompanying manifestations of the anxiety. As·*Raptus melancholicus* one designates the manifestation wherein otherwise retarded patients suddenly do something with great energy only to return to their previous external calm; but wherever I myself observed these manifestations, it involved catatonics.

Speech is quiet, slow, as brief as possible, often up to complete mutism. Only rarely does one observe an endless, monotonous whining. In the same way the hand-writing shows in its pressure curve, weak and greatly prolonged movements (*Kraepelin*).

Nearly all melancholics have *suicidal impulses* and would perish if they were not guarded.

In the simple cases of *melancholia simplex* the depressive *retardation* dominates the picture. The patients are sad, anxious, see only the bad side of everything, suffer from their inability to work, and announce that they are tired of life. Here especially a mild form of *depersonalization* is comparatively often noticeable in which the patients conceive the outer world as well as their own person as something different and strange. Peculiar illusions of persecution bother the patient (it is just as if the corridor were crooked, the light doubled, the whole house reduced in size). They can no longer get the right idea of their home and their relatives. *Compulsive ideas*, too, are more noticeable here than in the severer forms. Delusions and especially hallucinations may be lacking in the mildest cases.

If the retardation becomes severe so that the patients speak very little and no longer take care of themselves, the picture is then called *depressive stupor*.

In the severer cases delusions are invariably present and may stand in the foreground. At the same time the hallucinations usually but not always increase.

The depressive attack, also, because of the increase of the hallucinations or the thought disturbance, may assume a paranoid or delirious appearance (*melancholic insanity*). As an illustration of a morbid picture that would soonest deserve the name of paranoid, and nevertheless shows at once that it belongs to manic-depressive insanity, the following may serve as a characteristic picture:

Stock broker, born 1847. Three near relatives melancholic. Quiet, able, reliable. In 1889 sleeplessness, anxiety, increasing inability to keep books. After a while distrustful; then ideas that his letters were being taken, that poison was being given to him, and as a result of which he no longer could see well. People wanted to drug him, and have him endorse notes. He was said to be syphilitic; people knew it; everything was being taken from him. Attempted suicide. Then taken to insane asylum. A misprint in the newspaper and some utterances of others were supposed to refer to him. "Everybody has turned against me." Bad food was being cooked especially for him. He complained about everything and everybody and was very obtrusive. The physician gave him rheumatic pains in the shoulder; he

Do no work
Avoid blues by constantly talking
to folks of my bad points. The
struck in the sand attitude
I don't do anything because I
feel things are so bad that I
can't overcome them
Think of suicide as sort of
way out yet know I can't
do it

Have absolutely no heart; am
cruel to own folks by ——
At times I feel like busting things
Balk at dressing in morning;
Run away from people; again
the ostrich in the sand attitude.
Hate everything

FIG. 41 is the handwriting of the same patient who furnished the material for 37 (a) and (b), just as he merged into a state of depression. Here the patient shows a very scant productivity, and in contradistinction to his former euphoria he now describes the classical feelings of melancholia toward the end of a manic condition. Content full of feeling. Contrasted with his former writing mania, there is a retardation in the movements, shown by the slanting lines.

complained, cried and whined. Hallucinations could not be proven. Fairly rapid cure after one year.—Then complete health. He improved his business. In 1898, after an operation on his son, he was excessively concerned, anxious, sleepless; melancholic ideas of poverty which, however, were soon entirely supplanted by delusions of persecution. The least and the greatest occurrences indicated that he was being persecuted and that his life was in danger. He had to be answerable for everybody that did anything for him. On the whole he considered himself innocent, and only rarely had a melancholic idea of sinfulness. This time he saw "something horrible" on the floor, because of which he became afraid and violent. He thought that the physician injected poison into him with the stethoscope. On his birthday he awaited death; fear of a "nameless misfortune." His surroundings changed into animals that threatened him (but besides this there was still a certain understanding of what was real and possible). Then again he refers everything to himself. He is being persecuted, made fun of, is having all sorts of things put into his food. The pictures on the wall have a reference to him. With these one can put ideas into his head. This attack also lasted a year. Later for several years following, there was a plain hypomanic condition with unimpaired ability to work and clear insight. In 1915, again an entirely similar attack in which the patient died.

Mixed States. A. The three cardinal symptoms of mania and depression, exalted and depressed mood, flight of ideas and mental retardation, pressure activity and inhibition of the will, represent three pairs of contrasts. The corresponding functions of affectivity, of thought process, and of centrifugality are, as a rule, similarly changed in the disease as shown in types so far presented, and as they are in their minor development in the normal. But besides the positive fluctuations in the one field there may be negative ones in the other, and what is more they may occur in all of the six possible combinations which aside from the two main groups, melancholia and mania, result from the mutation of the three pairs. The most important of these *mixed forms* are: the depressive *"anxious mania"* (the affect is negative, while the thought process and certrifugality are positive), in which with depressed affect combined with ideas of sin, the patients speak and write much and complain that the thoughts come of themselves. In *"excited depression"* (affect and thought process negative, centrifugality positive), one has sought to include the picture of melancholia agitata. But this is incorrect; the agitation is nothing but the expression of anxiety and with it the other centrifugal functions are plainly retarded. The *"mania with impoverished thought"* (affect and centrifugality positive, associations negative) frequently occurs during the decline of a severe manic stage. Outwardly the patients seem easily moved, readily make a noise, feel good, but do not perceive properly; try to speak but cannot say much and repeat themselves. As a transition to this there often appear in the manifestation endless narratives of the same sort of thing, names of persons, or of places. From the inhibition of the mental and centrifugal functions and a positive affect, there originates the picture of a coagulated mania ("manic stupor"), in which the patients, though they have a cheerful expression, are immovable, unless at times at any opportunity they unsuspectingly play a trick.

B. Another kind of mixture of positive and negative deviation may also originate within the same psychologic function which we have artificially limited. Within the limits of thinking retardation and flight of ideas may occur side by side, whence originates heaviness of the mental stream combined with sudden changes, and frequent sound associations (as in certain stages of alcoholic effects). A mixture of despair and cheerful self-contempt is designated by *Kraepelin* as *grim humor*, "humor of the gallows." [118] A mixture of grandiose ideas and depression is also said to occur in manic-depressive insanity (the patient is persecuted by the emperor and king; he desires a romantic death and similar things, *Kraepelin*). *Kraepelin* presents a hand-writing curve which is normally strong and yet very much prolonged; this indicates high pressure with a retardation of movement. One of my female patients covered all available pieces of paper with writing but in a depressive manner with markedly sloping lines. Her affect, too, was a mixture of depression and exaltation. The pressure activity, combined with muteness, not at all rare in schizophrenia, is supposed to have been noticed here also. In one female patient I saw in two attacks a protracted pressure activity (long walks) with the absence of a feeling of exhaustion with negative signs of all other functions.

The mixed conditions of both forms are not rarely transitions of the individual phases, but may also appear as independent complete phases; they then constitute, even if the confusions with schizophrenia are disregarded, a more unfavorable formation of the morbid picture, run their course slowly and recur often, after they have barely calmed down.

A part of the symptomatology is common to both phases, as has already been shown us by the absence of coarser disturbances of perception, of orientation, and of the nervous symptoms.

In the psychic field mention should again be made of the condition of the *memory* which appears to be affected very little directly. During and after the attacks, the patients recall the essentials of what

[118] This is entirely different from the similarly designated mixture of anxiety and drinker's euphoria in Delirium tremens.

happened in the course of their duration, but there is rarely lacking a more or less extensive transformation of the recollections. The former manic patient can no longer imagine that he was so unpleasant, and in good faith represents most of his conflicts as justifiable reactions to unjust and awkward attacks, and often with such skill that he even convinces others. The severer the flight of ideas was, the

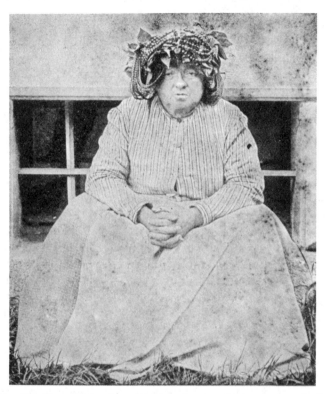

FIG. 42.—Mixed condition in a debilitated case. Inconstant euphoria. Motor retardation which crowds out the euphoric expression of the face but nevertheless permits the patient to decorate herself with necklaces made of mountain ash berries.

more difficult to be sure, is the orderly ekphoria of the experiences, and for this reason also obscurities and gaps appear. It is significant that individual manics believe after recovery, that they had really suffered from melancholia, because the few brief intercurrent depressions and the most striking inner difficulties are remembered much better and appear much more important than the cheerful total manic condition. To be sure these recollections may point to many a psychic and physical pain which we did not observe during the excitation.

There often exists in the healthy periods a lack of interest or a positive disinclination to devote any attention to the morbid processes, as a result of which forgetting is produced or at any rate simulated. Melancholics, who as a whole have a somewhat better recollection than the manics, may very easily repress very much, and often just the most important things. This even occurs when in the course of an attack they have definitely resolved that this time they will think of this and that during the free period, e.g. of the relation to the physicians. Often at the beginning of a later attack, the recollection of an earlier one turns up so vividly that the patients feel it very unpleasantly as a disturbing compulsion. The recollection of the *delusional forms* is usually defective and greatly falsified, under certain conditions totally lacking.

Insight into the disease is usually lacking and is never complete during the acute phases, although in case of more frequent repetitions the patients may themselves seek the institution as soon as they find it necessary. The manic invariably estimates his own worth much too highly, the melancholic infinitely too low. Frequently the patients have a relatively good insight of previous attacks, but not of the actual one, which they always consider "something very different."

In both phases the *hallucinations* are usually confined to sight and hearing, and often have little vividness. The patients themselves sometimes describe them as "manifestations." They are also not so obtrusive as e.g. in dementia præcox.

The *physical symptoms* of manic depressive insanity are not important. In euphoria the *turgor vitalis* is naturally raised; a patient who in a state of melancholia is a broken up individual may appear twenty years younger the next day when he has merged into a manic mood, and then present a vigorous bearing and good appearance. All vegetative functions adapt themselves to the situation. The exalted person usually has a good appetite and effective metabolism; sub-manics who eat regularly and do not exhaust themselves with incessant movements consequently usually gain; more severe manics, to be sure, lose, partly also because they do not take the trouble to eat enough, and instead use their food as material to satisfy their pressure activity instead of their hunger. I once had an experience by way of exception, where a manic could be saved from death only by being forcibly kept in bed, because his heart did not keep up with his activities, so that every now and then he developed *hydrops universalis*. There was no endocarditis. In melancholia the appetite fails, the bowels are also often sluggish; as a rule there is a loss of weight; *an increase of weight, with very few exceptions, indicates recovery.*

Pronounced increase in strength without accompanying recovery indicates a different, especially a schizophrenic, foundation.

In both phases *sleep* is poor, often so poor that a normal person would rapidly break down under it; the function of recuperation must take a different course in the disease than under normal conditions.

Examinations of *body temperature,* of the *blood, urine,* and *metabolism* generally have as yet yielded no regular findings. Noticeably often one finds sugar in the urine during the attacks.

Pulse and *respiration* correspond approximately to what one expects from emotional excitations and depressions of normal persons.

Menstruation often disappears, to·reappear toward the end of the attack.

The *reflexes* are sometimes increased; in the manic state they are said to be rapid, in the melancholic slower.—Manic "analgesia" is the result of changed attention.[119]

The *intervals.* Between the attacks most patients show so little that is pathologic that one speaks of "normal intervals." Nevertheless there is seen in many, especially when the disease has existed a long time, a distinct lability of the emotional condition, partly as a reaction to external conditions with irritability and exaggerated excursions in the direction of euphoria as well as depression, partly, however, as passing fluctuations from within, which *Kraepelin* considers as rudimentary attacks. In individual cases—only a very small percentage of all manic depressives—this goes so far that the patients lose their ability for social functioning; they are no longer capable of adapting themselves sufficiently to others and lack all stamina for independent work. In contrast to this the ordinary "intelligence tests" do not show any evident decline. In the periodic manics there frequently develops in the intervals a protracted mildly manic temperament; in those patients with mainly or exclusively melancholic phases there develops a protracted depressive mood of minor grade. Of these types there are all transitions to those who from youth onward appear mildly manic or melancholic and then are preferably afflicted with phases having similar signs.

Course. In the majority of the cases the disease becomes manifest through the first attack between fifteen and thirty, but at times may first show itself in the eighties. Individual cases go back to childhood; but every child which in youth seemed a little cyclothymic does not by any means later become manic-depressive; the anomaly may lose itself.

In general the attacks repeat themselves at varying intervals; im-

[119] See p. 56.

mediately after the expiration of one, another may appear, or decades may elapse from one to another. Naturally under these conditions it may also happen that in the course of a single life only one appears. But there are patients with whom for many years one can count on a more or less regular succession. If the intervals are about equal and not too long and the attacks of the same kind, one speaks of *periodic mania* and *periodic melancholia; as cyclic* (or *circular*) *insanity* are designated the types in which mania and melancholia with or without free intervals follow in regular succession.

For the *quality of the attacks* also we do not know any rule. The longer one can oversee the patient's life, the more rarely one finds series which are made up of the same kind of attacks. On the whole melancholia increases with age, while mania decreases. Severe manic attacks are likely to occur in the same patients with severe melancholic attacks, while submanias and submelancholias correspond in turn. For a long time many patients have attacks that resemble one another very exactly; one even speaks of a photographic exactness of the repetition. One of my "paranoids" each time took up again the delusions formed in an earlier attack to develop them further (inventor, reformer).—The single attack, aside from the mixed conditions of the transition, usually keeps itself within the same category. But in severer attacks with otherwise clear states in respect to both phases, confusion states lasting fifteen minutes or hours are not entirely rare, in which on the one hand, the patients whine senselessly, throw themselves on the ground, take no consideration of decency, and are inaccessible to any advice, and on the other hand, senselessly rage and struggle. According to *Kraepelin* patients with mere depression are more frequent; those with mere manias are the rarest.

The *individual attacks* usually last many months, a half year to a year, the melancholic probably on the average somewhat longer than the manic; upward deviations to several years are frequent, up to ten or more years very rare. By way of rare exception, individual patients have a tendency to complete their attacks in one or two weeks. Prodromic symptoms frequently take the form of general discomfort which is taken to be neurasthenic, and strangely enough not rarely in the forms of neuralgias which may have all the marks of a definite nerve inflammation, e.g. sciatica or intercostal neuralgia. A patient of *Schuele* hallucinated a gray bird every time at the beginning of the attack. Mania is preceded sometimes but not always by a really depressive introductory stage. The ascent is gradual, in severe attacks not very rarely in two periods, as after about two or three weeks' duration a remission occurs, which, however, is soon followed again by a severe aggravation. Then the disease usually remains at its height for a long time. Recovery sets in gradually and with fluctuations, in melancholias frequently so; better days appear, which after a while recur more frequently and show a more evident decrease of the symptoms. During the falling off of the mania the inhibitions then taking place simulate a "dementia" for the inexperienced. Not so rarely the character takes on an unpleasant nagging. After the manic attack there often follows a more or less severe depressive after-stage, or at least a feeling of exhaustion.—After melancholic phases the patients often feel "better than ever," are more active and pleasant than before, and that not only for months, but even for years. The rare sudden fluctuations occur especially in cyclic cases, in which the patient may change the phase from one day to the other. But transitions from, and toward the normal conditions, may at times also appear suddenly by way of exception.

Concerning the general *prognosis* little can be said as yet. The individual case recovers. Very rarely does a patient stay over in the asylum, because the intervals become so brief that a discharge cannot be considered. Every now and then a case makes his home in the hospital and remains there willingly even when the intervals are longer. Longer series of attacks seem to have a tendency to decrease the intervals with age. But in general the admissions decrease quickly in the forties, in spite of a slight increase between 45 and 50, and after the period of involution we see only a few of our regular customers from early manhood. Therefore many later remain free at least from more severe attacks.

The quality of the attacks sometimes seems somewhat more severe in old age; the manias are less strong, the melancholias rather confused; probably the delusional forms also increase a little.

During the acute phase *death* may occur, among melancholics chiefly as the result of suicide, otherwise from intercurrent diseases; some suicides take their families with them ("family murder"), in order to save them too from misery. Manics die at times from exhaustion or from injuries which they will not permit to be treated.

Manic-depressives have a certain tendency to suffer relatively early from *arteriosclerosis,* or other *brain atrophy.*

Protracted Displacing of Mood. To manic-depressive insanity belong the high and low spirits, which on the one hand do not last long, and on the other do not attain the degree of a morbid mood. For the latter reason they rarely come under psychiatric observation in spite of their frequency; nevertheless now and then a fluctuation of the mood rising to a pathological degree demonstrates the connection with the entire group, which moreover is made closer by heredity. The following forms can be distinguished:

1. *Constitutional ill-temper or depressive disposition* ("melancholic mood"), a protracted dark emotional coloration of all life experiences, difficulty in making resolutions; lack of self-confidence.

2. *Constitutional excitement or manic disposition* ("manic mood"). The manic temperatment of such people disposes to overhasty acts and to a thoughtless manner of living in general, when it is not restrained by a particularly sound understanding and a particularly good morality. For that reason we find here on the one hand snobbish, inconsiderate, quarrelsome and cranky ne'er-do-wells, who have no staying powers in their transactions, but on the other hand "sunny dispositions," and people endowed with great ability, amounting sometimes to genius, and not rarely gifted with artistic ability who possess a tireless energy. Such a man, e.g. was the founder of "Physiognomics," Lavater.

3. The *irritable mood.*

4. *Cyclothymics,* in whom periods of energetic euphoria alternate with despondent impotence. Among these too are found artists and other people who do great things. *Moebius* has given good reasons for counting Goethe with these. Whether H. von Kleist should be called manic-depressive or cyclothymic is arbitrary.

5. The *constitutional disposition may also change,* especially around the time of puberty. David Hess was depressive as a boy, then said to himself one time: "Now I am no longer melancholic," and remained until death in a manic mood; his sister, from youth up, was always "like quicksilver." Lavater too was sensitive in youth, "bashful," as was a famous still living scholar with a manic mood. A woman up to about her twentieth year seemed noticeably cheerful, lively in the pleasant sense, then for a time mildly depressive. Her membership in the manic-depressive group was proven by a melancholia lasting several years which began at forty-one, after which for ten years she was lively and very energetic, bore heavy blows of fate admirably, to be melancholic again at 54 for three years.

As *"milder forms"* periodic conditions are also to be mentioned, which take a course under the picture of neurasthenias or stomach neuroses or headache.

Conception. Manic-depressive insanity is a lasting anomaly that produces fluctuations in the sense of mania and melancholia and also readily shows itself in other ways as a lability of the sensibilities, or in the form of habitual shiftings of the mood. Everything that goes with this is shown by the examination of the family disposition which points to an equivalence of all the outlined disease pictures.[120]

So far everything is readily comprehensible; but there are certainly moods of a different origin which we cannot as yet distinguish as such from the manic-depressive. Therefore in regard to the differentiation we are not altogether certain where one of these other causes might cooperate, and, on the other hand, this fact must make us hesitate to endeavor to explain the attacks merely on the basis of predisposition. Some of these moods are undoubtedly purely psychogenic; others have a physical foundation, as in paretic or senile processes, in dementia præcox, and in disturbances of the inner secretion (Basedow manias and melancholias). Physical diseases, especially cardiac and vascular disturbances, produce depressions; incipient fever, chemical remedies like alcohol and tuberculin generate conditions, which have at least a great resemblance to mania. Now is it necessary for the appearance of such effects that there be always or at least in many cases a manic-depressive disposition? Is cerebral atrophy often or always or never the sole cause of the accompanying depression in senile forms? Are the cyclic forms of schizophrenia all mixed forms of the two diseases? [121] We cannot answer all these questions.[122]

If all along we have placed the affective fluctuations in the fore-ground, it was with the understanding that they are only the most conspicuous expression of the more general psychic disturbance. For it is true that the more important symptoms such as flight of ideas, pressure activity, associative and centrifugal inhibitions, which alone, besides the actual mood, are usually tangible, are indicated in every strong affect and may, therefore, be conceived as exaggerations of the "emotional effect." But opposed to this is the fact that the three symptom groups need not at all correspond quantitatively to one another even in the ordinary cases, thus the centrifugal retardation, e.g. even with painful mood that remains the same, may oscillate not only from one case to another, but also in the same patient. It is, for example, usually relatively more severe in young people than in cases of the involutional period; but above all the mixed states prove that the derivation of the entire picture from an affective fluctuation does not tally at all, or only to a slight degree. Then, too, especially in the thought disturbance many symptoms transcend the emotional effect,

[120] Compare the relation to the syntony of normals, p. 174.

[121] There are certain forms which symptomatologically give the impression of manic-depressive-schizophrenic mixed forms, but are a unity at least in the family disposition.

[122] Concerning the psychogenic release of true manic-depressive attacks, see pp. 132-489.

which on closer inspection are more frequent in the apparently simple cases also than would appear from the descriptions; only one cannot as yet grasp and describe them properly. Complaints about the obtrusive crowding up of a mass of ideas, the interference with the arbitrary direction of thought, the obscurities that belong to the flight of ideas and which in individual cases with a mere indication of flight of ideas or retardation may go as far as confusion and dream-like states, the hallucinatory and paranoid symptom complexes, paresthesias and "neuralgias,"—all of these prove a positive number of disturbances which must be of the greatest importance for the explanation, but which as yet have eluded our comprehension. Behind the customary expressions, dispositions, exhaustibility, irritability, inner secretion, there lies concealed in manic-depressive insanity very little, or nothing at all, that is matter of fact or even intelligently connected.

Extent. Kraepelin's idea of manic-depressive insanity is pretty well circumscribed. The transitions of the various forms among themselves and especially in the same patient, and the hereditary conditions prove the homogeneity of all the different pictures. The group cannot be sharply delimited from many mere psychogenic distempers in psychopaths, and from the melancholias not to be included as yet. A natural boundary also probably does not exist between the habitually moody and the "psychopathic personalities," especially between our irritable cases and the excitable among the psychopaths.

Of the conceptions of other classifications several correspond to individual forms of manic-depressive insanity or they disagree with it. The "mania" and "melancholia" of German psychiatry naturally belong to our disease, but all diseases with this name of non-German authors do not; they include a large part of the excited and depressive forms of other psychoses also, especially of schizophrenia. Probably everything designated as periodic neurasthenia, recurrent dyspepsia, etc., also belongs entirely to manic-depressive insanity; also attacks of hypochondria, and *Friedmann's* neurasthenic melancholias. The "acute" and the "periodic paranoia" correspond in part with our manic and depressive delusional forms, for the greater part, to be sure, with schizophrenic hallucinoses, similarly the majority of the amentia cases of the classifications other than *Kraepelin's*. Some of the litigants are manic-depressive or cyclothymic; if one has a good anamnesis, they are easily recognized; as distinguished from the paranoid litigants they have times in which they keep themselves very quiet, and even see the senselessness of their previous conduct and regret it; also the delusional system does not remain homogeneously centered. A part of the patients coming to the physician because of *compulsive thoughts* are depressive types.

"Melancholia" requires a special consideration. It is self-evident that very many of these afflictions fit in the above class. But, as was indicated, there are other depressions and it does not seem reasonable to bunch all the apparently independent depressions of the period of involution and class them with manic-depressive insanity. Formerly *Kraepelin* actually endowed the *melancholia of the period of involution* with a nosological independence as melancholia katexochen which, however, can no longer be sustained in the differentiation of that time. But the reasons for the separation were nevertheless very weighty. These forms have in great part a much more protracted course. They grow very slowly, often for one or two years, readily remain in their height for several years and again require a long time to decline. The retardation is frequently concealed by a great restlessness; really agitated forms are frequent even though probably rarer than in the senile melancholias. Then they regress much less than the others. Single attacks are very common in these cases. To be sure, if one wishes, one can conceive of the thing in this way; that with increasing age and most especially in the period of involution, the disposition for depressive attacks and for agitated and slowly developing forms increases, so that with a slight predisposition an attack occurs merely at this age and usually in the described form. But one often gets the impression that something else is involved; this is true also in the so-called "climacterium virile," a depression common to men, which runs its course in this form but is usually mild, which appears at the end of the fifties, even at the beginning of the sixties, rarely makes an asylum necessary, but nevertheless plainly reduces the joy of living and the ability to work, and usually presages another disease (arteriosclerosis!), but disappears in two or three years without leaving a sign. As long as we do not know the "nature" of the affective psychoses, only hereditary investigations have any prospect of throwing light on the subject. At present this separation is just as impossible, as an inner grouping of the cases which undoubtedly belong together in the wider classification.

Purely psychogenic depressions which occur in psychopaths who are not manic depressive and attain the height of a disease are very rare.[123]

As a definite *cause* of manic-depressive insanity we know only the inherited disposition where the different forms of the disease may substitute one another. The one member of the family is cyclothymic,

[123] See p. 537.

the other periodically melancholic, the third circular, etc. But in some families one or the other of the two phases predominates. I knew a family in which for five generations quite a number of members had committed suicide at the time of involution. One can take for granted that about 80% of all these patients are tainted, if the conception of "taint" is not too limited, and in large part in such a way that equivalent anomalies are found in other members of the family.

The *endowments* of the patients are often noticeably good, especially along artistic lines also, which is probably connected with their sensitiveness. One also finds more manic-depressives in the upper classes than in the lower.

According to *sex* about 70% of the patients are women.

Kraepelin found among the Javanese little tendency to depression, instead more to excitation. In the large insane asylums of Costa Rica with Indian inmates and in Jamaica with colored inmates, one does not count at all on suicide, although I was told in both places that many years ago one had occurred. The Jewish race is evidently strongly disposed to manic-depressive insanity. Within that race also the frequency—entirely aside from changing delimitations—varies greatly, in German Switzerland it is very small, in middle Germany it is higher. [124]

It is also supposed that brain lesions generate the disease, especially the delusional forms, which we still have to include in manic-depressive insanity. But up to the winter of 1919-1920 we know of no injuries to the brain incurred during the war that could have led to manic-depressive manifestations.

Individual attacks in large part come from within. War did not seem to release them. But one cannot doubt that now and then (I estimate about 10%) they can be released psychically; thus in a woman of good family, who probably in a moody state married an insignificant man, and during many years always had a manic attack every time the attempt was made to have her join his family—until the husband died.

Manias also occur at times after the *puerperium* in women who otherwise, as far as their lives can be investigated, have no attacks; then as *menstrual insanity* where they last only from eight to fourteen days. In one case of my observation an attack did not occur at every menstruation but the attack never came without menstruation.

[124] It is disproportionately high among the Jewish admissions of the Manhattan State Hospital, N. Y., which contains a rather mixed element of Jews. Cf. *Brill & Karpas,* Insanity Among Jews, N. Y. Medical Journal, Oct. 3, 1914. Also Kirby; Race and Psychopathology, N. Y. State Hospital Bulletin, March 1909.

Milder depressions are not rare in *pregnancy* but as a rule disappear with the birth.

It is often possible to make a *diagnosis* from a symptomatic investigation if one obtains a good account of preceeding attacks with healthy intervals. But if the anamnesis is lacking or if it is a case of a first attack, *then manic-depressive insanity can be recognized only by the elimination of other diseases. There are no specific signs of the affect psychoses; everything occurring in manic-depressive insanity can also be seen in other diseases.* If, however, *in spite of exact observation* no specific symptoms of another psychosis is found in such "mood," one may decide on manic-depressive insanity. But since a catatonia or a paresis may run a course for some time without distinct specific signs, one must not, at least in the first week, decide with certainty on manic-depressive insanity. Signs, which symptomatologically should be called catatonic, are said to occur here also; but at all events this is rare.

Special difficulties are presented by the *paranoid* and *delusional forms;* there only protracted and careful observation will make it possible to drop the suspicion of dementia præcox. On the other hand, differentiation from *paranoia,* for which the form was not so rarely mistaken, is usually made easy by the evidence of the depression.

Cases of dementia præcox are often mistaken for *mixed forms.* Only a more prolonged and exact observation with a weighing of all the circumstances, and sometimes a good anamnesis, will guard against this error. When in doubt one should remember that the pronounced mixed forms, especially the manic stupors also, are much rarer than similar schizophrenic conditions.

Incipient *paresis* can be differentiated by the physical signs and the senselessness of the delusions and by the examination of the spinal fluid. But hypochondriacal ideas, even in case of a good intelligence, can well strike the physician as somewhat senseless, since in such matters the healthy person also often has very peculiar notions.

Manic excitements can be differentiated from the *epileptic* even in a brief examination by the flight of ideas which does not occur in epilepsy, and by the absence of the signs of epilepsy, especially the slow mental process, the obscurity and peculiarities of speech.

Some *hysteric symptoms* may occur in manic-depressive attacks, especially when they are also present in the intervals. Pronounced and stubborn but isolated hysteriform symptoms point with probability to a complication with organic or schizophrenic diseases. Manias that belong to hysteria probably do not exist; but it is possible that there are such depressions.

A differential diagnosis from psychogenic depressions is symptomatologically not possible as yet. But on weighing all the circumstances, especially the family anamnesis also, one will,—especially after the recovery—make the diagnosis with considerably certainty.

Treatment. The *predisposition* might be eradicated by forbidding the begetting of children in manic-depressive families. It is a question whether this would be wise because a large part of these families maintain themselves in spite of all and even do distinguished things. The seriously sick naturally should not marry, not even in the free intervals; at all events I would not like to advise anybody to select a manic-depressive mate, as the difficulties for the healthy partner are often greater than for the one afflicted. But I must state that in spite of this, things go well in individual cases; the able and pleasant afflicted partners, when necessary now and then, take treatment in an insane asylum, and in the intervals may be excellent companions.

Also for the prevention of the individual attack not much can be done, because it usually comes about without external occasion. Nevertheless the avoidance of excitements and excesses of all kinds is good in other respects also, if it can be achieved.

With pronounced manics nothing can be done except to send them to a hospital. There the attack most easily runs its course in spite of all irritations because of the confinement. As far as possible irritants should be kept away; isolation, which still gives the patient a chance to entertain himself somehow with trifles, is the therapy which should be applied whenever possible. *As distinguished from schizophrenia a "degeneration" resulting from isolation is not to be feared.* If it is not feasible, then the supervised continuous bath is the best place for the patient to stay. Occasionally artificial feeding may be necessary.

The *milder cases* which one cannot resolve to send to a hospital are a trial. They have the tendency to ruin their fortune, their honor, their health—a girl of good family, in six attacks only came to the hospital after she was pregnant—they bother others, enter into litigations, and through sexual relations, engagements, etc., make also others unhappy. Under certain conditions a legal guardianship, where that is possible, can prevent much harm. But the guardian has a difficult task and his most effective intervention probably is to bring the patient to an asylum. In addition there are rare cases who particularly in the submanic stage, in spite of difficulties with the environment, have made a fortune by their initiative and inventions. But in general it is very risky to let submanics go their way; they always seek more excitements and just these should be avoided.

For *melancholia* also supervision in a closed hospital is the right thing. On the outside many of the patients perish from suicide, and even from starvation. But just in such depressions without other difficulties the family physician will not always be able to disregard the objections of the patient and the family to institutional treatment. But he should only assume the responsibility if the external conditions also warrant it. Against the danger of *suicide* strict supervision should be prescribed; but it does no good merely to say this generally, even though it be done most impressively. It must be made plain to the relatives that at least two attendants must relieve one another, that both attendant and patient, e.g. will go to the toilet and that at such times also supervision is to be carried on; because if the patient wants to take his life, he uses just those occasions of which one later says: "But it was only for a moment." Usually the windows must be secured, and when possible the patient should live on the ground floor. In the milder cases an orderly who sleeps very lightly may sleep beside the patient, perhaps placing the bed so that the patient can get away only over him. Especially dangerous is the period of convalescence when the impulse to suicide is still present, at least in the form of attacks, and the patient's energy is no longer very inhibited, while the vigilance of supervision usually lets up. Where a continuous supervision is not found necessary the physician must see the patient more or less often, usually daily, according to the fluctuations, to inform himself minutely from those about him concerning his condition in order to be able to intervene at the right time.

Supervision is made much easier by protracted *bed treatment*, which is also indicated for other reasons in severe cases, but which becomes a torture in milder cases who have the ability and feel the necessity of moving about in the open and even busying themselves.

In *anxiety melancholias* one can make the attempt to shorten the attack with an opium cure: opium or now pantopon in increasing doses within three or four weeks up to 1.0 Opium (0.2 Pantopon), or a little more; from one to two weeks after this high dose has been reached, one should go down just as slowly whether or not the attack has improved. Because if one has not accomplished anything then, the remedy is no longer effective but may make an opium addict of the patient.

Against *sleeplessness* hypnotics (not opiates) will have to be given now and then. The patient who usually does not want to eat, must be fed sufficiently, perhaps by the tube. Against the frequent constipation mild laxatives are to be used and what is more important—

to prescribe daily attempts, exactly regulated as to time, to go to the toilet.

"Distraction" can attain some mitigation only in the mildest cases; they usually do harm; the most beautiful music can have no good influence if the patient reacts to it with mental pain. Also all other kinds of complicated conversations are usually harmful, even if they can divert for a minute, because afterwards a reaction usually sets in. Here a careful testing is the right thing. The effect is best attained by work which does not tax the patient mentally or demand any decision from him. *In general it is very important to relieve the patient of all decisions, even of those that are simple, and involve trifles, until an extensive improvement has taken place.*

In *pregnancy melancholias* the question of abortion is often put. There are individual cases where the measure has had good results.[125]

In contrast with the schizophrenias *early discharge* from the asylum is to be guarded against. Many of the patients get worse outside; even in the asylums one has the experience that they do worse if they are placed too early in a better ward.

XII. PSYCHOPATHIC FORMS OF REACTION (SITUATION PSYCHOSES)

In case of any kind of disturbances within the psyche the affects also must function differently than otherwise and may then generate morbid syndromes.[126] Congenital anomalies, brain injuries, brain processes of all kinds, disturbances of nutrition, toxins, infections, and finally chronic emotional effects themselves constitute in their multi-colored manifoldness and in the most different combinations the foundation on which the abnormal reactions occur. Where definite processes, like the schizophrenic, or coarser organic brain changes, be at the base, the reactive syndromes are classed with the symptomatology of these diseases from which they usually derive specific peculiarities (schizophrenic delusions, although originated in the same way as the paranoid, differ from the latter; schizophrenic twilight states from the hysteric, etc.), where the abnormal reaction is based on a congenital disposition, the attempt has been made to distinguish it—often in connection with the disposition—as a special "disease" (*neuroses, paranoia*)   In such cases it is usually the abnormal domination of the affect, i.e. its excessive influence on the selection of the associations, sometimes also only the relative weakness of the logical faculties,

[125] Comp., however, p. 225.
[126] Comp. p. 126.

perhaps also of the affective inhibition (e.g. moral) which make the origin of morbid symptoms possible. But qualitative deviations of the affects as well as the intelligence, special sensitiveness in a particular direction, crankiness in thinking, etc., may also be the essential basis of the abnormal reaction form. However, the affectivity with its unlimited possibilities of variation is always the decisive factor while the narrowly confined intellectual functions are overwhelmed or only participate in a secondary rôle.

Most syndromes can best be kept distinct by means of the underlying mechanisms. Many are simply *exaggerated affective effects:* attacks of rage (e.g. Prisoner outbursts), attacks of screaming, stupor, momentary confusions, and fright neurosis. Here the easily aroused dominating affectivity or inadequate ability to deliberate is the main condition (Primitive race, "the nervous," oligophrenics, schizophrenics, epileptics). It is a case of *"primitive reactions" (Kretschmer).* But also in those not otherwise disposed to such reactions, some complex among other things may generate a particular sensitiveness: unrequited love, incessant "pin pricks," unworthy attitude, etc. More rarely ambivalence is the cause; thus in excessive anxiety for certain people, or in too violent or too protracted grief for some lost relative, where usually the unconscious feeling of some advantage derived from the loss causes the exaggeration by way of a sort of feeling of sin. As a rule patients of the latter sort are persons of more sensitive natures.

Another mechanism is the *false connection* to which among other things many *sexual abnormalities* are to be ascribed: A pupil in a classroom has his attention called to onanism by another pupil and at once makes an attempt. The teacher sneaks up and pulls him by the ear. At this moment the orgasm takes place and the result is that the patient can never obtain sexual satisfaction unless he himself or his beloved holds his ear (*Aschaffenburg*). In an analogous way the various form of *fetichism* originate, naturally only in a psychopathic disposition, probably in connection with weak sexuality.—An eleven year old patient of *Frank* suffered since his fifth year from incontinenta alvi, especially in the forenoon at half past ten. Psychoanaylsis revealed that six years ago at this hour, having to go to the toilet, he went to his mother in the kitchen, where hot fat was sprayed on his chest. In his fright he defecated in his clothes. Cure resulted from this explanation.—Other chance associations produce e.g. headache, always after some particular occurrence, because the first time headache appeared after it. This kind of connection may originate, especially in children, even without the essential cooperation of an affect; then it is merely a case of *habituation* or *association reflexes.*

Unbearable situations or those wished to be otherwise may be delusionally transformed by the disease (*delusional reaction*), or circumvented in reality (*"Flight into disease"*). The latter procedure in case of an existing schizophrenic process sometimes makes the disease manifest, but above all it leads to the *neuroses*, which is accomplished by the fact that the unbearable ideas with their affect are split off from consciousness and "repressed" into the unconscious, where they make themselves noticeable by supplementing morbid symptoms.

Delusional Reaction: In an *hysterical or schizophrenic twilight state* the patient hallucinatorily marries the lost lover; in *delusions* of *grandeur* unrealizable wishes are gratified. In *paranoia* and *paranoid delusions of persecution* the cause of one's own failure is projected into the environment, the blame is taken from the ego and besides the latter is relatively elevated by means of ascribing malice to the other people. In *litigiousness* one seeks, on the one hand, to fulfill wishes that in reality can be fulfilled with difficulty or not at all, and, on the other hand, one conceals the opposing rights of others and the difficulties of achieving one's own demands; one also overvalues one's own rights and, along with this, the importance of oneself and thus justifies one's own sensitiveness and joy in oppressing others. In the litigious delusion of paranoia, of the paranoid, of the submanic attack, this affective effect extends to the complete falsification of logic; the kind of reaction, the "choice of the disease," depends here on the psychic constitution of the patient and very little or not at all on the occasion.

Difficulties of intercourse with the environment lead to delusions of persecution in those who are hard of hearing.[127]

A special attitude is taken by the mechanism of *induced insanity:* the taking over of a patient's delusions by a previously healthy person as a result of persuasion and especially suggestion. But there too an affective predisposition must be assumed, which permits the acceptance of delusions having a definite direction.

By means of *flight into the disease* one achieves definite aims through the disease; by an attack of rage one achieves a yielding; by a fainting spell, a new hat; and by the more protracted disease one gets a pleasant sojourn in a sanatorium. By means of all these one can at the same time compel consideration, secure care and tenderness, obtain power over others who have to adjust themselves to the disease, extort an allowance, evade tasks from the simple household duties up to the terrors of the trenches. But above all one circumvents inner difficulties; one keeps off self-reproaches from consciousness; by means

[127] See p. 533.

of a symptom one identifies oneself with the beloved, or represents symbolically the union with the beloved who does not care for the patient.

Such *external* aims of the neurosis are very simple; the inner purpose, the fictitious accounting to oneself is often so complicated that we cannot go into details here. Only this should be mentioned, that naturally the neurosis is usually a poor solution from the subjective point of view also, as is shown by the fact that neurotics themselves condemn the evasion of difficulties by this means, because they do not admit the purpose of the device either to themselves or to others. Even the attack of rage which under these circumstances represents a primitive reaction, sensible in principle, often overshoots the mark so much that it becomes most unpleasant for the patient. In order to get the hat, one must have a real fainting spell; to be excused from work, one has unpleasant symptoms; the pensioned neurasthenic has to renounce all joy of living. Whoever becomes a thief out of revenge against the father or commits arson because of an unbearable situation, gets into jail; whoever achieves the companionship of the beloved symbolically is as little satisfied as the hungry dreamer who thinks he eats, and whoever satisfies his ambivalent feelings by imagining a sexual attack, which, though it arouses sexuality at the same time causes disgust, only gets hysterical vomiting out of it.

When we speak of flights into disease, as a *sort of purpose* of the neuroses, this should be understood with some reservation. A more primitive reaction passes away and has no subsequent significance. *But it becomes a neurotic symptom, difficult to combat, if it is released for definite purposes.* If physical, purely reactive symptoms, like paralysis of the vocal chords or the leg, trembling when in danger, diarrhœa or fainting from fright, vomiting from disgust, do not disappear with the releasing affects, or when they always recur without an adequate occasion, then there is involved something different in principle from simple reactions; *there is a positive quantity added, which as a rule consists of some necessity for being sick.* If the term "wish" is applied to this, it is to be understood in the widest sense. The most decent person occasionally has an impulse to take what does not belong to him or do something sexual that is not permissible; but it does not enter his head to act on this. Not at all seldom the pathogenic wishes are entirely unconscious, while in the patient's consciousness the opposite impulse is not only important but solely dominant or solely present.

The "morbid gains" are usually easily found on closer inspection. They are plain in the war and income neuroses, in the twilight states of commitments for examination; in "mass hysterias" or "imitative hysterias" they are based, among other things, on the desire, on the one hand, to be in the swim, and, on the other, to be distinguished from the mob. In school epidemics freedom from school is a special consideration, but in addition also the making oneself important and the imitation of everything conspicuous.

Naturally there are diseases of a neurotic kind, for the origin of which, at least in principle, an advantage is not necessary. Many primitive reactions, the suckling who perishes from anorexia in an unsympathetic environment, the homesick nurse-maid, the dog that starves on his master's grave, the girl that always gets pains in the loin when she lies in the grass after she had lain in the open during an illegitimate birth, the false connections of the sex impulse, the fever that appears after the injection of water when this is taken to be the accustomed tuberculin,—all these are illustrations. *But in the ordinary neuroses one always finds on close inspection an advantage from the disease.*

But there must be something besides that permits the nervous to take refuge just in disease, while there are other means of evading the difficulties. To be sure, it should be remarked that this evasion lies close at hand in our super-Christian age with its petting of weaklings, and is particularly encouraged by many families especially in the bringing up of children. But it is probable that still other forces bring the hysteric to the expediency of disease; thus many intellectual constellations, then the experience that with his strong affective reactions which at times appear even to the layman morbidly exaggerated, he often accomplishes his purpose, and perhaps there is a certain weakness toward the idea of disease. All of this *Kohnstamm* brings together under the name of weakened *"health conscience,"* which says as much as a long explanation, and which therefore I would not like to dispense with, though many object to it because "hysterics are again having some odium attached to themselves." *This objection is based on an entirely wrong conception, which one cannot sufficiently guard against. There is not involved a defect in the sense of "morality" or a weakness of the conscious psyche which one can make responsible and blame, and it is a serious theoretical and still more serious practical mistake, merely on the basis of neurotic symptoms, to reproach a patient with not wanting to get well.*

A few additional references should be made to the *individual mechanisms of the neuroses.* Besides in the "neurotic excitations" we find merely *exaggerated or primitive reactions,* e.g. in heart symptoms, paralyses of the legs, or the vocal chords, in hysterical vomiting, in diarrhœa from fright, and in fainting spells. Hysterical twilight states are usually to be conceived as exaggerations of the emotional effects that make way for desired associations and exclude the undesired. Others are repetitions of emotionally accentuated experiences, that are undertaken, partly because they are ambivalent and have a pleasurable component (twilight states as repetitions of sexual attacks), *partly because they are bound up associatively with definite affects.* Moreover, many syndromes that come in the form of attacks are released in accordance with the scheme of the *association reflexes*, whereby the momentary necessity for the disease withdraws as a pathogenic factor; the sight of a cap of a certain shape releases palpitation or an anxiety attack, because the critical person wore such a cap. Any chance event "recalls" a sexual attack, whereupon this is lived through in a more or less caricatured form in a twilight state. Such connections may be known to the patient, without on that account losing their reality. Very elementary also is the simple *"reflex enforcement" (Kretschmer):* the trembling reflex may be released under circumstances which would not be possible in the normal. For the neurosis, as for the affect and for suggestion, there are available many, especially physical mechanisms, over which the conscious will has no influence. Many symptoms, like nervous palpitation, fainting spells, throat spasms (globus), and perspirations, are released by the setting in motion of preformed mechanisms, thus also the "hysterophilic syndrome." [128] Certain others, such as headache, insomnia, and impeded thinking, originate otherwise especially easily under the influence of ideas. Hence a syndrome consisting of depression, sleeplessness, loss of appetite, impeded thinking, and palpitations during all mental or physical "work" (I purposely avoid the term "exertion") is so common in damage suits following accidents. *In a characteristic manner the craving for an income determines the disease, and the fear of being without means of support* determines its finer shadings (the patient not only has a desire for support but also the fear of having to be without work and income). Other reactions must first have existed in the imagination, in order to become capable of assuming an hysterical form. It is not easy directly to suggest to oneself and others vomiting, diarrhœa, perspiration, or palpitation, but it is quite possible if appropriate situations, such as having eaten something disgusting, feeling heat, and of terrifying situations are pictured in detail. Thus even the nervous person will most easily get those symptoms from imagination (auto-suggestion), that he has already experienced (pains in the back as a repetition of earlier rheumatism), or he will utilize an existing trouble, any other-

[128] See p. 543.

wise insignificant deficiency in an organ (stomach!), in order to make a disease of it (*"physical complaisance"*). Some physically conditioned disease is (especially in the case of children) afterwards continued psychically, most frequently perhaps whooping cough, chorea, and blephorospasms. Instead of being "utilized" directly, a predisposition may also be strengthened or actually made by some added factor: Desire to urinate when the pouring of water is heard in case of a bladder that is strongly retentive of urine, coughing of children with whooping cough when another child coughs, coughing spell as a result of sudden embarrassment in case of a latent irritation in the larynx.

A number of nervous symptoms are *symbols* (paralysis of the organs of swallowing, because one cannot "swallow" the father's demands), others are transformations, perhaps *"subliminations"* of suppressed desires (one of *Pfister's* patients was an enthusiastic practitioner of nature healing only when he practiced coitus interruptus), or *identifications* with persons whom one envies or loves.

A chance look may release a neurotic symptom, but only when it connects itself with a complex. The sight of a skin eruption will only induce the hysteric in spite of her disgust to have the eruption itself when it reminds her (in the unconscious) of the paternal syphilis.[129]

Sometimes the affect becomes *displaced* from one idea to another; the boy who years ago stole apples without having any pangs of conscience torments himself morbidly over the matter after he has begun to masturbate. The thought of stealing apples is more endurable than that of onanism; the latter is therefore repressed but its affect attaches itself to the idea of theft and gives to this a morbid severity. In such and similar ways do *compulsive ideas* originate.

Another process functioning alone or more frequently in connection with other mechanisms is the one mentioned above [130] of the apparent *accumulation of affects.*

Not all exertions or tendencies of the wishes and fears are pathogenic to the same degree. *The most important are the sexual and those that involve the self-importance of an individual.*

A connection of the neuroses with sex, especially of the hysterical forms, has been assumed for thousands of years, as the old name hysteria shows. To be sure at first one thought only in the coarsest sense of the lack of satisfaction of the *animal sperma desiderans* (= uterus), then about the middle of the preceding century of conditions of irritation that had their origin in the (female) genitals (*Romberg* was the leading representative of this view). But even

[129] See p. 136.
[130] See p. 38.

previous to this, some (*Lepois* in the 17th century) had conceived
the disease as a nervous disease and later as a brain or mental disease,
and especially since *Briquet,* who carried it out systematically, this
view gained ground rapidly, until in the last decade of the 19th century
it became the most general. But with this all, until the most recent
times, the essence of hysteria for most people was lust and lying,
although one was visibly concerned "to deliver the poor invalids from
the odium of the sexual origin of their sufferings."

But then the sexual reappeared in the form of the *Freudian doctrine,* which placed youthful sexual experiences and repressed sexual
desires and perversities at the root of the disease. This theory has
both ardent opponents and supporters. The following is certain:
Since the instinct of hunger is usually satisfied indirectly in civilized
man, the sex instinct is by far the most important. There is good
reason for the opinion of the poet and people in general that the
love aim is the highest. But our cultural conditions demand very
unnatural limitations of the impulse, and—what is much more important—it is *in itself* ambivalent and bound up, with strong inhibitions and even affects of anxiety.[131] It thus leads to a number of
external and internal conflicts, of which, however, the latter have the
tendency to take place partly or entirely in the unconscious, the place
where the neuroses are generated. Sexual dissatisfaction, but not
merely in the earlier physical sense (in an exceptional case one may be
satisfied by a love affair or by a marriage without coitus), is an important factor in the creation of the neuroses. Now whether for the
predisposition to a (chronic) neurosis such a sexual factor is also
necessary under all circumstances cannot yet be decided. It is significant that the severest effect of fright in the absence of a particular
predisposition rarely goes beyond the acute vasomotor-neurotic complex, and that the more careful examination of neurotics reveals as a
rule (traumatics and war cases excepted) sexual conflicts, and that
the disease may often be explained by these. In the symptomatology
of schizophrenia also, sexual conflicts play an important part; in
women usually the essential part. On the other hand, a traumatic
neurosis seems to us so plainly derivable from a struggle for an income
that at present there is no reason in the case of these diseases to inject
also a sexual predisposition. It is also certain that neuroses can be
cured without directly considering sex. If a satisfying life-work is
provided, then naturally a counter-protection against injuries from sex
is also obtained.

[131] Bleuler, Der Sexualwiderstand. Jahrbuch f. psychanlyt. und psychopath.
Forschungen. V, 1913, S. 442.

In spite of the fact that some of *Freud's* particular assertions will
not be maintained in the face of further experience, it is very wrong
to belittle this investigator, as was the fashion, and it is unscientific
to allow the emotions to play such an important part in the matter.
Just as the doctrine of hypnosis and suggestion, opposed in its time
in almost the same emotional manner, and in part, with the same
arguments, nevertheless laid the first part of the foundation of a
scientific psychopathology, so *Freud* has produced a great many funda-
mentals which have already given the science an entirely different
structure—and this even in his opponents to the extent that they
go into psychology at all.   Without them psychopathology would
not have progressed.   Much of what *Freud* offered was, as is usual
in such cases, not absolutely new, but he was the first to work it
out into such clearness as to furnish a practical idea as the foundation for further studies.   To these belong the rôle of the unconscious,
the request on principle of comprehending psychologically all psychic
symptoms and the demonstration that this comprehension may be
often gained by the observation of all psychic connections, also in
the unconscious activities, in the dream, etc.; the clear conception of
repression, of the ubiquity and significance of inner conflicts, of the
unlimited after-effects of earlier affective experiences, of the transference of the affect to conception originally foreign to it, of the intellectual conception of condensation, of the greater emphasis, even though
not yet full explanation, of the ideas of conversion (transformation
of repressed affects into physical symptoms), and of abreaction; then
the departure from the custom of ignoring the sexual life as much
as possible even in scientific matters, and the emphasis (even though
slightly exaggerated) of the significance of sex.

Besides sex, *the complex to put oneself over, to distinguish oneself, to obtain power over others* is important.   Many a neurosis serves
this complex primarily by compelling those who are about to act in
accordance with it.

If the self-estimation is not recognized by others, there develop from
this the many *attitudes of spite* that lead to changes of character [132]
or to disease; the young woman mentioned above [133] was badly treated
by her husband; after a scene she states that he should be told he had
made her sick; she developed an obviously nervous fever of short
duration and then a severe expectation neurosis, from which she herself suffered unspeakable pains, and which only now after forty-four
years is beginning to disappear.   That was the punishment for the

[132] See p. 128.
[133] See p. 128.

husband.—But this method of reacting is used not only toward people, but also toward God or fate; the "purpose" is then just spite.

A peculiar way of making oneself important is finding *joy in misery:* one always sees to it that one is the victim of injustice, usually only in little things but one magnifies it into a big affair, mild persecution mania, nervous symptoms, reasons for changing one's position, etc.

Other symptoms again are *compensations for feelings of inferiority*. An individual poorly endowed in certain directions wants to cover his mistakes and appear to be extraordinary in just that respect and for this reason seeks refuge in the neuroses.[134]

Conversely the *suppression of artistic impulses, talents in general, selection of the wrong vocations,* sometimes lead to neuroses and morbid attitudes.

Besides all sorts of complexes, which are by chance created by the situation (bad treatment in a subordinate position), may release neurotic mechanisms. But it is important that clear unambiguous endeavors, wishes and their definite suppression rarely lead to neuroses, but almost only to *ambivalent* complexes.

Not entirely unimportant, unfortunately, is the *iatrogenic* origin of neurotic manifestations. The physician solemnly diagnoses "enlargement of the heart," whereupon the patient is frightened and breaks down until the X-ray photograph resorted to by another physician relieves him of his nightmare. The stomach neurotic is not rare, to whom a particular food had been forbidden, because of a digestive disturbance "due to a weak stomach," who then in terror consults a string of physicians and has some dish forbidden him by each in turn, until he is at the point of starvation and with or without a physician's assistance makes up his mind to eat what he pleases.

The essential part of the mechanisms that generate neuroses almost without exception functions in the unconscious, as is indicated by the fact that the control of our conscious personality does not extend nearly so far as the neurotic influences (activity of the glands, production of a twilight state, etc.).[135] The hysterical psyche yields the control much more to the impulses lying in the unconscious, or otherwise expressed: these are relatively stronger in the hysterical psyche than in the normal person.

Thus the psychology of the affectivity and the unconscious give the key to the understanding of the neuroses and of many psychotic

---

[134] Comp. especially the works of *Alfred Adler.*

[135] Therefore *Babinski's* limitation of hysteria to his pithiatism, i.e. to conceptions which are accessible to the (conscious) will, cannot be accepted.

symptoms; the corresponding mechanisms are present in every person, "everybody is capable of hysteria." The healthy person also has wishes in his unconscious, which conflict with his conscious personality, some of which now and then manifest themselves in "the psychopathology of every day life," i.e. in errors, forgetting, and in dreams.

But the healthier a person is, the stronger the affect must be, in order that its results can be exaggerated into neurotic symptoms. In this respect acute injuries relatively seldom produce an effect and primarily only an acute effect, chronic injuries more easily produce lasting symptoms; but the most readily effective disease producers are acute, serious experiences after a chronic impairment of resistance and the gradual accumulation of restrained affects. *But when a protracted or general neurosis is developed from a transient symptom, then there usually exists not only some conscious or unconscious wish to be sick or to transform reality by means of the phantasy, but a psychopathic predisposition also.* Even pronounced fright neuroses during earthquakes and similar catastrophes were seen only in psychopathic people, and there too they passed away. *The wish alone, be it ever so strong, cannot at all produce a neurosis.* During the last war thousands had the wish to be freed from the hell by some disease, but the disease did not appear—in most cases certainly not because of moral and other opposing considerations. *One,* i.e. the unconscious, *must know the path to definite symptoms in order to travel along it.* By means of trembling during fright from a shrapnel explosion many were shown the path; from now on the unconscious remembrance of it could again release the trembling reflex, as often and as long as was necessary. All the chronic impacts also could finally—even though not frequently—*hystericise* the person with healthy nerves, i.e. make it possible for him to produce hysterical symptoms, *perhaps* along the path of mere physical nervous weakening, but in any case by means of the fact that the future patients experience in themselves the sensation of a number of morbid or "nervous" symptoms, for the release of which they have now found the path of association. The concept of hystericising thus contains the dispositional factor, which manifests itself in some weakening of the resistive capacity, and in road building between the idea and the symptoms.

The above material distinguishes only certain types. In reality the most different dispositions, mechanisms and syndromes intermingle and influence each other. Therefore it is impossible on principle to produce a division of the neuroses into properly defined entities, be it according to disposition, releasing causes, mechanisms, or syndromes. In this case one must clarify the various possibilities, and then see in the particular case which of them is realized. Relatively pure cases are e.g. the monosymptomatic hysterias of children, many of the trembling neuroses, many compulsion neuroses. For the remaining the disposition and mechanisms should be described, which is not possible to a sufficient extent; besides, one should also know the more frequent groupings of dispositions and symptoms and their connections, which unfortunately has not been adequately attained. Nevertheless we understand fairly well why hysterical symptoms frequently occur in "nervous" characters: without excessive domination, facile irritability, and lability of the affects, no hysteria can develop.

Also the frequent combination of hysteriform symptoms with pseudologia is at once comprehensible. Both syndromes want to sham something for themselves and others; they require an affectivity of strong effective force but labile, an easily influenced spirit and an exaggerated self-esteem. The (pseudo-) neurasthenic symptom complex, which represents a failure, is usually connected with a depressive fundamental mood, etc.

Just as among themselves, the psychopathic reaction forms cannot be sharply defined from other morbid groups also, and *especially not from the psychopathies* on the basis of which they develop, so that it is often arbitrary whether in a morbid picture one wants to emphasize the psychopathic disposition or the released reaction symptoms. There probably are constitutional, one-sided homosexuals; but in bisexuality chance connections and attitudes determine whether the homo- or the heterosexual components shall finally dominate. Many place the hysterical character in the foreground, others the symptoms; the anomaly of "the impulsive people" lies in some in the native characteristics, in others it is a reaction system. *Kraepelin* includes the compulsive forms in the original morbid states; we include them with most of the others in the reactions, etc. *At all events one should talk of hysteria and neurasthenia only, when on the top of the "nervous" or "psychopathic" foundation there is a distinctly acquired morbid attitude, or when one wishes to impress the patient with the possibility or expectation of an improvement.*

Among the psychopathic reactions we distinguish: the symptomatic intellectual forms of *paranoia, of the delusions of persecution of those hard of hearing and of induced insanity, the reactive changes of character, the reactive impulses (states of wandering, kleptomania, pyromania, the neuroses, and among these hysteria (pseudo) neurasthenia, the expectation neuroses, and the compulsion neuroses, but we want to call attention again to the fact that it is merely a question of an artificial separation of syndrome groups, which, genetically and symptomatically, usually intermingle and pass over into one another. But the same syndromes also occur on the basis of process psychoses, especially in schizophrenia and in a more limited manner in epilepsy; only when they apparently occur "independently" can they be considered as neuroses.* For practical reasons two groups are circumscribed etiologically: *the prison psychoses* and the *traumatic neuroses.*

In the compulsive forms the *prospects* are not very good.[136] In the following we speak only of hysteria and neurasthenia: Their curability depends primarily on the severity and extent of the psychopathic predisposition. If the disease is only a partial symptom of a twisted character which cannot get along either with people or with fortune, naturally little can be expected; for even if the symptoms were cured it would still leave a very sick person. More serious moral defects alone also hinder the cure. Especially in children a distinction should be made as much as possible between the generally abnormal with hysterical syndromes and those with a good constitution, who suffer from nervous symptoms only under the pressure of circumstances. The former are almost incurable; the latter with proper treatment usually regain their health quickly and in later life rarely become sick again.

Concerning the curability of the two neuroses in themselves, or to speak concretely, of those cases not associated with other abnormities, there is a difference of opinion according to whether one does not include the nervous disposition in the conception. At all events the symptoms are all curable even though all are not really cured. The neurosis does not lead to dementia. The worst obstacle to a cure exists when the patient, consciously or unconsciously, does not want to be cured. One simply can neither directly stimulate the inadequate energy so that the patient takes up the struggle of existence even under unfavorable conditions, nor can one often improve the situation so that no reason for being sick exists. But most patients are improved by treatment or are freed from their symptoms. Naturally the disposition is not cured, if, as is usual, it is congenital. Hence relapses are very common, whereby still other reasons cooperate (life cannot be constituted according to our desires, especially when the desire consists in wanting to shine without continuous achievement). It must not be forgotten that if the energy, wrongly applied for purposes of the disease, is led into channels that are proper and commensurate with the patient's endeavors, such people with their undivided application of their ability can accomplish more than the healthy. What hinders their activity is simply split off, and the far-reaching domination of

[136] See special discussion.

the vegetative functions by the psyche instead of being used for the production of physical morbid symptoms is used in the service of the new task. While formerly they could not sleep, they now do not need to sleep much; the system of metabolism that permitted the hysteric to retain his weight with a very small amount of nourishment may with a slightly different application become a very useful inexhaustibility of strength.

The *general diagnosis* of the psychogenic reactions is based, in the first place, on the recognition of the psychogenic mechanism which is usually not difficult. *The most important and also the most difficult part of the diagnosis, consists in the exclusion of a somatic (or psychotic) foundation by means of a careful investigation. The same mechanisms dominate schizophrenia, are frequent in epilepsy and all organic brain diseases, and may be released by any sort of physical diseases. Therefore one must know as exactly as possible what can be reactive and what cannot.* It is impossible to enumerate the details in this place; but this is hardly to be regretted because one could not get finished with it anyway, and only he who besides some experience in the appearance of the morbid pictures possesses the general conceptions of the nature of the reactive symptoms can manage to get along. But even the most experienced will occasionally have to leave a diagnosis open for some time. If one finds signs of schizophrenia or of paresis, then to be sure the matter is settled, but if a physical disease also exists, it may be difficult to recognize the kind and the significance of the psychogenic elements. One should keep in mind that the neuroses leave the ideas intact and do not produce obstructions without a comprehensible affective foundation. Hysterical indifference is very rare, and may be usually differentiated from the schizophrenic by means of its perspicuous genesis and its yielding to influence. Rigidity of a pronounced affect will probably hardly ever be hysterical. With the neurotic and especially with the hysteric one usually has a pronounced affective rapport, be it positive or negative. Whoever does not show the physician any deeper feelings in the course of a protracted examination is no mere nervous case.

The *general treatment* will be mentioned here only to the extent that it concerns the neuroses. The *disposition* can be influenced in very few cases. Where conditions of weakness of any sort are present, one will naturally combat them. It is more readily conceivable to remove the conditions out of which the syndromes grew or were nourished. Above all, wherever possible, a life work should be provided for the patient in which not only the external conditions are to be considered but also the internal which induced the patient to decline a life work. The will or the desire to be sick should, if possible, be overcompensated by positive endeavors which presume health.

For the rest, one can attack the *symptoms* by direct suggestion with or without *hypnosis;* or one can conceal the suggestion in any other remedy or procedures, if possible in such as under the given conditions really have a curative effect in any incidental matter (climate, mountain climate, water,[137] etc.). If the patient feels better externally, he gets along. Spontaneously or with skilfull instigation he makes plans for the future; briefly, he changes his attitude so that a subsequent reduction of physical energy cannot do so much harm. For (apparently) localized symptoms local treatment should not if possible be undertaken, because it would frequently strengthen the patient's idea that the disease is localized there; still less will one lower oneself to resort to fictitious operations. Miraculous remedies, from any sort of mystery pills up to a pilgrimage, may naturally also help. In the form of *Dubois'* "Persuasion" one can combine the suggestion of which both physician and patient are unconscious with a sort of training and enlightenment. This depends on the taste of the patient and still more on that of the physician. *Psychoanalysis* which brings the morbid mechanisms into consciousness or causes an "abreaction" of them cures many cases. Where it can be done, one will "subliminate" the pathogenic impulses, divert them into similar but useful channels and supplant associations having a morbid effect by more favorable ones. *Isolation* is often important or at least separation from an environment which is impressed by the patient's suffering or shows sympathy with him; especially in the case of severe hysterias of children, this measure is usually a necessary condition of the cure. On the other hand, the deliberate ignoring, the refusal to be impressed by apparently the severest symptoms, is an excellent remedy. A hysterical attack and many another symptom is really an exhibition. If one takes care that the spectators disappear at once when the exhibition begins (preferably by isolating the patient), then the entire arrangement is usually deprived of justification for existence, and it is given up in the shortest time. In general if by changing the inner or outer circumstances one can make the neurosis futile, naturally much

---

[137] Drugs as direct remedies against neuroses are to be avoided as much as possible. They divert both physician and patient from the true conception of the disease. If they have no effect, they have for that reason already done harm. If by chance they are effective, the cure is bound down to them and they have to be continued mildly until a change of conception renders them ineffective. It goes without saying that morphine should not be given. For incidental purposes one will naturally not want to dispense entirely with chemical remedies: Bromide for sleeplessness, iron for accompanying anemia, etc.

is gained.—Where physical resistance has been reduced, one will try to increase it, be it to deprive the disease of its foundation, or effectively to support the suggestion of health.

If matters improve, then a thorough *training* must follow in which a sensible manner of living must not be forgotten and thereupon a proper initiation into life. *What one does in the neurosis is a detail; the only decisive thing, is how one does it, and how one stands to the patient.* Some think that for this reason they have to become friendly with the patient, others consider this dangerous; if only there is a personal relation to the physician, one can overwhelm or impress or persuade the patient or use suggestion on him; here too the remedy is a detail. It goes without saying that for psychotherapy generally and for the application of every individual remedy special innate qualities are necessary, in which respect unfortunately many a quack is superior to the trained physician; added to this there must be professional experience, exact observation of the individual patient and his manner of reacting, and the weighing of the many accompanying conditions that have to be considered.

Prevention. The *congenital neurotic disposition* cannot be readily combatted except by the avoidance of the marriage of "neuropathic" people. A disposition acquired by disease or by unfavorable life experiences usually disappears without our intervention. One cannot evade the inner and outer *conflicts* at will; on the other hand, they can be subdued by creating a purpose in life; to be sure the normal person does not have to do this consciously, and on the other hand many a severe and characterless psychopath will be unable to form one or hold to it. But in the cases that lie between these extremes it depends on the attitude and the circumstances, matters that to some extent can be controlled. One can create a purpose in life or have one pointed out by another person. Every task is interesting as soon as one has gained sufficient associations in connection with it. Here one should not forget that most hysterics, like women, are more easily interested in things having a directly affective element, especially in personal things. On the other hand, a rigorous disciplining of thinking by dealing with tangible realities can counteract the emotionalism. But the 'health conscience" above all is amenable to educative influences. Whoever from youth onward is accustomed to treat his feelings of ill health as an inferiority and disagreeableness, whoever in childhood experience no advantage but always only obstructions from disease, will not so easily produce a neurosis. One has to create a *"pride in health"* (Gesundheitstrotz) even during the training of childhood, and where this has been neglected the physician should make it up as far as possible; but this feeling must not be mistaken for the health nonsense of psychopaths, who want to keep well by means of some system and are therefore incessantly on the watch for symptoms of health and disease.

For the prophylaxis in the case of psychopathic children *Ziehen* gives the following noteworthy rules:

1. Total abstinence from coffee, tea, alcohol, spices and tobacco up to and including puberty.

2. Supervision of the sexual life.

3. Hardening by cool rub-downs and cool baths; habituation to pain and exertion; regular gymnastics (eventually also sports). Careful restraint of the development of the phantasy (supervision of reading, care in leaving them alone, etc.); favoring all objective occupations (collections of all kinds, construction, drawing; later also painting from models or from nature, open air games with other children, etc.). The daily routine in all cases should be regulated by a definite schedule.

4. Attendance of a public school is, as a rule, preferable to private instruction.

5. In case of unfavorable home conditions (unfavorable example of the parents, coddling by the parents, etc.), education outside of the parental home in a private school or in a suitable boarding place or in the country with a teacher, physician, or minister should be prescribed; in more severe cases the so-called pedagogical sanatoria (schools with medical supervision), like those first founded by *Kahlbaum*, should be considered.

6. Habituation to obedience and self-control by means of a calm severity. Passionate scolding is almost never successful. Corporal punishments also are rarely effective; nevertheless they are permissible to the same degree as in the case of normal children. Other punishments (deprivation of pleasure, etc.), are not only allowed but when sensibly applied are, as a rule, effective.

1. PARANOIA

As the clinic can only rarely exhibit paranoiacs, it is in place here to present somewhat more detailed examples for purposes of orientation:

Delusions of Persecution. Engineer, born 1855. Father was an unsteady farmer, who did not like to work, during manhood felt himself persecuted in a vague way and hanged himself during an attack of delirium tremens. The father's father was a drunkard. Three brothers of the patient are unmarried, unsteady like the father; two are relatively steady, one is a drunkard. One sister is married, normal, has children.—Patient was a capable, cheerful boy, but somewhat shy toward strangers. Mechanic's apprentice, then in a technical school, then a skilled mechanic. Hoped to become distinguished. The future partner of the machine factory S. was his schoolmate. At the final examination of the technical school the patient exhibited a drawing, which he expected would make a name for him, but he was keenly disappointed when it was praised and then forgotten. He was a good marksman but even for his prizes he received too little recognition. He thought of journeying to the Cape of Good Hope with his brother, got as far as Marseilles, heard there that no steamer would leave. The brother travelled by way of Genoa, but the patient returned home, took a position in a branch of the firm S. in England but felt uncomfortable after a second, larger firm, R., in his native town offered him a position that he refused. He believed that now the firm R. would be put out about it. When the offer was made to him that his present position be made secure for three years, he suspected that the firm wanted to take advantage of him, and left his position. Then there began a wandering existence for twenty years contrary to his will: when he had a good position, he heard remarks that he was ungrateful toward the firm S., that he was an engineer who did not know algebra, and similar things. In reality they were random remarks that he wrongly applied to himself and memory deceptions in which to accord with his delusion he changed something in words he had heard. Some one said, "You will soon see"; he referred this to himself as a threat. He was in all sorts of places in Europe and America, and several times returned temporarily to an old position, but he was always driven away by such remarks. He devised reasons why the firms R and S., with the assistance of the association of former engineering students and in other ways, pursued him to take revenge on him, and at the same time to make use of his talent. "They simply gave the assignment to an agency and had me persecuted."

People were supposed to have ascertained where he was going and sometimes even to have sent the news in advance. Once he defended himself in an insulting letter to the firm, which naturally understood nothing about it. Often he felt safe for a time in some new place, but if he had to write home, it began again because the postal authorities opened his letters and gave his address to his persecutors. In restaurants people put their heads together when he entered. Special arrangments were made to make him acquainted with women, who should tempt him to all sorts of excesses so that he could then be exposed as a high flyer. Often care was taken that he did not get a position until he had used up all his savings; this was done so that he would become dependent on his new employers. Because his money had to go anyway, he began to drink Rhine wine and smoke Havana cigars and habituated himself generally to drink more than was good for him. In America he got married but did not take his wife with him when he was again "driven away," and more or less forgot her. Several times he wanted to start his own business but never got beyond the purpose. With the laborers he conversed little; he was too proud to do it. Once, when he returned to Zürich he felt that he was being observed by a sanitary policeman. That was possible because he had sent his photograph to Zürich. He wrote an essay on a Utopia which was no better than similar efforts but of which he was very proud. A few months before his admission to Burghölzli in 1897 he was a construction draughtsman. His fellow employees began to smirk, sometimes to laugh, all on his account. His superiors annoyed him. Once a drawing was lost; he was pointed to as the guilty person. People peeped through the key hole when he washed his privates in the water closet, and told others about it. People "made a big fuss about a few youthful errors" and said everywhere that he masturbated. In this way he lost his honor and the possibility of making a living, because no one wanted to employ a person of that sort. He would be a scoundrel if he had tolerated this and so he shot his superior from ambush. In the hospital for the insane his conduct was normal externally. At first he was visibly frightened at the result of his shooting. After he had openly stated the above motive for several days and claimed to have acted in self-defense, he framed excuses which he evidently believed himself (gun went off accidentally, then again that he had been confused, etc.). On the whole he was distrustful, friendly, worked in the printing shop of the hospital and besides tried to make all sorts of inventions (a milling machine which was usable but already equalled by one just as good, a steam engine without a swinging piston in which, to be sure, something was still lacking). At first he tried to carry on his studies "as secretly as possible"; after a while he became accustomed to the society of the others.

He spun out his delusions in various directions. In the remissions he could also correct some things; thus he once thought "Messrs. R. and S. only wanted to watch him but not persecute him"; "they simply suffered from fixed ideas." But soon after he took up the old system again. New delusions also turned up: in his ward there was a homosexual. Now people nudged and winked that he too was perverse. Furuncles that he had on his neck had been injected into him by the orderly. In his ward there were by chance several former employees of his last firm. They probably had to observe him, etc.; the delusion also developed retroactively in the form of memory deceptions. S. had already persecuted him in school. Chapters of a certain law had been used against him (this at a time when this law did not exist at all). He thought the murdered superior had dismissed him in disgrace, while in reality the patient had resigned. At certain times the delusional system merged into the background; at other times he occupied himself entirely with it, at the same time developing it further.

Noticeably early the patient showed signs of psychical senility. With this there now came more pronounced ideas of greatness that could not very well be sustained logically any longer: A second court of justice would liberate him. One judge or another had promised him to take up his cause. An uncle had left him a house and later an enormous fortune. Finally he suspected that he was not his father's son. All of this was supported in the form of memory deceptions. Even previously, 1907, he had escaped, but in spite of the fact that he had been helped with money, he only got as far as France and there thought it best to return to the asylum of his own accord. Without feeling that in this way he had hurt his position, he thought he had now proven that he could be discharged, and he planned to become a store-keeper.

Pathology: An excellent man with a certain amount of inventive ability cannot execute his ambitious plans because he has too little enduring energy. He thinks that a good drawing that he exhibited and a few medals that he won at rifle shooting should immediately open the way to distinction. Conversely, when in Marseilles there was no boat to the Cape of Good Hope and, likewise, when after his escape from the asylum he had trouble in making his way, he lost his courage. In sexual matters he was just as weak; he was married but simply abandoned his wife, not with deliberation but just because it happened so. He refused an offered position, found out later that he should not have done this and then thought that the people who offered him the position began to annoy him. They had assigned his persecution to an agency. The delusion has developed into a system and was supported by incessant ideas of reference and newly created memory deceptions.—Now this plain case of paranoia also has two complications that belong to other diseases; in the nineties the patient had, during the course of his paranoia, a brain disease, probably a gumma, and at that time was not quite clear in his thoughts for a brief period. From then on his memory, on very careful inspection, was no longer as good as formerly. It may be assumed that for this reason the memory deceptions appeared so easily, which already after a few days attached themselves to his act of murder, at first motivated by himself in an entirely clear manner. The same may be said of his premature mental senility. Moreover he had committed alcoholic excesses in the weeks preceding the murder, and had undergone a mild alcoholically tinged delirium. At that time, but only then, did he hallucinate. It must be assumed that this unenergetic man would never have gone as far as to shoot his persecutor without this alcoholic excitation.

Erotic Delusions of Grandeur with Delusions of Persecution: Daughter of aristocratic but not well to do parents, born in 1848, brought up at home with a classical education, is said to have covered in three months the work of each year in college. Associated with scholars. She wanted to investigate a definite, important historical subject but permitted herself to be diverted and wrote something different. Then she undertook a new historical problem which she gave up to care for her sick parents. At the same time she had pleasant social intercourse with acquaintances and friends. At thirty-six she went to a brother, whose wife had died, to keep house for him, but paid him her board to be on an equal footing with him. Two years later she was again at home. In the meantime her feminine instincts were aroused: "I felt that at bottom I was disposed to be very domestic; although I again plunged into society, nevertheless I did not know what to do with myself." She wanted to become a nurse but in some way did not get along with the authorities. In a sort of desperation she let herself be driven into marriage with a less aristocratic but evidently very refined man. As late as eight days before the wedding the future couple discussed a separation. However, the marriage was consummated but was soon followed by a legal separation. Later when I remarked to the patient that her husband had acted very generously in the matter, she thought: "According to what I saw, he did. According to what I heard later but cannot prove, he did not." As the patient was a Catholic and thought of marrying again, the separation gave her qualms of conscience. Probably a little later she formed the delusion that the archbishop had annulled her marriage. But before she was separated she believed that men of high rank wanted to marry her. They themselves, as well as other people, had proven this by their "hints." But nothing happened because intrigues against it had been undertaken and she was being slandered. She defended herself against this. Insanity was suspected. A psychiatrist evidently on the occasion of the separation, had given an opinion to that effect. She wrote to him that he was a scoundrel and she then believed that he had thereupon given a second opinion, declaring her sane. She was then put under guardianship and was afraid of being committed.

Even during the trial she fled to foreign countries and wanted to have herself certified to by a psychiatrist; but when she ascertained that he was known in a city where one of her supposed admirers lived, she was convinced that with the help of the courts he wanted to surrender her. She then went to a Swiss University where, as she thought, she was slandered as crazy and syphilitic and in other respects. As she feared being interned, although there was no reason for it, she once fled to another university and obtained her Ph.D. *magna cum laude*. Thereupon she looked for positions but found none, travelled around everywhere, in other parts of the world also, always felt herself pursued, especially when she sent off a letter; she wrote a pamphlet on German justice embodying her delusions. Meanwhile she again imagined proposals of marriage from prominent people, intercepted telegrams, opinions, and acts of people of the highest rank, of which nothing in reality existed. Everything influenced her being either in a friendly or hostile manner. After a while the patient calmed down somewhat but always believed herself pursued by everybody that had had anything to do with her. She produced articles and, which was significant, liked to write about secret societies.—Characteristic of the case is the fact of the predominance of scientific interests over the erotic until she had kept house and had reached the critical age. Only then did she have a desire for a home of her own but at the same time also for an elevation in rank; an unfortunate marriage not based on any erotic feelings; delusions of being desired in marriage by people of distinction, imaginary failure of a marriage because of intrigues and slanders. In spite of the patient's very high intelligence and her education, she was absolutely incapable of correcting the most senseless delusions even when confronted with them, as, for instance, that a psychiatrist in a university to which he did not belong demanded her dismissal, that in America she could be brought into an insane asylum by a nurse without any further formalities, etc. But with this all she was capable of obtaining her Ph.D. *magna cum laude*.

The way she herself described the origin of her combinations from hints is very pretty: "I heard the whole thing bit by bit; now one gave me a hint, then another, and I put this story together like a mosaic."

Persecutory Delusion and Litigiousness. Author, born 1857; college education; since his twenty-fifth year hard of hearing and then deaf. He worked on a newspaper, had a good income, was generous toward his brothers and sisters but saved nothing for himself. In early youth there were also a few signs of frivolity. Because of the expense of his education, he had given up his claim to his share of his father's estate, as a second brother had done. Toward the end of the nineties he became more sensitive. He no longer got along with the sister with whom he lived and with his colleagues on the newspaper; resigned and tried to obtain a position in a foreign place but failed. He then made adventurous, if not exactly gigantic, business plans that were quite foreign to his previous calling and became poor. Then there began a struggle for existence, i.e., for a legacy that was supposedly so large that he could live on it if he had to. He tried to retract his waiver of his father's estate. When the father made a will he nevertheless left him one third of the estate that he would have had without question; he went home, raised a riot, and wanted to compel the writing of another will. He attacked the existing will with all sorts of pretenses, maintained that the father had promised him not only his own share but also that of a deceased sister; he stole papers from his father. After the father's death, which followed soon, a brother-in-law made an arrangement with him that he would pay him more than his share if he would be satisfied and give up the papers. But the patient did not give up the papers and soon demanded more (because he could not live on what had been promised him). In court he accused his sister and brother-in-law of fraud, duress, concealing the estate, perjury and other crimes. As the courts did not decide in his favor, they too were attacked, partly in countless petitions and appeals, partly in the newspapers; the latter in such a manner that he convinced people of note of the injustice of the judiciary. He also got into litigation with his own lawyer, refusing to pay him his fee.

To be sure, here and there he lied; but on the whole he believed in the justice of his cause. He did not notice that he never proved anything. He readily moved in a circle: The brother-in-law got his share; proof: otherwise he would not have raised a riot; the brother-in-law raised a riot; proof: otherwise he would not have obtained anything (naturally the nonsense of these conclusions is concealed in a mass of words). Facts necessary for the purpose were simply invented (memory illusions). The letters that did not suit the patient he declared to be forgeries; he knew at once who dictated them.

In this case the disturbance of thought extends to mathematics. The patient is not capable of figuring a problem of practical importance to himself: If six brothers and sisters have to divide a fortune of 50,000 Fr. in such a way that three obtain only the legal minimum, how much does each obtain? He mixed up everything about the legal minimum and total, and always mistook the ideas in such a way that something big for himself always turned up. A discussion lasting several days could not enlighten him. Other conceptions also, that were simple for him, became unclear where it coincided with his purpose. Thus he would not keep apart the laws of inheritance and the laws of sales. He could not identify the same events when they concerned himself or an opponent. His unconscious but solely decisive "logic" was an affective one: He was in want; his brothers and sisters were better situated; he needed the inheritance much more than'they. The understanding was present only to support the realization of this wish. He formed ideas without any reason whatever (chiefly memory deceptions but also suppositions concerning relations); what contradicted his ideas was simply not brought into logical connection. He was entirely incapable of discussion. It was a certainty for him that the court and his brothers and sisters defrauded him; for him everything followed from that. He could not, conversely, prove the crime from the facts. For him the crime was the axiom from which he started. He could not see the viewpoint of others who demanded proof. For him everything was "logically demonstrable, proven, self-evident, not requiring proof; he has experienced it on his own body."

After the appointing of a guardian and the rejection of his suit the patient still remained active for some time; convinced, among others, a well-known, distinguished author of "the fact that he had found no protection in psychiatry," but seemed to have calmed down somewhat after a while. At all events, unlike the pure litigant, he has given up his court actions. It is significant that he prefers to write about super-men à la Napoleon.

The Wagner case; Delusions of Grandeur and Persecution; Multiple murder and Incendiarism.[138] During the night from the third to the fourth of September, 1913, the Headmaster Wagner, thirty-nine years old, murdered his four children and his wife while they were sleeping; the following night he set fire to several houses in another village where he had previously been a teacher, and was shooting at the male inhabitants, of whom he killed nine and seriously wounded eleven. Even as a boy he was easily insulted, ambitious, conceited. Later he had poetic plans for reforming the universe. His sexuality in respect to the animal impulse was strong, but he had a "disinclination" toward marriage and evidently no parental instinct, even though he loved his children in an ordinary human way.

His highly developed self-esteem had been deeply depressed by a futile struggle of many years against onanism. Later (1901), under the influence of alcohol, he had let himself be carried away to sodomy,

[138] After *Gaupp*, Zur Psychologie des Massenmords, I. Bd. 3. Heft der Verbrechertypen. Edited by W. Gruhle and A. Wetzel. Springer, Berlin, 1914.

and then had a dreadful feeling of sin with incessant fear of contempt and arrest, which soon brought about delusions of reference and the conviction that the inhabitants of the village knew of his crime and spoke about it.

His accusations against himself he transferred to his family; all "Wagners" should be exterminated; then his hatred extended to all mankind, above all to the inhabitants of his district who had treated him badly. He condemned himself doubly, in part as a man unworthy of this life, but in part as a genius whom he honored as at least equal to the greatest poets, but whom he also ranked as equal and superior to Nero, and, on the other hand, compared with Christ. Transferred in 1902 to another place, he enjoyed relative quiet for six or seven years without, however, ever ceasing to build up further his delusional system. But then, according to his opinion, the remarks and contempt continued there also. The result was the plan, even then developed in every detail, to murder his family as much because of reasons of race-hygiene as from pity, and then set fire to the village where he was first employed, and destroy it with all its hypocritical inhabitants. The first necessity was the extermination, the "redemption" of his children; but the revenge against, and contempt for, the village occupied him no less. His wife he had to kill because of pity. For a person like him there are special laws. He had not only the right but the duty to do this. His plan was a "humanitarian matter." For four years he postponed the execution of the bitter task. But when he was later transferred to a third locality and there felt himself the centre of bar-room gossip, he executed his plan systematically. In his feelings, as in his self-estimation, he was completely ambivalent: he could not witness the killing of a chicken, did not like to see blood generally. In the insane asylum also he was so soft during the visits of relatives that he denied them to himself, and with all this, he had made and also executed the bloodiest plans.[139]

The modern morbid picture of paranoia was created by *Kraepelin;* according to him it is characterized by *"the furtive development, resulting from inner causes, of a lasting, immovable delusional system that is accompanied by the complete retention of clearness and order in thinking, willing, and acting."* Formerly many kinds of diseases were designated by this name. Toward the end of the last century it was believed that the essence of the disease was to be found in the more or less isolated disturbance of the understanding; as every delusional idea and every hallucination represents such a disturbance, most mental diseases could be included in this, and this was preferably

[139] Comp. p. 531, his remarks on the brutality of weakness.

done. On the basis of this stereotyped conception acute forms with delusions and hallucinations were also included. As such acute syndromes usually belong to schizophrenia which later readily exhibits chronic delusions, the theoretical confusion of acute and chronic conditions, different in principle, could not appear as senseless at the patient's bedside as it really was. But the morbid pictures of *Kraepelin's* paranoia and the acute forms of insanity that were included belong together about as much as typhus and a fracture of the leg, both of which hinder walking and keep the patient in bed.

There was a better development of the paranoia concept among the French, who in penetrating studies clarified the psychology of the forms of delusions but could not exclude dementia præcox, and sought classifications according to the content of the delusion.

The essence of paranoia is the *delusional system,* i.e. a structure of delusions that all have a certain logical connection and contain no inner contradictions, even though the logic is not in all cases compelling. That the delusion nevertheless strikes the normal person as not only insufficiently supported, but also as senseless, is due chiefly to the false premises and the shutting off of criticism. Year in and year out, no matter in what corner of the world they are, the patients are pursued by a conspiracy of people, or they would have made great inventions, the practical elaboration and utilization of which is being hindered, or they are high servants of the crown, prophets, etc., who want to establish their claims.

Only the persecuted patients are as yet known more exactly; our description, therefore, is only to be carried over to the other forms with care.

The false premises are morbid *references to the self, and memory deceptions.* In a certain direction the patients have an exaggerated readiness of association; they bring a number of entirely indifferent or unimpeachable occurrences into relation with themselves. Children run after the wagon in which the paranoiac is riding; they mock him or show the high position that he will hold. Some one coughs; that is a sign that he must be on his guard or that he does not belong here or that another should be on his guard for him. Some one yawns; that means that he is lazy; if two people are together and laugh, then they are laughing about him. In the newspaper there is an expression that he has used recently; therefore the entire article is stolen from him. A higher official has looked up at his window; he has an important mission for him or he knows that he is the future sovereign. The minister preaches about Judas: the whole congregation knew that he (the patient) was the person meant. On the street everybody looked at him significantly. Between the event and the interpretation in the sense of the self-reference delusion there usually intervenes a latent period of from hours to years, most frequently of about a day. While the healthy person usually works over his experiences subsequently (consciously or more commonly unconsciously) in the sense of a many sided connection with reality and a correction of possibly wrong conceptions, the paranoiac connects his perceptions during the latent period with the delusions and falsifies them in the same direction.

Sometimes the patient's assertions seem so senseless that one has to ask to what extent sensory illusions are involved. Beside the most commonplace occurrences the patients are also accustomed to tell some that are altogether impossible. To illustrate: In spite of the fact that they came into the theatre without a sound, the entire audience looked around at them; the minister spoke of things that he could not possibly know from ordinary sources; a respectable person stuck his tongue out at them. Of course here and there real illusions may play a part as in every healthy affect. But whenever I could investigate carefully I found that sensations and perceptions were absolutely correct, but the patient transformed them, of course often immediately after the perception, and later in his thinking he operated only with these transformed pseudo-perceptions which he took to be real. Hence there are already involved here added *memory deceptions* which, to be sure, occur also in normal people. There are people who only subsequently falsify their recollections in the sense of offenses.

The complicated *memory illusions* which represent complete transact seem clearer to us.[140] At this and that consultation which really took place, the physician is supposed to have said that the patient was sound, that the expected elevation in rank would occur in one year. The waiter brought the patient a glass of brandy; later he is convinced that the brother-in-law who is accused of poisoning served him. His wife met a certain man on the stairs; later he believes she made signs to him in passing that were understood and replied to. Between the event and the complete transformation there usually intervenes a considerable lapse of time, at least a night, often much more, a year, even a decade. Supported by continually repeated "experiences" of this sort, the patient must come, in an entirely logical way,[141] to the conception that people have something particularly in mind about him, he goes further and knows also *what* they have

---

[140] See pp. 105-106.

[141] In the paranoid form of dereistic thinking the logic must also be included, but it is here essentially supported by the fact that the elementary impulses run in the same direction; the wish to be something special is already at the root of the disease.

in mind. They want to persecute him or prepare for his future elevation, and he knows *why* they proceed in this manner. The latter he
has naturally not been able to conclude in a compelling manner; but
as the chief factor is a certainty for him, inferences based on probability
which he considers certain suffice for him. A general criticism is impossible. To be sure, occasionally he may admit that one or another
of his partial ideas is not sufficiently proven or even that it is false.
But for that reason everything else is nevertheless a certainty beyond
a peradventure.

*Outside of the delusional system and everything that refers to it,
his logic and train of ideas are sound according to our means of investigation.* If he is otherwise intelligent, he can be a minister, architect,
or high school teacher and, aside from indirect difficulties resulting
from the delusions, can do very well in his calling. In everything connected with the delusions, paranoiacs are very *gullible* about corrob-
orating statements and, on the other hand, readily distrust everything
that does not suit them. It seems that this feature also frequently
shows itself outside of the delusion, be it because, beginning with the
disease, it has become generalized, or because it belongs to the patient's
individual character.

In the other functions also one can recognize no primary
disturbances.

Sensations and perceptions are sound. *Hallucinations* are nearly
always lacking; but one must not say that they are entirely excluded
because that is not the case even in normal people; but in paranoiacs
there are occasionally strong excitements or also ecstasies that may
run their course with hallucinations. When this is the case hearing
and sight are probably affected most; in severe acute conditions perhaps also smell and taste.

Memory, aside from the illusions, is good. Memory hallucinations
will probably not occur. Naturally the one-sided interest of the
patients also produces a one-sided preference for individual categories of memory material.

Orientation as to place and time always remains normal, except
perhaps in the very rare psychogenic twilight states.

Attention corresponds to the preoccupation with the delusions; if
these are once taken for granted it is normal. At any rate, one can
call the readiness of association for everything that can be utilized
by the delusion a one-sided tendency of the attention. A monotonous
trend of ideas is mentioned, but that is not always the case; nearly
all paranoiacs permit themselves to be diverted at least sometimes,
and many still have other considerable interests outside of the delusion.

The *affectivity* appears on direct observation to be primarily normal. Naturally one who has just discovered that in a new place of refuge he is also persecuted is depressed or irritated. The megalomaniac who has just received a sign of his calling from Heaven or the president feels well satisfied. But this corresponds to the normal affective reaction as far as the affect alone is considered. It is said that the patients are irritable; I do not know that this is true in the ordinary sense. The normal person also is irritated by incessant annoyances, on the average much more than most of these patients, who tolerate a remarkable amount of disagreeable things. Then there are paranoiacs who were already irritable before the disease broke out which is therefore not at all the cause, perhaps, however, the result of the temperament. But one also finds calm dispositions among paranoiacs; I have not as yet seen any sanguine dispositions.

Paranoia is said to destroy *morality*. Strictly interpreted, that is not the case. The moral feelings as such are not touched. But the whole morbid logic is so one-sidedly influenced by the delusion that the patients often cannot either recognize or feel the just rights of others. Furthermore, their own cause is so very much the only important, I might say the only sacred, thing in the whole world, that a few lies and acts of violence also disappear in the face of it, and are furthered and sanctified by the great purpose.

An *inner classification* of the paranoia forms can as yet be made only according to the content of the delusion,[142] which is naturally again conditioned by the natural disposition and other internal and external presuppositions. The forms most frequently met by the physician are those involving *injury*, which again are divided into *delusions of persecution*, the commonest form, *paranoid litigiousness*, and *delusions of jealousy*.

The *persecuted* one sees hostile people who will not let him advance in life because of jealousy or any other selfish reasons. At the same time they bother him, slander him, deprive him of his positions, try to poison him (no physical persecutory delusion). Wherever the patient goes, he is met again by persecutors, disguised or not, or at any rate by the results of their work, in the form of letters, incitation of the people in the neighborhood, or expressions of contempt.

The *litigious paranoiac* has as a rule at some time lost a law suit, or at any rate as a result of it has not *quite* obtained his rights as he expected. He now tries again, loses once more, goes to every higher

[142] A natural systematization would have to be based, in the first place, on the peculiarities of disposition on which the paranoia is founded and then on the reconstructing psychical mechanisms.

court but is not satisfied even by the last, but again finds reasons to enter upon a new method of trial. At first they are ordinary causes of action, but then new material motives are added: On the one hand the judges will not stand for everything, respond with penalties against the accused, let unjustifiable complaints lie, or do not investigate the way the patient expects. On the other hand, the latter becomes irritated, accuses the judges and finally all officials that have dealings with him of prejudice, violation of the law, and conspiracy. He denounces his own lawyers and those of his opponents, whereupon an action is begun by the other side. Thus the material is far from being exhausted; on the contrary, it is constantly increasing until commitment or a guardianship gives the judges rest, at least for a while. Whatever unpleasantness occurs to the patient is felt as a grave injustice which the whole world must set right or avenge. What they themselves do to others they do not notice at all. The worst scoldings and slanders from their own side they cannot evaluate and are completely astounded and indignant when the opponents react to them. In their logic the laws contain almost only what can be turned to their advantage. What is characteristic here is that from the one case all others invariably originate. With this the litigious paranoiacs are usually not only clever pettifogers, but they also acquire an extensive knowledge of the laws, which to be sure they interpret one-sidedly. Whoever, after wading through countless tons of documents, makes a slight mistake in an opinion or in a report, may be sure of being attacked by them because of it.

The litigious delusion may appear in organic connection with a purely paranoid system of delusion and in this way give proof that it should not be separated from paranoia: A mechanic, fifty-three years old, sued for divorce from his second wife, who was a drunkard, and won his case. In describing a scene with his wife, who irritated him, he had used an expression in court that anyway he was a "bad actor." In the judgment, in translating the slang expression into more elegant diction, it was stated that he had himself admitted that he was a "brutal man," and from this it was inferred that the wife alone was not altogether at fault and that he should contribute to the cost of action. The expression angered him and he demanded a reversal of the judgment; he did not recognize the divorce at all, visited his wife repeatedly in a demonstrative manner, went through all possible and impossible appeals, denounced the authorities, neglected his work and finally made considerable debts. Thus he had bought a suit with the assurance that it would be paid for, then he himself instigated the dealer to press him for the money; on being pressed, he proposed the courts, and when the creditor came to him to attempt to obtain a friendly settlement, he threw him out of the house. Thus the patient had to be brought to the hospital. He was a jovial, fundamentally really a good-natured man, who would like to have succeeded a little better in the world without, however, having the strength to accomplish this (the usual inner discord of the paranoiacs). In one respect, to be sure, he had accomplished something; "he, the simple laborer," had been able in the town meetings and at the elections to have his opinion prevail against respected citizens—but he still remained the simple laborer while one of his opponents rose to the highest position in Switzerland; another achieved the second highest position (painful wound to his vanity). Toward his wife he had the attitude of the drunken husband. In reality he still loved her; on the other hand, she conducted herself in such a way that he had to obtain a divorce, and in spite of his age he thought of a better marriage (second conflict). Hence the complex sensitiveness toward the judgments in the case that he won; hence the non-recognition of the divorce he himself asked for. In his consciousness, to be sure, the reason was different. His distinguished political opponents want to revenge themselves on him; they induced the judges to render such a decision so that every woman who would like to marry him would have occasion to inquire of them concerning his brutality, and so that they could thus lower his standing and hinder him in remarrying. But as the man was euphoric and not distrustful, his delusion developed in a somewhat unusual direction: As he had everywhere been treated with noticeable indulgence, even when in his actions and in his incurring debts he over-stepped the bounds, his opponents did not really mean to do so badly by him, or they wanted to prevent their part in the matter from being exposed in court. Therefore he believed that behind his back they paid all his debts, and in order to try them again and again, he made debts, sold his furniture that had already been put up as security, etc.

The *jealous* patients are probably for the most part women (alcoholic jealousy delusion does not belong here). They find evidence everywhere that their husbands deceive them with many other women; with the old laundress as well as with the beautiful daughter of the neighbor they have affairs, give them money, etc.

Hypochondriacal delusions also are said to occur in paranoia; as yet I have not seen them.

The forms of delusions of influence are never wholly free from an admixture of more or less pronounced ideas of grandeur. All such patients have an exalted feeling of self-importance; they consider themselves extraordinary in some particular line. The persecutory delusion is partly connected with it, because they arouse the envy of others whose path they cross, etc. On the other hand, where the grandiose delusion dominates, the feeling of persecution is only rarely lacking; sometimes, especially in erotics, it approximates the main delusion in significance.

Among the megalomaniacs we must first mention the *inventors* who appear in every branch of mechanics. Often some of the ideas are not at all bad, but some weakness in their planning is overlooked while it is just on this that the entire failure depends. Before Zeppelin and the Wrights, dirigible airships were decidedly favorite objects of invention; a half century earlier it was perpetual motion.

Allied to the mechanical inventors are the *discoverers* in all scientific fields. Here one already sees more frequently confused things. Entirely free in their combinations are the *prophets* in religious and political fields who often find many followers and obtain a certain amount of importance (Illustration: *Lombroso,* The Man of Genius).

With these probably should be classed the above mentioned multiple murderer Wagner. Potapkine, who infected pretty nearly the entire population of his village (in the province of Orel, Russia) with his teachings about a return to a primitive state, or at least influenced them so that numerous punishments for anti-religious acts were administered.[143]

The *geneologists* or interprétateurs filiaux of the French, the *paranoiacs with the delusion of high descent,* realize the everyday dream *of so many children, which has also found expression in the fairy tale;* they have merely been stealthily handed over to their poor parents or given to them to bring up; in reality they are children of the nobility but for some fantastic reason, made more or less plausible, they are not brought up in the circumstances to which they were born. Only a certain time or event is awaited for them to be returned to their proper social position.

The *erotics* believe themselves loved by persons of the opposite sex of higher rank, often of the highest; they pursue him with every possible kind of messages that they are ready for the honor, or they enter his residence by stealth or force, where they demand to be treated as husband or wife. That they do not succeed in this is naturally due to the intrigues of others, to wickedness which is usually thought out more or less definitely in detail in the paranoic manner.

All these forms are markedly egocentric; the entire delusional system turns about the patient, his wishes and his fears. But other

[143] Monatsschr. f. Kriminalpsychol. II. 1905/1906, S. 493.

forms can also be thought of. Thus I know a minister who for many years has the delusion that the children of his neighborhood are maltreated by their parents. From what I know the case can only be brought under the head of paranoia. The delusion would be comprehensible if one supposes that the patient suffers from repressed sadism or masochism.

The *course of paranoia* is always most chronic. Some of the patients, but not all, were on closer inspection noticeable even earlier for selfishness, misinterpretation of the acts of others, and sensitiveness. The prodromal stage is practically never observed by physicians, and the relatives also can usually give no good account of it, as the patients at this time are nearly all inclined to be very reticent. For the customary descriptions in the books the paranoids much rather than the paranoiacs have served as models. No dependence can be placed on the statements of the patients themselves because just in these connections they are deceived by a vast number of memory illusions. At all events many cases require a greater number of years to develop, in that the persecuted at first become only distrustful and are still capable of recognizing at least a kind of uncertainty in their conclusions, but after a while there comes to them the certainty which is then never lost. Similar is the case in many forms of grandiose delusions, whose haughty over-estimation of self and of their secret hopes are slowly and easily hatched out as ideas of greatness. But in both kinds an "illumination" can suddenly permit the disease to become manifest. In litigious patients it is usually to be dated from the first court decision; but the delusions and the entire litigation are usually developed completely only in the course of years.

Paranoia frequently breaks out first in later manhood—according to *Kraepelin* in two thirds of the cases after the thirties—but there are also cases which become sick around the twenties.

In all forms, periods (usually long ones, lasting months and years) of stronger delusional formation and corresponding reaction alternate with quieter phases, in which the patients are more capable of getting along with other people and of being active in their calling. Most of these excitations and mitigations seem to come from within outward; others, chiefly in the persecuted, are connected especially often with a change of residence, after which the patients at first feel safe; but after a while the old delusions become attached to the new surroundings; often a letter that the patients have written produces the change. They considered themselves concealed; now their address has become known through the addressee or through the indiscretion of the postal authorities, and the chase begins again. Thus many travel from place to place during their whole lives, always going as far as possible from the one just inhabited, and in this way get all over the earth. In the insane asylum at Washington, I was told that the capitol of the Republic especially attracts paranoiacs from the whole earth because they expect help from the President of the United States.

There is surely no cure for paranoia. Those cases described in the literature of the subject can without doing them violence be considered as schizophrenia; least of all the case of Bjerre.[144] On the other hand, improvements appear with age, either because the patients finally come to see that they carry on a useless struggle, or because during the involution the energy declines, so that they are less active, and because of their passivity get along better with those about them.

Conduct. As was said, most paranoiacs during the years of incubation are more or less reticent—more expansive characters with an inclination to delusions of grandeur may be exceptions. At the height of the disease we have to keep distinct how they conduct themselves in their ordinary business and social life, and how they carry on their delusion. Conduct is about normal as far as it is not influenced by the delusion. The degree of influence varies greatly from one patient to another. In the one the delusion takes up the largest part of their time and interest; almost in every social gathering some partial delusion crops up and makes the patients noticeable. At the other extremes there are calm, quiet natures that continue to work in their calling even though with difficulty; they change their place of residence now and then or do something else incomprehensible on the outside, but they may remain unnoticed by most people, sometimes even by those near to them; but in the same patients also the conduct changes as a rule in the course of months and years.

Within the limits of non-paranoiac activity the patients conduct themselves normally. They never lose control. But in the pursuit of their purposes they also conduct themselves on the whole like other people who would have to achieve a similar object. Prophets, to be sure, often indicate their mission by appropriate dress, hair and beard. But most of the patients are extremely inconspicuous. Real excitations which would be pathologic in themselves through their severity and through the disruptions of the train of thought occur, if at all, only as brief episodes. On the other hand, many of the persecuted, for comprehensible reasons, are ordinarily cranky, irritated, and irascible. In the pursuit of their aims nearly all show a certain, often a high degree of passionateness. Many persecuted patients react with eva-

[144] Zur Radikalbehandlung der chronischen Paranoia. Jahrbuch für Psychoanalyse usw. Bd. III. S. 795. Deuticke, Leipzig and Wien.

sion, threats, scolding, insulting letters, and appeals to the authorities. Those suffering from grandiose delusions often use the press in a prolific manner. In general many paranoiacs actually become "graphomaniacs." Actively persecuted patients readily become persecutors (persécutes persécuteurs).

If the patient can no longer resort to legal measures, he seizes on "self-defense," either shooting his opponent, or, not rarely, assaulting a distinguished person in the hope that publicity will compel an impartial investigation and thus at last bring the true facts to light. In rarer cases, in improvers of the universe and prophets, acts of violence belong to the delusional system, as in the Wagner case; the religious paranoiac David Lazaretti died in 1878 in a battle with government troops.

Frequency. In hospitals, paranoia is a very rare disease, so that some psychiatrists doubt its existence; not one percent of admissions can be assigned to it. But outside it is not such a great rarity. It is always some special occurrence (an assault, a trial) that brings the patients to the psychiatrist.

According to *Kraepelin,* paranoia chiefly afflicts men (70%); my experience also coincides with this.

The *diagnosis* of paranoia is not always at all easy in practice. The patients know which of their ideas are considered morbid by others and can conceal or weaken them so that they can be defended. The delimitation in principle from mere psychopathy is often absolutely impossible where the delusion has centered itself on a class of ideas that are beyond proof, as in the case of founders of religion, politicians, and philosophers. Indeed, one can even enter into disputes concerning the morbidity of scientific discoveries and mechanical inventions that are entirely new, even if so many real inventors were not considered "crazy," as far as they are not really sick in some way. For even a crazy man may sometimes invent something worth while. Moreover, an idea may, by chance, correspond with reality and nevertheless be a delusion.[145] For the diagnosis two things must be considered:

1. The logical proof of the idea by the patient, which in the morbid cases shows incorrigible mistakes in the premises as well as in the logic, to the extent that certain parts of a discussion are inaccessible, and important and self-evident counter arguments simply cannot be appreciated. But with this, the momentary affective state and the

---

[145] It happened that a paranoiac believed himself poisoned with corrosive sublimate and corrosive sublimate was really supposed to have been found in the beer in the chemical laboratory, because, as was ascertained later, the reagents were contaminated.

patient's general intelligence must be taken into consideration. The affect accounts for defective logic in normal people also, and a weak intelligence even without paranoia will not be able to grasp complicated relations.

2. The cancer-like extension of the delusion to ever widening areas and the far-reaching domination by the delusion of the entire personality in its behavior and its strivings. Some one may write a proof as convincing as it is disputable that the seat of the soul is in the sympathetic system; but he is not a paranoiac as long as he does not ascribe an abnormal significance to this "discovery" and does not find new evidence for it everywhere where none is to be found.—The individual ideas of reference and the memory illusions, even when according to their content they are possible, often prove on closer inspection to be distinctly morbid, inasmuch as what corresponds to the delusion is often carried out with utterly impossible definiteness and impossible details, while what does not belong to the delusion is not related at all, is not even perceived by the patient, is not experienced, and on demand can be supplemented only in a defective, unclear, and uncertain manner.

Anatomical findings that might belong to paranoia have not been found.

Limitation. The litigious paranoiac can usually be readily distinguished from other litigationists by his immovable consistency and especially by the circumstances that all his complaints can be ascribed to the first unfortunate litigation. The *paranoid* is usually recognized easily by the logical impossibility of the delusion and the inner contradictions, then by the hallucinations, the disturbance of the affect, and by other schizophrenic signs. Only in case of a very furtive beginning can these peculiarities be so little developed that one is in doubt for a while, or even incorrectly diagnoses paranoia. The *manic-depressive* delusional forms can be recognized first of all by the affective disturbances, the flight of ideas or the retardation of thought, by the inconsistency of the delusions and by the entire picture. The not very rare belated forms of paranoia are to be differentiated from the senile paranoid forms by the strong, consistent delusional system, and by the absence of symptoms that indicate cerebral atrophy. Therefore the *differential diagnosis is in paranoia also a negative one: Delusional systems, besides which no signs of another disease can be found, are to be considered paranoic.*

With these differential diagnostic observations the *delimitation of the morbid pictures is at the same time essentially disposed of.* "Abortive" cases of paranoia are supposed to have been seen.

(*Gaupp.*)[146] Now there certainly are katathymic delusional formations that correct themselves. But I would not call these diseases paranoia because a proper demarcation of the concept is attained only then when the incurability, which is an important sign of nearly all cases, is included in the denotation of the concept. The abortive cases probably also lack the important sign of the general extension of the ideas. Some of the abortive and "milder" paranoias (*Friedmann*) are probably mild manic-depressive delusional forms. The "periodic" paranoia belongs partly to our schizophrenia, to a less extent to manic-depressive insanity.

The *paranoia completa* (Délire chronique à évolution systématique of Magnan) belongs to the schizophrenia group (paranoid or paraphrenic).

The *alcoholic paranoias* are toxic psychoses sui generis, if they exist at all, and are not to be included in the paranoid groups.

The formulation of a paranoia *originaria* (Sanders), which is said to begin in childhood, is probably based on the mistaking of memory deceptions.

There are besides *paranoia-like diseases* which as yet have been too little observed; they are perhaps involutionary diseases; there is also the delusional formation in those hard of hearing,[147] and in oligophrenics: Many feeble-minded only come to the asylum because of the development of ideas of persecution, which are not quite systematized but which also do not degenerate to the complete nonsense and the symbolic foolishness of schizophrenia. Usually, but not always, there are hallucinations of hearing at night, sometimes also those of sight, rarely of the other senses. It does not go as far as the catatonic symptom complex and just as little to a severe progressive dementia. The affective rapport especially is preserved; the patients also retain their external bearing in so far as the direct reaction to the persecutions in the form of attacks of rage and scolding does not make them unsociable. Occasionally also disconnected grandiose ideas appear besides, or in place of, the delusion of persecution. It is not improbable that this is a case of paranoia upon which the oligophrenia puts its particular impress, in that it prevents a logical development of the delusional system. But with this conception also the difficulty of differentiation from *Pfropf-paranoid* remains.

Conception of Paranoia. The delusional system of paranoiacs is a psychic formation that gives the appearance of a simple exaggeration

---

[146] Ueber paranoische Veranlagung und abortive Paranoia, Zentralbl. fur Nervenheilkunde und Psychiatrie 1910, S. 65.

[147] See p. 533.

of normal processes.[148] The normal individual reacts in the same way but not *continually* so. Everybody has false references to oneself as well as insufficiency of logic as soon as he is in an affective state.[149] The manifestation becomes pathological only because it cannot be corrected, and especially because of the tendency to spread generally, and the unintermittent continuous working of the affective mechanism once put in operation. The only known symptom of paranoia, the delusional formation, proves to be a reaction form to certain external and internal situations. At all events, it is not a direct result of any process in the brain or of a constitutional degeneration, and one must assume that at least in the milder cases the disease would not have broken out without releasing an external situation, or at least would not have assumed the same form. For the origin of the disease determines the symptomatology in manifold ways.[150] To be sure, one will presuppose that here too there are such serious dispositions that even everyday and unavoidable difficulties would have set free the disease; such patients under any circumstances become paranoiacs, while others become sick only in the face of serious conflicts.

Invariably we see at the root of the disease a situation to which the patients are not equal and to which they react by means of the disease: The young man feels in himself the impulse to achieve and be something worth while, but because of an intellectual or especially characterological weakness he does not get as far as he would like. He is not sufficiently indifferent to ascribe the failure to fate and to let it rest on himself; still less has he the strength to admit his own mistakes to himself and make them clear to himself. Then according to the everyday method he blames the environment and merges into the delusion of persecution, or in case of a more cheerful disposition he fulfills his wishes in phantasy and works himself out of reality into the delusion of grandeur.

The young woman who wants to get married but who lacks the natural instinct to love and attract a man finally thinks herself loved without any action on her part, and as in the fairy tales devised for children supposedly sexless, she is loved by one who at the same time brings her promotion in rank (which is obviously felt as the chief thing). Since reality cannot be shaken off altogether, here too ideas of persecution are usually added, while besides the real delusion of persecution the ideas of greatness persist, unclearly and perhaps gen-

---

[148] That is the reason why not only in practice, but in principle also a sharp line between paranoia and the normal and mere psychopathy cannot be drawn.
[149] See p. 95.
[150] Comp. above the illustrations.

erally undeveloped, as mere efforts toward greatness. Thus there is probably no paranoiac (and paranoia-like) delusion of greatness without delusions of persecution, and no delusion of persecution without ideas of greatness or at least aspiration to greatness, and the difference between the two forms becomes relative. I therefore believe I may here include the delusion of grandeur in the consideration, although it has as yet been very inadequately investigated. The "exalted feeling of self" which is ascribed to paranoiacs of various kinds is, therefore, probably a necessary condition for the origin of the disease. But I should like to add that according to everything I know, this feeling must be opposed by a feeling of insufficiency, probably repressed, before the paranoia can originate. Whoever collapses without this *inner* conflict has no occasion for a delusion of persecution, and also probably cannot produce the energy to separate himself from reality. The multiple murderer Wagner himself felt the difficulty of his situation and expressed it in a remarkably correct way:

"You will therefore understand when I go into ecstasies over the man who is robust in body and soul, when the *strong, the indifferent, the fighters, the criminals and the beasts impress me. I think of them all as the opposite of myself.* In this writing I am not using what I have read, as I am in general a very independent spirit. I was not tempted by the 'fashionable philosopher,' and on this occasion I want to remark to the Nietzsche followers that the key to a comprehension of his writings is weakness. The feeling of impotence brings forth the strong words, *the bold sounds to battle are emitted by the trumpet called persecution insanity.* The signs of the truly strong are repose and good-will. The strong man, about whom we palaver in our literature, does not exist. Furthemore, there is no such thing as the strong man in the rôle of a tamer of the populace. The strong individuals are those who without any fuss do their duty. These have neither the time nor the occasion to throw themselves into a pose and try to be something great."

It is probably not an accident that in all closely observed paranoiacs, all of them persecuted, I found a peculiarly *weak sexuality* which may point to an insufficiency of the impulses generally or to inner inhibitions.

The disposition for paranoia would therefore consist:

1. in a very dominating affectivity which, however, in contrast with the hysterical disposition, is persistent and stable and

2. in a strong feeling of self which, however, is opposed by some inferiority, and

3. in external difficulties that increase or provoke this inner conflict (which probably wanted to be repressed);

4. there must exist a maladjustment between the understanding and the affectivity so that in certain matters the latter obtains the lead. But this maladjustment without the other peculiarities would only lead to katathymic delusions or hysterical moodiness, etc., but not to paranoia. Many investigations are still needed before we can see more clearly. But at all events there is not merely one but several dispositions that correspond to the above conditions and out of which the picture of paranoia may grow.[151]

The disposition for paranoia does not have to be the same as the "paranoid character," which likes to relate the actions of the environment to itself and interpret them in an evil manner and with this seriously undervalue the rights of others as against its own.[152]

Ferenczi finds the causes of paranoia in the repression of homosexual impulses; his line of proof is, however, altogether insufficient.

Formerly the French included paranoia among the *monomaniacs*, in the belief that there was involved a very circumscribed disease of the psyche. A debate as to whether or not monomaniacs exist is useless, as it depends on the conception, while in this case the facts are fairly clear. Likewise there is no sense in discussing whether the intelligence of the paranoiacs is retained because outside of the delusion they think correctly, or whether the patients are demented because in the delusions they produce nonsense and cannot correct it.

Behind the paranoia there was also supposed to exist a *process disease* (brain degeneration). In favor of this could be mentioned: 1. the not rare appearance of prodromes, before the releasing and symptom determining situation takes place, 2. the incurability and unyieldingness of the delusional system. 3. the beginning which usually takes place in advanced age, and 4. the remissions and exacerbations occurring from within independently of conditions. But for the incurability we have an example in the traumatic cases of how psychogenic causes when they are permanently effective produce a lasting morbid picture; furthermore, in the expectation neurosis which does not become cured without treatment. In an analogous way one can make it at least probable in paranoia, that the causes, the inner and outer splitting, cannot be removed. That the disease frequently appears in later years could be caused by the fact that only then do these conflicts become definite. The youth may always still have

---

[151] Comp. also p. 177.

[152] *Carriers of the paranoid character* are psychopaths of various kinds, but especially frequently latent schizophrenics and blood relations of schizophrenics.

hopes of getting up in the world, even though here and there he has failed. And the fluctuations from within require a still more exact confirmation, as perhaps external factors or purely psychogenic results of the inner "elaboration," of understanding oneself, can none the less determine such changes. There are cases of delusional formation similar to paranoia that run quickly into a cure which, however, do not usually [153] come to the physician's attention. Because when only transient and chiefly exogenous reasons are present, they must become cured before the deception develops into a disease.

Treatment. Nothing can be done for the disease. One has to make the best of it. Some of the patients are best left to themselves. The more one wants to help, the worse it is. One must interfere when they become violent or waste their fortune, in the former case by commitment, in the second case a guardianship may suffice at times. When possible one should avoid protracted institutional treatment because this only makes the patients all the more embittered against the whole world.

2. THE DELUSION OF PERSECUTION OF THE HARD OF HEARING

The hard of hearing and the deaf and dumb frequently do not sufficiently understand those about them, consequently they become irritable and distrustful and, with or without excitement, they come to false conclusions about the environment. In some cases, especially in elderly women, this develops into a more connected paranoia-like morbid picture, usually with ideas of persecution which rarely, however, attain full certainty and show more the character of anxious apprehension. Memory deception, illusions, and occasionally probably also hallucinations, confirm the delusion and increase the difficulties.

The disease runs a chronic course with fluctuations and is incurable, although through skilfull behavior of the environment it is still amenable to influences.

Allers observed similar cases among prisoners of war, who could not understand the language of their environment. It is significant that here recovery took place as soon as the patients understood and were understood.

3. LITIGIOUS INSANITY

Litigious insanity is in the first place a syndrome, which occurs in various diseases, such as schizophrenia, manic-depressive insanity,

[153] Comp. p. 529 *Friedmann, Gaupp.* I myself know several typical intermediate cases of this sort.

certain abnormal character dispositions, and also in paranoia. If one simply speaks of litigious insanity, the paranoiac is meant by it. In spite of the fact that this form of paranoia shows some peculiarities when compared to the others, I prefer to adhere to *Kraepelin's* former conception and treat it with paranoia, not only because of the inner connections, but also in order to avoid double description of the very numerous common features in both morbid groups.

4. INDUCED INSANITY (FOLIE À DEUX)

It happens that paranoid or paranoiac and rarely hypomanic patients not only can make those with whom they live close together believe in their delusions, but they so infect them that the latter under conditions themselves continue to build on the delusion; at all events they remain blind when confronted with the contradictions from reality, they have the same deceptions of memory and eventually even illusions and hallucinations as the one who became afflicted first, and pass through paranoid or hysteroid excitements. This is called *induced insanity*.

But the individual followers of a prophet who represents an undemonstrable view will be declared insane only in the worst cases, although usually none of them can be considered responsible or capable of action in matters connected with the induced view.

The primary inducing patient is in such cases an energetic character. Those induced are mostly his blood relations, more rarely it concerns husbands, which throws light on the significance of familiar dispositions. They often take active part in the development of the delusional system, also enhance one another in the development of symptoms (the same psychological process as in cumulative criminality). But above all they cooperate in the morbid reactions to the outer world, such as the querulousness, cursing or violence, or they withdraw together, restricting contact with the world to the most necessary minimum.

Through timely interference, i.e. a separation from the diseased focus, most of the induced cases can rapidly be cured. There are exceptions, however, which then lead one to suspect that they too suffer from an independent disease in which only certain manifestations, like the content of the delusion, were determined by induction.

In reference to paranoia-like epidemics, there are some showing such *hysteriform* symptoms as: ecstasies, convulsions, major hysterical attacks, chorea magna, visions, and other hallucinations of an hysterical character, and automatic preaching. Not rarely both series of symptoms exist together.

5. THE REACTIVE MENTAL DISTURBANCE OF PRISONERS

It is only natural that some mental disturbance should become manifest in prison; this is especially true of dementia præcox. Some are directly set free as a result of the confinement as delirium tremens, in the alcoholic; others first become recognized during detention, or break out there, as in the case of paresis where the connection between confinement and psychosis can at most lie in the fact, that the latently existing psychosis leads to the crime or to let oneself be detected, and then becomes manifest in prison.

Besides these, there are definite syndromes which are directly precipitated by the confinement and carry the mark of this origin in the course and in the individual symptoms. They naturally originate on the basis of certain dispositions, which may, however, differ very markedly. In some kinds of psychopathies and pronounced chronic mental diseases, above all in schizophrenia, then in epilepsy but also in others, the various pictures might appear, each depending on the psychic constellations. Among other things these strongly depend, on the situation of the imprisonment. Those syndromes which mimic acutely an insanity, as the Ganser symptom complex, are naturally in the first place diseases of detention pending trial, while the chronic pictures belong to the imprisonment following the sentence.

It is not yet possible to describe all forms. The following may be mentioned: (a), (b), and (c). *Exaggerated affect reactions at the confinement.* They begin mostly soon after the confinement, partly as an explosion of the gradually accumulated worry, and partly on the occasion of any irritability. They manifest themselves especially frequently in an attack of rage and cursing with blind destruction (Prison crash), or in an anxious *depression* with vague delusions of sin and persecution. In most cases these conditions pass over rapidly, the prison crash usually in a few hours. An affective disturbance which lasts longer and which occasionally appears even after longer confinement is the *stupor*, which has an hysterical character.

(d) A simulation of insanity, as imagined by the layman, which is controlled by the unconscious, is the *Ganser twilight state*,[154] and the *clown syndrome;*[155] the *puerilism* seeks to represent a childish dementia.[156]

(e) In long continued confinements we observe in the first place *psychogenic depressions* and *excitable states* as a reaction to the un-

[154] See p. 545.
[155] Bleuler, Das Faxensyndrom. Psychiatr.-Neurol. Wochenschrift, 12, Jahrgang 1910-11, S. 375.
[156] See p. 545.

pleasant situation, to which also belongs *Vischer's* barbed wire disease of war prisoners,[157]

(f) A *querulousness* with more or less pronounced delusions, in which the patients imagine themselves unjustly treated and hence react with all plausible statements and protests, and under conditions also with violence.

(g) One of the most frequent syndromes in long detention is the *imprisonment complex*, which originates in quite the same manner in various dispositions: Either gradually or with a sudden inspiration, with or without hallucinations, the patients imagine themselves innocent,[158] liberated or pardoned. But as they are not liberated in reality they develop delusions of persecution about the environment, the public prosecutor, and the courts. The delusion attains tangible certainty through hallucinations of the different senses, especially of hearing, and strikingly often also of smell (poisoned gases are blown in into the cell), and taste; these are supported by deceptions of memory and dreams of severe maltreatment which are taken for reality. The participation of the two components, liberation and persecution, may appear in very different ways. In one case one delusion dominates, in another the other. The syndrome resembles very much the paranoid and can only be differentiated from it with certainty by the outcome. As a rule it disappears after the patient has been discharged from prison or transferred to the insane asylum.

Next to the confinement querulousness *Kraepelin* mentions as a prison psychosis the "delusion of persecution with local coloring" (regularly with hallucinations) and Ruedin's so-called *"presenile delusion of being pardoned,"* which until now has only been observed in life prisoners after they have been confined for a long time. As the first is mostly associated with ideas of liberation and the second with ideas of persecution, the two states may be conceived as variants of the prison complex, determined by different outer and inner conditions. The presenile delusion of pardon is incurable.

Kraepelin's prisoner's insanity (Gefangenenwahnsinn) appears soon after the the arrest, and shows a mixture of depressive and grandiose ideas, which do not however become fixed, and a slight clouding of consciousness. It becomes cured after discharge or after transference into an insane asylum.

Treatment. The general prophylaxis consists naturally in a possible avoidance of conflicts and in restricting of solitary confinement,

---

[157] *Vischer*, Die Stacheldraht Krankheit, Zürich, Rascher 1918.
[158] Even in other cases the crime or the sentence are subsequently completely shut off from memory.

the special prophylaxis in an intelligible consideration of the situation and the peculiarities of the prisoners, who are all, as it were, psychopaths in all directions. The pronounced psychosis heals, in so far as it is not an exacerbation of an otherwise existing chronic state, at any rate in the most acute forms. Most of the others recover regularly by transference in a better milieu (hospital) which takes more consideration of the disease than of the "object of punishment." Psychoses pending examinations, which serve the (unconscious) purpose of attaining a discharge, or cessation of the trial as a result of insanity, do not naturally recover easily during the procedures. The most important conditions for the recovery are absent in cases of the specific diseases of life prisoners.

6. The Primitive Reactions

Under primitive reactions *Kretschmer* [159] includes the exaggerated or false simple affective reactions like screaming, attacks of rage, affect stupor, reactive depressions ("homesick"), the rare manic-like reactive states, and similar reactions. Whether one should also add to it vasomotor syndromes and other physical symptoms matters very little here. These reactions already occur in animals, then in children, in insane and neurotic patients of all forms, and among the most varied psychopaths, and what is more, they occur also in such who in other matters, e.g. intellectually, stand very high. Like in the prison crash, they frequently appear as independent transitory diseases. Such cases are usually ushered in with deep disturbances of consciousness with or without hallucinations. They last a few minutes, at most a few weeks, and leave behind a pronounced or absolute amnesia and full insight. *"Exogenous Reaction types."* These originate on the different psychopathies but only on the basis of actual mental diseases (schizophrenia, epilepsy, organic states, etc.). As they are relatively complicated, they can also be united into one concept with the reactive depressions and exaltations.

7. Reactive Depressions and Exaltations

Reactive *depressions*, which become aggravated to a mental disease, are quite rare in the light of present views. In so far as they come to the psychiatrist, they are mostly partial manifestations of other diseases, especially of manic depressive insanity, and naturally of psychopathies and neuroses. Also seniles who are incapable of helping themselves can react with melancholic states of short duration.

Reactive *manias* we do not know.

[159] Der sensitive Beziehungswahn. Julius Springer, Berlin, 1918.

8. THE REACTIVE IMPULSES (IMPULSIVE INSANITY OF KRAEPELIN)

Various *impulsive actions,* which, among other things were also described as *impulsive insanity* and formerly as *monomanias,* have changed into reaction forms in the great majority of cases. Still one observes externally the same acts as a result of organic brain disturbances, of epilepsy, of alcoholic poisoning, and similar diseases, and, moreover, the actual reactions sometimes act first on the basis of such disturbances of consciousness. Others are based on psychotic dispositions, especially schizophrenia. As independent morbid pictures they develop on the soil of all kinds of psychopathies.

Those that are most frequently observed almost only among men as states of *wandering* (Fugues, Poriomania) are of an epileptic nature, or are due to cerebral traumas; others occur in schizophrenias. Pure reactive impulses may be habitual or may appear only once in a life time; the latter especially in puberty.

The most common is undoubtedly the impulse to set fire (pyromania), which we observe most frequently among young people who find themselves (subjectively) in an unbearable situation, above all among half grown servant girls, who were torn away from their own family and can find no emotional contact with the new place. Notwithstanding the impulsive element in regard to the main object, the will to set fire, the pyromaniac often premeditates his act and does it with a certain refinement, so that some are not immediately detected. In such cases it mostly concerns a crime committed only once, but it may, however, be repeated a few times, or even many times. The perpetrators of the act cannot give, as a rule, any adequate reason, unless the prosecutor examines it into them; the act is so little their own that even if they are otherwise of a normal nature they cannot even display the proper regret. The nearest explanation is the one that by setting fire to the house in which it was unbearable for them they wished to force some change for themselves. Regardless of the fact that this could have been effected in many other ways [160] the explanation cannot at all be applied to all cases, e.g., where fire is set to houses of strangers.

In some cases the unbearable situation lies in a *sexual affair* or in unhappy sexual aspirations.[161] Others experience direct sexual excitements through setting or watching the fire. *Alcohol* also plays a

[160] A very intelligent girl in the same situation destroyed dishes; this was accomplished according to the Freudian unconscious manner, partly during short attacks of fainting, until the connection became clear to us.

[161] Another form of unburdening is the suicide (Comp. Jaspers, Heimweh und Verbrechen. Diss. Heidelberg, 1909).

great part. Some set fire only while drunk or during some time of every inebriation, without showing any other recognizable causes. To be sure *menstruation* also furnishes a disposition for it.

The act is sometimes preceded by distinct moodiness with anxiety, "homesickness," digestive, and similar disturbances. During the accomplishment of the act some seem to be in a kind of twilight state, while others reflect and go through a conscious struggle between their impulse and their morality. In some the impulse comes suddenly and is at once put in operation, leaving no time for an actual reflection.

To be sure, pyromania appears in very diverse dispositions. Some of these people do not even seem very morbid and can later lead a normal life.[162]

More rarely one observes young servant girls who when in the situation mentioned above *kill* the children entrusted to them, and the impulsive *poison mixers*, likewise only of the feminine sex, who are apparently governed by entirely different motives.

Kraepelin counts also among his impulsives some of the *anonymous letter writers* of which some are readily recognized as hysterical phantastic persons, who at the same time find sexual gratification from their pen activities.

More common are the *kleptomaniacs*, at present especially in the form of *shop-lifters*. The latter (it seems that only the feminine sex is afflicted in this way) succumb to the refined stimulus of the displays in stores and steal both necessary and unnecessary articles; it would often seem that it is done only during the menstrual period. The *kleptomaniacs in the old sense* cannot even otherwise resist the impulse of appropriating things, and here again it is done regardless of whether they can make use of the things or not, they hoard them, give them away, destroy them, and under conditions they even return them to the rightful owners. The morality of such people may in other respects be quite good. In some cases a connection was demonstrated between the act of stealing and sexual feelings, but on the whole we do not know the genesis of kleptomania. Disturbances of consciousness and especially hysteroid twilight states sometimes accompany the crime. One can then just as well speak of stealing during hysterical attacks as of kleptomania.

It is quite obvious that one must guard against too frequent diagnosis of kleptomania. One must demonstrate not only an impulse in the usual sense but a *morbid impulse*. The easiest diagnosis is made

[162] Comp. *Schmidt:* Zur Psychologie der Brandstifter, in Jung's Psychologische Abhandlungen. Deuticke, Leipzig-Wien, 1914, and Brill: Psychic Epilepsy, Long Island Medical Journal, January, 1907.

in the cases where even quite useless objects are stolen, or where the thief has made no use of the things stolen, or returned them in some way.

As a last category *Kraepelin* mentions the *buying maniacs* (onio-maniacs) in whom even buying is impulsive and leads to senseless contraction of debts, with continuous delaying of payment until a catastrophe clears the situation a little—a little but never altogether, because they never admit all their debts. According to *Kraepelin,* here, too, it always involves women. The usual frivolous debt makers, who in this way wish to get the means for pleasure, naturally do not belong here. The particular element is impulsiveness; they "cannot help it," which sometimes even expresses itself in the fact that not-withstanding a good school intelligence, the patients are absolutely incapable to think differently, and to conceive the senseless conse-quences of their act, and the possibilities of not doing it. They do not even feel the impulse, but they act out of their nature like the caterpillar which devours the leaves.

Here one might also add the *morbid collectors,* who senselessly sacrifice much time and money to a hobby and without any other moral weaknesses they very easily get to stealing.

9. THE REACTIVE CHANGES OF CHARACTER

The reactive changes of character only attract attention when the change may be designated as an aggravation. In most cases they appear in childhood, but may then continue throughout life unless corresponding measures or fundamental changes in the environment bring about recovery. But even later age is not immune to such transformations. If one does not conceive Michael Kohlhaas as an actual paranoiac and one wished to follow instead Kleist's description he would be one of these types.[163]

10. THE NEUROTIC SYNDROMES [164]

A. Hysterical Syndrome. "Hysteria" [165]

As the hysterical symptom complex one designates the more massive neurotic symptoms and those with conspicuous psychic connections,

---

[163] For further details see pp. 127-128.

[164] Concerning the general conception, origin, prognosis and treatment, see the introduction to Chapter XII, p. 493.

[165] Cf. the observations concerning the "Neurosen," pp. 493-494 f. For further details on hysteria see especially *Lewandowsky,* Die Hysterie, Berlin, Springer, 1914. For the prolific symptomatology with discussion of the older or more of the somatic conceptions, see *Binswanger,* Die Hysterie, Wien, Hölder, 1904.

that is to say, on the pure psychic sphere there are the psychogenic twilight states, and on the physical sphere, the anæsthesias, hyperesthesias, paralyses, convulsions and contractures, the formations of pimples and blisters, psychogenetic hemorrhages, if such exist, psychogenetic vomiting, and the many other analogous manifestations. In common with the ("pseudo") neurasthenias,[166] the hysterical symptom complex presents the paresthesias and the abnormal influences of the vegetative organs, including that of the vasomotor system.

The psychic and the physical hysterical symptoms, e.g., a contracture and a twilight state, seem to have no direct association at first sight. Nevertheless one can build up a useful concept only for all the mentioned symptom complexes, for they are produced through the same reactions in equally predisposed people, and although it is true that the psychic manifestations can occur alone, equally directed psychic anomalies occur next to the physical, always at least by way of indication.

Physical Symptoms. The expression "physical" in the symptomatology of hysteria as well as in the other neuroses has a different meaning than usual. In the hysterical anæsthesias it is a question of a pure shutting off of incoming impulses not even from the psyche, but from the momentary consciousness (something like in paying attention to a process, one does not perceive another), and in changed functions of organs it is a question of the psychic influence of these organs, like pain producing tears, shame causing blushing, and anxiety stimulating the intestinal activity. In other words it is a question of things which in other connection one calls psychic, but which are best designated as "psychogenic physical symptoms."

Charcot has assumed that a number of physical symptoms, especially the anæsthesias, and the absence of the palate and conjunctival reflexes, are constant symptoms of hysteria (not of the hysterical disposition), and he therefore designated them as "stigmata," thinking that one can diagnose through them the existence of hysteria even if no other symptoms were present. This is undoubtedly false. He who is careful at the examination not to influence by suggestion seldom finds the stigmata; however, the existence of psychogenetic anæsthesias naturally proves that there is a great auto-suggestibility and with it the possibility or the probability, that other psychogenetic symptoms also exist.—Some also spoke of *psychic stigmata* and understood thereby the psychic peculiarities leading to hysteria, especially the affective lability but also the peculiarities of character, which were falsely called hysterical.

[166] See p. 558.

The psychic origin of *anæsthesia* and *hyperæsthesia,* among other things, is proven by the fact that they correspond in their demarkations to the patient's ideas of anatomy.   Thus a hand, a forearm, a cuff, or a side of the body exactly limited in the middle line, is anaesthetic; and all that, must under ordinary conditions not at all show the consequences of anæsthesia.   Notwithstanding anæsthesia and analgesia of the hand, the patients do not injure themselves [167] and can do delicate works.   Kinesthetic anæsthesia does not give here any ataxia; indeed, in most cases the patients know nothing of the disturbance, until the doctor's examination calls their attention to it (except where the anæsthesia has a direct object, as in some traumatic forms).   The other results of stimulation of the anæsthetic areas are very diverse, the pain reaction of the pupils remains intact in most cases, but the reflex changes of the blood pressure can be absent; even shock through severe irritation of the anæsthetic abdominal organs may not appear.   Analgesia is often associated with slight or absent hemorrhage in minor injuries, and in raising of the galvanic skin resistance.   On the other hand the cutaneous reflexes are mostly not changed, especially those that are inaccessible to the will like the cremasteric reflex.   Also the reflexes of the mucous membranes behave differently (the absence of the pharyngeal reflex in the normal and in psychogenic patients seems to depend on the kind of examination as well as on the mode of reaction of those examined). That the symptoms may under psychic influences easily change in intensity and extensity is quite evident from the above.

The anæsthesias may effect any of the qualities such as touch, warmth, pain, sight, taste, etc., but not very frequently are they all effected together.   Besides neuroses, mostly monocular and with retained pupilary reaction, there may occur color blindness or a narrowing of color.   Characteristic of psychogenic origin is especially the "tubiform" field of vision whose surface magnitude does not increase with the distance.   Hearing is very seldom effected in peace time hysterias.   If definite boundaries are not fixed through suggestion of the examination, the hysterical disturbances of sensibility change very strongly in limitation and intensity as soon as one varies the tests somewhat by distraction and various combinations of suggestions.

The local hyperæsthesias need no description.   Especially to be mentioned are the general painfulness in movements (*Moebius* Akinesia Algera (Comp. Expectation Neurosis), clavus, torticollis hystericus, neuralgias, vaginismus, pruritus, etc.).   Some of the pains are at all events to be traced to some sort of cramps, so also the frequent

[167] Comp. as a contrast Morvan's disease.

globus hystericus, the sensation of a ball ascending from the pelvic region to the throat, and vaginismus. Valley's painful spots like the hysterical zones can be suggested to the patient. The famous "ovaria" is probably a product inspired by the doctor, even if the concerned pressure spots seem to have certain peculiarities.

The *tendon reflexes* are mostly exaggerated, if they are not diminished by an accidental cause, like stupor, weakening of the legs through long paralysis, and through similar factors. The *reactions of the pupils* are normal as a rule, still one rarely finds exceptions, which are not yet quite understood; contracted and rigid pupils are probably based on a contraction of accommodation.

The *reflexes of the skin and mucous membranes* are uncommonly changeable; anæsthetic places are not all always without reflexes.

Of motor symptoms one should mention *pareses, paralyses*, and *contractures*. The paralyses are again not anatomical but affect muscle groups which belong together psychically, that is, a part of a limb, but the paralysis is especially of definite functions (as astasia abasia, or paralysis of deglutition; with the exception of aphonia, disturbances of speech (stuttering) is rare, more frequently one observes some sort of tics).

Of the *organic functions* the *sympathetic and vasomotor system* (heart!) are frequently and deeply altered.

Trophic disturbances may also occur, in the form of pimples, blisters and bleedings (Stigmatized ones); at all events there is a *psychogenetic fever* as was demonstrated among other things by the experiences of lung specialists who injected *aqua destillata* instead of tuberculin and obtained a rise of temperature.

From the *gastro-intestinal canal* one observes besides the globus, also anorexia and vomiting as favorite symptoms; but any other function may be concerned.

Lewandowsky stresses here syndromes under the name of *hysterophilic ailments*, or diseases which occur independently on an unpsychogenic basis, but can also originate on a psychogenic path, e.g. migraine, epileptiform attacks, asthma, membranous enteritis, and occupation cramps.

On the *purely psychic sphere* one would mention in the first place the following permanent symptoms, which though essentially belonging to the disposition are also reenforced by manifest hysteria: Lability of the *affects*, moodiness, momentary reactions in all relations, with exaggerated affective outbursts in various directions. The latter display mostly something of the theatrical; one has the feeling that the real affective force displayed does not quite correspond to the amount of crying and tears, and that the threat of suicide heard from so many on every occasion, though often put in operation, is seldom accomplished. Laughing and crying spells without any clear motivation are not rare. It is also remarkable how lightly, on the whole, the hysterics carry their troubles; in many of them it is evident that they are actually pleased to play the part of being sick. That may go so far that they wish to acquire real diseases,[168] or that they are willing to injure or castrate themselves, or permit an amputation (*furor operatorius passivus*). Under certain constellations hysterics may temporarily or lastingly appear indifferent, poor in feelings, just like in an effective torpor.

The *suggestibility* of hysterics is familiar. But there was a time when these patients were described as being particularly impermeable to suggestions from others; against this, they were said to be especially auto-suggestible. The truth lies in the fact that they have a strong positive and a strong negative suggestibility.

The *attention* corresponding to the affectivity is very variable. In severe diseases the patients find it hard to collect themselves. Otherwise it mostly depends on the interest; in the different relations it may be excellent or also very bad.

The *memory* is easily falsified by the affectivity; the not rare connection between hysteria and pseudologia phantastica produces a stronger similar disturbance. "Distraction," while experiencing something and also in reproducing it, will influence the function of memory. Furthermore, amnesias are left sometimes by violent excitements, and regularly by twilight states.

The *intelligence* can be good or bad. But judgment is often clouded by the affect.

The *sexuality* of hysterics can be judged still less than that of others; we see all extremes; especially among the female hysterics there are many who are frigid in coitus or even take a negative attitude to it, whereas psychosexually they may be very sensitive.

The *attack like* symptoms regularly associate themselves with some affective experience, to which belong also physical injuries, especially such as are subject to compensation. In the hysterical *twilight states* the patients, in the most pronounced case, imagine themselves in an entirely different environment, in the desert, or in heaven, they have remarkable adventures, they are kidnapped by robbers or in states of ecstatic euphoria they are received in heaven, etc. They often repeat exciting scenes which they have actually experienced, such as sexual attacks and similar experiences. Other twilight states fulfill wishes

[168] "The one who simulates, wishes to appear *sick*, the hysteric *to be* sick."

that cannot be granted in life, or at least exclude a great unpleasantness with everything connected with it. Twilight states with disconnected confusions are also supposed to occur; at all events one sees anxious hallucinatory states with all sorts of terrifying grimacing faces and animal figures, in which logical connection cannot immediately be discerned.

Seemingly pure nonsense is produced in the *Ganser syndrome,* whose sense is to represent a psychosis, and whose clear purpose, to the observer, is to escape punishment or at least a long sentence. Systematically the patients do many things in the reverse way; they attempt to put in the key with the ward up or with the ring; when it is in the lock they turn the wrong way; they rub a match with the wooden side or on any part of the box except where it should be rubbed; to the question, how much are 2 × 3 they say: 5 or 7 or any number under 10, only not the correct one, they read on the clock 12 for 6, 3 for 9, they have two noses, etc.

Related to the Ganser syndrome is the *"hysterical puerilism"* which in some inconsistent manner plays the little child and can continue for weeks. The patient calls himself Johnny, speaks in infinitives, or not at all, counts coins clumsily and incorrectly; at best he counts only the pieces but not the value; he draws childish figures, plays the whole day like a little child, lets himself be distracted by any triviality, looks for his mother, and eventually states that he is 12 years old, etc. At the same time he does also other things incorrectly and in the reverse way, things that children would correctly understand, he does not recognize his relatives, and shows a very inadequate flow of associations. There may also be analgesia up to absence of the corneal reflexes. The syndrome has thus far been described chiefly in punished military persons.

Analogous in symptomatology, even if on account of outer conditions it runs a half or entire chronic course, is Wernicke's *Pseudodementia.* The patients, most of whom met with accidents, mimic mental weakness; they are unable to answer the simplest things, they rarely produce nonsense, but they do not know, or are not sure; they use childish excuses, which resemble those of organic patients; they do not know the date because they have not seen the calendar. To the question of 5 × 6, they simply put together the 5 and 6 to make 56. In serial statements they easily make mistakes, they turn things around and leave gaps. The *impressibility* is bad. Besides, one finds psychogenic anæsthesias, and vasomotor manifestations; the Romberg test is frequently very characteristic; they let themselves fall without any effort to balance themselves. The mood is often dull and depressed. Recovery does not come at all or one must wait for it a long time. Since the war with its accumulation of traumatic forms with all sorts of variations and mixtures, the name pseudo-dementia was extended to pictures, which besides the symptoms mentioned also show the Ganser syndrome, psychic-apractic and many other psychogenic symptoms. *What is characteristic for all these formations aside from the changeableness is the disappearance of the memory for elementary knowledge and experiences, which remains intact in the organic disturbances.*

Also oriented twilight states occur in hysteria. They frequently last quite long, even months; according to character the patients are different people; to be sure they follow a certain plane (e.g., stealing or traveling; many *wandering states* also belong here), but without any regard for the future and frequently in contradiction with their own character. At the same time they behave in an orderly way, and correctly grasp the environment in its simpler relationships, so that they do not always impress one as ill. In these as well as in the clouded twilight states, thefts, arsons, and similar crimes may be committed.

The hysterical twilight states of various kinds are often initiated by a moodiness of many hours; they last from minutes to days, rarely longer, and are regularly followed by complete amnesia.

Following twilight states or as equally justified manifestations *stuporous states* with flexibilitas cerea may sometimes appear. We then see *somnolent states* lasting from seconds to years ("Narkolepsy" when they suddenly fall upon the patient and do not continue long; such attacks may also be of another nature, to wit, epileptic). Reaction depressions, too, may occur in hysteria, but here they are only of short duration (days, weeks) moreover there may be transient attacks of anxiety with physical symptoms, like a choking in the throat, and the highest oppression.

Even without the actual twilight states ideas can sometimes become so vivid that they are taken as *hallucinations;* it mostly involves visual disturbances. Where auditory deceptions occur to a great extent without disturbances of consciousness, it is not a question of pure hysteria.

Mainly in hysterical people do *waking dreams* occur, which temporarily so control the patient that they have to be designated as morbid, because they hinder him from taking account of reality.

How far purely hysterical *delusional formation* can go is not yet determined; at all events, they depend on the psychic milieu. Even in our state of society a hysteriac can imagine herself gravid, present all signs of pregnancy, including colostrum, except the enlarged uterus, and cause her husband, a highly regarded practitioner, to take into the house the obstetrical nurse for a definite term. But if she should expect a Christ as her delusional child, the patient would be a schizophrenic if that happened in enlightened communities. In the same way, those patients are schizophrenics who in our country or in our times state that instead of a child they carry a toad or a snake.

One also speaks of *hysterical mania, melancholia,* and *insanity.* It is possible that sometimes through a certain treatment the affective relation to the environment may resemble an insanity; furthermore, manic attacks in people who at the same time have a hysteroid disposition (hence in a combination of both diseases) run a course with vivid visual hallucinations which remind one of hysteria, but what is otherwise so designated and especially what was formerly so called daily are schizophrenics according to my experience. The few times that I thought that I had to drop this rule; I made a false diagnosis.

As *hysterical attacks* one describes general motor manifestations with all kinds of movements (not spasms of individual muscles), buffoonry, and rigid states; the arc of a circle, supporting oneself on head and heels, is favored. Beside the more or less incoordinated movements, one frequently finds stronger or weaker hidden and caricatured representations of any kind of experiences or wishes, so that such attacks could just as well be added to the twilight states. Looking from case to case the manifestations have no definite character, but the individual attacks in the same patient may absolutely resemble one.another. They can last any length of time, and repeat themselves any number of times, a thousand or more in one day, but the pulse and general condition are influenced only remarkably little.

Next to such motor attacks there are also simple *fainting* and *dizzy* spells, which are probably due more to vasomotor origin.

Even more than in any other neuroses *sleep* is here very irregular, sometimes it is absent, sometimes very good and exaggerated, and sometimes it comes inopportunely.

Hysterical Twilight States.—42 years a bookkeeper. Always somewhat nervous. Not brought up by the family. *Not understood* by the family, but she does a good deal for them; she is also otherwise charitable. Her fiancé died of paresis in Burghölzli shortly before the wedding. Since then she kept up some contact with the hospital. Lately she had to keep house for and nurse her brother, who obtained a divorce and was also ill; she also had to care for a child suffering from diphtheria. To recuperate, she took a trip to a friend in Germany, but there got into a mess of trouble. After she had once taken a glass of wine against her habit, she began to dig up some graves in the cemetery, but later knew nothing about it. But she merged into other confused states and for that reason she came to the clinic, where at first she had attacks at different times of the day. She imagined herself in the cemetery, heard the dead, and saw now adults and now children. They came to her, some even into her bed, whereupon she left the bed so as not to make it uncomfortable for them. Dead children called to her that she should dig them up. While during her good periods she knew nothing of the twilight states, she recalled them well during her unclear periods. A single suggestion during the twilight states had the effect that she could also recall them in her waking state; to be sure, in the course of the next weeks they again lost in clearness. Later she had an attack every night regularly between 12 and 1 (ghost hour). Once she called the dead, telling them that they can all come, the room was large enough, there was room for all. Then she said: "Now they are all here." Thereupon she went to sleep. In another attack she kept herself awake, saying that all the dead were strangers and that all acquaintances were missing. Through one hypnotic treatment the twilight states were cut short and the headaches which continued disappeared later only after many seances. The very first hypnosis had been complete and deep. But after another patient next to her was hypnotized who did not merge into deep hypnosis, it was then impossible during this period of hospital residence to get her beyond this stage of hypnosis. Later she had various hysterical physical symptoms, once an hysterical torticollis; a surgeon mistook it for a caries and wanted to apply a plaster bandage and keep her in bed for several months, which would have cost her her position. A few hypnotic treatments cured it. For some years she has obtained consolation and relative good health from Christian Science.

Hysterical Physical Symptoms. A girl, who was brought up in low moral surroundings and was subjected to various sexual attacks, suffered among other hysterical symptoms from vomiting after tasting milk. It turned out that it originated from the fact that a stable servant, from whom she had to get the milk, wanted to force her to *receptio seminis in ore.* She had abdominal pains when she sat on the damp grass and attributed it to "catching cold." But during the performance of an abortion she lay on the cold grass, hence the association, which was revealed only on examination. She had to vomit after the visit of a friend: the latter once related to her that she too went through an abortion. The patient herself had attempted an abortion with tobacco suds, after which she had a terrible spell of vomiting. She had pains frequently in the right biceps "due to over-work" in ironing "during bad weather": On account of masturbatic compunctions she once squeezed her arm between the bed and the wall. The pain really came after masturbating, with a definite complex of ideas. All these and the rest of the symptoms permanently disappeared (now twenty years) after the connection was made clear to her in hypnosis. A part of the girl's statements could be verified by investigation, and especially also by an examination of court records, and without exception proved to be perfectly correct.

Hysterical Convulsive Symptoms. A nurse girl, 20 years old, brought up in respectable surroundings. Good intelligence, but quite early in life not frank and somewhat moody. At 12 years meningitis (?). From about this time she committed minor thefts at home. She was discharged from two places for dishonesty; then she was with a procureress in Paris and then got a position as nurse girl. At 17 years hysterical attacks with violence; then again muteness and even deafness. In the night she got attacks of screaming and convulsions. She was discharged from an insane asylum as cured after three months, and then she was learning dress-making for five months, where she behaved faultlessly. When she again had twitchings she came to an aunt whom she was to help in business, but she ran about instead and and brought home phantastic stories, how she conducted a secret bureau under the direction of negroes, and similar tales. She stole considerable sums of money, formed an alliance with a young man, to whom she told stories about having a fortune, but which, as always in such cases, at this time it was still in the hands of her aunt, the countess. She simulated a burglary attack and was examined in court. Then for many days there was absolute closure of the jaws and rigidity of tongue, which lasted 56 hours; she could, however, make herself understood by writing; there were twitchings in her limbs. By means of a few hypnotic treatments we definitely mastered the hysterical symptoms (now ten years). She was a year in very strict service, but held out bravely; then learned quickly the most important office work and has held for nine years a well paid office position.

Ganser State. 24 years coachman. Arrested on account of fraudulent security in horse dealing. After admitting participating in the crime, he gave false answers at the examination; he did not buy a horse, he was a servant, not a coachman, he did not know his family name, he was not married, had no children, was 28 years old. He gave the wrong year, and did not know where he was. On admission to hospital he answered in the same way, but on request he immediately gave correctly everything that he had in his pockets. Later he counted: 1, 2, 4, 7, 9, 11, etc. On the watch he mistook the big for the little hand. He wished to open the match box by pressing on the long side, then on the cover and the bottom and finally pushes it together. Of interest is the following: If questioned in the tone of an examination, one always received false answers during the twilight state, e.g. he was not married; but when asked in a sympathetic and pitiful tone about his poor wife, then he was just as definitely married, praised his wife, and told about his marriage journey, but when immediately thereafter he was again questioned in the examination tone he again forgot everything.

Even in such criminal cases the Ganser symptoms can represent a shutting off of an unpleasant situation, a simulation of oneself, and not only a simulation in the presence of the judge. After a few days the patient became clear, but had a retrograde amnesia for the crime and the arrest. After the latter was explained to him he attempted suicide; then he resigned himself to his fate.

Hysteria with Pseudologia. A 16 year old girl, mother prostitute, father vagabond. She herself was therefore brought up by strangers. Intelligence distinctly below the average. She was never very easy to manage, and as she advanced in age she became more spiteful, more garrulous, and more addicted to lying. She began to tell how she was maltreated by various prominent people; she gave so many details and spoke with such conviction that five of them were detained for examination. Contradictions in her statements soon created suspicion as to the truth of her assertions. Thus it came to trial. Here she not only repeated the stories but added much that was new; she told how she was maltreated during the attacks, how her ribs were broken, how the defendants at the examination were forced to sit on iron chairs, their hands tied to the back, how strictly every one of them was punished, and how as a result of a complaint that she has nevertheless withdrawn a clergyman was taken to prison on account of poisoned bonbons, so that now he was a street cleaner. She also related how she set fire to a house and was caught in the act, and how in the ensuing struggle she sustained a broken leg, and she almost knocked out a woman's eye. At the same time she modelled both the content and expression according to the scheme of blood and thunder romances. During the examination she showed now and then hysterical absences, in which her eyes became veiled, her look remarkably rigid, she sat motionless for a few minutes, only to arouse herself later as from a sleep, and knew nothing of what happened during the attack. The gynecological examination showed an old defloration. In the course of a few years she became considerably better, although she remained sensitive and sometimes did some mischief. As she had little hope of being discharged from the hospital because of the danger of illegitimate children, she finally demanded continually an oophorectomy, and because no attention was paid to her, she experienced such violent ovarian pains before each menstrual period that one had to give in, and the operation was done under due process of the law. Since then she has been decidedly calmer and more balanced and after ten years of internment she could be discharged to a private family where she behaves well and earns through work a part of her maintenance.

The Limitation of the Concept of Hysteria, although it would not be very sharp, considering its characterization,[169] it would nevertheless be sufficient, if one were not in the habit from the olden times to stuff into it so many other things, and above all things that should not be taken into it. Thus one should not include in it the strong affectivity seen among savages, or the phenomena of becoming perfectly rigid from a knock on the door, or the twilight like loss of clearness, and similar states, or the *mass epidemics* (chorea Germanorum, tremor epidemics in schools), or simple primitive reactions in attacks of rage. Quite different are the monosymptomatic hysterias of children, where in most cases the false connection is as important as the purpose of the disease, the monosymptomatic war tremors, the traumatic hysterias, and the various psychical and physical symptoms of the peace time hysterias.

Traumatic Hysteria, as far as our present knowledge goes, is not different from the other forms of hysteria; however, in those following accidents in peace time, attacks of twilight states are rarer than in ordinary hysteria; indeed, the details of the general structure of the hysterical picture strongly depend on the influences causing the disease, so that relatively frequent different symptoms stand here in the foreground. In injuries of peace time, attacks, paralyses and twilight states are comparatively rare; the war brought an unfamiliar accumulation of paralyses with tremors, which are due to exertion and fright.

Example of a *traumatic hysteria without damage suit.* A marked imbecile got into a marsh from which he could not get out. Since then he was unable to cross more open places like rooms and streets. He feels his way by touching with his left foot forward, and after considerable fumbling he slightly drags along the right foot. With it he assumes a bent swaying attitude, balancing himself with his arms. The disease would almost be monosymptomatic if at the same time the patient had not given up almost altogether his active associations to the outer world; he cares little about anything and permits himself

[169] See p. 540.

only to be fed. Perhaps that was his morbid gain. The treatment produced very slight results.

Hysterias in children without marked change of character are mostly monosymptomatic.

The clumsy name *Hystero-epilepsy* originated at a period when epileptiform attacks were still looked upon as neuroses, and when they could not be differentiated. Beside the ordinary epilepsies with lesser striking hysterical symptoms, there are such who in addition show hysteroid attacks. Furthermore, there are hysteriacs, though they are extremely rare, who can imitate or produce an epileptiform attack. The first is an epilepsy, the second a hysteria. *What is usually called hystero-epilepsy is hysteria with severe motor attacks,* which were falsely added to the side of epilepsy. One also speaks quite unnecessarily of *hystero-neurasthenia* when there is a mixture of symptoms showing shades of both diseases, which naturally occurs frequently.

The limitation of *Neurasthenia* must start with this disease, which analogous to its original conception, though it *is not* a nervous exhaustion, still mimics such. He who seeks to attain the aim of the neurosis by representing the breakdown with symptoms that are objectively intangible is a neurasthenic, but he who constructs the disease into a demonstration is a hysteric, no matter how the utilized mechanisms differ. The war hysteric makes a permanent symptom out of his tremor or the difficulty of hearing due to grenade shock. The environment through too much or too little observation often causes the disease to express itself in one concept. But above all, it is a strong personal need for expression and a more active character with a circumscribed feeling of inferiority in real accomplishments, which decides the "selection of the neurosis" in the sense of hysteria. Whereas in hysteria all affects occur, and quite particularly a strong feeling of self, neurasthenia always has a depressive undertone, which also manifests itself in the symptoms (pains, hypochondriacal feelings and ideas, sensitiveness to the extent of transient ideas of injury). However, one is not so accurate with those distinctions in the presence of the layman. As the name hysteria designates something notorious, whereas "neurasthenia" transforms the defect into something distinctive, the courtesy of the doctor has from the time of *Beard* favored the latter designation in his practice.

Much that is bad has been attributed to the *"Hysterical Character";* prominently mentioned are egoism, lying, vanity, unbridled affectivity, and lasciviousness. What is true in this matter is, that hysteriacs are affective persons, which means that they are occasionally carried away by the excitement of the moment. Furthermore, it may be said that for comprehensible reasons there is a certain inclination to make oneself noticeable in some way, which exists in the hysterical disposition more frequently than elsewhere. As they have to play a part, it is preferably people with a tendency to exaggeration, concealment, and lying that become markedly hysterical; at all events, in hysteria such a disposition is utilized and exaggerated. *For the rest the moral part of the character in hysteria can be good or bad, just as in other people.* Side by side with the most inconsiderate egoists we encounter among hysteriacs people most capable of sacrifice, notwithstanding the fact that a certain impediment to altruistic activity lies in their kind of affectivity. Pseudologia occurs without hysteria, and even more frequently hysteria with pseudologia. Because both have a vivid affectivity, and a peculiarity of the mental process (for the present not describable), and because both represent deviations from the normal, they occur more frequently together than would be the case if it were merely accidental. For fellow beings whom they love, hysteriacs are often capable of much sacrifice. They can, however, also occupy themselves with an abstract humanitarian problem with zeal and success, wherein some, to be sure, go off on a tangent (zoophiliacs). Medically conceived, some saints are typical hysteriacs. If a hysterical woman forges documents in favor of a charitable institution, it is in all probability vanity and not egoism that comes into play. In certain relations *Ziehen* is right when he says that hysteriacs rarely show objective interests. This is especially the case among women, but the hysteriac has still greater need for a *personal* relationship than the normal woman.

The necessary conditions for the Origin of hysteria can perhaps be characterized in the following way, as far as the distinct features are concerned: (1) under given circumstances the patient is not able to realize his strivings on normal paths, (2) a weakness of the health conscience [170] determines the *tendency* to create for oneself a makeshift on the path leading to the disease. (3) The *capacity* to produce for oneself neurotic symptoms, i.e. to produce a stronger development of the *schizoid capacity for splitting* of the personality. This shows itself in the capacity to split off,[171] in the inability to abolish altogether

---

[170] See p. 496.

[171] The difference between the hysterical and schizophrenic splitting cannot be described in brief. We see it in the examination of schizophrenia. In the latter next to the affective splitting there is still a primary or at least a splitting of the associations, which is independent of the affects, and which e.g. may lead to the falsification of simple concepts, which never happens in hysteria. But even the more affective splittings in schizophrenia, which can be comparable to those of hysteria, are more lawless, worse determined, more massive, and

suppressed strivings, and in the coexistence of contrary strivings. Feelings that are not perceived by consciousness can still be utilized by the psyche, in that, e.g., a number called out to the patient but not heard by him may appear as an optical hallucination. In the hysterical twilight state one can write automatically, and even preach. The "untrue" part of the strongly affective expressions, like in that of schizophrenia, probably consists in the fact that split off ideas, which are incompatible with the affect in question, continue to functionate in the psyche and inhibit it to a certain extent, or even alter it. (4) A strongly domineering but labile affectivity, which in a given moment gives the mastery to one single striving and at the same time directs the association of ideas in an abnormally strong manner in its sense. (5) A mild manic temperament with vivid wishes, and the need to assert one's personality.—The difficulty of adjusting oneself to the inner and outer circumstances, and the weakness of the health conscience are at the bases of all neuroses (and of many schizophrenic appearances). The "capacity to create for oneself neurotic symptoms" is a broader concept than that of the capacity to split the psyche. To this belong also memories of former diseases and a physical complaisance,[172] a readily excitable vaso-motor system, conscious and unconscious accidentally acquired connections,, ideas with reflection mechanisms such as secretions, spasms of the smooth muscular tissue, trembling of the voluntary movements, etc. All these possibilities can help to produce neurotic symptoms in general; but only in hysteria (and neurasthenia) does the special splitting capacity play a particularly big part, regardless of its close connection with the other indicated mechanisms. For the formation of hysteria the labile-manic temperament is especially necessary.

Notwithstanding all transitions *Two Groups of Hysteria* can be distinguished quite sharply. In *one it is the disposition,* of which the most important element is the personal need for self-expression; this gives rise to the development of the symptoms. The pronounced hysteriacs in the ordinary sense suffer from this form; they show the "hysterical" or rather "nervous" and labile character also during the times when they are free from symptoms, as well as the marked change in the manifestations, which originate from complexes rather than causes. In reference to the disease, it matters here very little whether one observes today a disturbance of sensibility, or a paralysis, or an

then again not so pure and sharp as in hysteria, so that the worst contradictions can actually exist together in the psyche. The schizophrenic psyche is infinitely more split than the hysteric. A hysteric affect lays claim to the entire conscious psyche; what contradicts it, is totally split off from consciousness.

[172] See pp. 498-499.

attack, or a twilight state. The *second type* is represented by most of the war hysterias. Here the most important factor in the origin is the affective event of the cause which creates a definite symptom. It is mostly produced by the path of *Kretschmer's reflex enforcement* in the widest sense, and by a desire which also needs the capacity to produce a symptom, bring it to the surface, and at the same time give it permanence. The first type occurs especially in women while the second type in men. The forms in which association reflexes (constipation following enemas, blephoraspasm following inflammation of the eyes) are the essential factor, and the aforementioned exaggerated reactions of primitives,[173] I would detach from hysteria, although the transitions to it are very easy.

The *Recognition* of hysteria is given in the discussion above (its differentiation from pseudoneurasthenia is not important). The most important element is the general diagnosis of the neurosis, the psychogenetic reaction form, and the demonstration of the absence of another disease in which the hysterical mechanisms cooperate (schizophrenia, epilepsy, brain diseases, etc.), or of a physical disease which gives cause to hysterical symptoms, as e.g. ulcer of the stomach, or phthisis. In detail one might call attention to the following: The *hysterical attack* is sharply distinguished from the epileptic,[174] if hysteria could not occasionally give rise to a real epileptiform attack in the same way as in the case of affective epilepsy (to be sure, this has not yet been definitely confirmed), or if a hysterical patient could not imitate, consciously or unconsciously, an epileptiform attack, which is naturally quite possible in hospitals. Hysteria does not follow the tonic-clonic phases, nor the temporal limitations of the epileptic attack. The movements may have any kind of character. Injuries occur only if required by the purpose of the disease. Babinski's sign is always absent, rigidity of the pupils almost always. The vaso-motor system rarely cooperates: the pulse remains good; the attack may sometimes be followed by an hysterical sleep but not by an exhaustion.

The strictly systematic acts in the twilight states makes the diagnosis of hysteria very probable, *but it is made definite only after careful exclusion of specific signs of other diseases.* One should especially look for the many prompt reactions of hysteriacs. Wherever the twilight state as such has a purpose, that is, wherever an insanity is played, the relation to the surroundings is unusually characteristic, especially when questioned. The patient acts as if he understood nothing, but under conditions he answers promptly, and even if falsely, the answers

[173] See p. 537.
[174] Comp. the latter.

are none the less definite, whereas in most of the other unclear states the patient must search for the thoughts. Frequently the patient acts as though he does not see the examiner despite his faultless grasp of the environment; one can quite easily notice that he does not *wish* to answer, inasmuch as in spite of the fact that externally he meets one half way, either in a hostile or negativistic behavior, he makes no effort to grasp the questions and to search for an answer.

Like a great many others, I care nothing about the absence of the so-called *stigmata*.

To the experienced physician certain hysterical types often betray themselves with great certainty by little signs which cannot all be enumerated; thus female patients who immediately speak of their suffering with erotic smiles and elaborate the examination into a little scene are regularly hysterical.

For *Prognosis* and *Treatment* see pp. 505 and following.

B. The So-called Neurasthenic Syndrome. Neurasthenia and Pseudoneurasthenia

The name neurasthenia was originally taken literally. In the form of neuroses so designated it was assumed that there was an exhaustion of the nervous system as a result of a long continued exaggerated activity; later the same was also assumed as a result of normal activity in a congenital morbid exhaustibility. However, there are exhaustive diseases; but because they do not represent neuroses in any sense they rarely come to the psychiatrist, not frequently to the neurologist, and even the general practitioner sees them less often than is supposed. *Overexertion and exhaustion certainly are only rarely causes of neuroses, and never of psychoses,* as the war has at last shown to those who did not wish to see it. A general decline of strength is no neurosis. People who toil hardest, who with a few hours of sleep and at that frequently interrupted through attention to the children, regularly do a day's work of 16 or more hours, year in and year out, only exceptionally become neurasthenic. And the (pseudo-) neurasthenics who come to the doctor have in most cases worked less than he. What usually produces the so-called neurasthenia are affective difficulties. These can, however, become enhanced by overexertion; to be sure, one does worse in his vocation when one is exhausted; but these are secondary matters, just as in the case of congenital exhausti- bility of the nervous system with which one wishes to save the concept in the everyday constitutional cases; for as soon as such patients become enthusiastic about any idea they are able to accomplish temporarily or persistently as much or even more than the average man. *Hence neurasthenia is usually a pseudoneurasthenia, and only that name should be used for it, if it were not too long.*

Neurasthenia in the actual sense of the word will be discussed here, only in order to make possible the differentiation of pseudoneurasthenia from this side.

Actual Neurasthenia, Chronic Nervous Exhaustion

Nervous exhaustion included by *Kraepelin* in the *activity neurosis, ponopathies* can naturally manifest itself in various ways, and according to its nature it is also mixed with various symptoms of physical exhaustion. Of neuropsychic manifestations one notes especially frequently the following: increased exhaustibility, difficulty in psychic activity (subjectively a bad memory), moroseness, irritable mood, and a tendency to look upon all possible trivial symptoms as serious diseases. Some of the old *hypochondriacs* are exhaustive neurotics. On the physical side we find: dull pressure in the head up to localized pain, also a feeling of physical weakness, all sorts of paresthesias, a strong fluctuating pulse, poor appetite and imperfect digestion; as a rule, poor sleep; one also notes besides, now this, now that symptom, all of which have been mentioned under pseudoneurasthenia.

If properly treated, it runs a *course* of weeks or months, usually with fluctuations, and ends in recovery. To be sure, relapses are not rare, especially where the causes cannot be removed.

Besides mental and physical exertion, one may also think of insufficient sleep as one of the *causes*, although insufficient sleep may also be the *result* of a true or false neurasthenia; one should also consider the predisposing factors, be they in the constitution, in physical diseases, or in similar disturbances.

The *differential diagnosis* is especially difficult when it is a question of schizophrenia (where, disregarding the actual schizophrenic symptoms, due consideration must be given to the absolute or relative indifference to the future and to the treatment), of cyclothymic depressions, where the exhausted patients are more accessible to soothing words and distractions than depressive cases, of the beginning of paresis, and of latent phthisis.

Treatment: The patient should be removed from the causative relationships; he should take better care of himself (sleep), *but he should not be educated to worrisome self-observation and to continued laziness;* despite the physical genesis of the disease, psychic influence is important (encouragement, and education, eventually with hypnosis). In marked excitement and insomnia moderate doses of bromide

(15 to 45 grains) are excellent, administered every evening. To avoid relapses, the external conditions should be regulated whenever possible; here an improvement of the affective situation is usually as important as the reduction of the work.

The (Pseudo) Neurasthenia

Whereas the just described true neurasthenia with its physical origins, with its preponderating physical manifestations, and its curability by simple care and strengthening no more belongs to the psychoses than a "typhus" in which the psyche participates, pseudo-neurasthenia, on the other hand, with its psychic genesis of the disease itself and of all its symptoms and its purely psychic suggestibility, is as much of a mental disease as hysteria. It is comparatively more frequent than the nervous exhaustion and represents, as mentioned, a definite form of flight into disease, which for itself and others shams (unconsciously) the nervous breakdown, and for that reason shows so much resemblance to the exhaustion. Concerning the special neurasthenic mechanisms one should particularly mention the marked inner conflict in decisions and in work, and to be sure the too early insertion of the exhaustion valve (one feels exhausted even before it is necessary).

The following are its most important *symptoms:* psychic and sensory irritability, fearfulness, inability to concentrate, forgetfulness, persistent and transient states of anxiety, dizziness, insomnia, paræsthesia, topoalgias, headaches, often with pressure in the head, muscular weakness, tremors, occupational cramps, all kinds of digestive disturbances, sometimes also bulimia and polyphagia, constipation, eventually with membranous colitis, pollutions, spermatorrhœa, ejaculatio præcox, impotence, particularly frequent and almost never lacking are cardio-vascular symptoms like abnormal irritability of the heart, tachycardia, congestions, hyperæsthesias, etc. Although not constant, the mood is nevertheless mostly depressive, and the idea of the disease and its symptoms is always of a depressive tone.

Depending on the preponderating symptom complex, it was customary to distinguish psychic, motor, dyspeptic, angioneurotic or cardiac, and sexual forms, to which may be added the etiological group of the traumatic forms; many authors add also the phobias to neurasthenia.

The *causes* were already alluded to in the general observations.[175] The extent of the cooperation of sexual excesses, especially onanism and coitus interruptus, and to what extent that takes place on psychic

[175] See p. 493, etc.

paths, is not yet quite clear. To be sure, depleting diseases can on the one hand instigate the flight into the disease, and on the other hand it can indicate the sensations, the exaggeration of which may evince the actual morbid picture.

In the *diagnosis* it is necessary in the first place to exclude a physical disease; here one should think also of tuberculosis, lues, and poisons like CO, which produce similar pictures. Paresis and schizophrenia should also be excluded. The depressive phase of cyclothymia is mistaken by many for neurasthenia. The man who makes many notes, who is always afraid that he did not tell the doctor enough, or that his reports were too incorrect, is mostly a neurasthenic; for the disease would have no sense if it were not important.

The *prognoses* are very different; they depend on the individual's disposition and on the possibility of removing the outer and inner difficulties even after the treatment is over. The "constitutional" forms, who were incapable from youth to adapt themselves to reality, naturally present a difficult prognosis; others who did not know how to help themselves for the time only can be permanently cured by a few suggestions, or encouragement, eventually through the explanation that their fear of the results of onanism are unfounded.

The *treatment* does not differ in principle from hysteria, although "tonic" measure may here exert a somewhat better suggestive force, and in mixed forms with real exhaustion may have a direct causal effect.[176]

C. The Expectation Neurosis

Following one or many bad experiences in any kind of event (reading, writing, swallowing, urinating, after having been dazzled by a strong light, or surprised through a loud noise, etc., into infinity),[177] the patient predisposed in this sense becomes dominated by the idea that he can no longer accomplish the function in question, or that he must suffer pain through it, and this idea becomes a reality. This results in paralysis of a definite complex of movement, cramplike additional movements, or painful paræsthesias. Besides speech stuttering which under conditions should be included in this category, one notes a number of other forms of "stuttering" (stuttering in walking, writing, urinating, etc.) ; psychic impotence naturally also belongs here, likewise *Moebius's* akinesia algera. I would also add to it the numerous gastric

[176] See p. 506.
[177] The expectation neurosis can also be a relique of a physical disease, e.g. an organic paralysis of deglutition.

neuroses, where the patient cannot tolerate certain foods and avoids them until his menu card becomes reduced to an intolerable minimum or to the point of starvation, and then finally through energetic advice he allows himself to be convinced that he can eat everything—as a rule with good success. Unfortunately it is not rare to find an expectation neurosis as a result of a pessimistic statement of the doctor.

The expectation neurosis usually develops slower than the *traumatic neurosis*, to which it shows a certain resemblance, and also cannot be sharply differentiated from many hysterical syndromes. However, there are characteristic developments; thus, for example, the stuttering in walking in contrast to the hysterical abasia: the expectant neurotic can still make an effort to walk, but he then becomes lame or gets pain, whereas the abasic patient is altogether incapable of attempting to walk. Moreover, the expectation neurosis has a "monosymptomatic circumscription," which also expresses itself in the frequent return to full normality after the syndrome is cured. Sometimes it is also difficult to differentiate it from certain phobias, at the roots of which disagreeable experiences are not seldom revealed.

As a syndrome the expectation complex may appear in any other neurosis and also in psychoses; indeed, in schizophrenia it can dominate the picture for decades; in the latter case, to be sure, there is more than one expectation symptom.

Left to itself or in improper treatment the suffering usually becomes aggravated and continues indefinitely. But once the diagnosis is definitely made, it is possible to bring about a cure in a few weeks or months through a definitely laid out *psychic treatment* such as enlightenment, calming, and reeducating. Even in schizophrenia a cure (of the syndrome) is not excluded, although it is rare.

D. The Compulsion Neurosis

The common diagnostic sign of compulsion neurosis, according to *Kraepelin*, is a vivid feeling of domination or fear indicated by ideas that obtrude themselves. At the same time the incorrectness of the content is usually recognized.

In the *compulsive ideas* any kind of idea obtrudes itself; it may be a musical motive, the idea of a funny face, a ghost's hand, an odor, a voice, of which one cannot rid himself. It frequently concerns disagreeable things: something disgusting, immodest processes, blasphemous utterances, or it may be in the form of *questions* (questioning mania, reasoning mania). The content of the questions may be indifferent, e.g. how the furniture of a room was arranged, why a table is rectangular, what is the date of newspaper lying in the street; other questions concern the creation, infinity, God, the Virgin Mary; then also all sorts of sexual problems. Some compulsive ideas force themselves into some sort of action, as in the case of the *arithmomanias*, the obsession to count everything possible, or to make calculations with any number that presents itself.

The *obsessive fears (phobias)* concern some threatening misfortune, such as the fear of being struck by lightning (*Kerauno-phobia*), of being robbed, of being attacked by an animal, of meeting with an accident while riding, of injuring oneself and others with a sharp object which happens to be near (*aichmophobia*), of being killed by some object falling from above, of contaminating oneself with dirt, bacteria, bichloride of mercury and thus make oneself and others sick. Precisely those thoughts which are especially terrifying to the patient come up most often; thus one observes blasphemous ideas in the religious, and murders in the chicken hearted, etc.

Kraepelin also includes here the somewhat peculiarly appearing phobias of space, *claustro-, nyctophobia*, fear of traveling, and fear of tunnels.

The fear of responsibility expresses itself in the compulsion to examine repeatedly whether a match thrown away no longer burns, whether the doors of closets are locked, whether letters are sealed, or whether no mistake was made in the calculation (doubting mania, *folie du doute*). Other patients are obsessed with the idea that they must always be particularly careful not to overlook anything; they might e.g. hear some one calling for help. Others fear lest they should forget names and are thus constantly compelled to think of them and repeat them (*onomatomania*). Others are afraid of their working tools, or entertain some fear of beginning their work (*aboulie professionelle*).

The fear of guilt usually consists in the fact that the patient imagines that he might do or has done something wrong or clumsy; this is not only accomplished deliberately through commission or omission, but the patients also fear that they might destroy their beloved ones through a thought ("omnipotence of thought," which shows a predilection for the compulsion neuroses). Then there are phobias that the patient must hang himself on a certain hook or that he must steal. In the phobias of contact with people (*homilophobia*) the patient fears e.g. that people direct their attention to him; here belong the examination fears, the phobias connected with clothes and the fear of blushing (*ereuthrophobia*); a teacher had the phobia that the children would see the slit of his pants.

The patient usually reacts very strongly to these phobias; in part, by avoiding all opportunities of coming in conflict with the fear, and by acting in the sense of the phobia. Thus when there is a phobia of bacteria, they constantly wash their hands, and touch nothing that anybody else might have touched. In aichmophobia they look everywhere for needles, they open their letters thirty times in order to see whether one is not wrongly addressed, they cross the threshold twenty times forward and backward, and similar acts. One of *Kraepelin's* patients was compelled to mow the same place 73 times in succession. Others have definite defense movements and magic-like protective formulæ, which they must utilize on all such occasions.

The primary *obsessive impulses,* in so far as they lead to action, are more rare; *Kraepelin* believes that, principally, they are something different, for it is usually a question of fearing that one could do something. Still there is no doubt that obsessive impulses sometimes occur with action, even outside of dementia præcox. Many add here also the *maladie des tics, coprolalia, echokinesis, miryachit,* and other phenomena.

It is the *anxiety* which in all cases drives the patients to actions or to omit actions. Frequently the patients can somewhat control the obsessions, but they are then afraid of the anxiety (*phobophobia*).

How closely doubt and impulse are connected is shown by the following example: Already when in college the patient had the *impulse* to tell any one of his teachers that he is an ass or to write it on paper; later he had the impulse to set fire to the curtains and the provisions in his business, to embrace every feminine person, to stick a pointed instrument into every bald head, and to put glass into the pans. At the same time he had *doubts* whether he had already performed this nonsense; he had to pick up all pieces of paper in the street to see whether he had not written anything against the honor of others; he was to go to the stores to see whether he had not set fire to them, etc. He began to study medicine, but the thought obtruded itself that all patients could be well by the time he will have passed his examination, and he would then have to starve (he had an income). He changed to the study of theology and then he feared that he could perhaps show his tongue from the pulpit. Dozens of such ideas prevented him from becoming something, although he finally began to study law.

As a rule, the patients recognize the incorrectness or the nonsense of the obsession, and struggle *against* it, whereas the delusional patient struggles *with* his idea; still despite this insight there is some sort of belief; it is something like the man who "in daylight mocks at ghosts but is not desirous of hearing about them at night." At the height of the affect they may merge for a short period into an indisputable delusion.

Besides these obsessive forms, the special enumeration of which could be immeasurably increased, one also speaks of obsessive affects, obsessive inhibitions, obsessive feelings, obsessive hallucinations and similar phenomena. I do not quite know what there is tangible about it to understand.

The compulsive neurotics are mostly individuals of little energy who feel timid, and not sure of themselves, but they are diligent and conscientious people. The mood shows a tendency to depression and fearfulness. The *intelligence* is strikingly often above the normal.

The *physical* symptoms of compulsion neurosis are of all possible nervous and vasomotor manifestations; there are also hysteroid disturbances.

The *course* of compulsion neurosis is a very dragging one. Fluctuations in intensity can occur, the content can change, while the fear remains the same. Still the picture on the whole is very monotonous.

The *beginning* of the disease may already be indicated in childhood, very often at puberty; in the majority of cases it occurs before the age of 25 years. Sometimes it can be dated from a definitive event, something like forced washing by sympathetic instructors, or religious scruples at the first communion. At the period of involution a gradual improvement usually occurs up to a kind of recovery.

The first *cause* is the hereditary neurotic disposition which frequently manifests itself in the family in a similar way. As to its distribution among the sexes, the statements in reference to men fluctuate from 29 (*Janet*) to 60% (*Kraepelin*).

The psychic mechanism and with it the precipitating causes are still insufficiently known. One was always struck by the connection with sexuality, and *Freud* would trace all cases to sexual complexes. In any case affects from the original initial idea are often here transferred to other ideas. *Frank* [178] has also demonstrated that repressed affects may assume compulsive significance through new and similar experiences.

The compulsive syndromes occur in the most varied dispositions and diseases, especially in neurasthenia, manic depressive insanity, and dementia præcox, but *only when they seem to have originated independently on a psychopathic basis does one call the picture compulsion*

---

[178] Affektstörüngen, Studien über ihre Atiologie und Therapie. Springer, Berlin, 1913.

neurosis.[179]　Corresponding to its genesis, it is often mixed with all kinds of other nervous and hysterical symptoms.

Outcome. In true cases of compulsive neurosis a cure is not easily attained. Patient education, mental gymnastics following *Oppenheim,* or *Dubois's* persuasion are supposed to have some success. I have seen some complete cures, at least from the practical side, by psychoanalysis (following *Frank*). It is a striking fact that "independent" compulsion neurosis is seen only in people who can permit themselves that disease, and that the symptoms always go only so far as the circumstances (and the doctors) permit; moreover, in the war, where it was disregarded, it is said to have disappeared. *Kraepelin* justly warns against tearing away these timid patients, lacking in energy, for an unnecessary long period from their vocations. They should better be accustomed to work and activity and trained to be energetic.

E.　The Accident Neuroses

The psychic disturbances which originate directly from brain injuries are organically determined diseases with local and general symptoms. The latter include especially marked irritability, intolerance to alcohol, and from mild to severe epileptoid moodiness and mental unclearness; in addition there are more or less localized headaches and other paræsthesias. These diseases are naturally not traumatic *neuroses.*[180]

By the latter name one understands diseases which psychically originate [181] through the excitement of the accident or otherwise as a result of the same, but they can naturally become connected with direct traumatic or toxic influence (carbon monoxide, in explosions). From the outwardly different forms *Kraepelin* has emphasized four pictures which designate the most important directions of the causation and with it also the symptomatology; to be sure, they cannot be sharply distinguished.

(a) The *fright* neurosis. This name the author now still uses only for the pathological reactions to the experience of a profound catas-

---

[179] The typical cases have so much about them that is schizophrenic in appearance and heredity, that one cannot suppress the suspicion that they are actual schizophrenics whose symptomatology exhausts itself in compulsive syndrome.

[180] See p. 240.

[181] Some, especially *Oppenheim,* assume for at least many cases a more physical basis, some molecular change of the nervous system through a physical or psychic "concussion," resulting from an extremely strong stimulus, indeed one even speaks of *traumatic reflex paralysis.* Following the war experiences these things are quite secondary.

trophe (earthquake, mining accident).[182] Besides stuporous inhibitions there come about various grades and kinds of disturbances of consciousness with excitements. Orientation becomes disturbed; in mild cases one observes distractibility, forgetfulness, and marked fatigue; in severer cases it may come to delirious states of an unclear character, often with quite senseless acts. Sleep is poor as a rule and disturbed by terrifying dreams. Palpitation and all the other signs of vasomotor lability, furthermore trembling and dizziness, complete the picture and usually continue longer than the delirious states. The latter last from hours to at most a few weeks; but even more chronic symptoms are wont to disappear regularly in a few months at the latest. For the period of the strongest excitement there is an amnesia in most cases. Under certain conditions the most profound fright is supposedly capable of producing a direct lethal effect.

The difference from hysteria consists in the fact that the morbid manifestations represent here only a strongly exaggerated but qualitatively normal reaction to a frightful experience, whereas hysteria produces its own symptoms. The hysteric has a reason for being sick and for showing quite definite symptoms, while the fright neurotic has not; that accounts for the qualitative difference and particularly also for the indefinite long duration of the hysterical reactions.

Recoveries of fright neurotics come as a result of time and rest, and calming measures, also raising of self-confidence, and similar means.

Concerning the *pseudo-dementia* following an accident see p. 545.

(b) Most of the psychiatrical accident cases of peace practice show the picture of *traumatic neurosis* [183] which *Kraepelin* characterizes as "a depressive or morose moodiness with woefulness, weakness of will, and all sorts of physical morbid manifestation partly of a general nervous nature, and partly local." The patients regularly complain of difficulty in thinking and of poor memory; but by objective examination the disturbance cannot be demonstrated, although thinking is retarded, and if the patients are put to mental or physical strains, even of only a mild degree, unbearable added manifestations rapidly show themselves, which in part are also otherwise present. The symptoms are as follows: pains, especially in the head, but also elsewhere, and palpitation with an objectively rapid pulse. Thus efforts to work are feared and at least as long as the patients are under observation all movements are restricted if possible, so that the patients sit around

---

[182] *Stierlin.* Uber psycho-neuropathische Folgezustände bei den Uberlebenden der Katastrophe von Courrières am 10 März 1906. Diss. Zürich 1909 oder Monatschrift f. Psych. u. Neur. Bd. XXV.

[183] The expression is unfortunately also used for "fright neurosis" and by *Hamburger* also for psychogenic pavor nocturnus.

more inactively, they walk only slowly, not only avoiding exertions but also firm attitudes and all excitement. Besides the army of vaso-motor disturbances, including dermographia and dizziness, the severer cases are regularly tortured also by an objectively demonstrable insomnia.

Tests in continuous arithmetic, especially those done in *Kraepelin's* laboratory, show that a true increase of fatigue (in contradistinction to organic brain disturbances) does not exist, but that a greater part of the behavior is explainable through a lessened effort of the will. The same shows itself also in registering motor activities.

For the further multiform symptomatology we must refer to the textbooks on accident diseases.

The traumatic neurosis is wont in most cases to drag on for quite a long time, or it may even be incurable, unless a satisfactory settle-ment, possibly in one sum, puts an end to the misery.

(c) *The Damage Suit Litigants.* In some individuals who suffered injuries through accident, the struggle for an income becomes active. Not only do they imagine themselves wretched, but they also con-sider themselves unjustly treated and defend themselves against it, as well as by exaggerations and falsifications, as by non-recognition of the court's decisions and by incessant appeals, in which finally libels and threats are not lacking.

The·damage suit litigant is probably incurable as long as an award in his favor is to be obtained, and when the litigation has continued a long time the prospects are probably rarely bettered through settle-ment in the paranoid character of these patients. The more important therefore is the prophylaxis.

(d) *Traumatic hysteria* can be described together with the ordi-nary hysteria; some peculiarities which correspond with the origin are not important in principle.

Conception of the Accident Neurosis. With the exception of the fright neurosis these diseases mainly originate from the "struggle for damages." The fear of the front (in war) has (consciously or uncon-sciously) a similar significance. In the accident neurosis in peace time the anxious idea to be sick and incapable of earning a living is in the foreground, which could in a measure be compensated by an award (or settlement sum): "If I should become well the compensation would be gone; the disease may also return, for it is so bad." Hence the constant care of oneself and the avoidance of every effort to regain the capacity for work. Through anxious expectation certain groups of paresthesias can then be produced with relative ease; among those are especially headaches, cardiac symptoms, and sleeplessness. The anxious avoidance of all exertion of will leads to a lack of energy and hindrances in thinking, so that the relatively uniform structure of the morbid picture in the principal components can be easily understood. In the damage suit litigants the desirous ideas are in the foreground; such people were happy to have met with "their accident" and now the deserved fortune is kept from them. This explains the reaction.

The enormous mass experiment of the war has furnished corroboration of this conception in the most striking manner for those who still had any need for it. It was known, even before, that without a "morbid gain" even a trauma produced no neurosis; that even injuries like a fracture conditioned a longer working incapacity in pension receivers than in others, but where no pensions rewarded the lasting disease (in the case of different laws, in the non-insured, in elemental catastrophies, in duel and sport injuires), there was never anything of a traumatic neurosis to be seen, and that where a monetary settlement was customary, the disease continued only until the money was received. In the war, therefore, where there was not only the prospect of a pension, but also of freedom from the horrors of the front, an enormous amount of material was observed, in whom the severer injuries produced no neurosis, although that alone was sufficient to incapacitate from service and furnish a pension, and that prisoners of war, with few exceptions that could easily be explained, remained free from neuroses. Significant are also the cures (and eventual relapses) through suggestive influences.[184]

To be sure, there are still other motives for a traumatic neurosis besides pension and fear of the front, but for some reasons they recede into the background in the present laws. All those morbid gains which produce the neurosis may sometimes also become active here; the injured may have a special interest in showing what a misfortune was produced by him who was the cause of the injury, etc.

In the damage suit hysteria we must have in mind still other determining cases besides the desirous ideas, be it a permanent disposition to hysterical expressions, be it in the factor at the basis of the kind of trauma, as, for example, fear producing a tendency to tremors.

But all three forms must be afraid to work because their income will be thereby diminished. This is so constant that a traumatic neurotic who makes an earnest effort to resume work and accomplish as much as circumstances permit must always arouse the suspicion that it is a question of an organic disturbance, or at least of a complication of the neuroses with some other malady, especially a brain injury.

[184] Comp. *Naegeli*, Unfalls- und Begehrungsneurosen. Stuttgart Enke 1917.

The statistics concerning the *frequency* of the accident neuroses give very different numbers. They may appear in perhaps from 1 to 2% of all damage suit accidents. With the kind of injury they have little connection, although traumas which affect the head will for conceivable reason preferably settle there. An essential cause lies in the disposition, which causes certain people to give up their own exertion, in order to live as parasites; frequently it is the environment, which systematically nurtures the desirous ideas, especially the wife.[185]

Unfortunately the chief cause of the disease is frequently the unskilfulness of the doctor, especially at the beginning of the treatment. If instead of supporting with all means the positive suggestion, the doctor pities these people, making the patients and himself important; if he considers the consequences as serious and prognosticates a long duration; if he "treats" too much, voluntarily advising against work, and indicates that serious consequences may first follow later, etc., then it is not to be wondered at when there is an outbreak of the "iatrogenous" neurosis or psychosis. Warning must be sounded against the not nearly limited advice, "to be careful of oneself," which sometimes defers the cure for a long time also in other diseases. If care is needed, it should be given in as accurate doses as any other remedy.

A worse effect is produced by the insurance societies and their investigators, who do not desist from worrying and irritating the insured patients; they exact foolish conditions, like the one that the patient must not work as long as he draws compensations. On the contrary, it is good if these people can *through work* add a little to their incomes and even earn a little more than in healthy days. Frequently the injured are first driven into the disease by unnecessary litigations for the rightful compensation. A possibly rapid, definite, and somewhat noble settlement will usually prevent the neurosis; the same may be accomplished by the opposite way, namely, the indisputable non-recognition of the right to compensation. Psychologically these two latter methods are naturally identical, for they both destroy the desirous concepts of the neurosis.

Although the pathology of traumatic neurosis is clear, it is not at all simple in individual cases to make the diagnosis, to decide upon the expert testimony, and the therapy. The insurance laws, the influence of good and bad advisors, as well as some other things, very strongly complicate the state of affairs. It is the duty of every physician to orient himself through special textbooks and courses concerning all these relations.

In cases where after definite regulation of the claims the will to

[185] Comp. the characteristic fairy tale of the fisherman and his wife.

work does not spontaneously remove the still existing hindrances, it requires skilful management to lead the patient back to work. It may e.g. be well to advise the patient to take up first some new occupation— as something lighter. If after this long idleness he is then unable to accomplish as much as those who are practiced in this work, and if he still tires rapidly, it is quite clear even to himself, and leaves no depressing effect, and the demand for the work, which he understands best, then comes without any further interference.

XIII. THE PSYCHOPATHIES

The psychic deviations from the normal which do not give the impression of pronounced insanities, which are based as a rule on heredity, but occasionally also on a former mild brain disease, are designated by various names, but are always vaguely differentiated. They are spoken of as degenerates,[186] constitutional cases, original anomalies, psychopathics, abnormal characters, etc. *The affective peculiarities are in the foreground in most cases. Even if there is an average or great intelligence, it has little regulating influence on the actions.*

We have here to deal with deviations from the normal in all possible directions and mixtures. *Hence psychopathy is only in so far a uniform concept as it embraces psychic deviations from the normal that are not limited in any other way; but it is always incorrect to say that "the psychopaths" have this or that quality.* According to the nature of the thing, they cannot have any definite limitations and no symptoms that are common to all. Every individual is really again something special. Nevertheless certain principal features and correlations frequently repeat themselves, so that for the purpose of the discussion some types can be particularly emphasized without doing too great violence to reality. But one must be quite clear *that it involves only artificially differentiated pictures, and that next to these pictures and between them there exists in reality an infinite shading of variations, transitions, and combinations.*

From what degree of the intensity and the grouping of the symptoms one wishes to designate the psychopath as sick is arbitrary, and from what degree one no longer wishes to consider him as a psychopath, but as insane, is not seldom the same. **Many psychopaths are really only in the social sense "not insane"; before the forum of**

---

[186] We avoid the name and concept of "degeneration"; comp. p. 201. A part of what is so called was recently brought into connection by *Naegeli* with the more fruitful concept of *mutation*.

natural science they suffer from the same anomalies as many insane, only in slighter degree; they are paranoid, schizoid, latent epileptics, cyclothymic, etc.

A great many of them do not really come to the doctor on account of their constitution, but on account of the false reactions conditioned by it, which frequently assume the form of ordinary neurotic symptoms, but still more frequently any other kind of irregularities which have not yet been emphasized. Some are really inseparably mixed morbid pictures of congenital and reactive anomalies. This is true of most of the sexual aberrations, which are false attitudes on an abnormal disposition, wherein now the one, now the other factor predominates.

Of the endless varieties we can here give an indication of only few types, in which limitation I adhere to *Kraepelin,* without, however, adopting strictly his classification of *original morbid states and psychopathic personalities.*

Kraepelin conceives the psychopathies as circumscribed inhibitions of development, which he puts in contrast with the general inhibitions (oligophrenias). Although such disturbances certainly exist, and the development in later age blurs some of these symptoms of the disease, the theory is probably premature and in any case does not embrace the entire group. In all domesticated creatures there are many, and all sided deviations from the normal, and certainly also in human beings; it is therefore probable that the majority of the psychopaths belong to this class of deviation. Besides, much too much may be explained through infantilism, and above all, the concept of the evolutional inhibition is still quite unclear as soon as one wishes to apply it to the facts, and in relations simpler than those of psychiatry it is really only rarely of use. These are only a few indications of objections to this theory.

The treatment of the psychopathies is not a very grateful task, for one cannot naturally change them; one must try to get along with them. At all events, excitable patients can be educated up to a certain degree of control and especially to a prophylactic avoidance of situations that are dangerous for them, and under favorable conditions fairly tolerable situations may be attainable for some. Rules can hardly be given, for the individual as such and the peculiarities of the environments must determine the behavior. It is quite obvious that unnecessary excitement should be kept away from such people, but they must absolutely know and feel that there is a limit to the tolerance of their excesses when carried to a certain degree, and that a transgression will automatically bring its counter measures whereby neither excuses nor subterfuges, in fact, no discussions whatever, will be permitted. It is usually best to ignore the smaller things, even if in cases where an actual education is not impossible it is sometimes very useful to start from little things; in any case, a neglect of consequences will always have to be reckoned with. As everywhere else it is particularly important to create an interest, an aim, for which the patients could strive, whereby definite traits of character, even if no virtues in themselves, such as vanity and pride, should often be made use of unreservedly, but should be developed within proper bounds. If the patient shows a hopeless apathy towards useful occupation, he can perhaps be interested in sport, art, in some scientific hobby, or in something similar; at the same time real work must never be neglected. In most cases it is impossible to educate the patients in the milieu in which they grew up; they must be taken elsewhere. But we have not as yet enough people who have the will and the necessary skill to assume this task, be it in a sanatorium together with others, which is not dangerous only if "the others" are not also moral defects, or in a private family. The closed institution can in some regards accomplish much more than the open one; it is used much too little. Some of the moral idiots are treated by the penal code, but this is neither to the advantage of the patient nor to society. But our views and laws and arrangements do not as yet permit any proper treatment of so many cases who could otherwise be well managed.

However, in many cases one should follow the important rule, to do that which is necessary, or promises some results, and not that which might induce feelings of revenge, coddling, or useless sympathy.

A. NERVOSITY

Under nervosity *Kraepelin* understands a "permanent injury to life's work as a result of an inadequate predisposition in the spheres of activity of the emotions and will. It is, on the one hand, mainly a question of a defect in the ability to resist emotional influences, and, on the other hand, of an insufficient power of will. This is regularly associated with a lack of equanimity in the development of the entire psychic personality." The development of intellect is frequently good, or very good.

The chief disturbance is in the sphere of affectivity; the patients react stronger to inner as well as to outer influences. "Everything gets on their nerves"; they are easily worried, or also easily pleased. It is, especially on this account that the unfreedom of the will originates. "They lack the trustworthy guide through a firmly formed channel."

In addition, one observes a progressive *fatigue* which does not at all seem to show itself in all positions. Some inspiration or any other favorable affective state can often keep away the fatigue for a long time, so that in some cases it must be questioned whether the heightened fatigue is not to be regarded as an emotional effect rather than a constitutional anomaly.

Thus the *capacity to work* is irregular and on the whole considerably diminished; nevertheless the patients are usually inclined to overestimate themselves.

The *memory* is often unreliable and uneven. The *phantasy* readily gets the best of the ideas relating to reality. *Sexuality* plays a particularly big rôle.

These conditions naturally show no barriers to either healthfulness or neuroses. *Moreover the prodromata of quite different mental diseases, especially paresis and schizophrenia, resemble these nervous manifestations, often to the extent of being mistaken for them.* In all cases one must therefore also think of these psychoses and exclude them through the anamnesis and the absence of their specific symptoms.

Besides these general persistent manifestations there are also many quite morbid features, idiosyncrasies, nervous dyspepsia, insomnia, hysterical signs, and similar symptoms.

Course: In most cases the disease usually shows itself already in childhood, frequently reaching its height in youth, but in many cases it shows later a gradual decline.

In his classification *Kraepelin* finds 65% men, probably because such anomalies disturb a woman less in her usual callings, and consequently the physician sees less of her, or because she is designated as hysterical.

Naturally the *treatment* is essentially a psychic training; at the same time the external conditions should be regulated as much as possible. Among medications bromide should be mentioned, which, in a great many attacks of moodiness and (apparently) exhaustions and irritating weaknesses, frequently gives quite good results after a few doses as well as after prolonged use.

B. The Aberrations of the Sexual Impulse [187]

Among the sexual aberrations *onanism* is so common that it is a controversy to what extent it is really abnormal. At all events it is considered morbid if it appears in early childhood (under certain conditions it comes spontaneously,[188] already during the first year), or

---

[187] Krafft-Ebing, Psychopathia Sexualis. Stuttgart, Enke, 14 Ed. 1912. English Translation of the Tenth German Edition, Samuel Login, N. Y., 1908.

[188] Not so rarely servant girls criminally stimulate the genitals of the little ones entrusted to them, in order to calm them or to gratify their own sex pleasures and thus habituate even normal children to onanism.

when it is practiced excessively, and when it is used as a substitute for the normal sexual relation not only on account of moral but also for other reasons ("onanism of necessity"). Moreover it accompanies regularly also the actual sexual abnormalities. It is not only performed through the excitation of the sexual parts but under conditions through a mere activity of the phantasy which leads to the orgasm ("psychic onanism").

Naturally onanism easily becomes harmful, because it gives every opportunity to excesses, because it deflects from the normal sexual aim, and above all because the feeling of guilt and the constant unsuccessful struggle against the "vice" consumes the psychic power, diminishes self-confidence, and gives cause for hypochondriacal and neurotic symptoms often of the severest kind.[189]

In the *treatment* of onanism, severe punishments, long sermons, and mechanical restraints are mostly harmful, and perhaps never useful, whereas diversion through play and work, arousing of other interests, and a healthy conviction of natural attachments have often made one' forget the bad habit relatively easily. If transient states of sexual excitation are at the basis of the onanism, e.g. in schizophrenia, one can sometimes ease the patient's struggle with daily small doses of bromide.

From onanism must be separated the state of being sexually in love with one's own figure and person, the *narcism*, which *Freud* considers as a normal passing stage of sexual development, and which is supposed to be found at the root of some psychoses and neuroses.

The normal attraction of the other sex can degenerate into a morbid impulse of *exhibitionism*, in which even where there is an opportunity for normal sexual relation, the patients find their true gratification only in exhibiting their genitals (eventually parts of the body otherwise covered) with or without simultaneous onanism. In imbeciles, the exhibitionism not rarely furnishes a substitute for the inacessible coitus. For reasons that are not quite obvious it frequently occurs in organic mental diseases, sometimes in epilepsy in the twilight states.

Fetichism is a pathological exaggeration of the normal transference of erotic feelings to parts of the body and objects of the beloved person (hair, "braid-cutters," pieces of clothing, especially shoes). The objects in question are not always acquired in a legal manner but are often needlessly stolen simply because the theft seemingly contributes to the sexual gratification. They are said to stimulate sometimes by looking at them, but in most cases they are brought into contact with the genitals and used for onanism. Normal coitus is usually not desired; some, however, use the fetich to make themselves potent.

[189] Comp. p. 209.

Voyeurs find their gratification in watching coitus in others, the *Renifleurs* by inhaling the odor of urine and the *Coprolagnists* through intimate contact or even through swallowing of excrements.

Another form of displacement in the object is *pedophilia*, or the desire for relations with children of the opposite sex, which occurs perhaps most frequently as an acquired anomaly in senile dementia. (It is not rare also among imbeciles *faute de mieux*).

As *pederasty* one designates at present only the gratification of a man with male individuals through *coitus in ano*. It is less common than the talking about it would lead one to believe.

Sadism [190] is an exaggeration of the erotic pleasure in dominating and torturing which is especially so frequently displayed also by the male in animals. *Masochism* [191] is the caricature of (feminine) yielding and a certain erotic pleasure in suffering pain. The peculiarity becomes pathologic through the fact that it becomes exaggerated and is then no longer a concomitant phenomenon of the erotic act, but an independent aim. Individuals so afflicted find the only or at least the necessary means to gratification in causing, or in suffering, pain. The two abnormities are seldom found isolated; usually they are associated in the same individual even though as a rule one strongly predominates. Sadism and masochism are also designated as *active* and *passive algolagnia*.

The name *sodomy* like that of onanism has displaced its meaning. It now designates exclusively the relation with animals which is not really due to morbid alteration of the impulse but is regularly practiced *faute de mieux*, especially by half mature people, lonely shepherds, imbeciles, and also by some feminine persons who live intimately with their dog.

Transvestites feel well only in clothes of the other sex, without being homosexual.

In rare cases the sexual aberrations, as well as the force of the impulse, show a *periodic character* in so far as they appear from time to time, but usually only for a few days and then again make room for the normal (or sexually weak) behavior. More frequently they appear only under the *effect of alcohol*.

The various kinds of parasexuality are usually connected with a *premature appearance of the sex impulse* and hence can become known very early, frequently at the age of three or four. Most of them are incurable in part simply because such patients, following their feelings, actually consider their form of sexual impulse as the only pleasant one and therefore dread a "cure," as much as a normal person dreads castration.

[190] Named after the Marquis de Sade, a writer afflicted with this disease.
[191] Named after Sacher-Masoch who portrays this anomaly in his novels.

The *theory of sexual aberrations* despite its extensive literature is still quite obscure. The majority of its bearers are also otherwise psychopathic, but in the most varied directions. The moral qualities have no direct connection with the sexual abnormalities; nevertheless the psychiatrist naturally recognizes a selection in which the moral defects dominate.[192]

The *diagnosis* is usually easy. But one must not imagine that every sexually abnormal person himself knows his condition; one must bear in mind that all sorts of mixed and transitional cases may occur and furthermore that the limitation of the normal sexual activity must be stretched pretty far; in this sphere one must not be surprised at anything and consider nothing impossible.

Treatment. In milder cases something can still be accomplished through proper training, eventually through *hypnotism:* But even when the possibility of cures may not be excluded, they cannot be attained in most cases, because the technique is a very rocky one. If such a patient is not married, how shall one gradually initiate him into normal sexual intercourse, without exposing him to new, moral and other dangers? Where something is to be attained through self-control, one does well under all conditions to train the patient to abstain from alcohol, not only on account of the effect on the inhibition of the impulse, but also because alcohol sometimes first permits the perversion to come to the surface.

Special consideration must be given to *homosexuality,* or contrary sexual impulse, or uranism,[193] the sexual love for persons of the same sex.[194] It is gratified in various ways, sometimes through mere companionship or looking at the person, but much more frequently also through all kinds of excitations of the genitals; in contrast to this there is a feeling of indifference or disgust towards contact with the opposite sex. With such people all sexual desires, actions, as well as the day and night phantasies are directed to the same sex. As a matter of fact homosexual love shows the same signs as heterosexual love but shows, particularly frequently something strikingly ecstatic and exalted, and only very exceptionally is it lastingly monogamous, although it is by no means free from manifestations of jealousy.

[192] See below Homosexuality.

[193] From Venus urania; following this terminology *Ulrich* calls the male homosexual "urning," and the female "urninda." The corresponding name for heterosexuals, which is, however, little used, is "Dioning" from Diona, the mother of Venus Pandemos.

[194] *Hirschfeld,* Homosexualität des Mannes und Weibes, Berlin, Marcus, 1914. Cf. also Chap. XI, in Brill's Psychoanalysis, Its Theories and Application, 3d Edit., W. B. Saunders, Philadelphia.

Noticeably frequent the orgasm takes place without friction. Abnormal practices such as cuni-peni anilinctio and other kinds naturally play a greater part here than in heterosexual gratification; *pederasty* (immissio penis in anum) is more frequently rejected with disgust than desired. A mingling with the various other abnormities such as fetichism, sadism, masochism, etc., is not rare. The feeling of shame manifests itself particularly toward the same sex and often in a very exaggerated manner,—an indication how little it is to be separated from the positive impulse. The common existence of an exaggerated sexual demand is only a partial manifestation of the very changeable affectivity, which readily fluctuates between the highest pleasure and deepest pain; on the other hand the aggravation to anger and worry recedes comparatively in contrast to the positive and negative esthetic feeling, which causes delight at the sight of a loop colored in accordance with one's wishes, or makes it "unbearable" to be in a room which is not furnished according to one's taste.

The tertiary psychic and physical sex characteristics of the same sex are often slightly developed or even substituted by those of the other sex.[195] The following are to be noted: An inclination towards the feminine in all possible spheres, in work, decoration (preference for feminine attire), in taste, in thinking, in mimicry, and in gait; in the entire behavior of a large number of urnings it is something common to see a slight indication of the feminine up to a complete imitation of the woman; the reverse can be seen in the urninda. The man with a slightly developed beard, high pitched voice or broad pelvis and the virago are relatively more common among homosexuals than among those of normal sexuality; nevertheless these anomalies of the physical partial manifestations markedly recede in frequency when contrasted with the psychic manifestations. According to *Fleischmann* the latter are found in 24% of his male homosexuals, where he includes apparently very slight deviations from the average. Only in exceptional cases are the genitals abnormally formed.

All homosexual peculiarities show themselves very frequently from the earliest age. The boy likes girls' games, and hangs on his mother's apron strings, and the girl runs around with boys. Early sexual development is quite usual, in which the abnormal direction can as a rule be seen from the beginning.

The *ethical feelings* are just as differently developed as in those who are sexually normal; still, at least in asylum practice one finds comparatively many morally defective urnings next to those of high stand-

[195] "Androgynous" = men with feminine build of body and "Gynandrous" = women with masculine build of body.

ing. That they are on an average especially prone to lying is certainly largely the result of the false position into which they are forced by the general customs and views of human society, which are formed on heterosexual patterns.

Also in the intellectual spheres one observes in these people all nuances; abnormities in all directions are as common as among other psychopaths.

Most homosexuals are neurotic in some manner. Excluding the secondary sex characteristics of the other sex, one does not find physical "stigmata of degeneration" more frequently than in normal people.

Formerly there were disputes as to whether homosexuality is a vice; there is no need of discussing this. Whether it is a disease, belongs to the sphere of foolish questions, especially as long as the concept of disease cannot be limited and it is not known what consequences one should deduct from it.

More important is the investigation, whether it concerns a congenital or an acquired, and hence avoidable disturbance.

In favor of an acquired disease aside from many empty reasons about which one reads [196] are: some other sexual anomalies, especially fetichism, can hardly be explained differently than through an accidental association of one of the first sexual excitements with an unusual object. It is quite natural to assume a similar origin for homosexuality, for at present it is hard to imagine how nature happened to produce so frequently such an anomaly, which seems to contradict the manifoldly confirmed view that the germ glands determine the other sex characteristics.—It is moreover noted that mutual sexual activity takes place in prisons and in all other places where persons of the same sex live alone in close contact more or less deprived of the other sex. There are also schools where homosexuality is considered something more superior than the proletariat service of *Venus vulvigata* and thus seem to have a certain recruiting force.—Psychoanalysts wish to trace the anomaly among other things to a strong attachment for the mother, and as a matter of fact one can sometimes find indications that such patients find it particularly hard to detach themselves from the mother.

All these reasons are in no way valid; none of the modes of origin ever brought forth can hardly even be assumed in a great number of patients, except the attachment to the mother which has not yet been followed up in a sufficiently large material. If it should really be

[196] Here also belongs the hearsay concept concerning the acquisition of pederastic "habits" as a result of sexual oversatiation.

found regularly, it would still not yet prove that it is the cause, for it must also be confirmed somehow, and what is more, according to our present knowledge, in something that we cannot designate as a congenital "disposition." And even if it were certain that fetichism owes its origin to merely accidental occurrences, it still cannot be imaginable without a previously existing foundation, and precisely in homosexuality an analogous explanation will not quite fit, if only because a great number of those who are later sexually normal must have experienced their first sexual stimulations in connection with their own sex (boarding schools!).

If the reasons for the acquisition of the anomaly are quite insufficient, there are, on the contrary, very many weighty indications showing that the essential root of homosexuality lies in the congenital constitution, and what is more not only in the sense that the direction of the sexuality was not firmly established and that an accidental experience determined the false tendency, but in the sense that the homosexual foundation itself forms the constitutional factor. Here we have in the first place the fact that many more urnings carry along signs of the other sex in the physical sphere than would be justified by the assumption of an accidental determinant of sex directions. Moreover on closer inspection the direction of the sexuality can frequently be recognized already during the first or the second year of life, and at all events in the majority of the urnings it is already determined at a time when the sexual feelings in the narrow sense play no big part—according to most patients no part at all. Most urnings are finished products at the third or fourth year at the latest. Moreover one can hardly understand how through the mere feeling to be an urning an inclination should arise to assume in all other relations the customs of the other sex. The urnings have to do with men, and, following what one otherwise sees under pathological conditions, would therefore much rather identify themselves with men and avoid everything feminine, if a primary disposition to feminine behavior would not hinder them in this.

It is also characteristic that homosexuals are sometimes entirely ignorant of their abnormity until they pass pubescence when they become aware of it by accident, while in the acquired sexual aberration as a result of an outer experience the precipitating cause usually remains conscious, and above all nothing can be noticed during the many years of this latency period between cause and effect. How firmly nature determines the direction is shown by considerable experience. Thus most of the homosexuals grow up in an environment which suggests a direction of the impulse contrary to their own and are still not changed by it; whereas heterosexuals, who because of a lack of relationship with women occupy themselves with the same sex for many years, are happy to be able to return to women. If one follows up the families of homosexuals one will, to be sure, find only in about 8% the same heredity, but exceptionally frequently one will observe a special lack of fixation of the sexuality, which in different members takes different abnormal directions, but persists in the individual and very frequently is particularly strong. That some physical abnormity is at play is also proven by the descendants of homosexuality, which according to *Hirschfeld* is for the greater part deeply degenerated in various directions. It should also not be overlooked that according to all we know about the frequency of homosexuality it is not directed by outer circumstances, but is about the same everywhere; according to *Hirschfeld* it fluctuates around 2% of adults. Of course it also occurs among animals but not much can be inferred from this as long as no numerical points of support for the frequency are found. Against this there is another biologic reason, namely, the continual succession from the pure heterosexual to the bisexual and from this to the pure homosexuality through all possible intermediate stages, not only in regard to the direction of the impulse but also in regard to the physical and mental qualities in general, in so far as they are connected with sex. I would not know how the accidental connection of the sexual impulse could produce such equal shading.

That the *theory* is still in sixes and sevens can be gleaned from the discussion itself, and if like many others and especially those who had most experience, I feel inclined to seek the essential factor of homosexuality in the congenital direction of the impulse, it is on the other hand again very clear that in cases of a fluctuating sexual direction accident may have a deciding influence. And such a fluctuation exists; indeed a thorough study of the impulse life of man shows immediately that even the most genuine "Dioning" has his *homosexual components*, and no schizophrenic have I yet studied more accurately without striking against it. (But I cannot agree with Freud and Ferenczi, who maintain that these homosexual components are an essential part of the disposition to schizophrenia,—the heredities of homosexuality and schizophrenia are not related.) For the present therefore the only hypothesis that can be formulated with any probability is that uranism is a biological manifestation. If it is proven that 2% of the people are everywhere burdened by it, then it may perhaps be caused by an hereditary mechanism similar to the one that to 100 women 106 men are born. This could also be reconciled with the remarkable circumstance that homosexuality does not die out despite the fact that it hinders procreation to a high degree. The newest investigations concerning the changes of the physical and psychic sex characteristics by implantation of germinal glands of the other sex in castrated individuals may perhaps throw some light on the subject.[197] It can be imagined, for example, that in the bisexual disposition the germ glands too are hindered by the sex determining causes from choosing between two extremes but that there is a suppression of one factor by another, which is never complete and under circumstances can still change in accordance with the determination of the development of the individual's germinal glands. At all events the sex hormones also exert an influence on the psychic direction of the sexual impulse.

If uranism is a biological manifestation, it is different in principle from the so-called degenerations, which represent a more accidental fluctuation about the normal point. The other psychic anomalies frequently associated with it which we do not differentiate from the usual psychopathic symptoms, form no hindrance to the theory. However, if the theory of the biological nature of the anomaly which is almost only supported by the numerical constancy of the occurrence should not be confirmed, this naturally would not furnish any reason for changing the view concerning the congenital nature of homosexuality.

The *diagnosis* is self-evident in most cases. One must be careful, however, not to mistake for homosexuality an occasional inclination to homosexual acts, and not to classify the bisexual intermediary stages with one or the other extreme.

Treatment in the sense of attempting a cure is possible only in the milder cases, that is, in bisexuals ("pseudo-homosexuals"), who can be educated by hypnotism or psychoanalysis to the extent of resorting to normal activity and even live in happy marriage.

The pronounced cases had to be considered incurable up to the present. Recently, however, *Steinach* cured a case by castration and implantation of another human testicle. Naturally the method is still to be confirmed. Meanwhile the patients must be taught *to resign themselves to their fate.* To know their position and not feel obliged to struggle against it internally is in itself a relief for many. The physician can do even still more in regard to *calming* the patient. In the first place he can do something for the nervous symptoms which are provoked by the difficulty of the situation in general, and espe-

[197] See *Steinach und Lichtenstern,* Umstimmung der Homosexualität durch Austausch der Pubertatsdrüsen. München Mediz. Wochenschrift 1918, **145.**

cially by the struggle with sexuality, the fear of prison, the worry about one's honor and that of the family, etc. Persons of delicate feeling who are especially endowed ethically and religiously reproach themselves severely, which can be reduced to a bearable measure by enlightenment. Besides this, stress must be laid on the psychic treatment of the nervousness in general. Some nervous symptoms seem to come directly from the enforced sexual abstinence (which I do not recognize as a cause of disease in healthy persons). Here too it is in the first place a question of the attitude taken. He who is inclined to assume chastity as something obvious suffers little or not at all. He who strikes his head against the wall, who consumes himself in the internal struggle, who looks for excuses in himself not to remain chaste will naturally be made neurotic by it. In the sense of this reflection the doctor must educate his patient—if he permits himself to be educated.

As to the value of diversion by any occupation that would fill one's life, or by sport, philosophy or art, it is the same as in other neuroses. To be sure, it is more difficult to educate a homosexual to abstinence than the average dioning. For their sexuality is in most cases abnormally excited and their nervous system reacts more strongly. *I know homosexuals who had themselves castrated and are now happy to be released from the struggle and fear of the prison.* Many cannot conceive, however, how one can give up a pleasure of life which the rest of humanity conceives as the highest. In many cases entering a homosexual "relation" signifies in the first place a release from the struggle and the neurosis. But the difficulties hardly ever remain away even if they came only as a result of a desire for change and all sorts of faithlessness. It is also not always easy to slip through the meshes of the law, although according to *Hirschfeld* only one out of 10,000 falls into the hands of the public prosecutor; more, however, get into the clutches of blackmailers. To be sure, some find their satisfaction in relationship with a friend without committing anything punishable. Emigration to other countries where the urning activity is not punished is only rarely to be recommended.[198]

The *punishment* meted out to homosexuals in the United States, Germany, in Austria, and in most of the cantons of Switzerland is to be designated as unjust from a physician's point of view.[199] It is also inconsistent, unworthy, and what I reproach it most with is the fact that it is of no use, but hurts also those who are sexually normal through the prying into sexual relations, and breeds the immeasurably

[198] Concerning the for and against see Hirschfeld.
[199] The same may be said of England and the United States.—Editor's note.

greater evil, namely, blackmailing. The law should only proceed against seduction, the significance of which, in my experience, is highly exaggerated, for in most of the seduced that I have seen there was nothing to spoil.

Naturally the urning is not irresponsible as such, notwithstanding the fact that the normal person frequently defends himself by pleading irresistibility of the sexual impulse. Nevertheless, here where the impulse is not only abnormal in its direction, but in most cases also in quantity, and where a mass of other psychic anomalies cooperate, the limit of responsibility is often permanently or temporarily passed, and mitigating circumstances are therefore always in order in the presence of a misunderstanding law-giver who began with wrong premises.

C. ABNORMAL IRRITABILITY

The irritable types react to influences from without in a very acute and exaggerated manner, which takes the form of attacks of rage lasting mostly a few hours, despair with suicide, anxiety attacks, or also stuporous states. During the attack reflection is altogether inadequate. Some cases are practically in a twilight state; the memory is later markedly clouded; jealousy and alcohol are especially frequent causes for the precipitation of the morbid exaltation.

D. INSTABILITY

The unstable types are distinguished by a lack of persistency of the affective functions accompanied by an exaggerated resoluteness of will as a result of inner and outer momentary influences; they represent persons who are readily changeable by their milieu. Many of them become frivolous criminals. They range from the actively irritable to the apathetic temperaments.

A 24 year old merchant. His father was a good man, but too bombastic, and wasted the family fortune. The mother was irritable, moody, and weak-willed. Her father was fickle-minded and also squandered his fortune; he was a bigamist. The patient himself received an irregular sort of schooling, but was a good scholar; after his father's death he had to be apprenticed in a business house where he purloined a considerable amount of money from the stamp bank. He then got into a reform school, where he did well and because he had a good voice he was also allowed to take singing lessons. Already at puberty he left here and there unpaid bills. A little later he spent more than a year with an aunt whom he could pump in a remarkable manner, so that she had to withdraw into an attic and start again to earn her living by handwork, while he kept for himself a bedroom and parlor and lived very high in general. He was in some business houses and apparently had a number of engagements as an opera singer, but could not remain anywhere, partly, but not always, because he contracted debts with which the police were concerned. One complaint was dropped because he acted more like an irresponsible fellow than a fraud; in some others where he seemed to have obtained money fraudulently it did not even come to court. By presenting to the authorities a forged contract he even deceived the orphanage (at the age of 23 years). Finally he became engaged to a girl also of a somewhat light character, from whom he received big sums, partly under false pretences, partly by other means, in the expenditure of which she sometimes participated. She finally had to bring charges against him. Thus the patient came to be examined. We found a very good intelligence, but a slight moral defect which prevented him from feeling sorry for his bad deeds. *Nevertheless his past life showed that he made repeatedly good resolutions and worked well for short periods in new places, until he was again overcome by temptation, which was usually the case after a few weeks or months.* Outwardly he had an elegant appearance and usually felt sure of himself. But his affectivity showed at the examination an over-hastiness and a marked inability to bridle his will to the demands of the task and hold it at the necessary height until the task was solved. Just as in life, it also showed itself in very simple tests in which he never could concentrate his attention long enough, and never could follow resolutions to the end. In his written work he sometimes began quite well but then lost the thread, or he became unnecessarily brief and stopped without having finished. About his financial matter he was not himself sufficiently informed. Whether he signed a note for 600 or 700 francs he did not notice. Neither he nor his bride could tell with any accuracy how much he got away from her. Even a simple example in arithmetic at first rattled him, although he was good in calculations. When he was forced to throw light on his crime he not only became uncertain and mixed up everything, but quite uselessly he began to lie senselessly and against his own interest. For his fraudulent acts, which are even now considered more in the light of recklessness towards a much too gullible person than as an actual crime, we had to consider him as responsible, but as unfit to take care of his own affairs. This was done with the hope that the firm hand of a guardian might lead him into better paths.

To be sure, instability is not rarely mixed with other anomalies, so also with all grades of moral oligophrenia. Such a case is recognized by the following letter which is given as an illustration to show how deductions can be drawn from written expressions:

Dear Mother:

Am since last Thursday in the hospital for the insane, Burghölzli (Zürich), Ward B. Your loving letter before you left Hinwil was received and it has pleased me very much mother dear to hear that in spite of my foolish pranks you have not given up hope, I thank you very much for it, and I feel sure that better times are in store for us. I am pleased to be up here, the food and attendance is excellent, I can also amuse myself nicely so that time passes very quickly. I hope that I shall soon be allowed to work. As I see from your letter you have a sore foot, I wish you a rapid recovery so that you shall soon be allowed to visit me. The visiting days are Sunday, Tuesday and Friday from 10 to 11. When you come bring along Mr. Huber, I would like to see him again, you know that he expected from me only what is good. Dear mother *send* me next week a package with apples, some chocolate, and some cigarettes, Camels 20 for 25 cents, one is allowed to smoke when one has something to smoke, please don't forget it, let me know how everything is at home. On the way from the station to this place I saw Rosa Meier over on the Pfauen, she saw me too, perhaps she told it to you. I hope dear mother that at least by next Friday you will be able to walk again so that you can come to see me. I always have a good desire for fruit.

In the hope of seeing you and a package, I am with greetings,

Your loving son Arthur.

The style is clear, intelligible, simple, and considering the degree of education very good. The orthography, however, is not so good. This difference usually signifies that the writer is not incapable of learning and understanding, but that he did not have the required zeal at school. The same is shown in Arthur also in other things; thus he does not know the number of the Swiss cantons which one hears so often that even very strong imbeciles can automatically repeat them, but he is well able to recount in succession the cantons through which one has to pass in a certain journey.

The expressions "loving letter" and "dear mother" in the text denote that he is seeking an affective relation with his mother; this is also shown in "I thank you very much for it," and in the mention of the sore foot and in the wish for recovery. To what extent Arthur actually loves and misses his mother cannot be quite definitely concluded from the letter alone; however, one rather gets the impression as if a real emotional relation existed for her, and from his other behavior towards her, we know, that he really still loves his mother in a certain sense.

But how far does this love for his mother, his penitence, and the good resolutions reach? He knows that he has committed foolish acts; he is pleased that his mother did not give up hope in spite of that, he is very grateful to her for it, and he feels sure that better times are in store for both of them. It is important to note here that it does not at all enter his mind that it is up to him to bring about these better times, that he has to work with himself, and that he has to take on a training forced upon him by fate and the asylum; he sees only the pleasant side of things, and that he will later fare better. About this place he has nothing to say except about the excellent food, and that one can amuse himself well. He then gets to his mother's sore foot; he wishes her a rapid recovery but expressly for the purpose that she should be able to visit him; here he does not lack the necessary associations in which he immediately tells her the exact visiting times. But at the same time he would also like another entertainment; he wants Mr. Huber; his mother is not enough for him so he thinks of telling her that this man does not belong to the bad company in which he otherwise "gets." Then he would also like apples, chocolate and cigarettes; but he cannot wait until the mother recovers the use of her foot; she should send him these things and he even underlines the word send. How impatiently he expected this package is shown in the hope he expressed later, that the mother should be able to come next Friday, whereas he expected the package to be sent even before. He would then like to show a bit of interest about things at home, but here all further associations are lacking; he does not inquire about anything special, whereas about the cigarettes he adds the brand and the price. He then feels like telling of a meeting, but only as an occurrence without any reference to his present position, whereas that could have furnished an excellent opportunity to show whether he really was ashamed or not of seeing Rosa Meier who met him on the way from a reform school to a hospital. He then again returns to the hope of his mother's recovery; but expressly only in the connection that she visit him soon, and the visit only in order to furnish him the fruit, and not as a fulfilment of his yearning for his mother. This connection is repeated again in the last sentence and is particularly emphasized, with which the letter as well as its purpose is ended.

From all sides the writer thus returns again and again to the idea of the pleasure. A certain affection towards the mother is expressed, also the recognition that he has actually hurt her by his behavior, and that he will change for the better. But all this has only a passing and secondary significance. The main thing is the pleasure, he thus shows himself more and more changeable in affects, and towards the most important things superficial, without persistence, always returning again to his pleasures. With obliging and grateful mimic, he always asks for something on every visit; now it is for some trifle, now for his discharge. About the main thing, the improvement and the measures and time required for it, that does not enter into his head. As the young man is not without moral feelings, as his misbehavior was due to weakness, and not to direct impulses, and as he is in some ways manageable in the asylum, the prognosis is not yet very bad at his age, but only on condition that he will be confined in the asylum for a long time. Corresponding to his instability, he has until the present never stuck to work without being forced; everywhere he ran away; a certain stability must be forced upon him in part from without, and in part it may be expected by maturing his character which is still somewhat childish.

E. Special Impulses

Among the impulsives *Kraepelin* includes the not quite regular groups of squanderers, wanderers, and dipsomaniacs.

Frequently in spite of good intelligence, the *squanderers* simply cannot at all manage pecuniary matters. Sometimes with great cleverness they contract debt over debt, ruining themselves and frequently many other people with whom they come in contact.

The *wanderers* according to *Kraepelin* are restless people who do not feel contented anywhere; they therefore cannot endure staying in any place and move from place to place. It must be added, however, that the pathologic wandering impulse is neither a uniform disease nor even a uniform syndrome. Besides the types just mentioned there are many others, e.g. the jolly business schemers; furthermore people who find it pleasant in every new place, but who "soon become bored" with it; sensitive types of the most varied categories, who get into trouble everywhere and hence run away; poriomaniacs, who through hysterical, schizophrenic, and epileptic moods and unclear states, are driven into the open.

The *dipsomaniacs*, too, represent no uniform category.[200]

Kraepelin then also adds the *gambling mania* and the *collecting mania* and brings the whole class in relation to affective epilepsy.

---

[200] Comp. p. 351.

F. The Eccentric (Verschrobene)

The psychic life of the eccentrics lacks uniformity and correct judgment. Awry conceptions of relationships, incorrect logical operations, peculiar views and frequently also modes of expression bring them outwardly near to the latent schizophrenics, from whom they cannot yet be easily distinguished, although it is certain that such types can also be based on congenital anomalies. *They are the only representatives of the constitutional aberrations in whom the affectivity is apparently not altogether or preponderatingly disturbed.*

G. Pseudologia Phantastica (Liars and Swindlers) [201]

All the pathologic liars and swindlers suffer from an exaggerated activity of their phantasy with unsteadiness and planlessness of the will. Always in the sense of their high flowing tendencies, vanity in any direction, irritability, ambition, and sexuality, they think themselves so well into fancied positions and rôles that, forgetting the unreality of these structures, they allow their actions to be determined by them. If they have no strong moral feelings at their disposal they must naturally degenerate into panhandlers and swindlers. For conceivable reasons a reenforcement with hysterical symptoms is very frequent but not necessary.[202] It is remarkable that on two occasions I have seen the syndrome appear as a forerunner of actual psychoses (paresis and dementia præcox) in so pronounced a way that for a long time I overlooked the main disease.

Illustration: Henneberg's [203] patient who studied theology and law for some time and also solved a price problem, assumed the title of "Dr. of Jurisprudence," quickly opened many business bureaus, bought a big rapid press, all with money obtained fraudulently. He dictated many fictitious business letters which he did not, however, send out, and wasted much money for theatre tickets, which he gave away as seemingly free tickets.[204]

H. Constitutional Ethical Aberrations

(Enemies of society, antisocial beings, moral oligophrenics, moral idiots, and imbeciles. Moral Insanity.)

Enemies of society, asocial and antisocial beings represent, to be sure, pathologically no uniform class. The inclusive term is only

[201] See pp. 108-9.
[202] See Hysteria.
[203] Zur forensichen und klinischen Beurteilung der Pseudologia phantastica, Charité-Annalen, XXV. Jahrg. 375. Ref. Zentralbl. f. Nervenheilkunde und Psych. 1902, XXV. Jahrg. S. 282.
[204] For further example, see pp. 108-9.

held together by practical and social viewpoints; various predispositions may lead to crime. A good picture of the varieties of criminals
is given to us by Aschaffenburg.[205] The *chance,—affect,—and opportunity criminals* are really not such bad people; they go off the track
under the influence of a situation which they cannot control because
of changeable feelings, lack of reflection, *slight* moral weakness and
similar defects. It is for this reason that *Aschaffenburg* conceives
them as *criminals* of the *moment*. The *chance-criminal* does harm as
a result of carelessness, the *affect criminal* can kill or injure his ad-
versary as a result of just indignation or rude excitement, while the
opportunity criminal may steal from the bank when he finds himself
in any financial distress. The real criminals in increasing degree of
dangerousness commit individual crimes with cold reflection (*pre-
meditated criminals*); the *recidivistic criminal* allows himself to be
drawn into many such acts, but is able, however, to work again in the
intervals with relatively good will and can generally behave quite
honestly. The life of an honest man is altogether incompatible with
that of the *habitual criminal;* nevertheless it is due more to negative
motives that the latter remains a criminal, e.g. distress, when he has
been out of work; but he prefers the not to steal to the not to work.
The *professional criminals* have positive impulses to crimes as such,
which they perform like the violinist his art; they live on crime only.
There are many specialists among them, e.g. the house burglars, the
pickpockets, etc.

It is quite obvious that the first three classes *frequently* show some
lack of morality, while the others lack something of it. However the
ethical defect is not the only, and frequently not even the essential
factor in their aberration; they are just as abnormal in so many other
directions: they may be unstable, weak, labile, irritable, eccentric,
unclear, debilitated, etc.

The degree of dangerousness depends among other things on
whether, and in what degree, the anomalies, especially the moral defects, are associated with positive bad impulses and especially with
activity. The merely heartless person will cause pains to others if
he can gain some advantage thereby; but he who takes pleasure in
the pains of others will make a direct effort to torture his fellow
beings, even if it is of no use to him. One can steal out of sheer laziness and out of a lack of moral feelings, or out of positive pleasure in
gaining a livelihood in this way. In every case all these people in
time take an attitude against society, which defends itself against

[205] Das Verbrechen und seine Bekämpfung II. Aufl. Heidelberg, Winter, 1906.
S. 179.

them by reprisals. Many finally conceive themselves as pioneer fighters for freedom and justice against a hypocritical and violent order of society. *A dread of orderly work* or at least a lack of a persistent capacity for work is common to almost all the various kinds of criminal natures.

The *intelligence* of the antisocial beings is very diverse; it is more frequently bad than good; many of them are more eccentric than stupid. That a lack of moral affectivity will cause difficulties to thinking in ethical spheres is self-evident. There is perhaps a uniform quality which manifests itself as moral impulse and as moral understanding, in the same way as the impulse for music or mathematics is preferably associated with special endowments. A good moral understanding and a good development of social feelings would then have to occur together or be absent together.

The moral defect is as a rule congenital and also inherited, even though as a result of brain injury there may arise not only irritability, but also a certain lack of consideration for others and even a pleasure in teasing. In milder cases the patient may improve somewhat in proper environments, but hardly after the twentieth year. However, one should not forget that in children even repeated criminal acts, quite apart of those caused by the milieu (stealing among the Spartans, or at the command of foster parents) need not always be a sign of a bad development of the moral feeling. Such people who are simply spoiled by the milieu are in a measure still educable.

A great many asocial beings show already in youth the type of mind that they will represent later. A great many of them are backward in school even if the intelligence is good, because they do not adapt themselves sufficiently, and show too little diligence or attention. In rare cases one finds unusual accomplishments in a single direction. Many are lazy, inclined to steal, and to lie, they are cruel to animals and human beings, they are full of demands, and either through intention or neglect they spoil their own belongings and those of others, they are vain, unreliable and egotistic. They cannot yield to authority, and run away when something does not please them; punishments are not feared; as a matter of fact neither cake nor the whip produces any visible effect. In putting through some bad pranks they develop cunning and energy, they rapidly learn from others the bad things, but with difficulty or not at all the good ones, and instinctively seek bad company. A premature sexual impulse in normal or perverse direction is almost always the rule.

How logic becomes weakened in the same sphere with the moral feelings is given by *Hanselman* in a typical example: An apprentice comes home late at night and soils his bed and Sunday suit by vomiting and is reproached for it by his master. He then related it and added impudently: "A master who calls me lousy is no man for me; he has not learned any manners." Here we see at first quite a different estimation (in the main affective, but also intellectual) of his own action and that of the master, then a lack of associations in a manner peculiar to oligophrenia: The patient does not understand that the situation demanded the calling down. The first error gives force to the meaning of the other. As severe as such going off the track seems, yet it does not alone prove the deep antisocial disposition. The suggestion of the environment, the attitude towards society and its organs can in itself produce such logical jumps. (Compare the war attitude of whole nations.)

Many of these children are physically malformed in some way; they show many "stigmata of degeneration."

Aside from the types described in other places as the unclear, unstable, and pseudologs, who often become criminals, there is one group under the various types of asocial and antisocial beings that can in some measure be differentiated. I refer to those in whom the feeling tone of all ideas concerned in the weals and woes of others is stunted (*moral imbeciles*) or is entirely absent (*moral idiots*); both groups together would be designated as *moral oligophrenics*.[206] Sympathy with others, instinctive feelings of the rights of others (not one's own) is absent, or is inadequately developed. At the same time the other kinds of emotional feelings can be perfectly retained, or likewise can only be affected in a certain degree, for the absolutely apathetic, the "unemotional" naturally do not become dangerous criminals. However, the degree of danger varies greatly; it depends on the existence of bad impulses, and the vividness of the activity.

Until now I have never seen moral oligophrenia without finding a qualitatively similar defect in the nearest relatives, mostly in one of the parents, although it is not always easy to show it. Moral defects appearing after brain injuries or in mild schizophrenia have quite a different character.

[206] As *moral insanity Prichard* designated some time ago diseases in which the "moral" factor in the broad sense of the English expression, seemed to be affected. Such patients acted wrongly although no confusion of thought was demonstrable. This included in the first place the submanias (folie raisonnante of the French), then also the obsessive impulses and other diseases. German psychiatry adopted the name in the sense of a defect of the moral feelings. Both the name and the concept have become discredited because they had been manifoldly abused practically and theoretically. The concept should not, however, be dispensed with in psychiatry, because it designates a definite disease; but everybody agrees that a substitute should be found for the name.

Peculiarly enough there are still some people who for doctrinary reasons maintain that there are no such moral defects without intellectual weakness, which must be the basis of the badly developed morality. Well, one can naturally find in every man, and still much easier in one otherwise already in some way defective, some slight deviation from what one calls normal. But such intangible finding actually proves nothing; just as little is proven by the fact that among the criminals who *allow themselves to be caught* one finds a great many moral defectives. It is quite certain that the moral state has no relation to the height of intelligence, that there are intellectual oligophrenics with a well developed moral sense, and that one meets moral idiots in whom one can demonstrate neither any other kind of pathologic disposition, nor a mental disease, nor any explainable intelligence defect; but one must not look for the latter in prisons only.

Moral idiots form the neucleus of *Lombroso's* concept of the "born criminal." The latter embraces, however, in unclear association also other criminal natures, e.g. the excitables and unclear ruffian or people with epileptoid characters. The author has moreover asserted many strange theories, like that of the *"reo nato,"* who is a sort of latent epileptic, atavistic, and like the child. But only a small part of the born criminals in any way resemble epilepsy; about atavism in man we know nothing, and it is absolutely false to confuse the tendency of a murderer with that of a primitive warrior, that of the thief with that of the normal from an environment which has another sense of property. Nor is it true that the born criminal is like the child. The normal child has altruistic feelings as soon as it can express itself in this direction; the only thing it does not understand sufficiently is the complication of the relations, so that the feeling tone must be absent in some situations where it would manifest itself without anything further in adults who examine the magnitude of things from all sides.

Despite these weak spots and its poverty in logic *Lombroso* deserves great credit for having set going the study and treatment of the criminal in place of the simple repression of the crime. Thanks to him, there is at least a more general demand for a change in the criminal codes, which are quite inadequate for the present needs, and the way is being paved for a general improvement.

I. THE CONTENTIOUS (PSEUDO-LITIGIOUS)

The fighting maniacs stand between those who feel in the right and forever appeal to the law, on the one hand, and the paranoid litigants, on the other. This middle form cannot be differentiated from the former, but is quite definitely separated from the other by the facts that although it leads to false conceptions it never attains the form of a real delusion, that the disease does not continue to progress, but that it is simply the temperament that leads to many fights which need not necessarily be connected with one another and cannot be given up, when the patient finally recognizes the uselessness or some of the dangers of a certain fight. Unimportant as well as important differences equally involve the whole person, for the patients are too sensitive to have any feeling and understanding for the rights of others. All acts of others running counter to their own demands they conceive as malicious, or as personal insults. Their character shows an enhanced feeling of self, "a mixture of sensitiveness, regardlessness and arrogance" (*Kraepelin*). Their own affair they feel as the very affair of justice and they consider it a "duty" to carry it through.

The understanding of the patient varies, but most of them have a narrow field of vision, and with it a certain cunning and strong alertness. Like in all affective people the memory is disturbed in the manner that the experience becomes changed in the sense of the patient's feeling of self.

The "development," if one may speak of such in this disease, varies. Through constant fighting with certain neighbors who give tit for tat, the patients naturally merge into an incessant state of irritability which makes their anomaly look worse. Transference into more favorable or especially into new circumstances gives them peace for some time. To be sure, they regularly neglect their callings. Probably for external reasons it almost always involves men; women of similar character live through it in quarrels within the family.

The theoretical difference from the paranoid forms is very characteristically compared by *Kraepelin* with the difference between the traumatic patient, who as a result of a single experience remains so constituted that he must feel sick, and the hypochondriacal patient who now discovers that, and now this sign of disease.

The recognition is in most cases not difficult, but its differentiation from the normal is not easy. Some of the people so designated show *manic moods of a chronic* nature. These differ, however, from others, mostly by a certain kindness which becomes mixed in all quarrelings. They are able under conditions to speak quite well of their enemies and become reconciled to them after the worst kind of brawls.

XIV. OLIGOPHRENIAS (PSYCHIC INHIBITIONS OF DEVELOPMENT)

The study of the associations and memory have shown us that the brain or the psyche holds so firmly the individual experiences [207] as well as their connections, that whatever is experienced simultaneously or in immediate sequence forms a uniform memory structure which can again be ekphorized through every individual engram. Thus certain classes of engrams, simultaneously acquired, form associations with one another. Associative connections of a different kind are also formed between new and former experiences and then between the same ekphorized engrams, and thirdly, the memory pictures are brought into connection with one another in memory and thought.

The formation of engrams varies comparatively little. Most animals have a memory, but in principle it is obviously only for those experiences which they can use. Idiots form engrams of everything. But the development of the associative connections fluctuates within the widest limits,—we may say, from the animal and idiot, to the genius, for intelligence depends chiefly on the manner of the possible associations.

Hence in the pronounced psychisms of inhibited developments we deal, as it were, only with a want of associations.[208] Wherever the poverty of the same inhibits the progress of the person, depending on the degree of disturbance, we speak of *idiocy, imbecility,* or *debility,*—morbid pictures, which *Kraepelin* comprises under the name of *oligophrenias.* The parallel expression "psychic inhibitions of development" is a misconception. Intra- and extra-uterine brain diseases as well as other things may result in the same poverty of the possibilities of associative connections as in inhibition of development in the structure of the brain.

One must, however, sharply distinguish from the brain developments, the development of the psyche, or the acquisition of experience material in childhood, without which the most endowed structure would remain sterile. With the help of the associative connections, the individual engrams of the sensations are raised to concepts and ideas by the childish psyche. This "psychic development," the gathering and

[207] Individual experiences range from the simplest sense perceptions (green, flat form, the position on the plant, etc., which make up the concept of leaf) to individual actions which in their totality form a complicated scene.

[208] The possibilities of psychic connections must naturally depend in some way on the number of the anatomical elements in the brain; *however, one does well not to bring into relation the process of association with the anatomic "association systems" of the brain.*

arranging of experience material, naturally becomes insufficient when the receptive organ is disturbed. *All oligophrenias are, in this respect, inhibitions of development.*

Moreover, some also think, more or less clearly, that just as the physical strength continues to grow after birth, the same holds true for the psyche as far *as its disposition is concerned;* that normally it progresses during the whole of childhood while in the oligophrenics it "remains still." If we disregard the training of functions, this idea is quite confused, and, in part, certainly false.

Such a development has nowhere been comprehended on a purely intellectual sphere. On the other hand, we are familiar with the fact that the emotional lability and the flightiness of volition observed in the child become transformed into the more stable feelings and definite objective desires of the adult. To be sure, there are some quite rare forms of diseases designated as *"Infantilism"* which retain the infantile characteristics, but such grown-ups show a very marked distinction from real children. Besides, infantilism as such does not by any means represent a clear cut picture of a disease. It is often mixed with signs of mental debility, with sexual abnormities in which the sexual aim manifests itself in playing instead of in the sexual act, and in an unchildlike impulse to "play" the child.[209]

To be sure, one frequently speaks erroneously of a deficiency in intellectual development. But if an imbecile attains the level of an eight year old child and stops there, it does not signify that this "stop" is essentially due to the fact that the ontogenetic development progressed from birth to this point and stopped, but it means that the capacities possessed by the patient from the very beginning suffice to elaborate the material into such a complication as one would put before an eight year old schoolboy. Again it is quite another matter if a hitherto normal child becomes afflicted with some brain disease and then cannot learn anything more complicated, remaining, as it were, at a standstill. But here we deal with a child who was permanently intelligent, who became permanently stupid.

Oligophrenias differ from all other mental diseases through the fact that as a result of insufficient assimilation of empiric material, scanty and inadequate ideas and concepts are formed in childhood, and that as a result of a permanently existing poverty of the associative connections, even the actual empiric material cannot be adequately elaborated.

Although in the oligophrenias we deal with a general disturbance of the cerebral cortex, the weakness of *intelligence* alone stands out

[209] Cf. *Hirschfeld*, Sexualpathologie, Weber, Bonn, 1917, p. 29.

as the principal symptoms of these diseases. For the weakness of intelligence is not only of the greatest practical importance, but the very cerebral anomalies that come into consideration represent in a certain relation quite a uniform simplification of the intellectual apparatus, whereas other functions like the instincts and affectivity need not necessarily be affected, or even when deviating from the normal they radiate into the most dissimilar directions and show nothing that is typical of imbecility. As a matter of fact, affects like euphoria or anger are the same in the genius, in the idiot, and in the animal, at least as far as we can observe, whereas the intellectual functions show colossal quantitative differences.

The oligophrenias comprise not only the congenital disturbances but also those that were acquired in early childhood. Despite the multifariousness of all these diseases there are many good practical reasons why even science should not be satisfied with such a summary judgment. The weakness of the associations and the existence of the disease during the bringing up stamp the whole group with something characteristic symptomologically, and what is more, with something of common practical importance.

The oligophrenias are, in part, simple aberrations of the normal, and even in cases where a definite morbid process produces the mental weakness it may be hardly perceptible. The pathological group cannot therefore be separated from the normal into which it gradually changes through mental *debility* and *narrowness* or through *stupidity*. But even within these entities there are only fluctuating transitions on a psychic basis.[210] One designates as *idiots* in a general way patients of a higher degree who cannot acquire any school knowledge or who are absolutely unfit socially; as *imbeciles* patients who do not advance beyond the position of common school graduates, or those who can still mix in human society and can even perform some subordinate services, and as mental *debility* one diagnoses those who come to a standstill in the development after the public school or who in simple relationships can still maintain themselves somewhat independently; that is, they fail when confronted by the average demands. Debility is of little medical, but of greater forensic significance.

Other criteria with marked limitations are really of no value, for the simple reason that the various spheres of intelligence may attain different heights in the same patient. Idiots are supposed to be individuals who are unable to talk, or who are unable to execute a verbal

---

[210] The etiological anatomic division is quite different; here one can see a great number of distinct pathological pictures.

order, or who show pronounced physical deformities. It is quite superfluous to say of imbeciles: "That, as a rule, their understanding or
numbers hardly goes as far as ten, when the patient can learn to count
mechanically even up to 100." *Sollier* as well as *Ziehen* make a *moral*
distinction between the two classes in favor of imbecility. This is
contrary to all facts; imbeciles may be morally as high as they are
defective, and idiots as malevolent as they are kindly. The only
difference lies in the fact that the lighter grades, the imbeciles, rarely
come to the physician, while the idiots are always in need of care.

Some often obtain a scale of the grade of imbecility through a
comparison with children of a definite age. Thus a patient is said to
have reached a level of an eight year old child, and with the *Binet-
Simon* [211] test one can really delude one into the formation of such a
parallel. But one must remember that the child has an enormous
advantage over the imbecile, as it quickly learns more new experiences;
it has the paths for new understanding and all he needs is to bring
them in contact with experience. On the other hand, the imbecile
has the advantage of having numerically more widespread experiences
which thus enable him to move about more freely, as, for example,
to make a journey, or do some work, in which the child is still helpless.
The intelligence of the normal child is therefore never on the level of
the imbecile. Certain complications of thought are still inaccessible
to the child because it lacks experience, while in the case of the
imbecile the complications of thought are lacking because he is *deficient
in the capacity to absorb complicated experiences*.

Symptomatology. Idiocy can be recognized without any difficulty.
The treatment, too, is more in line with nursing and education than
medical interference. It would, therefore, be superfluous to give here
a more accurate description of severer forms, and *the subsequent
psychopathological remarks will be devoted, in the first place, to
imbecility*. Still whatever is said of the latter is also true of idiocy, if
the defects are markedly exaggerated, and of mental debility, if the
defects are minimized.

Perception and *apperception* are little disturbed directly through
the diminution of the association of ideas, whereas complications
naturally often produce severe injuries. The brain disease which is at

---

[211] The idiot was also compared to an animal, and was said to evince an
"animal-like dementia." Of course, both an animal and an idiot have smaller
capacities of association than the normal person, but the animal brain is a
simpler machine excellently adapted for the required situations, whereas the
idiot's brain is a more complicated but unsuccessful or spoiled apparatus which
has an insufficient adaptive capacity. A chronometer does not sink to the level
of an hour-glass just because it is badly constructed or because it is spoiled.

the basis of oligophrenia is very frequently connected with disturbances of the senses, especially that of hearing, which not only affects perception and apperception, but also extremely retards or makes even the whole psychic development impossible.

Oligophrenias which are not complicated by diseases of the sense organs often show some dullness of the *sensations;* in any case the perceptions are often correspondingly somewhat retarded. The threshold of differentiation is as a rule quite high in all spheres. Some patients never learn to know perspective or pictures in general; thus a compass is a globe, and an hourglass is a bottle. They do not understand scenes pictorially represented because they see only the detached elements. They see "a man holding the hand of the other who is in bed; here stands a man," but they cannot see the connection of the elements, namely, a physician at the bedside.

Association of Ideas. The oligophrenic has not the capacity to form the necessary number of associative connections—and what is something different—to keep them in mind simultaneously at a given moment. He thinks more in unelaborated sensible terms than the normal person, and he thinks only of customary things which frequently occur, and of simple matters which require few associations. He abstracts poorly, i.e. he forms only simple concepts, some of which are incorrectly abstracted, *but he is not able to form any abstraction in the specific sense.* Nor has the oligophrenic the capacity to separate ideation complexes once formed; that is, he has no ability to "reproduce in different order the material formerly acquired" (*Hoche*).

Ignoring that which is not of frequent occurrence and making better use of customary material causes a *kind of insufficiency of memory.* This is, however, only secondary and the actual defect lies only in the lack of associations. The latter may simulate under certain conditions an absolute memory defect, as when a spider jumps on the head of a nail many times in succession. This is not because the spider "forgets" that the nail head is not edible, but because it cannot distinguish this particular black spot from other black spots which usually represent flies. To react to it differently than to flies the spider would have to perceive its particular qualities or to associate it then with the details of the environment. Both conditions require many associations.

Yet to a certain degree the number of associations can be replaced by the frequency of the experience. Thus the perceived details of the nail-head or the individual sensations of the environment may suffice to form a distinction even where there are relatively few associations, if the sensations are constantly repeated in a way that now one, now another detail will become firmly associated with the edibility. To be sure, an animal rich in association will acquire right at the first experience all the connections necessary for the particular purpose. Accentuating the characteristic elements, the abstraction, as discussed above, is also facilitated by a repetition of the same experience, i.e. many repetitions of similar experiences will perforce develop the most characteristic elements. That accounts for the fact that the customary material is always more realizable even where there is no question of facility of memory in the sense of practice.

Another example would be the case of an oligophrenic who repeatedly allowed himself to be duped by the same or similar April-fool jokes. His associations centered only on the joke, but he did not connect his new experiences with the idea of the critical day. Under certain circumstances he was also unable to form sufficient abstractions to distinguish the jokes from what was intended to be serious. However, when the same joke was very frequently repeated, the deception finally did bring about the association, and the weakminded patient became suspicious, even where he should not have been.

The effects of the memory therefore depend on the number of associative connections, altogether regardless of the fact that ekphoria generally is easier, the more association paths it has at its disposal.[212] Moreover, the poorer the associative connections, the more repetitions are necessary before the psyche can utilize a complicated situation through memory. *Hence it is mainly the everyday events that come into being in the oligophrenic; he is unable to use in his reflection the uncommon material.*

The poverty of association impedes the *formation of concepts* because the latter naturally require a combination of many actual experiences, and what is more, they must be not only of the present but also of the past.[213] The more abstract a concept the more combinations must be made. That is why there is an absence of higher abstractions. Many concepts are also falsely formed because the essential is not differentiated from the unessential. For the essential element is either that which constantly repeats itself in the various experiences which are composed into a uniform concept, or subsequently that which attaches to itself the fundamental deductions. Thus the (popular) concept of "leaf" is held together by the flatness of the structure which grows out of a plant, whereby all the other attributes can change. In the concept of "poison" the common element is the destruction of life resulting from taking it into the

[212] Cf. p. 31.
[213] Cf. p. 13, etc.

body. Whoever does not connect together all the more important experiences of leaves and poisons can never have a correct concept of these things. What is more, a great part of the concepts is not independently separated by the child, but is brought about by language. This particularly necessitates many associations and accounts for the fact that imbeciles find it difficult to take over strange concepts and to correct their own in speaking with others.—The abstraction represents also *a separation of the ideas from the ordinary concrete material.* Because inhibited, the ideation material consists in only too much of concrete individual pictures instead of an elaboration of the sum of ideas. But if some general concepts are once formed, owing to their easy accessibility (similar to those in organic cases), they are very frequently used where they are inapplicable (e.g. "implement" instead of "shovel").

The *separation of the ideation complexes* can take place in the positive or negative sense: The detailed experience, as for example the green color in the concept "leaf," may be dropped, for there are green and other colored leaves, or it may be emphasized as the essential distinction, like the characteristic form of all oak leaves, through which the detail is recognized. The separation is effected through new experiences. Thus if one has seen green leaves only, then the form of the leaf as well as its position on the plant become firmly associated with the color green. One only imagines green leaves. But then one notices a red leaf. He who possesses many associations of ideas will still associate the idea of leaf with its form and position, but he now has besides two separated ideation complexes, one with the green and the other with the red color component. Following the usual laws, the second will inhibit the first in so far as it disagrees in the partial component with the idea green; the latter is therefore "separated." If, conversely, in many oak leaves the form is always repeatedly perceived, despite such differences in size and color, we then say that in the concept complex "oak leaf" the figure is accentuated and separated from the general concept of the leaf. On the other hand, the imbecile does not view simultaneously the structure of color, form, and position, and therefore shows a tendency to ignore some individual components and to overestimate others. If one of them, let us say the color green, made a special impression on him, then the red leaf will not stimulate in him the association of the green leaf. The two experiences continue side by side disunited without influencing each other, or he may ignore the color and then fuse them into one concept, but it does not come to his consciousness that there are green and red leaves. In both cases the structures as a whole remain stable. But to single out individual components from the sensation complexes is as important a fundamental condition of concept formation as putting them together. It is also an essential part of the process of abstraction and at the same time one of the fundamental conditions of reason.

The difficulty in differentiating the structure, owing to a lack of understanding of the important element, explains the apparent contradiction that on the one hand the patients often cannot associate to an individual quality despite the fact that frequently they repeatedly stick to a mere partial manifestation. The patient takes all men with yellow buttons as policemen because he was unable to form the correct concept of a policeman, and the buttons have especially impressed him; he can associate only to them; on the other hand, he is not able to distinguish between a beech leaf and an oak leaf because he is incapable of isolating the individual quality of the various formations of the borders.

Experimental Associations are so very characteristic in the oligophrenias that they can be used for diagnostic purposes. But a more precise examination can be done only in the torpid forms.[214] The retarded course of psychic reaction can be measured here, because even with perfect understanding of the experiment and without stupor the reaction time may be prolonged to double. The poor capacity for abstractions is shown through the fact that the patients find it hard, indeed, for the most part they are altogether unable, to respond to the stimulus with one word. Words and concepts occur in life only in association and can only be isolated artificially. This cannot be done by torpid oligophrenics, and accounts for the fact that instead of an isolated concept they express a whole idea. Thus the stimulus word "to light" brought the reaction "The baker lights the wood." But they do not even grasp the stimulus word as a separate concept, but something like the question: "What do you know about . . . ?" or "What is the meaning . . . ?" As the only similar experience happened in school they easily confuse the new situation with the one in school and often answer according to the rules, examples, and phrases studied there, even if the answer is quite incorrect (Winter—consists of snow). As they are unable to associate to a mere word, and must put everything in one connection, their inner associations are more numerous than in an intelligent person. The

[214] *Wehrlin,* Über die Assoziationen von Imbezillen u. Idioten. Diss. Zürich 1906. Also *Jung u. Riklin* Diagnostische Assoziationsstudien, Barth, Leipzig 1906. For the general application of the association experiment in mental cases as used by the Zürich school see Chap. VIII of Brill's Psychoanalysis, Its Theories and Application, 3rd Ed. Saunders, Phila.

content is especially rich in explanations and above all in definitions of the concept mentioned by the stimulus word. The following will illustrate it. Lamp—to light; prison—consists of cells, where one locks up useless people; head—part; war—when two countries fight each other. The explanation may also be given through examples: wreath—you see it at the Turn festival; sick—I was already sick; father—he threw me once down the stairs.

The poverty of ideas results from the many repetitions in content and form, which are frequently applied where they do not fit; the stimulus word may then be replaced by a synonym or it is slightly varied (cat—kitty). Frequently an expletive serves for a great many answers. This is especially true of the word "man" which in the intelligent person is, so to speak, a complex indicator, but serves here frequently to conceal the poverty of thought (head—the man; swim—the man can swim). More frequently than healthy persons, the oligophrenics find no associations at all, and this is especially the case in somewhat unusual words; no reaction does not always mean that it is merely a question of an emotional stupor. The vagueness and lack of clearness of the concepts and manner of expressions frequently come to light in the most dramatic manner: (wedding—serves for amusement; family—where many children are; grandmother—older mother; sweet—when a girl has sugar; tree—component part; star—a part of heaven). The insufficient removal of the idea from the concrete material is also sometimes seen, thus: To sing—consists of notes and song books. The slight bewilderment of the patient (emotional stupor) often expresses itself through various peculiarities.

It is naturally impossible to describe the whole oligophrenic disturbance of intelligence, and especially all its infinite varieties. Some examples should illustrate the defects of the various principle functions.

The Adhesion to the Concrete: The patient knows of Christ only what he saw on pictures. (Who was Wilhelm Tell?) "We have played him in the neighboring town; masked women and children were there too." Or: "One Tell is put up in Altdorf, and now still another statue in Burglen." (Do you know the three Confederates?) "O yes, there were three men who raise their hands high and stretch their fingers so." The difference between Catholics and Protestants consists in the fact that the Catholics have Christ on the cross standing on the streets. (Where does one go when he dies?) "In the cemetery near the church in Seebach. They have made there a new church." (What is this? [picture of hedgehog].) "Don't they prick? One was on our ground in the fall." Even in customary thinking the normal person mostly utilizes elaborated ideas which are distinguished from the concrete. He thinks of a certain person as a brutal character, whereby he does not have to know whence this idea originated; to the imbecile he is that person who gave him a beating at a certain place.

The Inability to Get Away from the Customary: (How can you divide an apple for three persons?) "You make four pieces, give one piece to each and one remains." [215]

Bad Formation of Abstract Concepts: "Helvetia is the woman who is copied on the coins, and always walks around Switzerland to kill those who wish to harm it." "Freedom is when one has no debts." "Religion is when one goes to church." *To be sure, such defects are not seen at their best in the provoked definitions, which even in the healthy person do not exactly correspond to what one wishes to convey, but in the occasional use of such concepts.* The patient speaks of justice, but understands by it only the deserved punishment and not also the merited reward; he speaks of religion and includes in it the fact that he came to his meal at the proper time. Or a patient speaks of states and territories and mixes them with cities, towns, and countries, showing that he has no *clear* concept of either a state or territory, and that his knowledge of a city or town is only fair.

Poor Abstraction Capacity: The patient has learned to calculate by means of match sticks but is unable to do the same problems with eggs. He writes: "In the garden the weather is always nice"; he is unable to imagine the idea of garden when he is not in it. A short story read, as, for example, a fable, he often relates in the subjunctive mood, because he cannot rid himself of the idea: I have read that. . . . If one questions him concerning a definite detail from a complex of ideas, the patient is then altogether unable to answer only this question. He is forced to bring in the whole connection and thus sometimes fails to answer the question either directly or by implication. (But how were you annoyed?) "Because I am just conservative. . . ." This was given to the question as to the relation of the conservatives to the liberals.

Just as oligophrenics are unable to disregard a greater complex of ideas, *just so are they unable to bring a new idea into new connections.* The patient can count, i.e. he can say correctly the numbers in succession, but despite all effort he cannot actually be made to count also his own fingers. One of *Kraepelin's* patients has learned to cook quite well in a bigger kitchen, but when she was later in another home of only three, four people, she served just as many

[215] Cf. also the example of the driver who didn't think to drive around a stone lying in the street but beat the horse, p. 82.

eggs as she formerly did for a whole round table. When the patients
are confronted with new tasks, or when they are transferred to a new
environment, the thoughts in many of them almost stop (emotional
stupor).

Frequently the patients grasp even all the details of the stories
they have merely heard, e.g. the story of Wilhelm Tell, but cannot
reproduce them without help, *because the logical connection has not
become clear to them.* Some form quite incorrect combinations:
Moses fed five thousand men on the Mount of Olives. (Who was
Peter?) "He crowed three times." Where vivid phantasies exist
very characteristic additions and distortions are often made up:
Gessler put a pole right across the street, Tell was to have walked
under it.—The people who killed Christ were uneducated.—The forbidden tree in paradise bore poisonous fruit, and Adam was punished
because he would not go to the tree.

Low grade imbeciles cannot understand a clinical examination
(They are here "to give information").

Next to great *Gullibility,* there is still a greater *inability to pick
up information.* Only in simple things do oligophrenics become wise
through experience. For they really do not understand the connections
and do not know what the problem is. Nor can they transfer one
experience to another even if the situation is similar. Instruction is
also hindered because the patients are not aware of the limits of their
knowledge, e.g. they believe that they know everything.

A servant girl considered it a bad joke when she was told to put
her savings in a bank. She thought that no one could be so stupid
as to pay her something for being obliged to take care of her money.
Another defective could not be convinced that a certain foreigner
was not weakminded because he mispronounced some sounds and
because he used expressions different from the vernacular used exclusively by children and imbeciles.

Many of these persons are altogether unable to grasp that an
answer must be correct.[216] They answer at random, nod affirmatively
to everything that they do not understand, etc.

Particular difficulties are encountered in *comparing* and *differentiating.* The more extreme defectives cannot at all understand questions
of differentiation, such as what is greater? which would you prefer?
To many it is impossible to put a question theoretically. Thus to the
question, If your mother were dead, who would give you food? the
answer was "But my mother is still living." Or to the question, If
you buy a coat for $36, how much change will you get from $50?

[216] Like children in their first years and primitive people.

the answer was "$15," upon which the patient insisted, because he once bought there a coat for $35 and received $15 change. Or, a two-dollar bill is less than a one-dollar bill and two halves of a dollar, because one "must change it and one then gets too little back."

Judgment and Understanding of things and relations are naturally insufficient, and that accounts for the mistakes which rapidly increase with the complication and unusualness of the objects to be judged. Except in the very simple combinations, such as stealing and getting a whipping, the patients are impeded when it comes to include the past and take account of the future. Higher points of view are naturally not formed and not understood.

Some milder imbecile can still acquire some *Vocation* with the necessary practical knowledge. A peasant may be able to do the farm work correctly, but in many things he is unable to say why it is done in this way. The *imbecile can do much more than he knows* in contradistinction to the normal child, where the reverse is the case (*Kraepelin*). At all events, the *capacity for practice* in all things is mostly very slight.

Hoche aptly enumerates the intellectual peculiarities of the imbecile as follows: "He is paltry, sticks to one thing, perceives concretely; he is inconsistent and dependent in the conduct of life; he overestimates his own personality, shows a strong development of the egoistic interests; he is gullible and shows a slight resistive capacity to the will of strangers and to his own, and eventually evinces abnormal impulses, etc." [217]

Not so seldom the intelligence shows itself quite unharmoniously. There are some gaps, which are not, however, very striking or then there are special gifts, as for music, mathematics, for the observation of the weather, for good optical perception and reproduction in drawing, painting, etc. An imbecile was able to draw the Strassburg Cathedral with hundreds of details which he has seen only once years before.

The *Mode of Expression* of imbeciles is naturally awkward and depends on the degree of the deficiency. Most idiots show a marked weakness even in simple grammar, and in the highest grades speaking ceases altogether. Some, even the more intelligent, never learn to talk, although they hear and understand (auditory muteness). Imbeciles speak in a circumstantial manner because they are unable to pick out and omit the unessential, and show a preference for familiar phrases.

Orientation as to Place and Time continues to be good, in so far as

[217] *Binswanger und Siemerling*, Lehrbuch der Psychiatrie, 3rd Ed. Fischer Jena 1911, p. 224.

the patients are able to perceive such relations. Many wander about far without losing their way. Not all these patients are in position to judge time correctly. In any case, most of those who are at all familiar with numbers have a concept of an hour, day, and year. If one should no longer be able to differentiate between day and night he would certainly also be so stupid that no kind of understanding could be had with him.

Bad is often the orientation as to position which they sometimes judge quite falsely and as to the meaning of their own person which

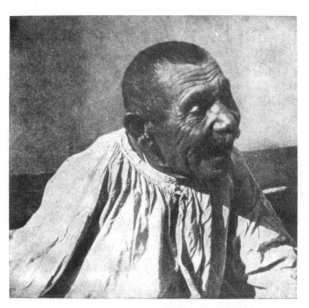

Fig. 43.—Imbecile, somewhat microcephalic. He could repeat whole sermons after once hearing them. Despite the strong vivacity and the many folds the facial expression is very simple, and coarse.

they easily overestimate. On the other hand, it is not correct to say that there are oligophrenics who have not yet separated their personality from others; if they speak of themselves in the third person, it is due, like in children, to quite different reasons.

The *Affectivity* varies extremely; everything that occurs in non-oligophrenics can also be found here. But in these aberrations from the type there are deviations from the average as well as extremes. There was a preference for classifying oligophrenics into dull (apathetic), and excited (erethic) types, the former of which are supposed to be in the majority. But there are just as many transitional forms.

The two types only represent those who on account of their emotional abnormity attract more attention and hence are more observed. To be sure, the affectivity easily gives the impression of being more erethic than it is, because of. the slight control exerted through the intelligence. The lability, which is not rare and which impresses upon some oligophrenics a childish character, may be due to many causes. Most of the etiological forms show a preference for a definite affective state. Thus the cretins without complications, all move about clumsily but are jolly people; most of the microcephalics are lively and easily excitable in all directions; those who have cerebral lesions are disposed to irritability and endogenous moods, etc.

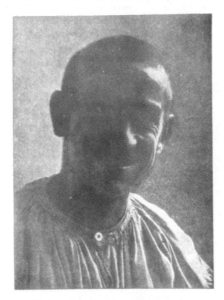

FIG. 44.—Imbecile showing foolish laughter. Although he expresses a certain amount of astonishment or expectation besides the effect of laughter, the expression is uncommonly coarse and uninhibited. It does not express any play of thought. The expression is the opposite of "spiritualized," it is the punch of figure type.

It is self-evident that the oligophrenics are incapable of gradating their finer feelings, for the latter represent reactions to finer modulations of complicated ideas which the patients lack. The facial expression is therefore undeveloped, just as in a clumsy looking drawing, but an additional factor in most cases is the inadequate motor coordination. Even the tone of speech expresses modulations of affects only in coarse outlines.—In some, not exclusively torpid oligophrenics, there is a marked insensibility to pain, which as a rule may be of central origin.

Very frequently, especially in actual brain diseases, one observes depressive or irritable, seldom euphoric moods, which often cannot be distinguished from those of epilepsy; sometimes they are accompanied by headaches and other paresthesias and even by lighter confusions. Moods resulting from outer causes are just as frequent. Some come to the physician on account of *attacks of rage,* which in part are comprehensible reactions to a situation not understood, but in part represent exaggerated answers to a usual stimulus.

Corresponding to the affectivity the *attention* is very varied; to be sure, it is most frequently normal. Many severe cases impress one with a strong hypervigility which makes them incapable of resisting the slightest distraction; every noise, every fly coming into their field of vision distracts them. It is conceivable that education as well as useful occupation are deeply hurt by it. In some the attention flags very quickly.

Just as in all aberration, there are marked inequalities in the disposition of the various *feelings* of the same patient. But it cannot be said that definite classes of feelings are especially lacking or developed. The *moral feelings* comparatively seldom suffer if oligophrenics who do not come to the attention of doctors are also included here; these feelings naturally cannot accentuate any of the more complicated concepts because the patients are unable to form the same. Attachments and love, even gratitude, are quite commonly seen, although they are markedly reduced as a result of a lack in oversight. It is also self-evident that, all things being equal, a low intelligence can only insufficiently control impulses and affective fluctuations. Cretins are as

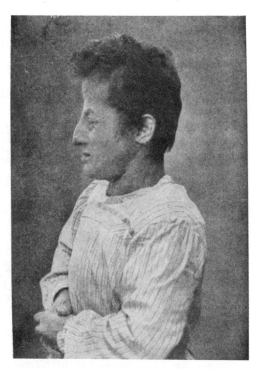

Fig. 45. — A 45 years pyrgocephalus (steeple-shaped skull) an erethic female idiot, without clear speech but who can, however, attend to her own wants.

a rule quiet and kindly disposed, but not really apathetic. With the majority of oligophrenics one has a very pleasant emotional relation, just like parents with children.

Sexual feelings and impulses are usually present. A great many of the patients masturbate. A complete absence of the sexual feelings mostly occurs in cretinism, but here it is not rare.

The *memory* in oligophrenics, like the affectivity, fluctuates from very bad to phenomenally good, but the majority are by far in the middle zone. It is not correct to say that as a class these patients have a bad memory. On the other hand, it is quite obvious that things which they do not understand, and differentiations which they cannot grasp, are badly retained in the head—exactly like in other people. Nevertheless just among imbeciles there are striking exceptions; some remember well things which they do not understand, and some after one hearing, retain in memory a whole sermon verbally and

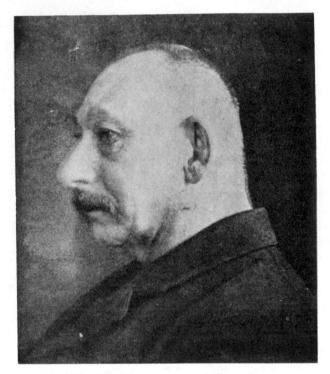

Fig. 46.—Microcephalic middle grade.

with good imitation of accentuation. Like in non-idiots, a particularly good memory for numbers, optical impressions, and similar things is readily connected with special talents in corresponding directions.[218]

Following moods, confusional attacks, and even after strong excitements, perfect or partial *amnesias* are not rare.

Of the *psychic accessory symptoms* only the actual excitements

[218] For the explanation of the apparent memory weakness as a result of insufficient use of experiences, see under association of ideas.

and moods are to be mentioned. But then there are *complications*, which in any case are often directly connected with the disease. Thus above all there is epilepsy, then all possible psychopathies and neuropathies, especially hysteroid manifestations; furthermore, there are katathymic delusions which may resemble an unintelligent paranoia but often connected with hallucinations, and under certain conditions can be cured. Whether the schizophrenia sometimes also observed is only accidental, having been grafted on oligophrenia, is not yet known.

Physical Symptoms. The deeper the oligophrenia the more frequent and the more pronounced are the physical anomalies encountered; idiots are only exceptionally well formed people. A part of the disease is directly connected with the disease of the brain such as micro-, hydro- or macrocephalus. As a result of cerebral and spinal cord diseases the limbs are malformed and paralyzed. Other symptoms are the accompanying manifestations of the brain disease.[219] Still others are loosely connected with the mental disturbances and are signs of the bad foundation in general; among those can be mentioned pyrgo-, and scaphocephalus, all possible "stigmata of degeneration,"

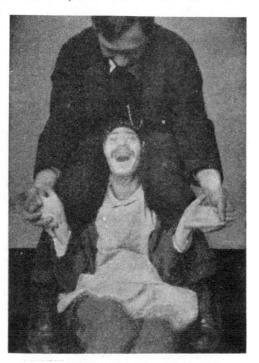

FIG. 47.—High grade microcephalic, 25 years old, the greatest head circumference 40 cm. Height 150 cm. In an idiot asylum he was anxious, irritable, uncleanly, crying, biting, and scratching. Subjected to better treatment he was a clean, erethic idiot. He understands requests and can express simple ideas in sentences, also slightly useful in the house.

smallness from the beginning of youth ranging up to dwarfishness, malformed and poorly developed teeth, deep horizontal fold in the forehead, chronic skin diseases, etc. A great many dystrophies are associated with abnormal functions of the endocrine glands, of which the thyroid, hypo- and epiphysis are especially important. Many of

[219] See pp. 367-8 for the cretin habitus and the signs of congenital syphilis.

these patients not only remain small, but resemble children even in their general physical formation. The ages of elderly idiots are mostly guessed as much too young; "they do not age."

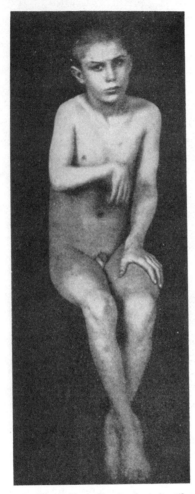

Fig. 48. — Cerebral infantile paralysis, showing the typical attitude of the right upper extremity. Slight atrophy of the right leg.

The *movements* are badly coordinated in the severe cases. *Speech* becomes unwieldy, frequently there is stammering and lisping, rarely stuttering. The distinctions between primary and secondary syllables are often insufficiently accented, and the soft palate closes badly (nasal sound). The perception and imitation of the refinements of speech in its various directions may especially be disturbed.

The *gait* of idiots, if at all possible, is awkward, and clumsy; the patients have not learned to use only the necessary muscles in quiet attitudes; they waddle and walk too heavily; elasticity and grace are absent. Where the labyrinth is deformed one observes the characteristic disturbances. Not rarely there is a finer or even coarser tremor sometimes during motion, and sometimes even at rest.

The knee reflexes are almost always exaggerated.

The Behavior. The most severe cases of idiocy are perfectly helpless. They lie or sit around like children; they are regularly unclean. Depending on the temperament, they play or are unruly, they are noisy, strike one another, or anything at all in the surrounding. Many of them, and still fewer of the higher grade idiots, have definite movements; they rock themselves, shake their heads, and make definite playful motions with their fingers, etc. These movements are frequently accompanied by definite grunting, crying, and grumbling sounds. Erethic idiots who cannot be educated are a great plague, especially if they are still capable of going about. They grasp everything, they soil and destroy things through carelessness and also intentionally.

Those standing on a higher level lack "bearing"; the hanging jaw, the open, sometimes gaping mouth, frequently evince a lack of psychic energy.

Even those who are fortunately not so often erethic and approach to the middle level of imbecility are not so easy to manage, because they forever harbor some design; intentionally or unintentionally, they are up to something, they run away, steal, and fight. Sexual crimes, exhibitionism, murderous attacks up to lust murders, are not so rare. The more quiet ones, if they can keep themselves clean and eat alone, can be managed like children.

The sex character shows itself in all of the various classes in a remarkable and pronounced manner. Feminine idiots wish to have attention and invent for this purpose every possible trick; they scratch themselves, so that the physician should have to treat them, etc.; even the best of friends are jealous of one another. It frequently happened that I had to pull out teeth simply because I performed this operation on one of the fellow inmates. Male idiots tease and fight readily, even though there is no enmity between them.

At play as at work many of them continually become more and more stimulated until they can no longer stop and finally merge into excitement like some children.

In so far as they are not hindered by criminal tendencies, imbeciles of higher standing with an orderly bringing up fit in the family and social order, and most of them can make themselves somewhat useful; in cases of special talents or in other good conditions they can even earn nice sums. One of my patients did very well as a "landscape painter" at a watering place by manufacturing always the same picture cards in great numbers.

Many imbeciles feel the need to show that they are not so stupid; that is, they have a strong *"intelligence complex"* which results not only from the inadequate self-cognition but directly from the feeling of insufficiency for which they compensate. To be sure, the intelligence complex, be it as an overestimation or as an idea of insufficiency, is also found in other patients and in healthy people.

Crimes are not seldom committed by imbeciles, and that not only by those brought up with difficulty and by moral defectives, but also by those who are otherwise kindly disposed; in their faulty valuation of things, slight occasions may often lead to murder and especially arson. (We have already spoken of sexual crimes.) A slight quarrel with the employer may provoke a suicide, a simple reproach for something wrong, an act of arson. An imbecile was displeased because his brother and sister-in-law were talking nearby, so he set fire to the house. How a lack of judgment and comprehension of the situation may lead to a violent act was shown by a mental weakling who has maintained himself independently for years. He went to a comrade

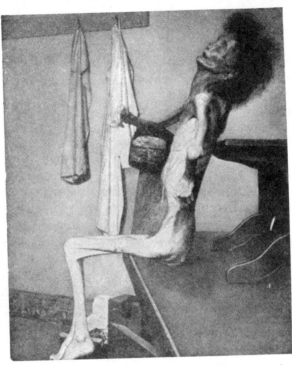

Fig. 49.—Female idiot with an enormously undeveloped muscular system; the skin was tightly stretched so that e.g. there was no longer any conjunctival sac. Height about 120 cm. She looked no different in life than she looks here as a corpse. She never attained the weight of 120 kilos. She could make herself slightly understood through speech. Imbecilic excitements on emotional bases. Was able to knit. Died at about the age of 40 years. Her twin sister is exactly the same.

who had an account in a delicatessen store and wanted to buy a sausage and bread on the former's account. The comrade naturally hesitated, whereupon the patient created a row and, as he was threatened with the police, he walked out and broke a show window. Mental weaklings naturally very readily imagine themselves in an untenable situation and may then commit the crimes described above.[220]

[220] See p. 538.

Course. Deeper congenital idiocies are mostly recognized very early. The children fix on nothing, do not grasp after objects, do not laugh, and remain backward in everything that is called psychic, and mostly also physical development. To be sure, in some cases the oligophrenia first starts after birth in consequences of a brain disease, especially encephalitis and meningitis. Many lighter forms fail for the first time at school, still others when they are about to apply the material learned in their apprenticeship, or even later on going out into independent existence, or in the army, where they attract attention not only through ignorance, but also through stupor, and desertion. Women easily become prostitutes, men alcoholics; both frequently get on the streets. A sudden event like the death of the parents, which puts the patients on their own feet, sometimes brings the disease to the surface; likewise other new tasks, a change of place with new relationships, may bring on a stupor, or anxiety rising to confusion with delusional ideas, and even hallucinations.

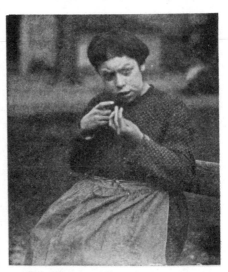

Fig. 50.—An idiot playing with her fingers. She is grown up but cannot talk. Somewhat stupefied features in the presence of the act of being photographed.

The marked diversity of the quantitative course depends on the disease lying at its foundation. Some are backward only in comparison to other children, but continue to catch up to some extent. Others continually become worse, especially at puberty, regardless of the other standard which results from the new tasks. Among these "progressive oligophrenics" one especially finds hereditary lues. Sudden or gradual aggravations may appear even later, the cause of which is not known; in any case there are slowly progressing cerebral degenerations of various kinds. The vital force of oligophrenics, especially of idiots, is poor. On the average they do not get old. They easily become ill—I have seen them as early as in their fifth decade—with pronounced brain atrophy.

The *causes* of *oligophrenia* can be divided into the following classes:

I. In one class it is a matter of various *family predispositions,* which manifest themselves in this way; it is said that oligophrenia is the last link of a progressive degeneration. This concept is not clear and not proven.

II. There are also *germ injuries* through alcoholism of the parents (procreation while drunk?), syphilis, and still other diseases.

III. General *diseases of the mother* and her pelvic organs may under certain conditions, even though quite rarely, bring about a malformation of the skull and the brain.

IV. *Brain- and general diseases of the fœtus* and the child, above all meningitis and encephalitis, as well as any brain injury.

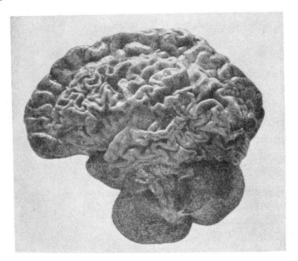

Fig. 51.—Half sided microgyria in a mild imbecile with hemiparesis.

The names (taken from *Weygand*) may give an idea of the special diseases:

1. Psychic defective states in early youth due to lack of education.
2. Psychic defective states due to an absence of some of the senses.
3. Psychic weakness due to an inhibition of disposition.
4. Idiocy on the basis of inflammatory brain diseases.
5. Idiocy on the basis of inflammation of the meninges.
6. Idiocy through hydrocephalus.
7. Amaurotic familiar idiocy and related disturbances.
8. Tubercular hypertrophic sclerosis.
9. Mongolianism.
10. Infantilism:
     Infantilism due to heart disease.
     Infantilism in intoxications and infectious diseases.

11-16. Glandular infantilism.
11. Status thymico-lymphaticus and idiotia thymica.
12. Thyroid disturbances (Dysthyroidism).
13. Dysgenitalism.
14. Hypophysis disturbances (Dyspituarism): acromegaly. Dystrophia adiposo-genitalis. Hypophysary dwarfishness. Epiphysary disturbances.
15. Adrenal disturbances.
16. Pluriglandular diseases.
17. Syphilidogenic idiocy and infantilism.
18. Alcohol and weakmindedness in childhood.
19. Athetoid Idiocy.
20. Chorea and weakmindedness.
21. Spasmophilia and epilepsy.
22. Idiocy and rickets.
23. Chondro-dystrophia and weakmindedness.
24. Steeple shaped skull and weakmindedness.
25. Dementia præcox in childhood.
26. Dementia infantilis.
27. Manic depressive insanity in childhood.
28. Hysterical degeneration and inhibitions of development.
29. Neurasthenia and infantile inhibitions of development.
30. Other diseases of the central nervous system in connection with psychic inhibitions of development.

Many of the forms concern more boys than girls.

Special Forms. Still two more states of idiocy are described, which do not altogether fit in with our cases of oligophrenia and should better be put under the original morbid states or under the psychopathic personalities.

I. **The Unclear Ones.** There are cases which are not at all so poor in associations, and still form unclear concepts. They have not as yet been particularly described. The unclearness seems to be connected with a lack of firmness in the association complexes, so that a concept, or an idea has at this moment this limitation and in the following moment quite another, without the patient being aware of it. Most of these cases are active natures, who are related to the manic temperament. They have a great many phantasies and are quite unsteady in their desires and actions.[221]

Illustration: Carpenter builder, owner of his own business. "He rarely answers a question clearly and directly, even where it would be to his advantage and where there is no reason for evading it. He

[221] Cf. pp. 26, 68, 68.

usually says something else from which one must figure out the answer. He designated it as a libel on the part of X. when the latter, as a witness, confirmed the fact that the patient smoked at his work, which he admitted himself. This indistinctness is one of the reasons for his absolute inability to judge himself and to realize his faults. After I have, for example, recounted to him all his rude actions towards his wife and he admitted them in part, he could still say that he was a good husband, that one like him she will never get. As a matter of fact, just as in the former asylum he is even still now 'pretentious' and pleased with himself."

When he came to the hospital he believed that he had **Fr. 25,000** in cash, while his wife had to exert the greatest effort to save the business from bankruptcy. He believed that it would be easy to put the business in a flourishing state, but could not say how. And then he again spoke in the same sense and wished to make us believe that he conducted the business better than his wife. To be sure, he had once himself confirmed the fact that his guardian had saved his houses for him.

He did not even know whether his machinery was mortgaged. He did not know how much he owed on his property. He signed notes and had no idea how he would pay them. He made a direct demand that his wife pay him back **Fr. 25,000** but could not substantiate it. On what legal grounds he would base his claim when he would sue his wife for the return of his business he had no idea. Once he went so far as to assert that there was no need of getting the business because the business was his. His foolishness in allowing himself to be sued by the Woman's Clinic for a small sum, he does not even realize now. As he was angry because his wife went to the clinic he refused to pay, but failed to understand the consequences, namely, that in so doing he did not hurt his wife, but the innocent clinic and above all himself. So also when he incited the workingmen against his own business merely to cause his wife difficulties. Just as foolish was his action in the hospital when he refused to give a history of his life, or to object to his temperature being taken when he was sick. And the worst of it is the fact that even now after, four years he is not able to recognize the mistakes he then made in anger.[222]

The lighter grades of this and similar disturbances are designated since *Von Guden* as *higher dementia*, according to *Hoche* as "parlor dementia." It concerns people who usually absorb the school material quite well, under certain conditions even excellently, and can even use

[222] Cf. also the Nature Healer, p. 69 and below.

it in certain combinations, but in spite of great activity they are failures in life. Their behavior is the reverse of the oligophrenics; they have much knowledge and can do nothing. Endowed with a good, even if not with a very exact memory, and with a more or less readiness of speech, they fool many a teacher; indeed, they may pass their college examination and even higher ones. Above all, they have a great ability to adapt themselves quickly to circumstances—but only externally. In certain relations they are instinctive psychologists and thus very able to "do" the people. One finds among them some very successful swindlers. If their oral and printed psychic products are more closely observed, one finds repetitions of ideas of others in newer arrangements and more confused formations of the same. A young man had gone so far in another college that he became a lecturer; when he had to examine officially a girl who was illegitimately pregnant he could not understand how this was possible; he took an umbilical cord for a fœtal ventral fin.—Another held political speeches, but among other things he was rigid and firm in believing that the only aim of the other party was "to make the people stupid." A third was a nature healer; he wrote a mass of pamphlets, had an enormous income and maintained so many disciples that they formed many sections of a society, which existed for years, to spread his truths. This patient wrote the following, among other things: "Transparency with the help of self-cognition and world cognition can only be produced in so far as the person is transformed into a love glowing condition." He wanted man to become transparent so that his diseases could be seen. "In the glow, bodies if they don't become transparent they are at least translucent, hence also in the glow of love." Such is the unclearness of the concepts and logic of such people.

II. Another form into which the higher dementia merges without any demarkation is the *relative dementia*. Not always, although frequently, there exists also here a certain unclearness of thinking. The most essential, however, is a disproportion between striving and understanding. There are people whose understanding suffices for a usual attitude of life, and often even for one a little above the average, who, however, are too active, and constantly adjudge to themselves more than they can grasp, and therefore commit many stupidities and suffer shipwreck in life.[223]

The psychic [224] *diagnosis* of idiocy is self-evident; of most cases

[223] *Bleuler*, Verhältnisblödsinn. Allgem. Zeitschr. f. Psychiatrie u. Psychisch-gerichtliche Medizin. Bd. 71. Reimer, Berlin, 1914.

[224] The diagnosis at the basis of the brain disease is here omitted.

of imbecility it is also easy; it first becomes difficult in the lesser pronounced forms and in cases of mental debility.

However, high grade cases have also been confused with schizophrenia. Disregarding the combination of both diseases (grafted-schizophrenia) one must consider the *kathathymic delusional formations of oligophrenics,* which can only be diagnosed from grafted paranoia by the absence of definite schizophrenic signs, and by the fact that it may disappear altogether.

The stereotyped form of movements of many idiots cannot really be mistaken for the stereotyped movements of catatonics, if one has seen both forms. They have the character, if not of a deliberate, yet of a willed act like the dangling of a leg; they do not give the impression as if they ran side by side with consciousness and contently are also easier understood and more elementary. The answers to the usual questions concerning birth, what he did when examined in school, what he was doing now, what his father was doing, frequently betray the defects by the slowness and unclearness of the understanding and by the circumstantiality of the answers.

The stammering and other speech disturbances of the imbeciles are not seldom mistaken for paretic speech. The elisions of the latter, the stumbling of syllables, and the addition of these signs in certain coordinating difficulties are nevertheless still easy to recognize. In contrast to this one rarely observes in the oligophrenics an inability to get away from the individual sounds; more often there is a gliding over, a swallowing of the sounds; moreover, the organic connection of the successive sounds is often absent; it is as if they begin to learn a foreign language.

Only idiots can be psychically diagnosed in early childhood; children who do not laugh, who do not grasp for shiny objects and in general react insufficiently are idiots. Severe cases of malformations of the head frequently enable even the layman to recognize the disease.

As acquired dementias may in some relations externally injure the actual thinking in a manner similar to those of oligophrenics, one of the most important diagnostic means is the proof of the insufficient acquisition of ideas and knowledge in youth. *By assuming a definite schooling and a full receptive capacity through the senses,* it is then possible to draw conclusions from the existing knowledge concerning the intelligence at the time of its acquisition, that is, one can find out to what degree of complexity material has been received during school time, to what degree it was understood and could be elaborated upon. But it should not be forgotten, as often happens, that the knowledge test is not the intelligence test but the material for it. A schizophrenic, an organic patient, or epileptic who is still in the stages when an examination can still be made will not lose the more complex and markedly abstract concepts which he has formerly acquired. The lack of such acquisition can thus demonstrate oligophrenia. But one must be experienced to know what to expect in this direction in the various circles of average people, and especially must it not be forgotten that a person may be above the average in one sphere and at the same time below the average in another.

In both cases one must consider the interest, and the attention applied to the learning. One can remain back at school not only on account of insufficient intelligence, but also when one does not pay attention, or does not exert himself. In the same low intelligence one who has the need in life to follow up the causal relations can know more than another who is indifferent in this relation.

Moreover the patient may suffer from an *examination stupor*, he may not be at home in a special sphere, he may be somewhat negativistic, or, as often happens at examination, he may have the bad will to make himself appear stupid, and *finally he may on the contrary pass excellently all such tests and fail completely in the one standard examination which goes throughout life.* The latter may be due to the following variety of causes: his weakness may lie more in the sphere of the affectivity or of the will, or he may have little understanding for just practical ideas, or his impulses may give him problems and lead him into situations for which even a good intelligence is not big enough. Similar situations are frequently observed in schizophrenia, where under certain conditions the patient will be able to do cube root with ease, and fully understand the whole procedure, but is incapable of dressing himself properly.

The cases of mental debility and the poorly endowed healthy person are distinguished from each other not by the amount of their knowledge but by the measure of their ability, by the ability to use their knowledge independently. It is not a question of intelligence as such but of intelligence as a guide through life. And only in the latter direction is the mental weakling necessarily defective.[225]

The decisive factor in all difficult cases is therefore the *anamnesis* which must be taken here with particular care.

In the deeper standing imbeciles the *Binet* tests (p. 596) are quite useful for some purposes. One can also request the patient to finish incomplete sentences, fill in *Ebbinghause's* unfinished text, explain

[225] *Wagner von Jauregg*, Gutachten. Wien, Klin. Wochenschrift, 1913, 26, p. 1947.

pictures, interpret proverbs, and repeat and explain fables.[226] Such tests are only useful when all circumstances are taken into consideration; *and as it is precisely the beginner who is sure to lack the perspective of all matters that come into consideration, one is explicitly warned against the careless application of the tests.* Moreover the *manner* of answering is much more important than the content. The test examinations furnish very good *occasions* for the state of intelligence to reveal itself under conditions, but it does not necessarily do so.

In all lighter cases, however, all these things are of secondary importance. All the theoretical tests can be passed faultlessly, while the patient is perfectly unfit to manage his own affairs. It is not a question to test theoretically and actually his understanding of his own business, but above all his whole past, in order to see how he behaved himself here. *Life is really the only sure touchstone.*

What is here said concerning theoretic examinations should only be considered as illustrations and suggestions for individual procedures. It is impossible to prescribe all that is to be examined in the individual case. It is not always of special importance what one talks with the patients, but how one observes and how one concludes. *Here as in no other place the physician must set aside his own reason, and depending on the condition of the case he must omit some tests and insert others. The most important thing is always the judgment of the observations and inquiries.* Despite all rules the intelligence test is as much a test of the doctor's intelligence as of the patient's intelligence.

But all that was said here refers only to the *original state of intelligence;* to use the "intelligence test," by which it is customary to understand only a rapid examination of school knowledge and at most also the knowledge of life, in cases of acquired forms of dementia, especially with the object of excluding a dementia præcox, is absurd; to try to make a diagnosis through it is impractical.

Procedure of the Intelligence Tests. The first thing to do in making an intelligence test is to try to get in contact with the patient so that he should not merge into an examination stupor or fall into a negative attitude; one therefore attaches the conversation to something quite natural, perhaps by questioning him about his health, his sleep, or his situation. And according to the patient's reaction a subject is chosen which he is most likely to take up. The differences between the sexes are also to be noted; on the whole, more practical and psychological knowledge is expected in women than theoretic and exact knowledge.

[226] For further detail see *Ziehen*, Die Geisteskrankheiten des Kindesalters. Reuter & Reichard, Berlin, 1915.

Too much cannot be expected of them in concepts relating to geography and geometry.

One allows the patient, for example, to tell about his family, what the father does, and similar things. One can then enter into his *school knowledge* by asking him how he was at school, what subjects he *liked best*, etc. In this way it can be ascertained whether he was left back. When he relates something from history, it is not most important to see how much he knows, but how he elaborates it, especially whether he recounts details in phrases which he has perhaps learned by heart, or betrays a review of things gained through independent grasp and judgment, or whether he repeats something that is of current opinion, etc. Just here it is often possible to find out to what extent the patient was able to work out the essentials and whether he has a sharp grasp of things or not. One also notices whether he relates things diffusely or whether he is able to condense them. To hang on the nonessential, on the perceptible, and in connection with the other symptoms also to omit the logical intermediate connections without noticing it shows imbecility. Especially suitable for differentiating between phrase-like repetitions and fully understood elaborations are questions from *biblical history* and from the *simpler dogmatic theology* ("Why did Christ die?"). In *geography* it is characteristic of many oligophrenics that they are well oriented as to their environment in so far as they have learned it through experience, but become unclear or do not know as soon as they are asked something that they should have learned from theory. Even elementary knowledge in cosmic geography such as how day and night come about, or darkness, etc., need not be expected with certainty from every healthy person; nevertheless even here the answers are characterized by good understanding on the one hand, and the opposite in the case of oligophrenics. In *calculating* one frequently finds that in practical life they have the capacity to get through with current buying and selling examples and card playing while they fail in simple theoretical examples. Rarely is the case reversed, in that the patients repeat only what was taught in school and reproduce it in the manner they studied it, but cannot apply it to practical life. The latter patients seem at first the more intelligent but they are more helpless in life. In testing in mathematics, like in everything else, one should begin with easy examples and proceed to the more difficult (first ask patient to count coins, addition and subtraction, then multiplication. The tables are usually a matter of memory and not of understanding. There are imbeciles who cannot solve $2 + 2$, but can easily solve, for instance, 2×2 and 14×14. Then go to division and finally to fractions).

The patient is then *allowed to read* something simple, e.g. one of the fables from p. 189. Oligophrenics are in most cases easily differentiated from later acquired psychoses by the schoolboy's way of reading, by the difficulties in rarer or more complicated words, etc. The reproduction of the content is not so easily judged because disturbances of attention easily play a part here; even a normal person, when excited, can read whole pages without grasping anything.

In most cases one can quickly orient himself to an extent that he can save himself the questions which are too easy or too hard for the special case. But in order to obtain as far as possible an exact measurement of the height and the manner of the understanding, it is necessary among other things to put questions which also seem somewhat difficult. The latter often causes people to say that we ask the patients things which even a healthy person cannot answer, and that we incorrectly diagnose mental weakness from this sort of not knowing. Regardless of the necessity for restriction, such questions should nevertheless not be avoided, because it is not only a question of knowing and not knowing *but of how the patient answers*. Does he not realize himself that he does not understand the thing? How does he conceal his ignorance? How does he help himself out of difficulties? Such observations rather than direct questions enable one to recognize easier the psychic height of the not severe cases of imbecility, and it is particularly the unclear cases which can be discovered best in this manner. What one *asks* is indeed really not so important as what one *concludes*.

Already from the oral examination it is possible to write a life *history* from which one obtains without anything further the degree of school education, also the conception of life, the wealth of the association of ideas, and many other things. The mode of writing with its awkwardness in letter formation and grammar and content is often characteristic of oligophrenia. The patient is then allowed to see simple *pictures*, and one observes whether he differentiates between current things and those occurring more rarely, which one knew only from description, such as strange animals, plants, etc.

Then one uses pictures which represent a situation and observes whether the patient grasped only the detail or the whole meaning.

If, as exceptionally happens, the examination has thus far failed to display the patient's capacity for *abstraction*, i.e. if it has not been discovered to what extent the patient is able to form abstract concepts and use them, an attempt should be made to talk to him directly about abstracts (work, sleep, jump, memory, glance, poverty, joy, beauty, bravery, state, redemption), but great care must be exercised in doing it. Even healthy persons are not able to define easily the common *definition*.

One can then start a conversation about things of life. How does he judge his relationship, eventually his crime? Does he know from where the material comes for his own trade? Does he know the significance of the individual manipulation? etc. Why did he run here and there from his work? What does he intend to do? How does he wish to get out of this muddle?

Very good starting points, indeed often the diagnosis, can be obtained through the *association experiment*.

One must guard in everything against taking glibness of tongue or ape-like reproduction for knowledge or even understanding; moreover one must watch for clearness of ideas especially in people who are endowed with a fluency of speech.[227] If the patient has no stupor one must verify the degree and extent of his attention, fatigue, etc. Furthermore, the affectivity must be accurately observed; one should also see in how far it controls the logic. For this purpose it will sometimes be necessary to bring up at the end of the examination, when there is nothing more to spoil, emotionally accentuated themes, such as hurling at the patient merited reproaches, etc.

The second, often more important, part consists in ascertaining his behavior at work and leisure, during the observation, and in his past life.

The actual oligophrenias are very frequent diseases; more than one per 1000 of the population belongs to them. Nevertheless the physician has really very little to do with them.

Treatment.[228] The unclear types and the relative dementias do not come so often to the physician. They are all incurable, but here and there still somewhat educable; but more than taking measures of guardianship can hardly be applied to them with any success. Early intervention by transferring the patient into an environment which will take account of his peculiarities and consequently keep him away from all wrong ways may produce a certain improvement.

Against the disease itself up till now only in cretinism (Thyreodin) can something be done, perhaps also in congenital syphilis.

Otherwise it is simply a question of *care and education*. Both must be understood in a special way. A certain amount of adaptability is possessed by almost all patients even also by the severer idiots. In consequence of unfavorable treatment, especially in cases

---

[227] Compare the example of unclearness, p. 615.

[228] Cf. also: Th. *Heller,* Pädagogische Therapie fur Ärzte usw. Leipzig u. Wien, 1914.

of beating or coddling, some patient may become a dangerous and harmful individual, the control of whom will necessitate many people, but who under proper treatment may act like a lovely child. Where dangerous tendencies exist commitment is naturally necessary. Of special importance in the lighter cases is the selection of the right vocation, which should better make too little, than too many demands on the abilities and energy of the patients. Many parents wish to go too high.

Also in later life it is especially important that the patients have a position in life suitable to their abilities and temperament; too high demands are always harmful. But even in the cases who are seemingly most hopeless one should not forget that in most cases some improvement is possible, very often much improvement, if the patient is put into the right hands. Some of the educational institutions for oligophrenics are very useful.

In excited cases of hydrocephalus a lumbar puncture or even a puncture of the ventricle may give temporary alleviation. The first operation can even be periodically repeated.

Where there is a tendency to sexual excesses, sterilization or castration may take the place of permanently confining the patient. But one must govern himself regarding this advice according to the views of the environment and follow the legal forms, such as the consent of all concerned, the guardian, or counsel ad hoc, etc.

FINIS

INDEX

Classics in Psychiatry

An Arno Press Collection

Feuchtersleben, Ernst [Freiherr] von. **The Principles Of Medical Psychology.** 1847

Georget, [Etienne-Jean]. **De La Folie:** Considérations Sur Cette Maladie. 1820

Haslam, John. **Observations On Madness And Melancholy.** 1809

Hill, Robert Gardiner. **Total Abolition Of Personal Restraint In The Treatment Of The Insane.** 1839

Janet, Pierre [Marie-Felix] and F. Raymond. **Les Obsessions Et La Psychasthénie.** 1903. Two volumes

Janet, Pierre [Marie-Felix]. **Psychological Healing.** 1925. Two volumes

Kempf, Edward J. Psychopathology. 1920

Kraepelin, Emil. **Manic-Depressive Insanity And Paranoia.** 1921

Kraepelin, Emil. **Psychiatrie:** Ein Lehrbuch Für Studirende Und Aerzte. 1896

Laycock, Thomas. **Mind And Brain.** 1860. Two volumes in one

Liébeault, A[mbroise]-A[uguste]. **Le Sommeil Provoqué Et Les États Analogues.** 1889

Mandeville, B[ernard] De. **A Treatise Of The Hypochondriack And Hysterick Passions.** 1711

Morel, B[enedict] A[ugustin]. **Traité Des Degénérescences Physiques, Intellectuelles Et Morales De L'Espèce Humaine.** 1857. Two volumes in one

Morison, Alexander. **The Physiognomy Of Mental Diseases.** 1843

Myerson, Abraham. **The Inheritance Of Mental Diseases.** 1925

Perfect, William. **Annals Of Insanity.** [1808]

Pinel, Ph[ilippe]. **Traité Médico-Philosophique Sur L'Aliénation Mentale.** 1809

Prince, Morton, et al. Psychotherapeutics. 1910

Psychiatry In Russia And Spain. 1975

Ray, I[saac]. **A Treatise On The Medical Jurisprudence Of Insanity.** 1871

Semelaigne, René. **Philippe Pinel Et Son Oeuvre Au Point De Vue De La Médecine Mentale.** 1888

Thurnam, John. **Observations And Essays On The Statistics Of Insanity.** 1845

Trotter, Thomas. **A View Of The Nervous Temperament.** 1807

Tuke, D[aniel] Hack, editor. **A Dictionary Of Psychological Medicine.** 1892. Two volumes

Wier, Jean. **Histoires, Disputes Et Discours Des Illusions Et Impostures Des Diables, Des Magiciens Infames, Sorcieres Et Empoisonneurs.** 1885. Two volumes

Winslow, Forbes. **On Obscure Diseases Of The Brain And Disorders Of The Mind.** 1860

Burdett, Henry C. **Hospitals And Asylums Of The World.** 1891-93. Five volumes. 2,740 pages on NMA standard 24x-98 page microfiche only